D1558611

Illustrated Tips and Tricks in Sports Medicine Surgery

Illustrated Tips and Tricks in Sports Medicine Surgery

Frederick M. Azar, MD
Professor
Director, Sports Medicine Fellowship
University of Tennessee-Campbell Clinic Department of Orthopaedic Surgery & Biomedical Engineering
Chief-of-Staff, Campbell Clinic
Memphis, Tennessee

Wolters Kluwer

Philadelphia • Baltimore • New York • London
Buenos Aires • Hong Kong • Sydney • Tokyo

Acquisitions Editor: Brian Brown
Development Editor: Sean McGuire
Editorial Coordinator: Tim Rinehart
Editorial Assistant: Amy Masgay
Marketing Manager: Stacy Malyil
Production Project Manager: Barton Dudlick
Design Coordinator: Stephen Druding
Artist/Illustrator: Bernie Kida
Manufacturing Coordinator: Beth Welsh
Prepress Vendor: SPi Global

9 8 7 6 5 4 3 2 1

Printed in China (or the United States of America)

Library of Congress Cataloging-in-Publication Data
Names: Azar, Frederick M., editor.
Title: Illustrated tips and tricks in sports medicine surgery / editor, Dr. Frederick M. Azar, MD, Professor, Department of Orthopaedics, The Campbell Clinic, Germantown, Tennessee.
Description: Philadelphia : Wolters Kluwer, [2018]
Identifiers: LCCN 2018015521 | ISBN 9781496375414 (hardback)
Subjects: LCSH: Sports injuries—Surgery. | Orthopedic surgery. | BISAC: MEDICAL / Orthopedics.
Classification: LCC RD97 .I45 2018 | DDC 617.1/027—dc23 LC record available at https://lccn.loc.gov/2018015521

LWW.com

Contributors

Jeffrey S. Abrams, MD
Medical Director, Princeton Orthopaedic & Rehabilitation Associates
Chief, Shoulder Surgery, Sports Medicine Princeton
Attending Surgeon, University Medical Center at Princeton
Princeton, New Jersey

Christopher S. Ahmad, MD
Professor of Orthopedic Surgery, Columbia University Medical Center
Vice-Chair of Research, Department of Orthopedic Surgery, Columbia University Medical Center
Attending Physician, New York-Presbyterian Hospital
New York, New York

Marcio Bottene Villa Albers, MD
Postdoctoral Associate
Department of Orthopaedic Surgery
University of Pittsburgh
Pittsburgh, Pennsylvania

Frank Alexander, MS, ATC
Athletic Trainer
Center for Shoulder, Elbow, and Sports Medicine
Department of Orthopedic Surgery
Columbia University Medical Center
New York, New York

Answorth A. Allen, MD
Attending Surgeon, Hospital for Special Surgery
Professor, Clinical Orthopedic Surgery
Weill Cornell Medical College
New York, New York

Annuziato (Ned) Amendola, MD
Professor of Orthopaedic Surgery
Duke University School of Medicine
Sports Medicine Orthopaedic Surgeon
Duke University Hospital
Durham, North Carolina

Victor Anciano, MD
Resident Physician
Department of Orthopaedics
University of Virginia
Charlottesville, Virginia

Allen F. Anderson, MD
Orthopaedic Surgeon
Tennessee Orthopaedic Alliance
Nashville, Tennessee

Christian N. Anderson, MD
Orthopaedic Surgeon
Tennessee Orthopaedic Alliance
Nashville, Tennessee

Michael R. Anderson, DO
Foot and Ankle Fellow
Department of Orthopaedic surgery
University of Rochester
Rochester, New York

Robert Anderson, MD
Director, Foot and Ankle
Titletown Sports Medicine and Orthopedics
Green Bay, Wisconsin
Founder, Foot and Ankle Institute
OrthoCarolina
Charlotte, North Carolina

James R. Andrews, MD
President & Chairman of the Board
Andrews Research & Education Foundation (AREF)
Medical Director, The Andrews Institute
Gulf Breeze, Florida
Chairman of the Board & Medical Director
American Sports Medicine Institute (ASMI)
Birmingham, Alabama

Andrew E. Apple, MD
Resident
Department of Orthopaedic Surgery
Tulane University School of Medicine
New Orleans, Louisiana

Robert A. Arciero, MD
Professor, Orthopaedics
Department of Orthopedic Surgery
University of Connecticut Health
Farmington, Connecticut

Danny Arora, MD, MSc, FRCSC
Orthopaedic Surgeon
Department of Surgery–Orthopaedic Surgery
Oakville Trafalgar Memorial Hospital
Oakville, Ontario, Canada

Champ L. Baker Jr, MD
Past Chairman of Board
Hughston Foundation
Staff at Jack Hughston Memorial Hospital
Phenix City, Alabama

Justin H. Bartley, MD
Sports Medicine Specialist
DaVita Medical Group
Albuquerque, New Mexico

Judith F. Baumhauer, MD, MPH
Professor and Associate Chair
Orthopaedic Surgery
University of Rochester School of Medicine and Dentistry
Rochester, New York

Asheesh Bedi, MD
Chief, Sports Medicine
Harold W. and Helen L. Gehring Early Career Professor of Orthopaedic Surgery
Director, Sports Medicine and Joint Preservation Center
Associate Professor, Orthopaedic Surgery
University of Michigan
Ann Arbor, Michigan

Matthew C. Bessette, MD
Sports Medicine Fellow
Department of Orthopaedics
Cleveland Clinic Foundation
Cleveland, Ohio

Matthew H. Blake, MD
Director of Orthopedic Sports Medicine
Department of Orthopedics & Sports Medicine
Avera McKennan Hospital & University Health Center
Sioux Falls, South Dakota

Ioanna K. Bolia, MD, MS, PhDc
International Research Scholar
Steadman Philippon Research Institute
Vail, Colorado

Joseph A. Bosco III, MD
Professor and Vice Chair
NYU Langone Orthopedics
NYU Langone Health
New York, New York

James P. Bradley, MD
Clinical Professor Orthopaedics
Head Team Physician Pittsburgh Steelers
University of Pittsburgh Medical center
Pittsburgh, Pennsylvania

Karen K. Briggs, MPH
Director, Hip Research
Steadman Philippon Research Institute
Vail, Colorado

Matthew Brown, MD
Fellow
The Orthopedic Clinic Association
Phoenix, Arizona

Stephen S. Burkhart, MD
President
The San Antonio Orthopaedic Group
San Antonio, Texas

Angus F. Burnett, PhD
Director of Clinical Projects
CMO Office
Aspetar Orthopaedic and Sports Medicine Hospital
Doha, Qatar

Charles Bush-Joseph, MD
Professor, Department of Orthopedic Surgery
Rush University Medical Center
Chicago, Illinois

J. W. Thomas Byrd, MD
Cofounder Nashville Hip Institute
Clinical Professor
Department of Orthopaedics and Rehabilitation
Vanderbilt University
Nashville, Tennessee

E. Lyle Cain Jr, MD
Sports Medicine Specialist
Andrews Sports Medicine & Orthopaedic Center
Birmingham, Alabama

James H. Calandruccio, MD
Associate Professor
Director, Hand Fellowship
University of Tennessee-Campbell Clinic Department of Orthopaedic Surgery & Biomedical Engineering
Memphis, Tennessee

Thomas R. Carter, MD
The Orthopedic Clinic
Emeritus Head of Orthopedics
Arizona State University
Phoenix, Arizona

Jorge A. Chahla, MD, PhD
Sports Medicine Fellow
Department of Sports Medicine
Cedars-Sinai Kerlan-Jobe Institute
Santa Monica, California

Zaira S. Chaudhry, MPH
Research Fellow
Department of Sports Medicine
Rothman Institute
Philadelphia, Pennsylvania

Michael D. Chiu, MD
Orthopedic Sports Medicine
Illinois Bone and Joint Institute
Chicago, Illinois

W. Stephen Choate, MD
Staff Orthopedic Surgeon
Ochsner Sports Medicine Institute
New Orleans, Louisiana

Michael C. Ciccotti, MD
Resident Physician
Department of Orthopaedic Surgery
Thomas Jefferson University Hospital and the Rothman Institute
Philadelphia, Pennsylvania

Michael G. Ciccotti, MD
The Everett J. and Marian Gordon Professor of Orthopaedic Surgery
Chief, Division of Sports Medicine
Director, Sports Medicine Fellowship and Research
Department of Orthopaedic Surgery
The Rothman Institute
The Sidney Kimmel Medical College at Thomas Jefferson University
Head Team Physician
Philadelphia Phillies and Saint Joseph's University
Philadelphia, Pennsylvania

Steven B. Cohen, MD
Professor
Department of Orthopaedic Surgery
The Sidney Kimmel Medical College at Thomas Jefferson University
Rothman Institute
Philadelphia, Pennsylvania

Brian J. Cole, MD, MBA
Associate Chairman and Professor
Department of Orthopedics, Rush Medical College
Chairman, Department of Surgery, Rush Oak Park Hospital
Section Head, Cartilage Restoration Center
Midwest Orthopedics at Rush
Chicago, Illinois

Eric J. Cotter, BS
Medical Student
Georgetown University School of Medicine
Washington, District of Columbia

Ryan P. Coughlin, MD, FRCSC
Orthopaedic Sports Fellow
Department of Orthopaedic Surgery
Duke University Medical Center
Durham, North Carolina

James B. Cowan, MD
Orthopaedic Sports Medicine Surgeon
Department of Orthopedic Surgery
Northwest Permanente
Portland, Oregon

Kathryn L. Crum, MD
Orthopaedics and Sports Medicine Specialist
Central Florida Bone & Joint Institute
Orange City, Florida

David M. Dare, MD
Sports Medicine Specialist
Raleigh Orthopaedic Clinic
Raleigh, North Carolina

Molly A. Day, MD, ATC
Orthopaedic Surgery Resident
Department of Orthopaedics and Rehabilitation
University of Iowa Hospitals and Clinics
Iowa City, Iowa

Thomas M. DeBerardino, MD
Professor of Orthopaedic Surgery, Baylor School of Medicine
Co-Director, Combined Baylor School of Medicine and San Antonio, Texas Sports Medicine Fellowship
Medical Director, Burkhart Research Institute for Orthopaedics (BRIO)
Sports Medicine Orthopaedic Surgeon at the Sports Institute and TSAOG Orthopaedics
San Antonio, Texas

Jeffrey R. Dugas, MD
Fellowship Director
Andrews Sports Medicine & Orthopaedic Center
Birmingham, Alabama

Andrew J. Elliott, MD
Attending Orthopedic Surgeon
Foot and Ankle Service
Hospital for Special Surgery
Clinical Assistant Professor of Orthopedics
Weill Medical College of Cornell University
New York, New York

Peter D. Fabricant, MD, MPH
Department of Pediatric Orthopedic Surgery
Hospital for Special Surgery
Assistant Professor of Orthopedic Surgery
Weill Cornell Medical College
New York, New York

Gregory C. Fanelli, MD
Associate, Sports Injury Clinic
Department of Orthopaedics
Geisinger Medical Center
Danville, Pennsylvania

Matthew G. Fanelli, MD
Department of Orthopaedics
Geisinger Medical Center
Danville, Pennsylvania

Larry D. Field, MD
Director, Upper Extremity Service
Director, Sports Medicine Fellowship Program
Mississippi Sports Medicine Center
Jackson, Mississippi

David C. Flanigan, MD
Associate Professor
Department of Orthopaedics
The Ohio State University Wexner Medical Center
Jameson Crane Sports Medicine Institute
Columbus, Ohio

Rachel M. Frank, MD
Sports Medicine, Cartilage Restoration, and Shoulder Surgery
Team Physician, University of Colorado Athletics
Assistant Professor, Department of Orthopedic Surgery
University of Colorado School of Medicine
Denver, Colorado

Freddie H. Fu, MD, D.Sc. (Hon.), D.Ps. (Hon.)
Distinguished Service Professor
University of Pittsburgh
David Silver Professor and Chairman
Department of Orthopaedic Surgery
University of Pittsburgh School of Medicine
Head Team Physician
Department of Athletics
University of Pittsburgh
Pittsburgh, Pennsylvania

John P. Fulkerson, MD
Clinical Professor of Orthopedic Surgery
University of Connecticut
President, the Patellofemoral Foundation
Sports Medicine Specialist
Orthopaedic Associates of Hartford
Hartford, Connecticut

Andrew G. Geeslin, MD
Orthopaedic Surgeon
Sports Medicine, Knee, Hip, Shoulder
Borgess Orthopaedics
Clinical Assistant Professor
Western Michigan University Homer Stryker M.D. School of Medicine
Kalamazoo, Michigan

Thomas J. Gill, MD
Professor of Orthopaedic Surgery
Tufts University School of Medicine
Chairman of Orthopaedic Surgery
Steward Healthcare Network
Director, Boston Sports Medicine and Research Institute
Boston, Massachusetts

Scott D. Gillogly, MD
Chief Medical Officer
Aspetar Orthopaedic and Sports Medicine Hospital
Doha, Qatar

Steven L. Haddad, MD
Senior Attending Physician
Illinois Bone and Joint Institute, LLC
Glenview, Illinois

Mia S. Hagen, MD
Assistant Professor
Orthopaedics and Sports Medicine
University of Washington
Seattle, Washington

Christopher D. Harner, MD
Professor
Vice Chair of Academic Affairs
Director of the Sports Medicine Fellowship
Department of Orthopaedic Surgery
McGovern Medical School
The University of Texas Health Science Center at Houston (UTHealth)
Houston, Texas

Robert U. Hartzler, MD, MS
Shoulder and Elbow Surgeon
TSAOG and Burkhart Research Institute for Orthopaedics (BRIO)
San Antonio, Texas

Richard J. Hawkins, MD
Chairman, Hawkins Foundation
Clinical Professor of Orthopaedic Surgery
University of South Carolina School of Medicine–Greenville
Adjunct Professor of the Department of Bioengineering
Clemson University
Greenville, South Carolina

Laurence D. Higgins, MD, MBA
Chief, Sports Medicine and Shoulder Service
Orthopaedics
Brigham and Women's Hospital
Boston, Massachusetts

Sherwin S. W. Ho, MD
Professor of Orthopaedic Surgery
Director, Orthopaedic Sports Medicine Fellowship
Department of Orthopaedic Surgery and Rehabilitation Medicine
University of Chicago
Chicago, Illinois

Tyler J. Hunt, BS
Boston Shoulder Institute
Department of Orthopaedics
Brigham and Women's Hospital
Boston, Massachusetts

Bradley P. Jaquith, MD
Sports Medicine Specialist
Tennessee Orthopaedic Clinics
Knoxville, Tennessee

Darren L. Johnson, MD
Professor and Chairman
Department of Orthopaedic Surgery
Director of Sports Medicine
University of Kentucky School of Medicine
Lexington, Kentucky

Christopher C. Kaeding, MD
Executive Director
Sports Medicine Institute
The Ohio State University
Judson Wilson Professor, Department of Orthopaedics
Executive Director, Sports Medicine Center
Columbus, Ohio

Brian J. Kelly, MD
Clinical Instructor
Department of Sports Medicine
Allegheny Health Network Orthopaedic Institute
Pittsburgh, Pennsylvania

John D. A. Kelly IV, MD
Director Shoulder Sports Medicine
Director Penn Throwing Clinic
Professor of Clinical Orthopaedic Surgery
Co-Director Sports Medicine Fellowship
Penn Perelman School of Medicine
Philadelphia, Pennsylvania

Raymond J. Kenney, MD
Orthopaedic Sports Medicine Fellow
Department of Orthopaedics and Rehabilitation
University of Rochester Medical Center
Rochester, New York

Moin Khan, MD, MSc, FRCSC
Assistant Professor, Surgery
McMaster University
Hamilton, Ontario

Jacob M. Kirsch, MD
Orthopaedic Surgery Resident
Department of Orthopaedic Surgery
University of Michigan
Ann Arbor, Michigan

Mininder S. Kocher, MD, MPH
Professor of Orthopaedic Surgery
Harvard Medical School
Associate Director, Division of Sports Medicine
Boston Children's Hospital
Boston, Massachusetts

Jason L. Koh, MD, MBA
Chairman
Department of Orthopaedic Surgery
NorthShore University Health System
Evanston, Illinois
Clinical Professor
Department of Orthopaedic Surgery
University of Chicago
Chicago, Illinois

Joseph D. Lamplot, MD
Orthopaedic Surgery Resident
Orthopaedic Surgery
Washington University in Saint Louis School of Medicine
St. Louis, Missouri

Drew A. Lansdown, MD
Assistant Professor in Residence
Department of Orthopaedic Surgery
Sports Medicine & Shoulder Surgery
University of California, San Francisco
San Francisco, California

Robert F. LaPrade, MD, PhD
Complex Knee and Sports Medicine Surgeon
The Steadman Clinic Chief Medical Officer
The Steadman Philippon Research Institute
Vail, Colorado

Natalie L. Leong, MD
Assistant Professor
Department of Orthopaedic Surgery
University of Maryland, Baltimore
Baltimore, Maryland

William N. Levine, MD
Frank E. Stinchfield Professor and Chair
Department of Orthopedic Surgery
NewYork-Presbyterian/Columbia University Medical Center
New York, New York

Bruce A. Levy, MD
Professor of Orthopedics
Department of Orthopedic Surgery
Mayo Clinic
Rochester, Minnesota

Christopher A. Looze, MD
Sports Medicine Specialist
MedStar Orthopaedics
Baltimore, Maryland

Michael D. Maloney, MD
Professor of Orthopaedics
Chief Division of Sports Medicine
Medical Director URMC Surgery Center
University of Rochester Medical Center
Rochester, New York

Bridget Mansell, MA, PA-C, ATC
Physician Assistant
Orthopaedic and Rheumatologic Institute
Cleveland Clinic
Cleveland, Ohio

Anthony A. Mascioli, MD
Assistant Professor
University of Tennessee-Campbell Clinic Department of Orthopaedic Surgery and Biomedical Engineering
Memphis, Tennessee

Matthew J. Matava, MD
Chief of Sports Medicine
Department of Orthopaedic Surgery
Washington University
St. Louis, Missouri

David R. McAllister, MD
Chief, Sports Medicine Service
Professor and Vice Chair of Faculty Affairs
Department of Orthopaedic Surgery
David Geffen School of Medicine at UCLA
Los Angeles, California

Eric C. McCarty, MD
Associate Professor
University of Colorado School of Medicine
Chief of Sports Medicine and Shoulder Surgery
Department of Orthopedics
Denver, Colorado

James D. McDermott, MD
Orthopaedic Surgeon
Fellowship Trained in Sports Medicine
Sports Medicine Institute
Spartanburg, South Carolina

Michael H. McGraw, MD
Sports Medicine Specialist
Orthopaedics East & Sports Medicine Center
Greenville, North Carolina

Dayne T. Mickelson, MD
Orthopaedic Surgeon, Sports Medicine Specialist
Proliance Orthopaedics and Sports Medicine
Bellevue, Washington

John R. Miller, MD
Assistant Professor
Department of Orthopaedics & Rehabilitation
Loyola University Medical Center
Chicago, Illinois

Mark D. Miller, MD
S. Ward Casscells Professor
Head, Division of Sports Medicine
Department of Orthopaedic Surgery
University of Virginia
Team Physician, James Madison University
Director, Miller Review Course
Charlottesville, Virginia

Claude T. Moorman III, MD
Edward N. Hanley, Jr, MD Endowed Professor and Chairman
Department of Orthopedic Surgery, Atrium Health
President, Atrium Health Musculoskeletal Institute
Charlotte, North Carolina

Gina M. Mosich, MD
Resident Physician
Department of Orthopaedic Surgery
University of California, Los Angeles
Los Angeles, California

G. Andrew Murphy, MD
Associate Professor
University of Tennessee-Campbell Clinic Department of Orthopaedic Surgery and Biomedical Engineering
Memphis, Tennessee

Jonathan Newgren, MA
Clinical Research Coordinator
Department of Orthopedic Surgery
Rush University Medical Center
Chicago, Illinois

Daniel F. O'Brien, MD
Resident Physician
Orthopedic Surgery
University of Connecticut Health Center
Farmington, Connecticut

Michael J. O'Brien, MD
Associate Professor of Clinical Orthopaedics
Tulane University
New Orleans, Louisiana

Gabriella Ode, MD
Orthopedic Surgeon
Department of Orthopedic Surgery
Atrium Health
Charlotte, North Carolina

Martin J. O'Malley, MD
Associate Attending Orthopedic Surgeon
Hospital for Special Surgery Associate Professor of Orthopedic Surgery
Weill Cornell Medical College
New York, New York

Nathan D. Orvets, MD
Shoulder and Elbow Specialist
Orthopedic Surgery
Northwest Permanente, PC
Portland, Oregon

Richard D. Parker, MD
President, Cleveland Clinic Hillcrest and Eastern Region Hospitals
Sports Medicine Specialist
Cleveland Clinical Sports Health
Cleveland, Ohio

Nikolaos K. Paschos, MD, PhD
Pediatric Sports Medicine Fellow
Department of Sports Medicine
Boston Children's Hospital
Harvard Medical School
Boston, Massachusetts

Brendan M. Patterson, MD
Assistant Professor
Department of Orthopaedic Surgery
University of Iowa
Iowa City, Iowa

Thierry Pauyo, MD, FRCSC
Clinical Fellow in Orthopedic Surgery
Boston Children's Hospital
Boston, Massachusetts

Djuro Petkovic, MD
Orthopedic Surgeon
Illinois Bone and Joint Institute
Morton Grove, Illinois

Marc J. Philippon, MD
Managing Partner, The Steadman Clinic
Co-Chairman, Director of Sports Medicine Fellowship, Director of Hip Research
Steadman Philippon Research Institute
Vail, Colorado
Adjunct Associate Professor of Orthopaedic Surgery
University of Pittsburgh School of Medicine
Pittsburgh, Pennsylvania

Matthew T. Provencher, MD, CAPT, MC, USNR
Complex Shoulder, Knee and Sports Surgery
The Steadman Clinic and Steadman Philippon Research Institute
Vail, Colorado

Catherine Richardson, BS
Clinical Research Assistant
Department of Orthopedic Surgery
Rush University Medical Center
Chicago, Illinois

Scott A. Rodeo, MD
Co-Chief Emeritus, Sports Medicine and Shoulder Service
Co-Director, Orthopedic Soft Tissue Research Program, The Hospital for Special Surgery
Professor, Orthopedic Surgery, Weill Medical College of Cornell University
Attending Orthopedic Surgeon, The Hospital for Special Surgery
Head Team Physician, New York Giants Football
New York, New York

Jason P. Rogers, MD
Sports Medicine Specialist
Greensboro Orthopaedics
Greensboro, North Carolina

Anthony A. Romeo, MD
Professor, Department of Orthopedics
Program Director, Shoulder & Elbow Fellowship
Head, Shoulder & Elbow Surgery, Division of Sports Medicine
Rush University Medical Center
Chicago, Illinois

Andrew J. Rosenbaum, MD
Assistant Professor
Director of Orthopaedic Research
Division of Orthopaedic Surgery
Albany Medical Center
Albany, New York

William H. Rossy, MD
Attending Physician
Department of Orthopaedic Surgery
Penn Medicine Princeton Medical Center
Princeton, New Jersey

Michael K. Ryan, MD
Orthopaedic Surgeon
Department or Orthopaedic Surgery and Sports Medicine
American Sports Medicine Institute
Andrews Sports Medicine and Orthopaedic Center
Birmingham, Alabama

Marc R. Safran, MD
Professor, Orthopaedic Surgery, Chief Division of Sports Medicine
Department of Orthopaedic Surgery
Stanford University
Redwood City, California

Anthony Sanchez, BS
Research Assistant
Center for Outcomes-Based Orthopaedic Research
Steadman Philippon Research Institute
Vail, Colorado

George Sanchez, BS
Medical Doctor Candidate
Geisel School of Medicine at Dartmouth
Hanover, New Hampshire

Felix H. Savoie, MD
Ray Haddad Professor and Chair
Department of Orthopaedic Surgery
Tulane University
New Orleans, Louisiana

Brian B. Shiu, MD
Clinical Asssistant Professor of Orthopaedics
University of Maryland School of Medicine
Baltimore, Maryland

Hardeep Singh, MD
Orthopaedic Surgery Resident
Department of Orthopaedic Surgery
University of Connecticut
Farmington, Connecticut

Julian J. Sonnenfeld, MD
Orthopaedic Resident
NYP/Columbia University Medical Center
New York, New York

Kurt P. Spindler, MD
Vice Chairman of Research
Orthopaedic & Rheumatologic Institute
Director of Orthopaedic Clinical Outcomes, Academic Director of Cleveland Clinical Sports Health
Cleveland, Ohio

Murphy M. Steiner, MD
Hand Surgery Fellow
University of Tennessee–Campbell Clinic
Department of Orthopaedic Surgery and Biomedical Engineering
Memphis, Tennessee

Cory M. Stewart, MD
Senior Associate Consultant
Orthopedic Surgery
Mayo Clinic
Eau Claire, Wisconsin

Eduardo Stewien, MD, MS
Head of Sports Medicine
Hospital Adventista de Manaus
Manaus, Amazonas, Brazil

Michael J. Stuart, MD
Professor, Department of Orthopedics
Chair, Division of Sports Medicine
Mayo Clinic
Rochester, Minnesota

Dean C. Taylor, MD
Professor, Orthopaedic Surgery
Duke University School of Medicine
Durham, North Carolina

Thomas (Quin) Throckmorton, MD
Professor
Shoulder and Elbow Surgery
Residency Program Director
University of Tennessee-Campbell Clinic
Department of Orthopaedic Surgery and Biomedical Engineering
Memphis, Tennessee

Fotios P. Tjoumakaris, MD
Associate Professor, Orthopaedic Surgery
Sidney Kimmel College of Medicine
Thomas Jefferson University
Rothman Institute, Sports Medicine
Egg Harbor Township, New Jersey

John M. Tokish, MD
Department of Orthopedic Surgery
Mayo Clinic
Phoenix, Arizona

Kimberly V. Tucker, MD
Orthopedic Surgeon
Adult, Adolescent, and Pediatric Sports Medicine Specialist
Atlantic Sports Health
Bridgewater, New Jersey

Dean Wang, MD
Fellow
Sports Medicine and Shoulder Service
Hospital for Special Surgery
New York, New York

Tim Wang, MD
Clinical Assistant Professor, Orthopaedic Surgery
Stanford University
Stanford, California

Chris S. Warrell, MD
Orthopaedic Sports Medicine Fellow
Andrews Research and Education Foundation
Gulf Breeze, Florida

Ryan J. Warth, MD
Clinical Research Monitor
Department of Orthopaedic Surgery
University of Texas Health Science Center at Houston
McGovern Medical School
Houston, Texas

Brian R. Waterman, MD
Associate Professor, Sports Medicine
Assistant Fellowship Director, Sports Medicine & Shoulder Surgery
Department of Orthopaedic Surgery
Wake Forest University School of Medicine
Team Physician, Wake Forest University Athletics
Team Physician, Winston-Salem Dash
Medical Center Boulevard
Winston-Salem, North Carolina

Brian M. Weatherford, MD
Illinois Bone and Joint Institute
Clinical Assistant Professor
University of Chicago Pritzker School of Medicine
Glenview, Illinois

Kristina L. Welton, MD
Fellow
Orthopaedic Surgery–Sports Medicine
University of Colorado
Boulder, Colorado

Robert W. Westermann, MD
Team Physician, University of Iowa Athletics
Assistant Professor
Department of Orthopedics and Rehabilitation
University of Iowa
Iowa City, Iowa

Riley J. Williams III, MD
Professor of Orthopedic Surgery and Attending Orthopedic Surgeon
Hospital for Special Surgery
Weill Cornell Medical College
New York, New York

Megan R. Wolf, MD
Resident Physician
Department of Orthopedic Surgery
University of Connecticut Health Center
Farmington, Connecticut

Brian R. Wolf, MD, MS
John and Kim Callaghan Endowed Chair and Director of UI Sports Medicine
Professor and Vice-Chairman of Finance and Academic Affairs
Department of Orthopaedics and Rehabilitation
University of Iowa Hospitals and Clinics
Iowa City, Iowa

Jarret M. Woodmass, MD
Clinical Fellow in Orthopedic Surgery
Massachusetts General Hospital
Boston, Massachusetts

Rick W. Wright, MD
Executive Vice Chairman
Jerome J. Gilden Distinguished Professor
Department of Orthopaedic Surgery
Washington University School of Medicine
St. Louis, Missouri

James D. Wylie, MD
Child and Young Adult Hip Fellow
Orthopedic Department
Boston Children's Hospital
Boston, Massachusetts

Ken Yamaguchi, MD, MBA
Sam and Marilyn Fox Distinguished Professor of Orthopedic Surgery
Orthopedic Surgery
Washington University School of Medicine
St. Louis, Missouri

Jane C. Yeoh, MD, FRCSC
Clinical Fellow in Orthopaedic Surgery
Department of Orthopaedics
University of British Columbia
Vancouver, British Columbia

Saif U. Zaman, MD
Attending Physician
Dekalb Orthopedics and Sports Medicine
Atlanta, Georgia
Jefferson Sports Medicine Fellow
Rothman Institute at Thomas
Philadelphia, Pennsylvania

Foreword

I developed the idea for the first book in this series, *The Harborview Illustrated Tips and Tricks in Fracture Surgery*, more than two decades ago. I thought that a book with succinct, bulleted text and numerous illustrations, radiographs, C-arm images, and clinical photos showing how we fix fractures at Harborview Medical Center would appeal to orthopaedic surgeons, especially those in training and community surgeons needing a quick review of tips and tricks before caring for patients with fractures. The success of the first edition, which was first published in 2011, led to international translations and an enlarged, updated second edition published in 2018.

Given the popularity of the first edition, during preparation of the second Fracture edition, Brian Brown (an Executive Editor at Wolters Kluwer Health) and I discussed the concept of extending this series to other orthopaedic surgical specialties. He and I approached Dr. Frederick Azar with the idea of creating a similar Tips and Tricks edition for orthopaedic "sports" and arthroscopic surgery. Dr. Azar's enthusiasm and that of his colleagues resulted in this publication.

M. Bradford Henley, MD, MBA

Preface

The purpose of this text, as the title suggests, is to provide focused information from the experts on how to approach technical problems in sports medicine surgery. To make the tips and tricks easily obtainable for a specific procedure, information concerning anatomy, indications, contraindications, and alternate treatment methods are kept to a minimum. Drawings, operative photos, and videos are used liberally to illustrate surgical techniques.

Although this was a large project in terms of the number of chapters and authors, with the help of Tim Rinehart and others at Wolters Kluwer and Kay Daugherty of the Campbell Foundation, communication with the authors was timely, chapter revisions were prompt, and production moved along smoothly.

My sincerest thanks to the many sports medicine "stars" who willingly shared their knowledge and expertise with us. Whether you've done a procedure once or 100 times, you might learn something new from the "tips and tricks" described—I know I did. I hope residents, fellows, and practicing orthopaedists will find this text helpful as they continue to care for athletes of all ages and abilities.

Frederick M. Azar, MD

In memoriam:

During the preparation of this text, we lost one of our most stalwart sports medicine supporters, Dr. Allen Anderson, to a tragic accident. For over 40 years, he provided first-class care to athletes of all ages and abilities. His skill and compassion were responsible for many an athlete resuming his or her sport at a high level. We will miss his warmth and friendship, as well as his expertise and knowledge, and are proud and humbled to include his chapter (written along with his son Chris Anderson) in this collection.

Contents

KNEE

FOOT & ANKLE

Chapter 1
Principles of Shoulder Arthroscopy

W. STEPHEN CHOATE
JASON P. ROGERS
RICHARD J. HAWKINS

Sterile Instruments/Equipment

- Scope
  - A 4-mm large joint, 30-degree fiberoptic scope is used for shoulder arthroscopy.
  - A 70-degree scope occasionally is used to optimize visualization from the posterior portal around "acute angles" and to limit portal crowding.
  - Subscapularis repair, Bankart or anterior labroligamentous periosteal sleeve avulsion (ALPSA) repair, coracoclavicular ligament reconstruction, and distal clavicle excision
- Standard arthroscopy tower
  - Monitors (2), light source, shaver motor, radiofrequency ablation source, printer
  - Viewing screens are positioned above and below the patient's head to improve working access in the lateral decubitus position.
  - A dual inflow/outflow arthroscopy pump, which tightly controls compartmental fluid pressure, is preferred for fluid management.
  - Inflow pressure is set at 35-75 mm Hg depending on bleeding and fluid extravasation factors.
  - Epinephrine-infused normal saline (0.33 mg/L) is used for irrigation fluid and has been shown to improve visual clarity, decrease total operative time, and reduce fluid volume utilization.[1]
- Intra-articular/subacromial instruments
  - Blunt camera trocar and dual port cannula. Inflow tubing is connected to cannula, but no outflow suction is used.
  - Graspers. Looped devices with and without teeth are useful for removing loose bodies/foreign material, shuttling suture, and mobilizing tissue.
  - Probe.
  - Bipolar radiofrequency thermal ablation (RFA) device. We prefer a 90-degree wand.
  - Motorized devices. Generally a 3.5- to 4.5-mm bone cutting shaver is adequate for bony and soft tissue debridement (eg, subacromial decompression, distal clavicle excision).
  - For sclerotic bone, a 3.0- to 5.0-mm cylindrical burr can be used on the reverse.

Anesthesia

- A combination of general anesthesia and interscalene regional blockade is preferred.
  - This reduces postoperative pain scores and the need for supplemental analgesics.[2]
  - Paralysis of the hemidiaphragm is a known complication of interscalene blockade and can lead to postoperative respiratory compromise.
- Hypotensive anesthesia is requested to limit blood loss and optimize visual clarity.
  - The goal is a <49-mm Hg difference between systolic blood pressure (SBP) and fluid pressure within the surgical compartment, which typically translates to an SBP of ~100 mm Hg.

Examination Under Anesthesia

- In all shoulders, we screen for selective or global capsular tightness that may require release (Fig. 1-1).

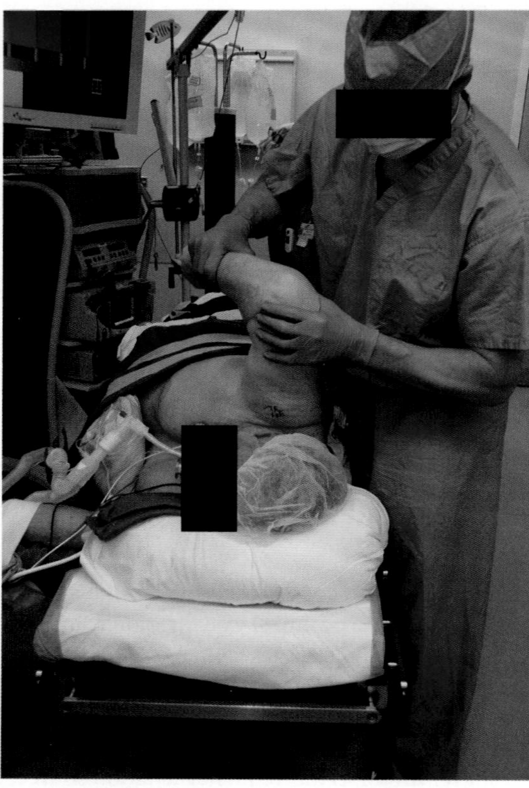

Figure 1-1 | In the absence of instability, examination under anesthesia is performed for the operative shoulder with the patient in the lateral decubitus position. Passive range of motion is tested in all planes to screen for capsular tightness.

- Translational and provocative stability testing is important to confirm instability direction and severity. This is best performed with the patient supine to allow comparison to the contralateral, unaffected shoulder. The scapula is more easily stabilized in this position.
  - Overaggressive load and shift testing, which can cause bleeding and compromise visualization, should be avoided.
- In shoulders with instability, we screen both shoulders for multidirectional laxity.

Patient Positioning

- General principles
  - Communication with the anesthesia team is essential to ensure safe head and neck positioning and a secure airway. The tube is secured to the nonoperative side.
  - Unobstructed access to the medial aspect of the operative shoulder is ensured.
  - A wide operative field is established; matching the edges of the sterile drapes will help protect against shrinking of the field during draping.
  - To protect against fluid extravasation and field contamination, the patient's arm is placed into the position of traction before the final occlusive layer is applied at the edges.
  - Ioban covers the axilla, especially in males, to limit wound contamination.
  - All exposed bony prominences are padded.
- Lateral decubitus position (LDP)
  - We prefer this position for nearly all shoulder arthroscopic procedures. Lateral traction increases the glenohumeral and subacromial spaces, which is useful for viewing and accessing labral/rotator cuff pathology. Access to the posterior shoulder is unobstructed. In addition, there is no increased risk for patient hypotension/bradycardia, which can cause cerebral hypoperfusion.
  - The beach-chair position (BCP) is used when conversion to an open procedure is planned.

- The patient is positioned laterally on a standard operating room table with the operative shoulder facing up. We are careful to move the patient to the top and operative side of the bed to facilitate access during the procedure.
- Foam padding protects the contralateral arm (radial and ulnar nerves), greater trochanter, fibular head (peroneal nerve), lateral malleolus, and heel. Pillows are placed between the knees and ankles.
- A vacuum beanbag is used to secure the pelvis and lower torso in position with a posterior tilt of 20-30 degrees to bring glenoid parallel to floor (Fig. 1-2).

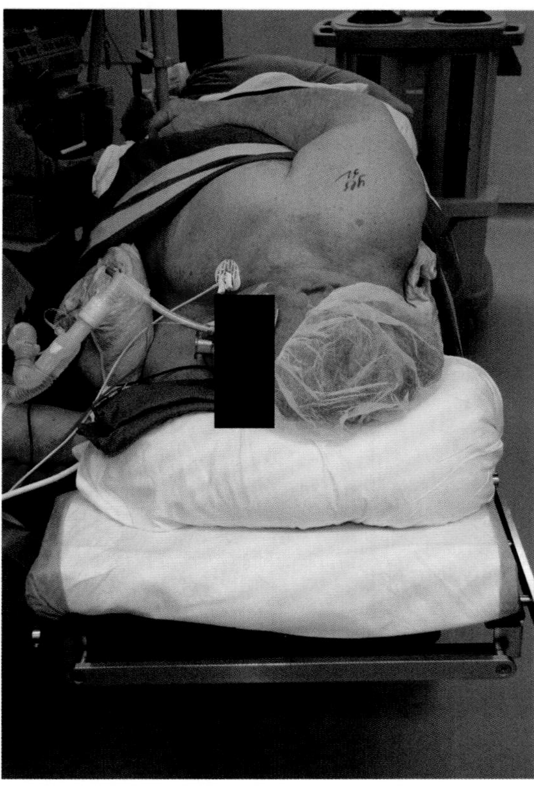

Figure 1-2 | An approximate 20-degree posterior lean of the operative shoulder brings the glenoid face parallel to the floor, which facilitates visualization and access.

- An axillary roll reduces tension on the brachial plexus and assists ventilation.
- Blue towels and tape and/or heavy straps are helpful to secure the beanbag around the upper torso and prevent malpositioning and posterior shoulder sag during the procedure (Fig. 1-3).

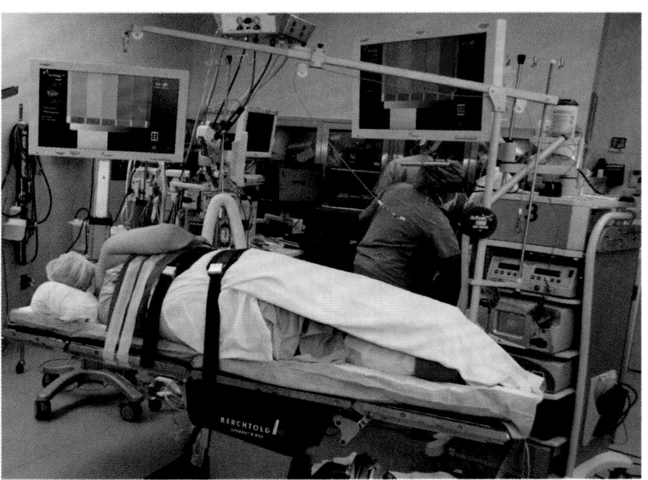

Figure 1-3 | Gradual posterior sag of the shoulder can be an issue during the procedure. In addition to seat belts to secure the body, we have found blue towels and silk tape helpful in securing the beanbag around the patient's upper torso, which minimizes the sag. The operating table is turned 90 degrees away from anesthesia to optimize access.

- Lateral arm holder
  - We prefer a weighted traction tower anchored at the foot of the nonoperative side of the bed.
  - The traction sleeve is positioned high in the axilla to limit slippage (Fig. 1-4).
  - Traction (10 lb) is moved between adjustable cables and pulleys to generate varying degrees of abduction and forward flexion.
  - Lateral distraction through an axillary strap in slight abduction (20 degrees) creates a lateral force vector that improves access for glenohumeral labral work (Fig. 1-5).

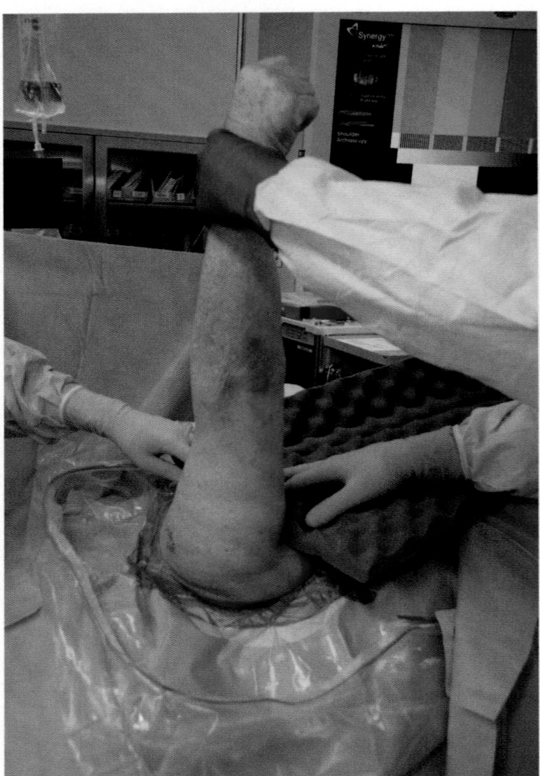

Figure 1-4 | The foam traction sleeve is placed high in the axilla to limit slippage down the arm and loss of traction during the procedure.

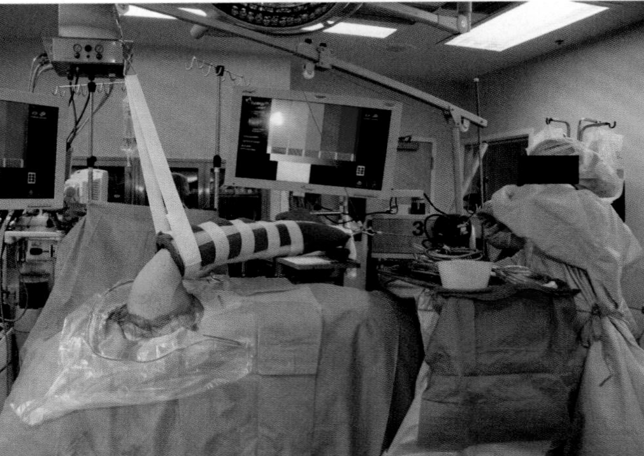

Figure 1-5 | The traction tower consists of cables and pulleys with weights that can be adjusted to provide varying degrees of abduction, forward elevation, and lateral distraction. This device offers the advantage of an axillary distraction strap, which is particularly useful when working in the glenohumeral compartment.

  - For visualization of the rotator cuff footprint and subdeltoid recess, the axillary strap is removed and the weights are adjusted to increase the abduction angle and longitudinal traction (40-70 degrees).
  - It is important to limit the traction time to preserve local and distal tissue perfusion.
  - A pneumatic lateral limb positioner alternatively can be used.

Surgical Anatomy

- Portal placement
  - Placement is dictated by pathology and the planned procedure.
  - Before the skin incision is made, portal location is identified with an 18-gauge spinal needle to localize entry point and trajectory. Future adjacent portals and skin distance should be considered to prevent crowding. If portal location is suboptimal, punching through a different fascial or capsular window through the same skin incision can be helpful.
  - Accurate identification and marking of bony landmarks are critical to ensure safe and effective portal placement.
  - Important landmarks include the posterolateral acromion, anterolateral acromion, superior "soft spot" between the acromion and clavicle, and coracoid process.

- For obese or muscular patients, drawing the surface anatomy before putting the arm in traction can assist in landmark identification.
- Posterior viewing portal
  - This portal is established first for a standard viewing portal. Proper positioning is critical for adequate visualization of both the glenohumeral and subacromial spaces.
  - The portal usually is made 2-3 cm distal and 1-2 cm medial to the posterolateral acromial edge; however, adjustments often are required for larger/smaller shoulders and pathology (eg, more superior for rotator cuff pathology, more distal and lateral for labral pathology).
    - The palpable "soft spot" between the infraspinatus and teres minor muscles is a reliable landmark for referencing the glenohumeral joint line.
  - The trocar tip is gently swept from side to side to feel for the humeral head laterally and then the glenoid "shelf" medially. The trocar is aimed toward the coracoid once adjacent to the "shelf" to enter the glenohumeral joint. The surgeon's free hand is used to triangulate.
    - Aggressive forced entry, which can lead to iatrogenic cartilage injury, should be avoided.
    - The risk of injury to the axillary (49 mm inferior-lateral) and suprascapular (29 mm medial) nerves should be kept in mind.[3]
- Anterior working portal
  - After the camera is established in the joint, an anterior "working" portal is created with an 18-gauge needle from outside in through the rotator interval.
  - Portal location is adjusted based on the planned procedure (eg, higher in interval for SLAP, lower and just above the subscapularis for Bankart). A spinal needle is used to confirm the trajectory for future anchor placement in unstable shoulders.
  - The skin is incised with care taken to avoid injury to the cephalic vein. The anterior interval capsular tissue is dilated with a hemostat to facilitate access in and out of the joint.
  - To avoid injury to the brachial plexus, portal placement should stay lateral to the coracoid process.
    - The mean nerve distances from the anteromedial coracoid tip are axillary, 30.3 mm; musculocutaneous, 33.0 mm; and lateral cord, 28.5 mm.[4]
- Additional portals may be necessary. Figure 1-6 demonstrates the typical portal locations used for shoulder arthroscopy.
- Intra-articular anatomy
  - Diagnostic arthroscopy should proceed in a systematic, stepwise fashion to identify all important structures.
  - Outflow from unoccupied portals is limited to prevent turbulence and secondary bleeding. A cannula, digital pressure, or lap sponge can be used to plug the portals. Increasing inflow pressure alone only worsens bleeding in this circumstance (Fig. 1-7).

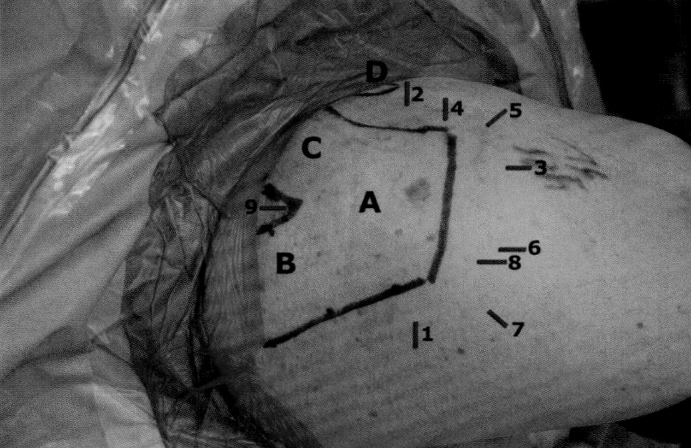

Figure 1-6 | The bony landmarks of the acromion (*A*), scapular spine (*B*), clavicle (*C*), and medial coracoid (*D*) are marked to establish reliable reference points for safe portal placement. The typical portals used for shoulder arthroscopy include posterior (*1*), anterior central (may move distal for true midglenoid portal) (*2*), anterolateral (*3*), anterosuperior (*4*), anterosuperior-lateral (*5*), posterolateral (*6*), posterior 7 o'clock (*7*), Wilmington (*8*), and Neviaser (*9*).

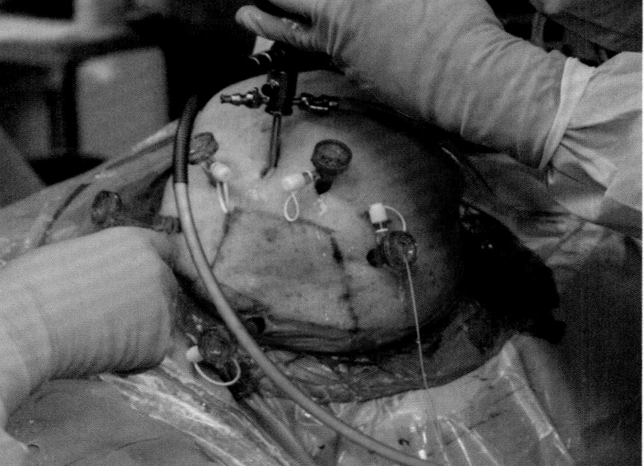

Figure 1-7 | When using multiple portals, cannulas are helpful for maintaining intracompartmental fluid pressure and preventing turbulence.

- Glenohumeral joint examination
    - Examination starts at the biceps root attachment. The labrum is probed and assessed for SLAP pathology. The long head biceps tendon (LHBT) is followed toward its groove, and the intertubercular portion is pulled into the joint for assessment. The medial biceps sling is examined, and, if disrupted, the rotator interval is opened to exclude a "hidden lesion" of the subscapularis (Figs. 1-8 and 1-9).

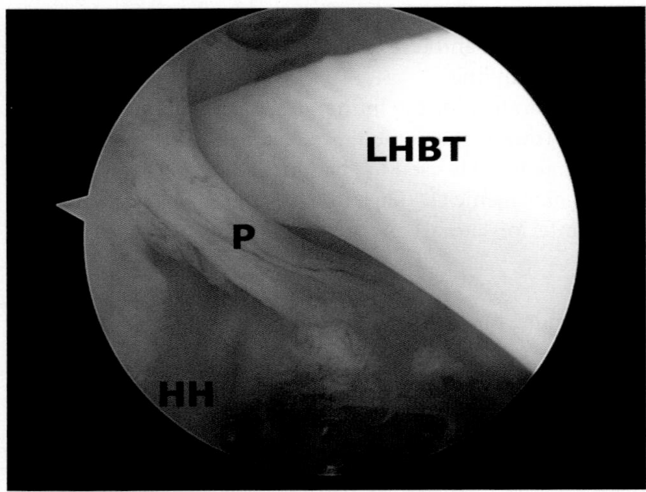

Figure 1-8 | The biceps long head (LHBT), reflection pulley (P), and rotator interval are inspected for tearing or tendon subluxation. HH, humeral head.

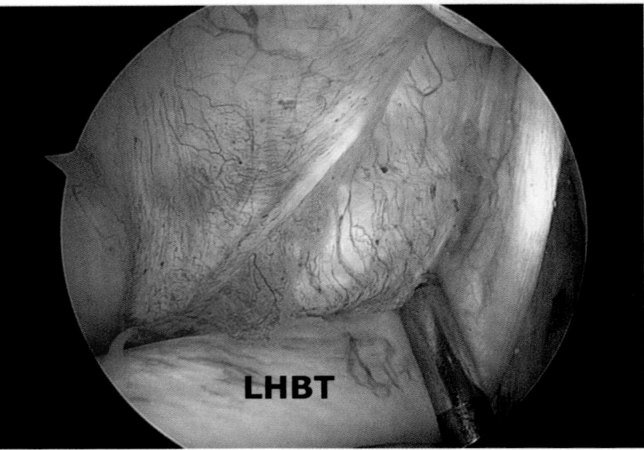

Figure 1-9 | A probe is brought through the anterior portal to pull the intertubercular portion of the LHBT into the joint for inspection.

- The superior and middle glenohumeral ligaments and adjacent subscapularis insertion are examined (Fig. 1-10).
    - A posterior lever push maneuver is used to expose the subscapularis footprint. In the setting of subscapularis pathology or revision surgery, the coracoid is exposed through the rotator interval to assess the coracohumeral interval.
    - Loose bodies may be found in the anterior subscapularis recess.
- The labrum and inferior glenohumeral ligament complex are inspected from anterior to posterior (Fig. 1-11).

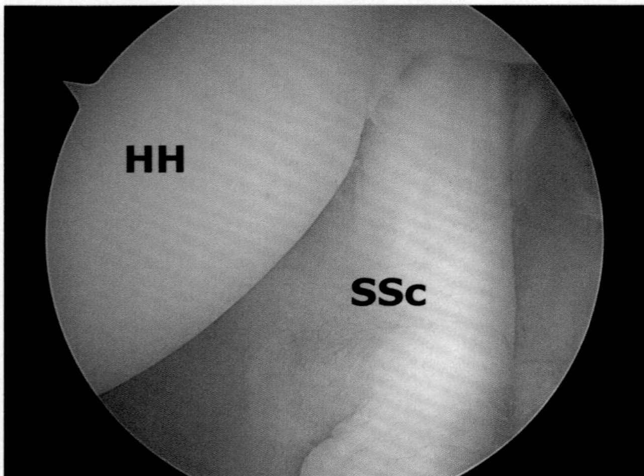

Figure 1-10 | Visualization of the subscapularis (SSc) articular insertion is enhanced with a posterior lever push maneuver. In some cases, a 70-degree scope is useful as well. HH, humeral head.

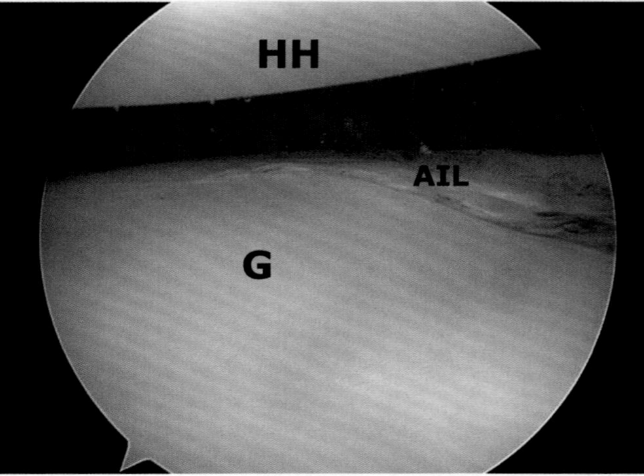

Figure 1-11 | View of the anteroinferior labrum (AIL) from the posterior portal in a left shoulder. HH, humeral head; G, glenoid.

- Care is taken not to fall out of the joint when viewing the posterior labrum from the posterior portal.
- Loose bodies may be found in the axillary pouch.
- Switching the scope to the anterior portal occasionally is required to more closely assess the posterior labrum and to obtain a "bird's eye view" centering shot of the humeral head and glenoid (Figs. 1-12 and 1-13).

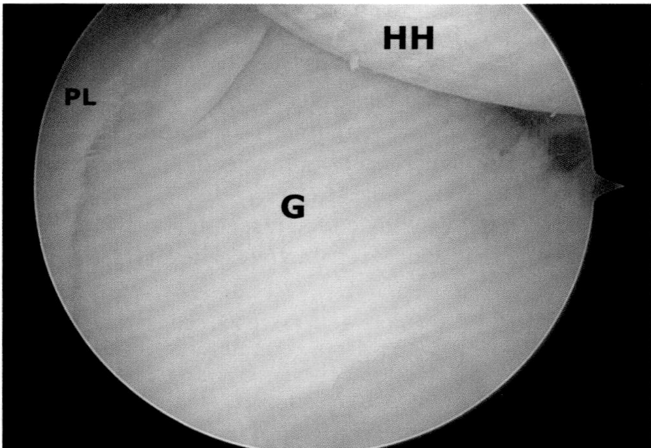

Figure 1-12 | "Bird's eye" view from the anterosuperior portal. Anterior decentering of the humeral head (HH) due to a soft tissue Bankart lesion. The tear extends into the posterior labrum (PL). G, glenoid.

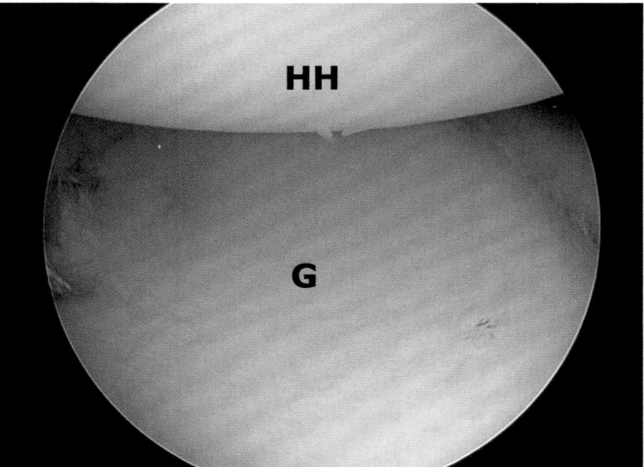

Figure 1-13 | Following labroligamentous repair, successful recentering of the head is seen. HH, humeral head; G, glenoid.

  - The undersurface of the rotator cuff is best viewed with the shoulder abducted (Fig. 1-14).
- Subacromial examination
  - The cannula and trocar are redirected into the subacromial space through the posterior portal. The trocar tip is used to localize the coracoacromial ligament (CAL), then swept laterally and posteriorly into the subdeltoid recess, staying away from the hypervascular medial bursal tissue (Fig. 1-15).

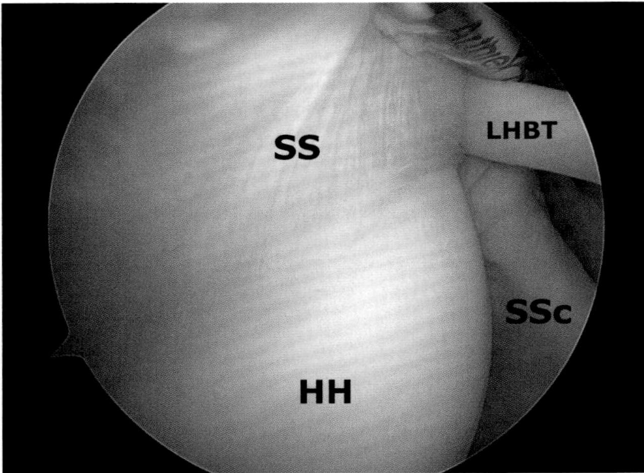

Figure 1-14 | View of an intact supraspinatus (SS) articular insertion from the posterior portal in a left shoulder. HH, humeral head; LHBT, long head biceps tendon; SSc, subscapularis.

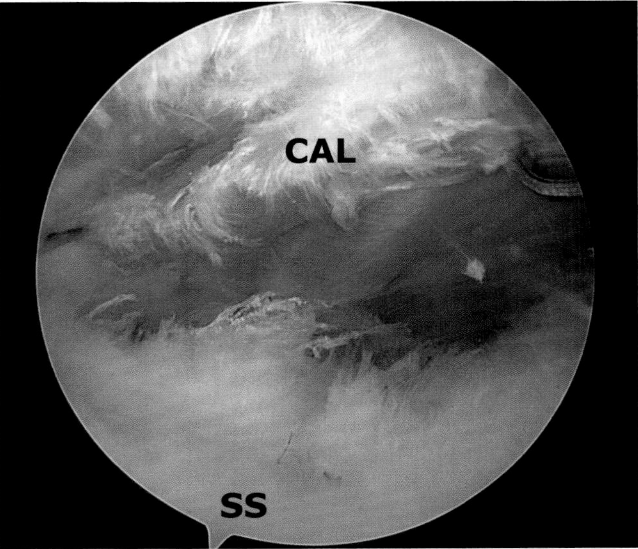

Figure 1-15 | The subacromial space is inspected from the posterior portal. The coracoacromial ligament (CAL) often is frayed and degenerative secondary to chronic outlet impingement, as is seen in this case. SS, supraspinatus bursal surface.

- A lateral working portal, placed ~3 cm from the anterolateral acromial edge, often is required to clear bursal tissue and create a "room with a view."
- Upon entry into the space, the camera is directed upward to view the acromial undersurface and the CAL. The RFA device is introduced through the lateral portal and "chopsticked" with the camera for localization (triangulation). The camera is pulled back slowly until the thermal device is in view.
- The camera is turned down, and a combination of the ablator and shaver is used to fully expose the rotator cuff and clear out the posterolateral gutter.
- The subdeltoid adhesions and bursal connections to the humerus are excised to increase access into the subdeltoid recess. The deltoid fascia is preserved.
- With the camera in the lateral portal, dissection of the scapular spine base assists in identification of the supraspinatus and infraspinatus musculotendinous structures.
- The rotator cuff, CAL, AC joint, acromion, extra-articular biceps, spinoglenoid notch, and suprascapular nerve can all be evaluated from the subacromial space.
- Only 56% of the LHBT can be viewed from within the joint. Tendon inspection from the subdeltoid space is important when clinical concern for biceps pathology is high (Fig. 1-16).

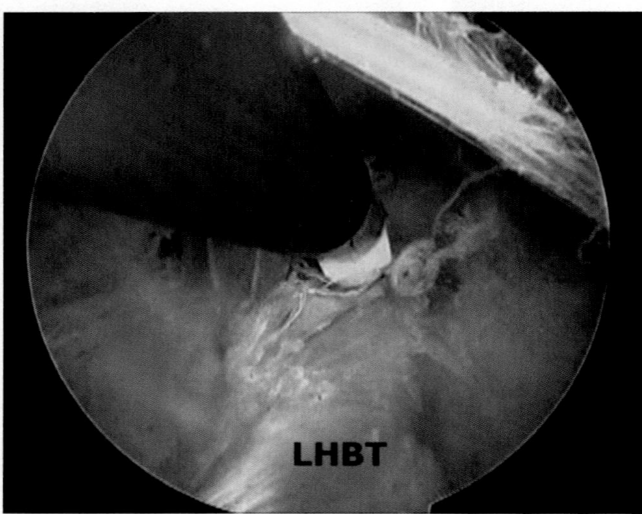

Figure 1-16 | With the camera in the anterolateral portal, the transverse humeral ligament is released and the long head biceps tendon (LHBT) is seen just above the pectoralis major tendon within the subdeltoid space.

References

1. van Montfoort D, van Kampen P, Huijsmans P. Epinephrine diluted saline irrigation fluid in arthroscopic shoulder surgery: a significant improvement of clarity of visual field and shortening of total operation time: a randomized controlled trial. *Arthroscopy*. 2016;32(3):436-444.
2. Hughes M, Matava M, Wright R, Brophy R, Smith M. Interscalene brachial plexus block for arthroscopic shoulder surgery: a systematic review. *J Bone Joint Surg Am*. 2013;95:1318-1324.
3. Meyer M, Graveleau N, Hardy P, Landreau P. Anatomic risks of shoulder arthroscopy portals: anatomic cadaveric study of 12 portals. *Arthroscopy*. 2007;23(5):529-536.
4. Lo IK, Burkhart SS, Parten PM. Surgery about the coracoid: neurovascular structures at risk. *Arthroscopy*. 2004;20(6):591-595.

Suggested Readings

Paxton ES, Backus J, Keener J, Brophy R. Shoulder arthroscopy: basic principles of positioning, anesthesia, and portal anatomy. *J Am Acad Orthop Surg*. 2013;21:332-342.

Snyder S. Diagnostic arthroscopy. In: Snyder S, ed. *Shoulder Arthroscopy*. 3rd ed. Philadelphia, PA: Lippincott Williams & Wilkins; 2014.

Chapter 2
Arthroscopic Bankart Repair

DANIEL F. O'BRIEN
MEGAN R. WOLF
HARDEEP SINGH
ROBERT A. ARCIERO

Indications[1-15]

- First-time traumatic shoulder dislocation with Bankart lesion confirmed by MRI
- Athlete <25 years old
- High-demand athlete
- Recurrent shoulder dislocations

Contraindications[16-22]

- Multidirectional instability
- Large Hill-Sachs lesion
- Humeral avulsion of the glenoid labrum (HAGL)
- Capsular deficiency
- Glenoid bone loss of 25% or more

Advantages of Arthroscopic Bankart Repair[2,23,24]

- Less surgical morbidity
- Less postoperative pain
- Reduced cost
- Improved cosmetic result
- Easier/faster rehabilitation

Equipment and Instrumentation

- Patient positioning
  - Balanced arm traction, 7 lb longitudinal traction, and 5 lb lateral traction
  - STaR (Shoulder Traction and Rotation) sleeve (Arthrex, Naples, FL)
  - Beanbag positioner, vacuum
  - Sterile blanket, rolled
- Arthroscopy
  - Fluid pump system
  - 30-degree arthroscope with standard arthroscopic instruments
  - Spinal needle
  - Arthroscopic elevator/spatula
  - 8.25-mm cannulas
- Repair
  - Three or four double-loaded 2.0-mm suture anchors

- Three No. 0 PDS sutures
- Curved suture hook
- Suture retrieval forceps
- Suture passer
- Arthroscopic knot pusher
- Closure
  - 2.0 nylon sutures
  - Shoulder immobilizer with abduction pillow

Patient Positioning

- The patient is placed in the lateral decubitus position using a vacuum beanbag positioner with the operative shoulder up (Fig. 2-1).

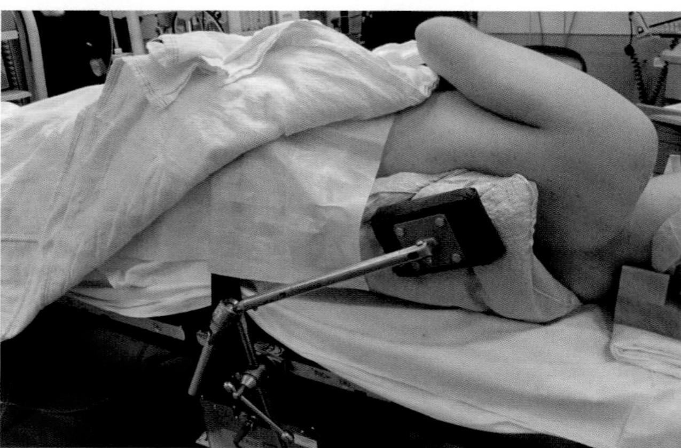

Figure 2-1 | Patient positioning. The patient is placed in a lateral decubitus position with a vacuum beanbag positioner. A hip positioner may be useful to assist in maintaining position through augmentation of the beanbag positioner.

- A corner of the beanbag immobilizer or a gel pad is placed at the junction between the thorax and axilla of the nonoperative shoulder to prevent nerve injury during surgery.
- Sterile draping of the surgical field is performed per surgeon preference.
- The operative arm is placed in a sterile STaR sleeve and attached to the balanced arm traction device with the arm externally rotated (thumb up) and abducted 20-30 degrees. Seven pounds of longitudinal traction and five pounds of lateral traction are placed (Fig. 2-2).

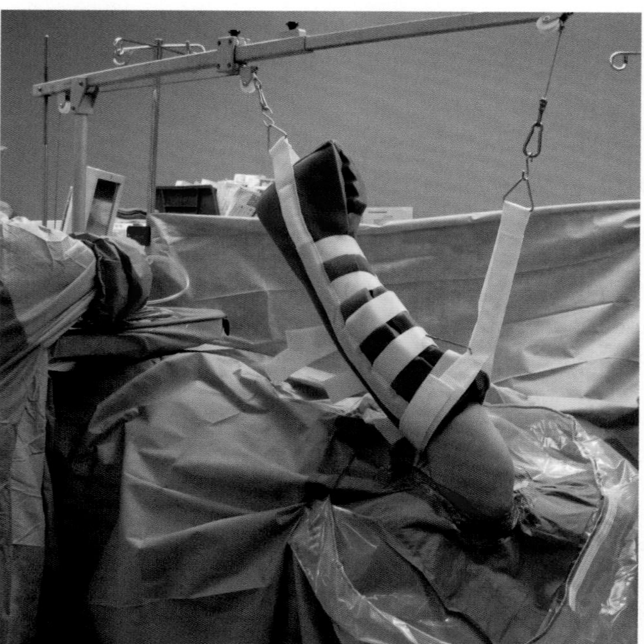

Figure 2-2 | The arm is placed into a sterile STaR sleeve and attached to the traction device. Seven pounds of longitudinal traction and five pounds of lateral traction are then placed onto the traction device to allow for optimal viewing of the capsulolabral complex of the glenohumeral joint.

Surgical Approach

- Bony landmarks of the shoulder are marked with a surgical marker, including the coracoid process, clavicle, acromion, acromioclavicular joint, and spine of the scapula for orientation before portal placement (Fig. 2-3).

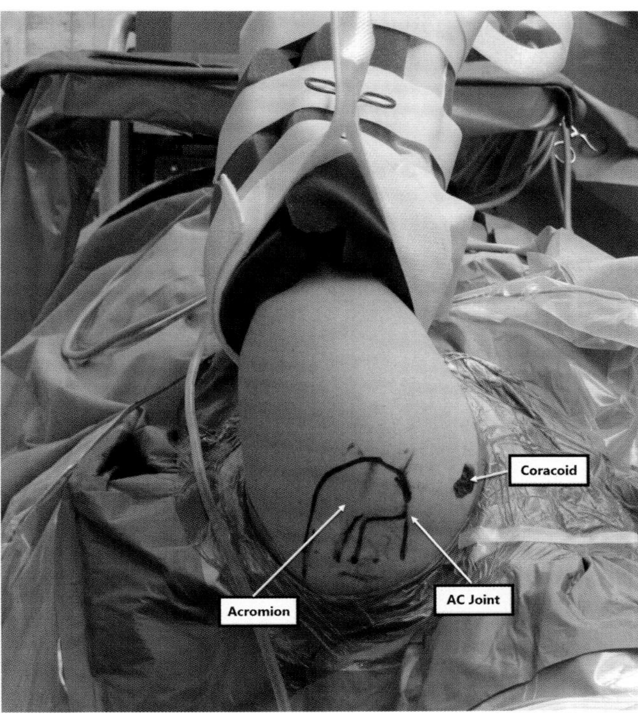

Figure 2-3 | Landmarks are palpated and marked with a surgical marker, including the spine of the scapula, acromion, acromioclavicular (AC) joint, and coracoid. These will be landmarks for proper portal placement.

- A standard posterior arthroscopic portal is created first (Fig. 2-4).

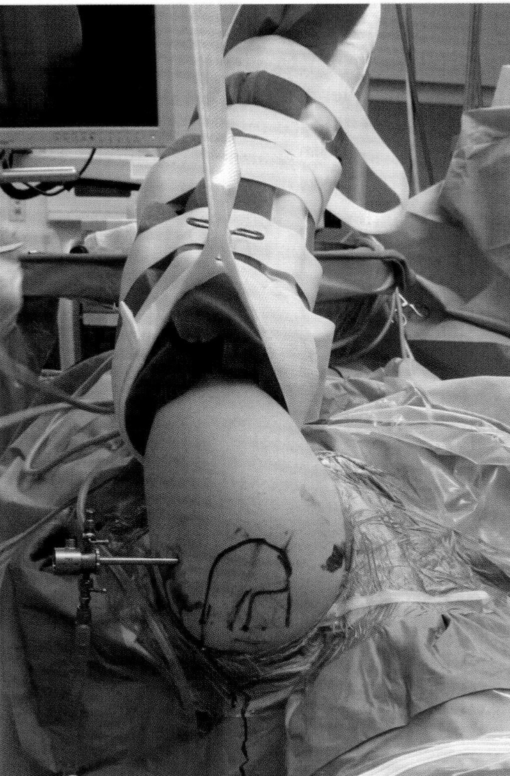

Figure 2-4 | The posterior portal is first placed by marking a position 1 cm distal and 1 cm medial to the posterolateral tip of the acromion. After a skin incision is made, a blunt trocar is placed directed toward the coracoid. The trocar is removed, leaving the sheath for placement of the arthroscope.

- The portal is marked 2 cm distal to the posterior angle of the acromion and more lateral to the traditional portal. This will ensure that the portal is not too medial coming into the glenoid.
- A small skin incision is made and the blunt trocar is inserted aiming toward the coracoid. The trocar is removed, leaving the sheath, and the arthroscope is inserted.

- A complete diagnostic arthroscopy is performed, and the Bankart lesion is visualized using the posterior arthroscopic portal.
- Under direct visualization, the anterosuperior and anterior portals are created using a spinal needle to allow for accurate portal placement (Fig. 2-5).

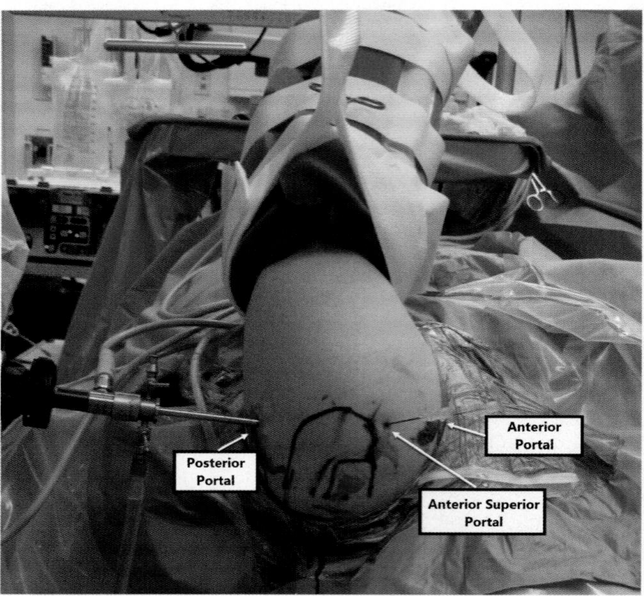

Figure 2-5 | The anterosuperior and anterior portals are created under direct visualization. The anterosuperior portal is placed just in front of the anterolateral edge of the acromion and lateral to the coracoid and should enter the joint just posterior to the biceps tendon. The anterior portal is placed halfway between the acromioclavicular joint and lateral aspect of the coracoid and should enter the joint just above the subscapularis, parallel to the glenoid surface.

- The anterosuperior portal will be the viewing portal. The spinal needle is placed just in front of the anterolateral edge of the acromion and lateral to the coracoid. Proper intra-articular placement is located just posterior to the biceps tendon. A skin incision is made and blunt dissection is carried to the capsule with a hemostat before the trocar is inserted to prevent nerve injury.
- To create the anterior portal, a spinal needle is placed halfway between the acromioclavicular joint and lateral aspect of the coracoid. This should pierce the capsule just above the subscapularis and directed into the joint, parallel to the glenoid surface. Place an 8.25-mm cannula in the anterior portal.

- The camera is removed from the posterior portal and placed in the anterosuperior portal for the duration of the procedure. An 8.25-mm cannula is placed in the posterior portal.
- A sterile rolled blanket is placed in the axilla to provide lateral distraction of the glenohumeral joint, which improves visualization of the entire inferior aspect of the joint (Fig. 2-6).

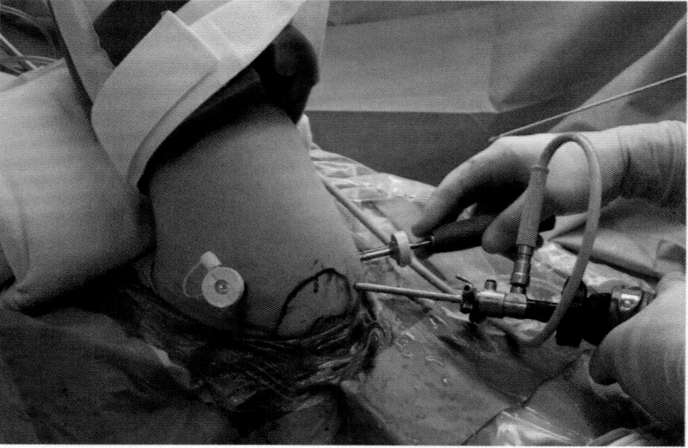

Figure 2-6 | 8.5-mm cannulas are placed into the posterior and anterior portals to be used as working portals. The camera is placed into the anterosuperior portal for optimal viewing of the inferior portion of the capsuloligamentous injury. A sterile towel roll is placed in the axilla to access visualization of the inferior glenohumeral joint.

Repair Technique

- The labrum and inferior glenoid are inspeccted using an arthroscopic probe through the posterior portal. The capsulolabral complex is often scarred to the scapular neck and can be medialized (the anterior labroligamentous periosteal sleeve avulsion, or "ALPSA," lesion). This must be fully mobilized and freed where the labrum is "floating" and the subscapularis muscle is exposed. A burr is inserted through the anterior or posterior portal to roughen the scapular neck until a bleeding bony surface is achieved, which assists in healing of the repair (Fig. 2-7).

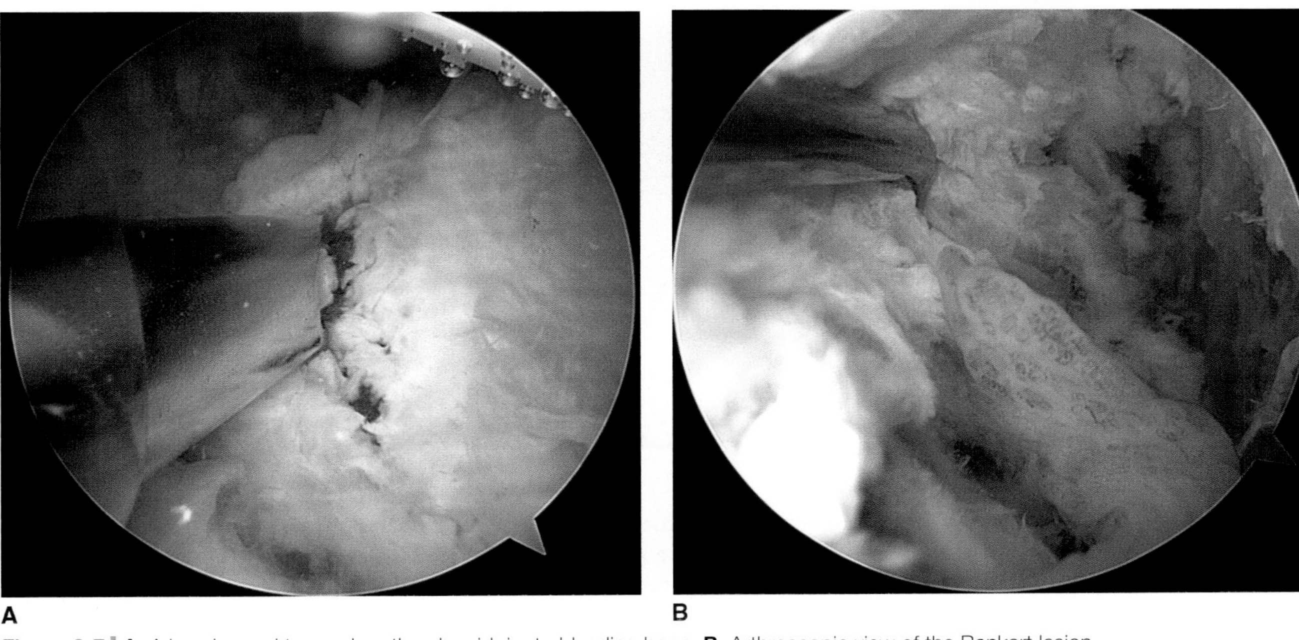

Figure 2-7 | **A.** A burr is used to roughen the glenoid rim to bleeding bone. **B.** Arthroscopic view of the Bankart lesion.

- A double-loaded 2.0-mm suture anchor is placed in the anteroinferior glenoid at the 5 o'clock position for the left shoulder or the 7 o'clock position for the right shoulder (Fig. 2-8). If necessary, a percutaneous portal through the subscapularis will permit access to the inferior aspect of the glenoid.
- A curved suture-passing device is used to pass a No. 0 PDS suture from the posterior or anterior portal through the capsulolabral complex at the 6 o'clock position.

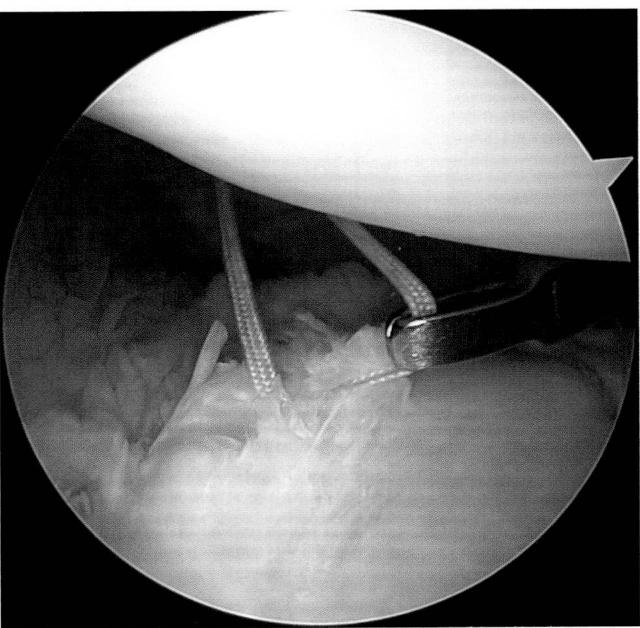

Figure 2-8 | The suture anchor is placed at the edge of the glenoid at the 7 o'clock position for the right shoulder viewed from the anterosuperior portal, allowing for enough bone stock for anchor stability. The grasper is located at the 6 o'clock position.

- The suture should be placed inferior enough so that the pierced capsulolabral complex is inferior to the previously placed anchor. This will ensure that the inferior glenohumeral ligament and labrum are given proper tension when the suture is tied (Fig. 2-9).

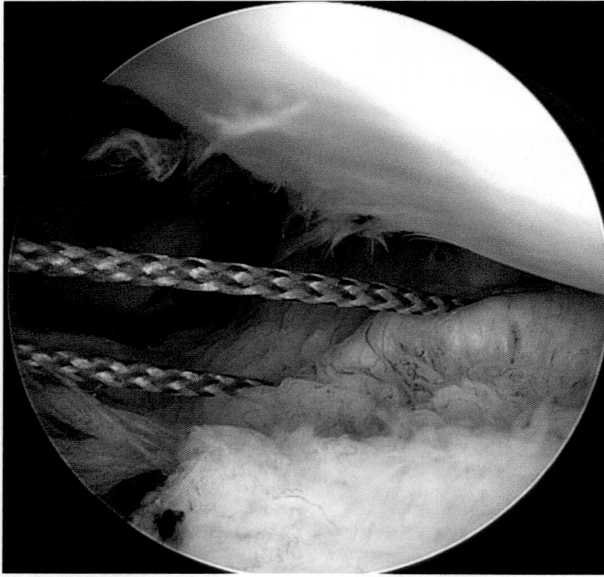

Figure 2-9 | Suture is passed inferior to the anchor to decrease the inferior capsular volume and ensure that the inferior glenohumeral ligament and labrum are given proper tension when the suture is tied.

- One of the anchor sutures is shuttled across using the PDS and through the capsule and labrum.
- This step is repeated to complete a mattress suture (Fig. 2-10), which is tied.
- The second suture from the same anchor is then passed, and a simple knot is tied. This will re-establish labral height and recreate a "bumper" (Fig. 2-11).

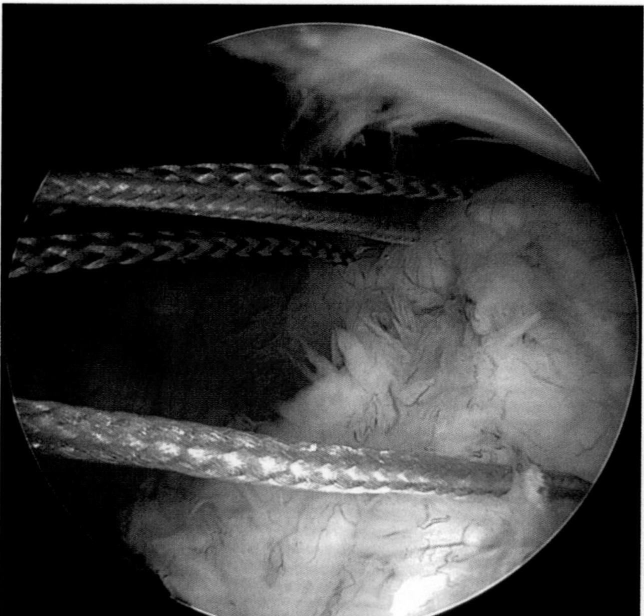

Figure 2-10 | The first suture is a mattress suture with adequate spread to create optimal tension.

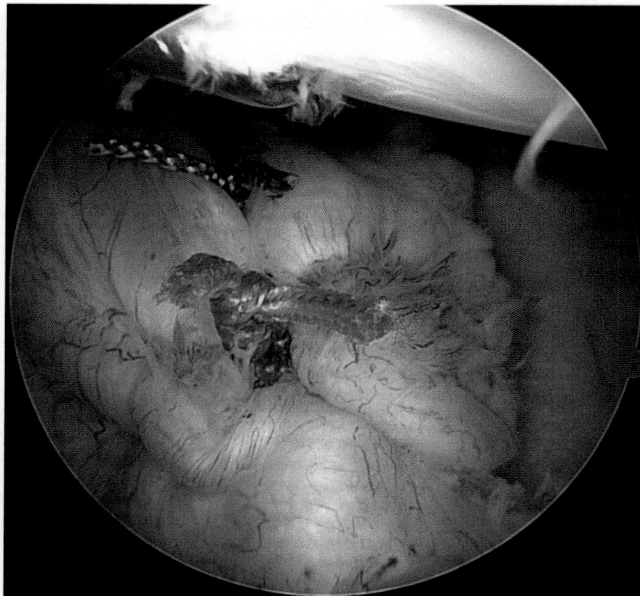

Figure 2-11 | A simple knot is tied in order to provide a capsular tuck for capsular redundancy.

- These steps are repeated, again using double-loaded suture anchors, placing suture anchors at the 9 o'clock and 10 o'clock positions for the left shoulder and 3 o'clock and 4 o'clock positions for the right shoulder for a total of three suture anchors.
- With these additional anchors, a capsular "tuck" is combined with the labral repair to ensure that the ligament is retensioned with the labral repair (Fig. 2-12).
- The repair is examined with the arthroscopic probe (Fig. 2-13).

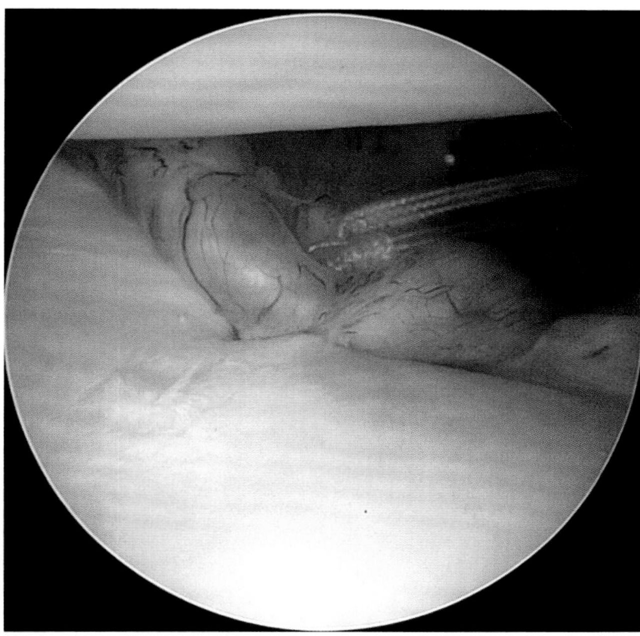

Figure 2-12 | A capsular tuck at the 5 o'clock position on the right shoulder viewed from the anterosuperior portal is combined with labral repair to ensure retensioning of the ligament and provides a bumper around the glenoid rim.

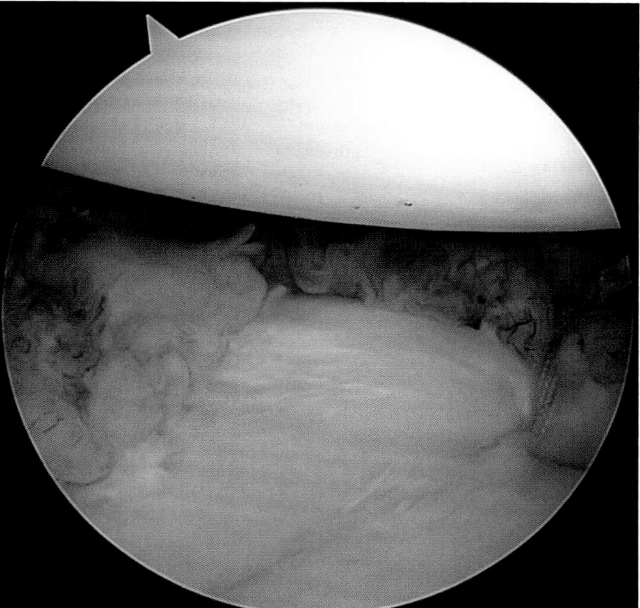

Figure 2-13 | The final repair is viewed arthroscopically prior to removal of instruments and closure.

Postoperative Care

- The patient is placed in a shoulder immobilizer with an abduction pillow for 4 weeks. The patient may remove the immobilizer only for pendulum exercises three times daily.
- After 4 weeks, the patient will begin active assisted range-of-motion exercises.
- Active range-of-motion exercises are initiated at 6 weeks.
- At 6 weeks, the patient is allowed to perform strengthening exercises.
- Return to sports training may occur at 5-6 months and full sports participation at 6 months.

References

1. Rowe CR, Patel D, Southmayd WW. The Bankart procedure: a long-term end-result study. *J Bone Joint Surg Am.* 1978;60(1):1-16.
2. Harris JD, Gupta AK, Mall NA, et al. Long-term outcomes after Bankart shoulder stabilization. *Arthroscopy.* 2013;29(5):920-933.
3. Simonet WT, Melton LJ III, Cofield RH, Ilstrup DM. Incidence of anterior shoulder dislocation in Olmsted County, Minnesota. *Clin Orthop Relat Res.* 1984;186:186-191.
4. Bottoni CR, Smith EL, Berkowitz MJ, Towle RB, Moore JH. Arthroscopic versus open shoulder stabilization for recurrent anterior instability: a prospective randomized clinical trial. *Am J Sports Med.* 2006;34:1730-1737.
5. Hovelius L, Olofsson A, Sandstrom B, et al. Nonoperative treatment of primary anterior shoulder dislocation in patients forty years of age and younger. a prospective twenty-five-year follow-up. *J Bone Joint Surg Am.* 2008;90(5):945-952.
6. Gumina S, Postacchini F. Anterior dislocation of the shoulder in elderly patients. *J Bone Joint Surg Br.* 1997;79(4):540-543.
7. Marans HJ, Angel KR, Schemitsch EH, Wedge JH. The fate of traumatic anterior dislocation of the shoulder in children. *J Bone Joint Surg Am.* 1992;74(8):1242-1244.
8. Robinson CM, Howes J, Murdoch H, Will E, Graham C. Functional outcome and risk of recurrent instability after primary traumatic anterior shoulder dislocation in young patients. *J Bone Joint Surg Am.* 2006;88(11):2326-2336.
9. Burkhead WZ Jr, Rockwood CA Jr. Treatment of instability of the shoulder with an exercise program. *J Bone Joint Surg Am.* 1992;74:890-896.

10. Liu SH, Henry MH. Anterior shoulder instability: current review. *Clin Orthop*. 1996;323:327-337.
11. Mohtadi NG, Chan DS, Hollinshead RM, et al. A randomized clinical trial comparing open and arthroscopic stabilization for recurrent traumatic anterior shoulder instability: two-year follow-up with disease-specific quality-of-life outcomes. *J Bone Joint Surg Am*. 2014;96(5):353-360.
12. Boone JL, Arciero RA. First-time anterior shoulder dislocations: has the standard changed? *Br J Sports Med*. 2010;44(5):355-360.
13. Simonet WT, Cofield RH. Prognosis in anterior shoulder dislocation. *Am J Sports Med*. 1984;12(1):19-24.
14. Bankart ASB. Recurrent or habitual dislocation of the shoulder-joint. *Br Med J*. 1923;2(3285):1132-1133.
15. Bankart ASB. The pathology and treatment of recurrent dislocation of the shoulder-joint. *Br J Surg*. 1938;26(101):23-29.
16. Wheeler JH, Ryan JB, Arciero RA, Molinari RN. Arthroscopic versus nonoperative treatment of acute shoulder dislocations in young athletes. *Arthroscopy*. 1989;5(3):213-217.
17. Arciero RA, Wheeler JH, Ryan JB, McBride JT. Arthroscopic Bankart repair versus nonoperative treatment for acute, initial anterior shoulder dislocations. *Am J Sports Med*. 1994;22(5):589-594.
18. Handoll HH, Almaiyah MA, Rangan A. Surgical versus non-surgical treatment for acute anterior shoulder dislocation. *Cochrane Database Syst Rev*. 2004;(1):CD004325.
19. Bottoni CR, Wilckens JH, DeBerardino TM, et al. A prospective, randomized evaluation of arthroscopic stabilization versus nonoperative treatment in patients with acute, traumatic, first-time shoulder dislocations. *Am J Sports Med*. 2002;30(4):576-580.
20. Aboalata M, Plath JE, Seppel G, Juretzko J, Vogt S, Imhoff AB. Results of arthroscopic Bankart repair for anterior-inferior shoulder instability at 13-year follow-up. *Am J Sports Med*. 2017;45(4):782-787. pii: 0363546516675145.
21. Chapus V, Rochcongar G, Pineau V, Salle de Chou E, Hulet C. Ten-year follow-up of acute arthroscopic Bankart repair for initial anterior shoulder dislocation in young patients. *Orthop Traumatol Surg Res*. 2015;101(8):899-893.
22. Chahal J, Marks PH, Macdonald PB, et al. Anatomic Bankart repair compared with nonoperative treatment and/or arthroscopic lavage for first-time traumatic shoulder dislocation. *Arthroscopy*. 2012;28(4):565-575.
23. Waterman BR, Burns TC, McCriskin B, Kilcoyne K, Cameron KL, Owens BD. Outcomes after bankart repair in a military population: predictors for surgical revision and long-term disability. *Arthroscopy*. 2014;30(2):172-177.
24. Tjoumakaris FP, Bradley JP. The rationale for an arthroscopic approach to shoulder stabilization. *Arthroscopy*. 2011;27(10):1422-1433.

Chapter 3
Open Latarjet Procedure

MATTHEW T. PROVENCHER
ANTHONY SANCHEZ
GEORGE SANCHEZ

Sterile Instruments/Equipment

- Self-retaining Kolbel retractor
- Hohmann retractor
- Mayo scissors
- Blunt retractor
- Periosteal elevator
- 90-degree oscillating saw blade
- Angled saw
- Chandler elevators
- Toothed grasping forceps
- Microsagittal saw
- Osteotome
- 3.2-mm drill bit
- Mayo scissors
- Single-prong self-retaining subscapularis spreader
- High-speed burr
- Fukuda retractor
- 4-mm Steinmann pin
- 2.5-mm drill bit
- Kocher clamps
- Implants
  - 3.5-mm cortical or 4.0-mm malleolar screws
  - Suture washers
- Drill

Positioning

- An interscalene block is recommended.
- The patient is positioned in modified beach-chair position with the head elevated 40 degrees.
- Two folded towels are placed under the scapula to flatten and stabilize it.
- The arm is draped free to allow intraoperative abduction and external rotation.
  - A pneumatic limb positioner (Smith & Nephew, Andover, MA) or a padded Mayo stand is used.

Surgical Approach

- An arthroscopic examination is performed.
- An oblique 5- to 7-cm incision is made from the tip of the coracoid process, extending inferiorly down the deltopectoral groove to the superior portion of the axillary fold.[1]

- A standard deltopectoral approach is used. The cephalic vein is protected and gently retracted laterally with the deltoid musculature.[2]
- A self-retaining Kolbel retractor is placed between the pectoralis major and deltoid to maintain exposure.
- If more exposure is desired, a Hohmann retractor can be placed over the top of the coracoid while the arm is in abduction and external rotation.

Coracoid Graft Harvest

- With proper coracoid exposure and the arm in external rotation and abduction, Mayo scissors are used to further expose the coracoid from its tip all the way to the base.
- The coracoacromial (CA) ligament is identified and sharply transected 1 cm laterally off its coracoid insertion.
  - It is important to harvest 1 cm of this ligament so it can later be incorporated into the capsular repair to produce the bumper effect.
- To improve exposure on the medial side of the coracoid, the arm is placed in adduction and internal rotation.
- The pectoralis minor is released with an elevator.
  - Care must be taken to protect the neurovascular structures inferiorly with a blunt retractor.
  - The release should not continue past the tip of the coracoid in order to avoid risk to the graft blood supply.
- A periosteal elevator is used to remove excess soft tissue from the undersurface of the coracoid (Fig. 3-1A).
- Palpation to identify and protect the axillary and musculocutaneous nerves is necessary throughout the coracoid exposure.
- A 90-degree oscillating saw blade is used to create a medial-to-lateral osteotomy of the coracoid at a line just anterior to the coracoclavicular ligament insertion at the coracoid base (Fig. 3-1B).[1]

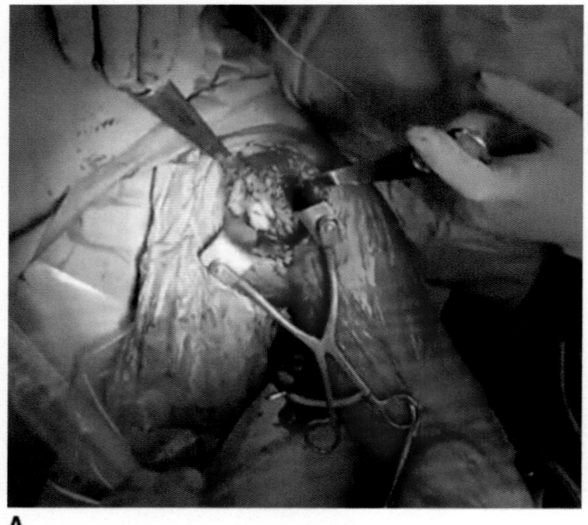

A

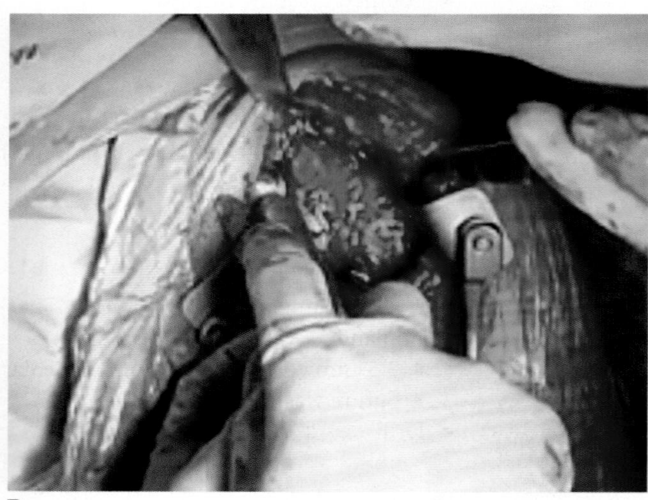

B

Figure 3-1 | A. The coracoid is first exposed in order to carry out a successful osteotomy. **B.** The osteotomy is performed at the "knee" of the coracoid.

  - The coracoid graft should be 22-25 mm long from the tip to base.
  - The osteotomy is made perpendicular to the coracoid process to avoid accidentally extending it to the glenoid articular surface.
- An angled saw is used instead of a half-inch osteotome because the saw is less likely to cause iatrogenic glenoid fracture.
  - Levering on the fragment with an osteotome can assist in completing the osteotomy but should be avoided if possible to avoid splitting the fragment.
  - Chandler elevators are positioned inferior and medial to the coracoid to protect vital neurovascular structures.

- The blood supply to the graft enters the coracoid at the medial aspect of the insertion of the conjoined tendon; care is taken not to disturb it while performing the osteotomy.
- After the osteotomy is made, toothed grasping forceps are used to gently hold the graft at the level of the incision and the coracohumeral ligament is released to liberate the coracoid.
- The musculocutaneous nerve is then identified and released from the posterior fascia of the conjoint tendon, just until it dives into muscle ~4-7 cm from the coracoid tip.
- The coracoid is brought out of the incision >1-2 cm to avoid any tension on the musculocutaneous nerve.
    - It is important to completely release all soft tissue adhesions on the posterior aspect of the conjoint tendon to allow ease of coracoid transfer.
    - The musculocutaneous nerve also is identified and gently released until all tension is freed all the way up to the musculocutaneous nerve insertion into the muscle.
- The arm is now returned to the neutral position.

Coracoid Graft Preparation

- A scalpel is used to remove any remaining soft tissue from the deep surfaces of the graft, with care taken not to harm the blood supply or CA ligament stump.
- A microsagittal saw is used to decorticate the medial coracoid surface and expose a broad, flat cancellous surface to optimize graft union.
- If the osteotomy resulted in a spike of bone (which means optimal length harvest), it is removed while making sure not to compromise the length of the graft.
- An osteotome is then placed beneath the coracoid, and a 3.2-mm drill is used to place two bicortical drill holes along the central longitudinal axis of the graft about 1 cm apart (Fig. 3-2).

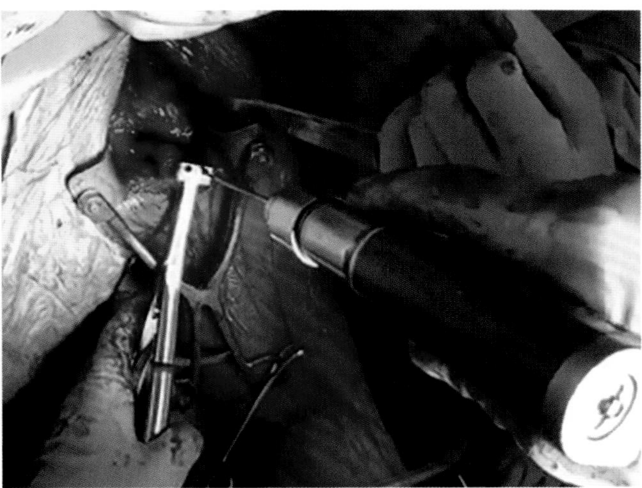

Figure 3-2 | Preparation of the coracoid process.

Glenoid Exposure and Preparation

- The arm is externally rotated, putting the subscapularis on stretch.
- The superior and inferior margins of the subscapularis are identified, and the subscapularis is split with Mayo scissors 3-4 mm medial to the medial aspect of the biceps tendon.
- It is then divided medially up to the level of the coracoid, but no farther because the subscapularis nerve supply enters the subscapularis about 1-1.5 cm medial to the coracoid.
- As first described by Walch and Boileau,[3] we prefer to split the subscapularis at the junction of the superior two-thirds and inferior one-third.
- Then, by opening the scissors inside the capsule perpendicular to the muscle fibers, the plane between the upper subscapularis and anterior capsule is better visualized.

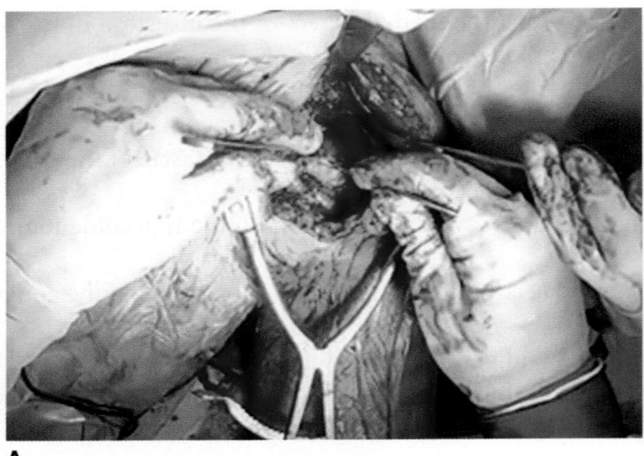

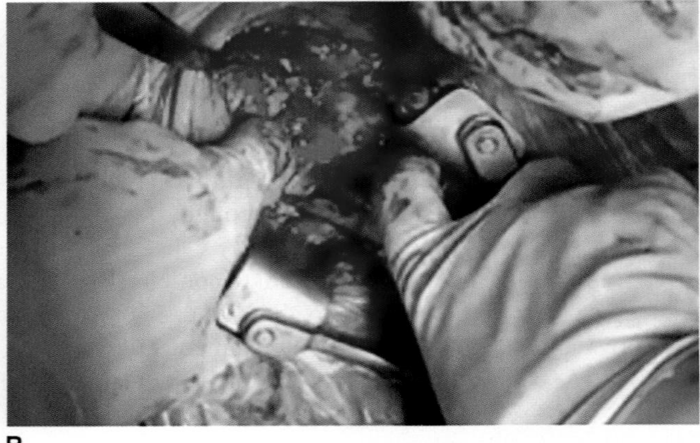

A B

Figure 3-3 | A. Division of the subscapularis at the junction of the upper two-thirds and inferior one-third. **B.** The scissors are then oriented vertically to expose the underlying capsule.

- Next, a single-prong self-retaining subscapularis spreader (or blunt Gelpi) is used to open the subscapularis split (Fig. 3-3A and B).
- The capsular cut is extended with a scalpel to the lesser tuberosity for exposure of the glenohumeral joint line and capsule.
- To preserve length, an "L"-shaped capsulotomy is made, superior first at the superior glenoid and ~1 cm medial to the glenoid rim.
- A no. 2 high-strength suture is then used to tag the corner (superomedial) of the capsule for later repair.
- Electrocautery is used to excise the anteroinferior labrum and periosteum off the region of the glenoid neck where the coracoid graft will sit.
- A high-speed burr is used to lightly decorticate the anterior glenoid neck and create a flat, bleeding cancellous surface for graft placement.
  - It is essential to form a bleeding bed of bone on the anterior glenoid and prepare the anterior aspect of the glenoid as perpendicular to the surface as possible.

Coracoid Graft Fixation

- Proper coracoid placement is arguably the most critical aspect of the Latarjet procedure.
- Allain et al.[4] noted that excessive lateral coracoid placement results in increased postoperative degenerative changes.
  - Additionally, failure to correct the recurrent anterior instability will occur if the graft is overly medialized.
  - The graft should function as an extension of the previously deficient inherent articular arc of the glenoid.
- A low-profile Fukuda retractor is inserted inside the joint to retract the humeral head.
- Exposure can be improved:
  - Superiorly by placing a 4-mm Steinmann pin into the superior scapular neck
  - Medially by replacing the Hohmann retractor with a Kolbel retractor
  - Inferiorly by placing the same Hohmann retractor between the capsule and the subscapularis, thereby exposing the 6 o'clock position on the glenoid
- De Beer et al. first described the congruent-arc modification to the traditional Latarjet procedure, which we recommend.
- In this modification, the coracoid is rotated about its axis by 90 degrees to lie on the inferior surface of the coracoid, which they found to be identical in radius of curvature to that of the native glenoid surface (Fig. 3-4).[5,6]
- The ideal position is between 3 and 5 o'clock on the glenoid.
  - Once the correct position is achieved, a 2.5-mm drill is used to create two bicortical anteroposterior holes parallel to the glenoid articular surface.
  - Kocher clamps on either side of the coracoid (one on the glenoid side and another on the alternative side) should be used during drilling to ensure a trajectory that will not compromise the bone.
  - Alternatively, commercial devices are available that stabilize the coracoid during drilling.

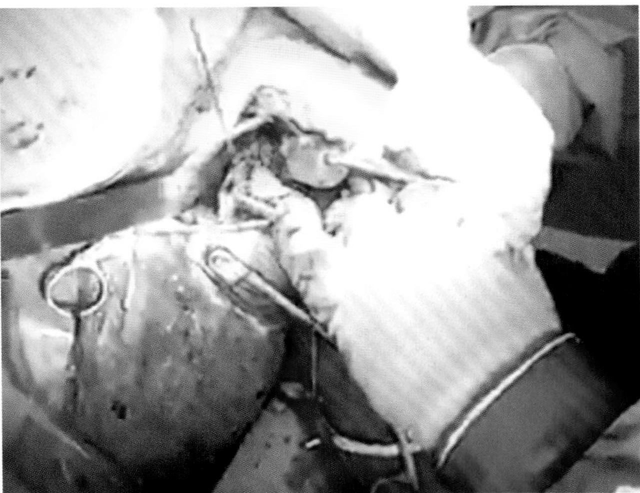

Figure 3-4 | Placement of the graft in the traditional Latarjet orientation.

- Fixation is achieved with two 3.5-mm cortical or 4.0-mm malleolar screws, typically 34-36 mm long, and washers with preloaded suture washers (Arthrex, Naples, FL) (Fig. 3-5).
  - The screws should be snug but not overtightened.
  - Any lateral overhang of the coracoid can be smoothed with a high-speed burr.

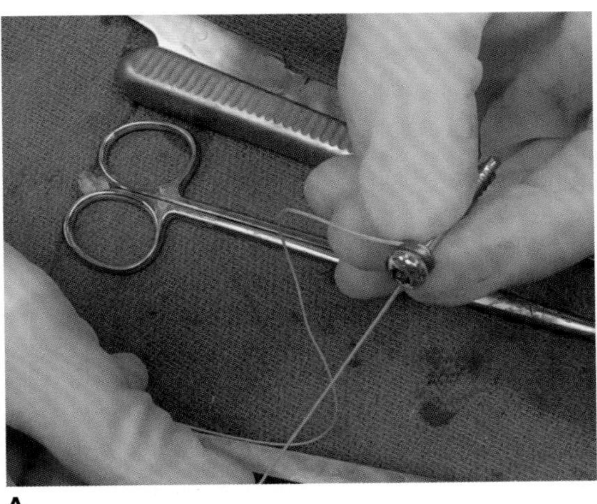

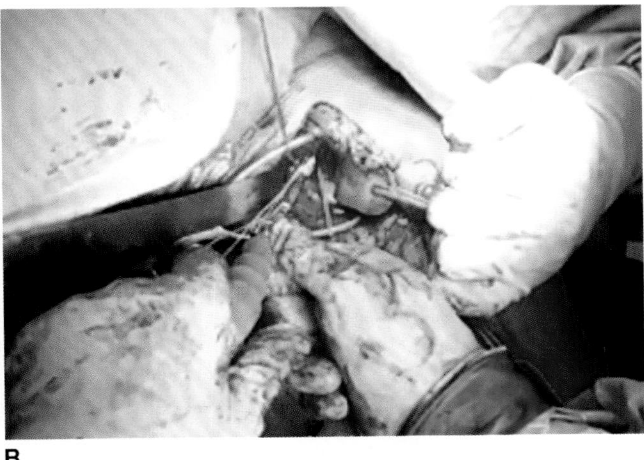

A B

Figure 3-5 | **A.** Fixation screw loaded with suture washers to be used in capsular repair. **B.** Coracoid graft securely fixed to the glenoid with two screws with no lateral overhang.

Capsular and Subscapularis Repair

- A well-repaired capsule should allow the graft to function as an intra-articular platform and help protect the humeral head articular cartilage from the abrasive bone block.[7]
- With the arm adducted to the side and placed in ~45 degrees of external rotation and the Fukuda retractor removed, the capsular repair is performed with the no. 2 FiberWires preloaded in the suture washers (Arthrex, Naples, FL), as well as with additional free high-strength no. 2 sutures to the capsule and the CA ligament (Fig. 3-6).
  - To allow imbrication of the capsular tissue, the sutures are placed in a figure-of-eight style.
  - For further reinforcement, the CA ligament remnant on the coracoid graft is incorporated into the capsular repair.

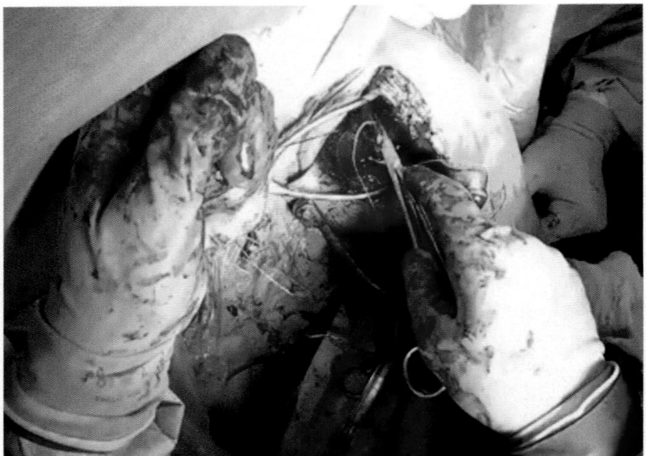

Figure 3-6 | Capsular repair using suture washers.

- Finally, with the conjoined tendon exiting medially and anteriorly through the split, the subscapularis is repaired over the coracoid transfer with high-strength no. 2 suture.
  - When repairing the lateralmost extent of the subscapularis split, care should be taken to avoid the long head of the biceps tendon.
- Following copious irrigation, the wound is closed in a standard layered fashion.
- Patient should be followed using serial CT imaging to ensure proper bone block union (Fig. 3-7).

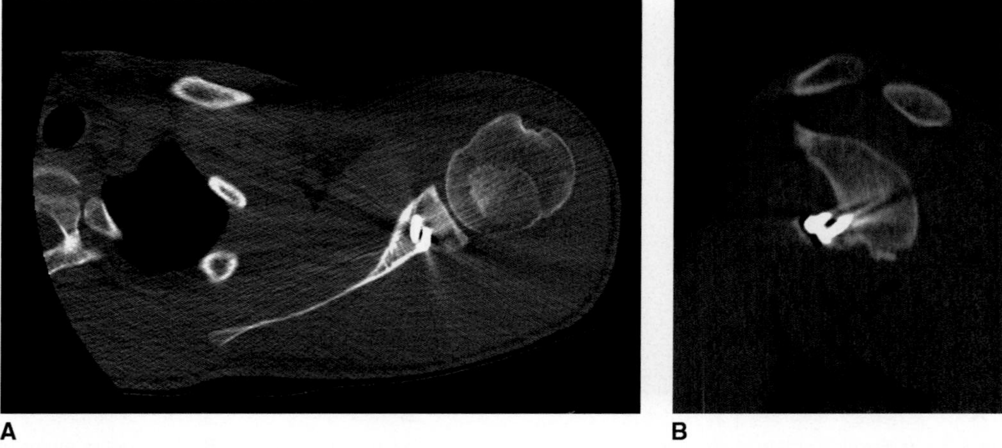

Figure 3-7 | Postoperative **(A)** axial view CT and **(B)** sagittal view CT images at 6 months demonstrate a healed coracoid bone block.

References

1. Young AA, Walch G. Open bony augmentation of glenoid bone loss–The Latarjet and variants. In: Provencher MT, Romeo AA, eds. *Shoulder Instability: A Comprehensive Approach*. Philadelphia, PA: Elsevier; 2011:197-208.
2. Young AA, Maia R, Berhouet J, Walch G. Open Latarjet procedure for management of bone loss in anterior instability of the glenohumeral joint. *J Shoulder Elbow Surg*. 2011;20(2 Suppl):S61-S69. doi:10.1016/j.jse.2010.07.022.
3. Walch G, Boileau P. Latarjet-Bristow procedure for recurrent anterior instability. *Tech Shoulder Elbow Surg*. 2000;1(4). Available at: http://journals.lww.com/shoulderelbowsurgery/Fulltext/2000/01040/Latarjet_Bristow_Procedure_for_Recurrent_Anterior.8.aspx
4. Allain J, Goutallier D, Glorion C. Long-term results of the Latarjet procedure for the treatment of anterior instability of the shoulder. *J Bone Joint Surg Am*. 1998;80(6):841-852.
5. de Beer J, Burkhart SS, Roberts CP, van Rooyen K, Cresswell T, du Toit DF. The congruent-arc Latarjet. *Tech Shoulder Elbow Surg*. 2009;10(2):62-67. doi:10.1097/BTE.0b013e31819ebb60.
6. de Beer JF, Roberts C. Glenoid bone defects—open Latarjet with congruent arc modification. *Orthop Clin North Am*. 2010;41(3):407-415. doi:10.1016/j.ocl.2010.02.008.
7. Boone JL, Arciero RA. Management of failed instability surgery: how to get it right the next time. *Orthop Clin North Am*. 2010;41(3):367-379. doi:10.1016/j.ocl.2010.02.009.

Chapter 4
Arthroscopic Posterior Shoulder Stabilization

FOTIOS P. TJOUMAKARIS
JAMES P. BRADLEY

Background

- Posterior shoulder instability is characterized by pathologic glenohumeral translation ranging from a mild subluxation (microinstability) to traumatic dislocation (macroinstability).
- Posterior instability of the shoulder is less common than anterior instability, representing 5%-10% of all patients with shoulder instability.
- Patients are candidates for surgical repair/reconstruction when conservative treatment fails. This may consist of rest, physical therapy, and possibly even a corticosteroid injection for rotator cuff–related symptoms.

Pathogenesis

- May be from direct trauma (direct blow to the anterior shoulder or landing on an outstretched, adducted arm). This could result in a dislocation. Position of risk is a forward flexed and adducted shoulder.
- Electrocution or seizures are an indirect mechanism that may result in posterior dislocation secondary to the contraction of the subscapularis and pectoralis.
- Recurrent posterior subluxation (RPS) is likely a more common pathologic entity from repetitive microtrauma to the posterior capsule, labrum, and posterior glenoid. This often occurs with repetitive overhead or throwing sports.
- Tears of the posterior labrum or capsule, humeral avulsion of the glenohumeral ligaments (reverse HAGL), and excessive posterior glenoid retroversion can all contribute to the pathologic laxity/instability.

Patient History

- Age, arm dominance, sport of choice (for athletes), and nature of traumatic event or symptoms are documented.
- Pain is characterized by discomfort in the position of provocation (forward flexed and adducted), vague discomfort during or after sports, or loss of velocity in throwing athletes. Pain often is diffuse and deep-seated in the shoulder.
- Any response to conservative treatment (closed reduction, sling use, immobilization, physical therapy, or corticosteroid injection) is documented.
- Any associated symptoms (periscapular pain, neurologic symptoms radiating into extremity, cervical neck discomfort) are evaluated.

Physical Examination

- Inspection of any rotator cuff or periscapular muscle atrophy or asymmetry.
- Palpation to document soreness of the anterior or posterior capsule, coracoid process, acromioclavicular joint, and greater tuberosity.

- Range of motion of the injured shoulder compared to the contralateral extremity.
- Strength assessment to evaluate the rotator cuff muscles and periscapular muscles in forward flexion, abduction, internal/external rotation, and extension.
- Provocative testing, including the Kim test, jerk test, circumduction test, and load and shift testing.

Radiographic Findings

- Standard radiographs often are negative.
- An MRI arthrogram is the gold standard imaging modality to detect injury to the posterior labrum and capsule.
- A CT scan can be obtained if bone injury/deficiency is suspected.

Surgical Technique

Equipment

- Large joint arthroscopy equipment (30- and 70-degree arthroscopes)
- Arthroscopic shoulder tray with the following additions:
  - Cannula insertion/dilation instruments
  - 6.0-/7.0-mm or 8.25-mm working cannulas
  - Suture-passing devices (ReelPass SutureLasso [Arthrex, Naples, FL]) or (Spectrum [Linvatec, Edison, NJ])
  - Arthroscopic periosteal/labrum elevator/spatula
  - 3.5-/4.5-mm arthroscopic shaver
  - 4.0-/4.5-mm hooded burr
  - No. 1 or no. 0 polypropylene suture
  - No. 1 polydioxanone (PDS) suture
  - 2.4-mm biocomposite short PushLock anchors (Arthrex, Naples, FL)
  - 1.3-mm SutureTape (Arthrex, Naples, FL)
  - Anchor drill with guide and trocar.

Anesthesia

- Interscalene nerve block typically is used with or without general anesthesia.

Positioning

- The patient is positioned in the lateral decubitus position on a beanbag (Fig. 4-1).
- Bony prominences are padded (fibular head/peroneal nerve, lateral malleolus, axillary roll, pillow between the legs to alleviate low back pressure).

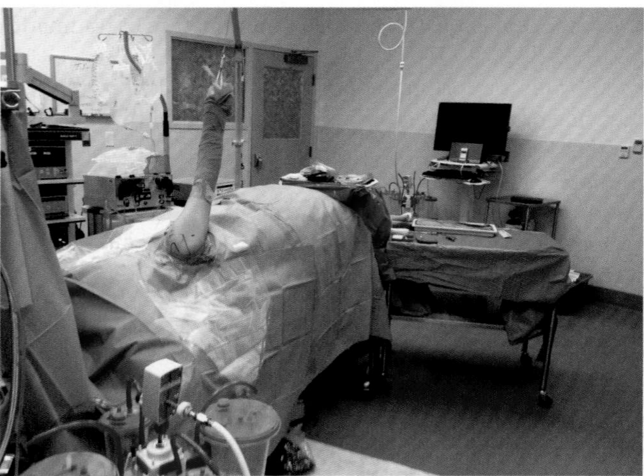

Figure 4-1 | The lateral decubitus position for arthroscopic posterior labral repair.

Approach

- Viewing is done from both the anterior and posterior portals in an all-arthroscopic fashion.
- Instrumentation is used from both the anterior and posterior portals.

Portal Placement

- 30 cc of saline are first used to insufflate the joint from a posterior injection portal.
- The posterior portal typically is created in line with the lateral edge of the acromion (1 cm lateral and 1 cm inferior to a standard posterior arthroscopy portal).
- Placement of this portal more lateral allows easier access to the posterior glenoid and can facilitate anchor placement.
- An anterior portal is established high in the rotator interval with an "inside-out" technique with a switching stick.
- The anterior switching stick is then replaced with a 6- or 7-mm clear cannula.

Diagnostic Arthroscopy

- A thorough arthroscopic examination is carried out with a 30-degree arthroscope to look for associated pathology (chondral damage, rotator cuff tear, biceps tear, anterosuperior labral pathology). The labral tear is identified along the posterior glenoid margin (Fig. 4-2).

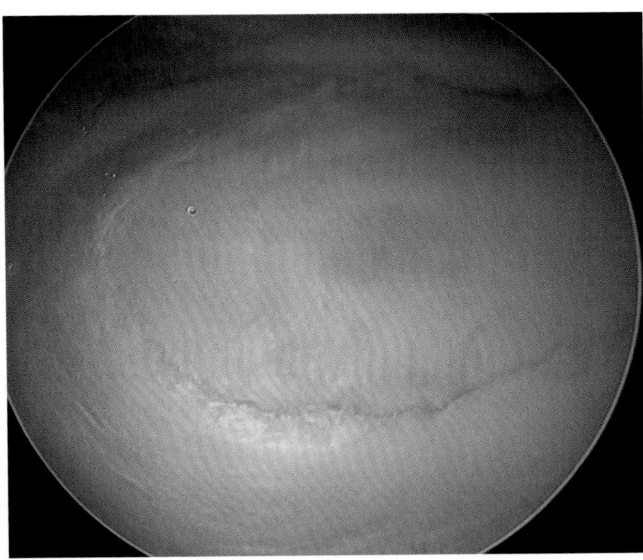

Figure 4-2 | Arthroscopic view from the posterior portal demonstrating a large posterior labral tear in a patient with recurrent posterior subluxation (RPS).

- Debridement can be carried out with a 4.5-mm full radius shaver using the oscillation mode.
- At the conclusion of the diagnostic arthroscopy, the scope is placed in the anterior cannula and the fluid inflow is switched to the side port of the cannula. A switching stick is placed in the posterior portal, this portal is dilated to 8.0 mm, and an 8.25-mm distally threaded clear plastic cannula is placed.
- If necessary, a 70-degree arthroscope can then be placed on the camera, which allows excellent vision of the posterior compartment of the shoulder.

Preparation of the Labrum

- An elevator can be brought either through the anterior portal before placement of the scope anteriorly or through the posterior portal to elevate the posterior labrum from the posterior glenoid rim/margin (Fig. 4-3).
- Care must be taken during labral preparation that the trajectory is adequate for mobilization so that the elevator does not slice through or amputate the labral tissue.
- The labrum should be mobilized gently and methodically off the posterior glenoid neck. The capsule is elevated until the underlying muscle belly of the posterior rotator cuff is seen, similar to anterior labral preparation during Bankart repair (Fig. 4-4).

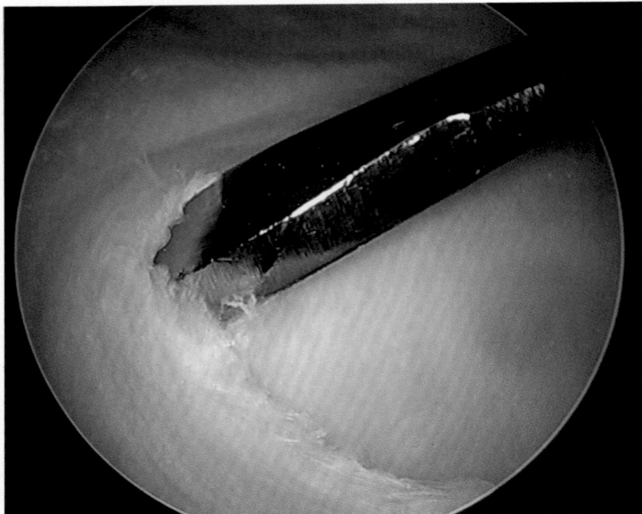

Figure 4-3 | A periosteal elevator is brought in from the anterior portal and used to elevate the labrum off the posterior glenoid margin/neck.

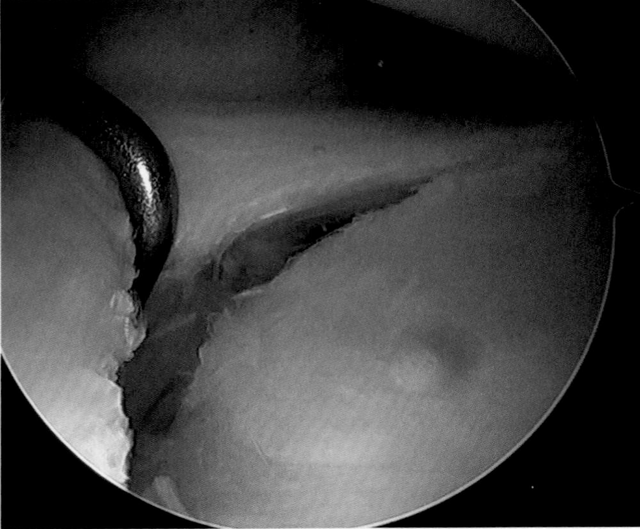

Figure 4-4 | The labrum is fully mobilized in preparation for knotless suture anchor repair.

Preparation of the Glenoid

- The glenoid is prepared with a hooded burr to protect the posterior capsule and labrum during bone debridement.
- A cancellous/cortical bed of bone is exposed to allow adequate labral healing and adherence.
- An arthroscopic shaver is used to remove the bone debris and prepare the edge of the labrum for repair.

Suture Passage and Anchor Placement

- Through the posterior portal, a suture-passing device is used to pass a no. 0 polypropylene suture through the labral and capsular tissue (Figs. 4-5 and 4-6).
  - For patients with macroinstability, a capsular shift and labral repair often are performed, and a larger pass of the suture hook is necessary to achieve adequate plication. For patients with RPS and isolated labral injury, the suture is shuttled primarily around the labrum only and the capsule is left unaltered.

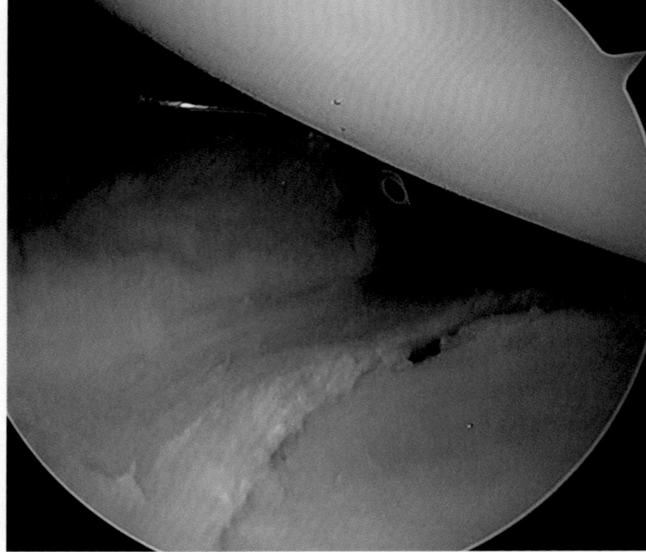

Figure 4-5 | A suture hook is used to shuttle suture around the labrum-capsule complex.

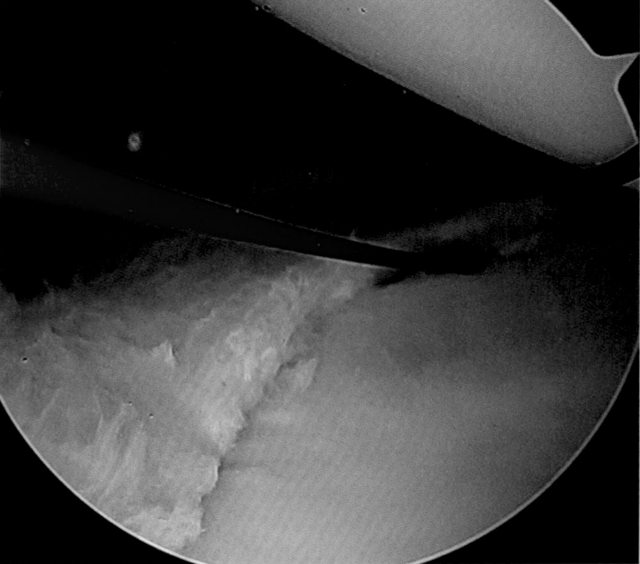

Figure 4-6 | A no. 0 polypropylene suture is used as a shuttle device once passed through the labrum and capsule.

- The shuttled suture is retrieved through the posterior cannula and a loop of SutureTape is placed in a knot of the monofilament polypropylene suture for passage.
  - The goal is to create a "cinch" stitch or luggage-tag–style suture that captures the labrum-capsule complex.
- The loop of SutureTape is delivered back out of the posterior working cannula, and the tails of the suture are delivered through the loop and pulled taut to secure the knot against the labrum (Fig. 4-7).
  - A knot pusher can be used to reduce the knot firmly against the labrum and reduce slack (Fig. 4-8).

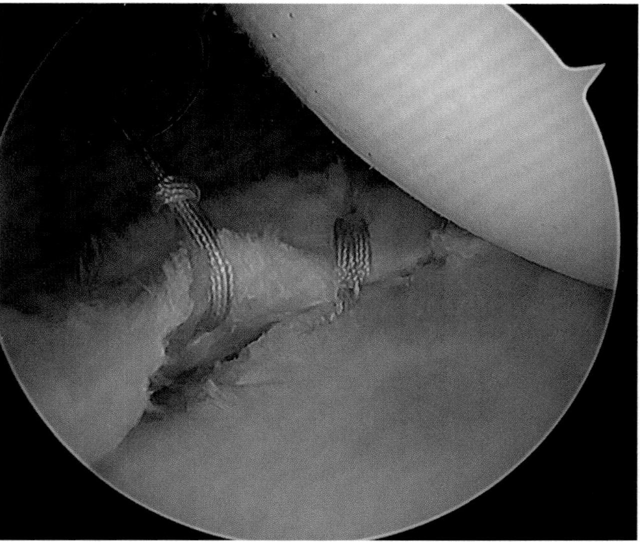

Figure 4-7 | The "cinch" stitch is demonstrated, similar to a luggage-tag construct.

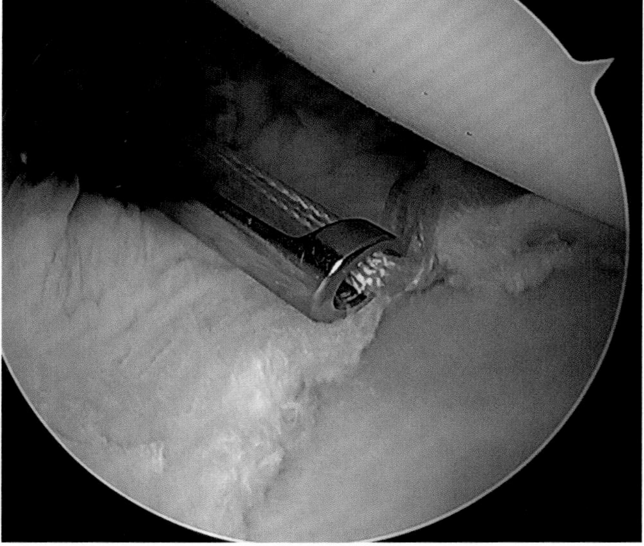

Figure 4-8 | A knot pusher can be used to reduce the "cinch" stitch to the labrum, removing any slack before placement in the anchor.

- The pilot hole for the anchor is drilled at the desired location on the glenoid face (Fig. 4-9).
  - An accessory posterolateral portal often can be used for anchor drilling and placement of a 5-mm or 6-mm cannula to facilitate suture passage and anchor placement.
  - The posterior working portal can be used in isolation if the portal allows a 45-degree tangential drilling angle to the glenoid. Otherwise, the drill may skive, causing articular cartilage injury.

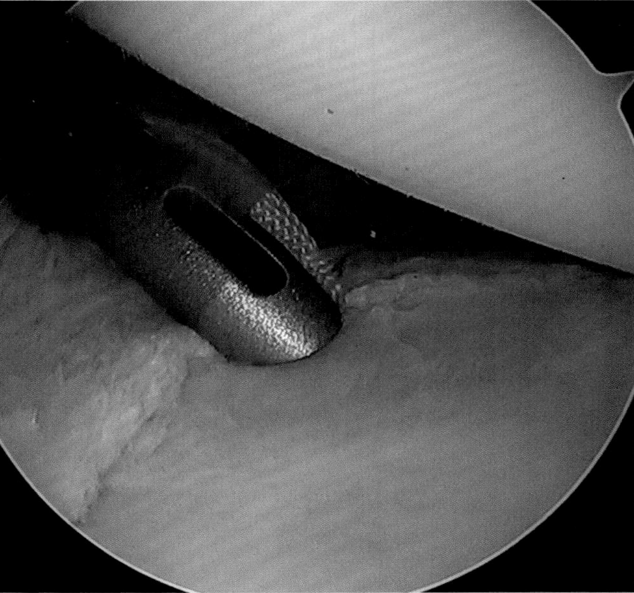

Figure 4-9 | Anchors are drilled through the posterior working cannula at a 45-degree angle tangential to the glenoid to avoid articular cartilage injury.

- The ends of the SutureTape are passed through the eyelet of the knotless anchor, and the anchor is impacted into place with tension applied across the sutures during anchor placement.
  - Anchors in the 8 o'clock to the 11 o'clock positions generally are placed through the standard posterior working portal, while the 6-7 o'clock anchor may be better approached through an accessory portal.

Completed Repair

- Anchors are placed 3-5 mm apart (depending on the size of the labrum/glenoid) until the labrum and capsule are secured back to the glenoid (Fig. 4-10).
- Knotless anchors have supplanted suture-tying anchors in our technique because of the decreased risk of knot abrasion, which can result in articular cartilage injury and internal impingement against the posterosuperior rotator cuff and capsule, particularly when placed above the equator of the glenoid.

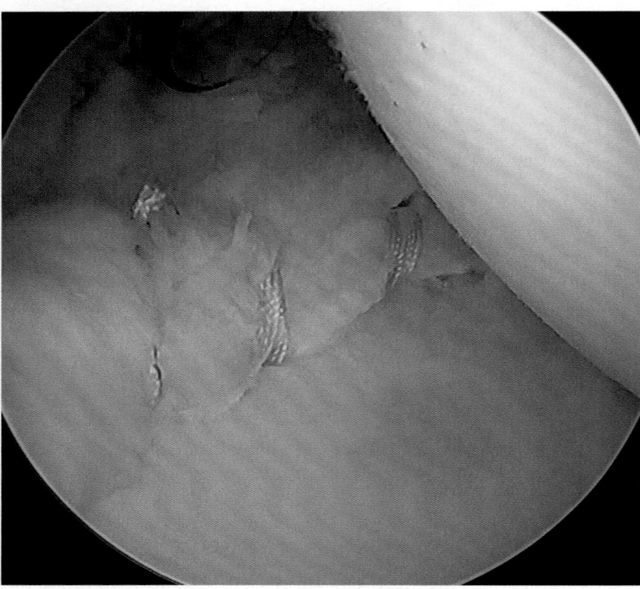

Figure 4-10 | The posterior labrum is repaired with the capsule incorporated to complete the labrum repair.

Capsular Closure

- The posterior portal is closed with a no. 1 polydioxanone (PDS) suture.
- The posterior cannula is withdrawn just external to the capsule, and a PDS suture is introduced just adjacent to the portal with a suture hook crescent (Fig. 4-11).

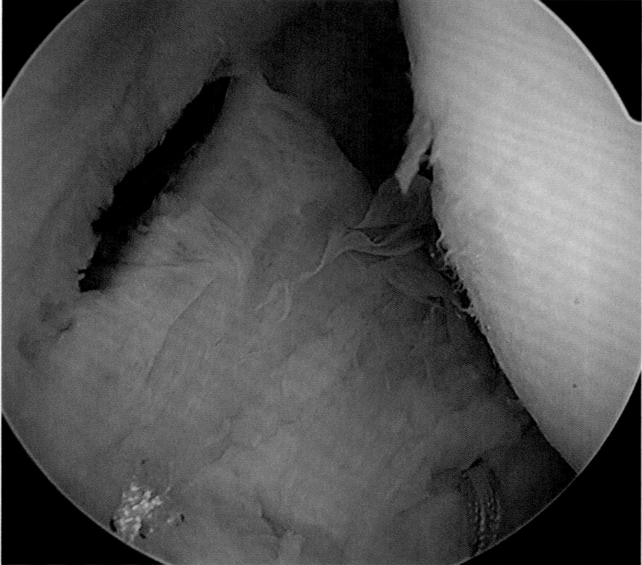

Figure 4-11 | To facilitate capsule closure, the cannula is placed just beyond the capsule to allow suture passage and extra-articular suture tying.

- A penetrating grasper is used on the opposite side of the portal to retrieve the suture, which is then tied with a sliding, locking knot in an extra-articular fashion, completing the repair (Fig. 4-12).
  - Additional sutures can be passed in a wider fashion if additional plication is required based on the predetermined needs of the patient from the preoperative plan.

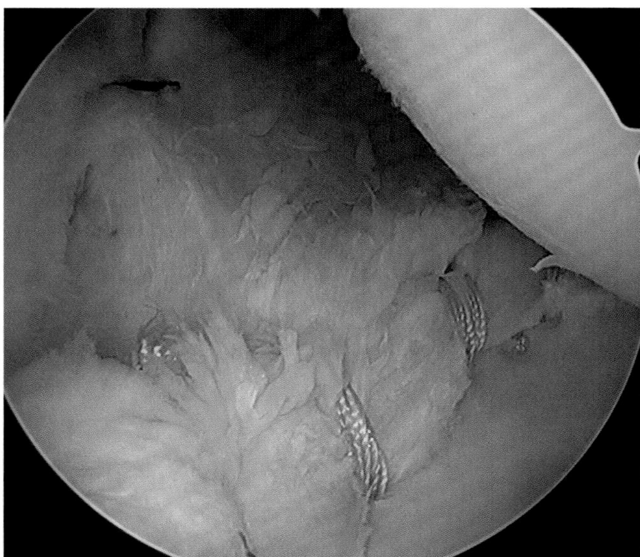

Figure 4-12 | View from the anterior portal looking posteriorly demonstrating labral repair and completed capsular closure.

Postoperative Management

- A shoulder abduction sling is worn for 6 weeks.
  - Active range of motion of elbow, wrist, and hand is allowed.
  - Passive shoulder motion in the scapular plane is allowed.
- Patients complete passive and active range of motion exercises by 8-12 weeks.
- Strengthening is initiated at 12 weeks.
- Throwers may begin a light-throwing program at 16 weeks.
- Return to sports for nonthrowing athletes is typically 6 months. Throwing athletes will progress to game readiness over 12 months.

Outcomes

- Outcomes of arthroscopic posterior instability repair are generally good.
- Studies document failure rates ranging from 0% to 20%.
- Documented return-to-sports range from 70% to 100% in most series using a modern arthroscopic technique.

Complications

- Recurrent instability
- Stiffness
- Infection
- Neurovascular injury

Suggested Readings

Arner JW, McClincy MP, Bradley JP. Arthroscopic stabilization of posterior shoulder instability is successful in American football players. *Arthroscopy*. 2015;31(8):1466-1471.

Badge R, Tambe A, Funk L. Arthroscopic isolated posterior labral repair in rugby players. *Int J Shoulder Surg*. 2009;3:4-7.

Bahk MS, Karzel RP, Snyder SJ. Arthroscopic posterior stabilization and anterior capsular plication for recurrent posterior glenohumeral instability. *Arthroscopy*. 2010;26:1172-1180.

Bradley JP, Baker CL III, Kline AJ, Armfield DR, Chhabra A. Arthroscopic capsulolabral reconstruction for posterior instability of the shoulder. A prospective study of 100 shoulders. *Am J Sports Med*. 2006;34:1061-1071.

Bradley JP, McClincy MP, Arner JW, Tejwani SG. Arthroscopic capsulolabral reconstruction for posterior instability of the shoulder: a prospective study of 200 shoulders. *Am J Sports Med.* 2013;41:2005-2014.

Bottoni CR, Franks BR, Moore JH, DeBerardino TM, Taylor DC, Arciero RA. Operative stabilization of posterior shoulder instability. *Am J Sports Med.* 2005;33:996-1002.

Goubier JN, Iserin A, Duranthon LD, Vandenbussche E, Augereau BA. 4-portal arthroscopic stabilization in posterior shoulder instability. *J Shoulder Elbow Surg.* 2003;12:337-341.

Kim SH, Ha KI, Park JH. Arthroscopic posterior labral repair and capsular shift for traumatic unidirectional recurrent posterior subluxation of the shoulder. *J Bone Joint Surg Am.* 2003;85:1479-1487.

Lenart BA, Sherman SL, Mall NA, Gochanour MA, Twigg SA, Nicholson GP. Arthroscopic repair for posterior shoulder instability. *Arthroscopy.* 2012;28:1337-1343.

Pennington WT, Sytsma MA, Gibbons DJ, et al. Arthroscopic posterior labral repair in athletes: outcome analysis at 2-year follow-up. *Arthroscopy.* 2010;26:1162-1171.

Radkowski CA, Chhabra A, Baker CL, Tejwani SG, Bradley JP. Arthroscopic capsulolabral repair for posterior shoulder instability in throwing athletes compared with nonthrowing athletes. *Am J Sports Med.* 2008;36:693-699.

Savoie FH, III, Holt MS, Field LD, Ramsey JR. Arthroscopic management of posterior instability: evolution of technique and results. *Arthroscopy.* 2008;24:389-396.

Williams RJ, Strickland S, Cohen M, Altchek DW, Warren RF. Arthroscopic repair for traumatic posterior shoulder instability. *Am J Sports Med.* 2003;31:203-209.

Wooten CJ, Krych AJ, Schleck CD, Hudgens JL, May JH, Dahm DL. Arthroscopic capsulolabral reconstruction for posterior shoulder instability in patients 18 years old or younger. *J Pediatr Orthop.* 2015;35(5):462-466.

Chapter 5
Arthroscopic Treatment of Multidirectional Instability

BRIAN R. WATERMAN
CATHERINE RICHARDSON
JONATHAN NEWGREN
ANTHONY A. ROMEO

Sterile Instruments/Equipment

- 4.0-mm arthroscope and camera
- Two or three 8.25-mm cannulas
- Wissinger rods
- Cannulated tissue dilators
- Arthroscopic shaver with 3.5-mm shaver and 4-mm hooded burr
- Arthroscopic rasps
- Angled tissue elevator
- Mallet
- Percutaneous drill sleeve and targeting spear
- Anchor-specific drill bit and battery-powered drill
- Multiple angled and straight retrograde suture-passing devices
- Suture grasper
- Ringed suture
- Knot pusher
- No. 1 polydioxanone suture
- Implants
  - 2.4- and 3-mm double-loaded suture anchors
  - 2.9-mm knotless suture anchor
  - 1.5-mm high-tensile, nonabsorbable tape

Physical Examination

- Physical examination is performed in the preoperative holding area to confirm presence of symptomatic laxity *and* instability (or apprehension) in multiple planes, as well as tenderness to palpation (eg, long head of the biceps).[1-3]
- After ultrasound-guided interscalene block and general endotracheal anesthesia are administered, bilateral examination under anesthesia is performed.
- Range of motion.
- Anterior: anterior load shift test.
- Posterior: jerk and Kim test, posterior load shift test.[2,3]
- Inferior: sulcus sign (in neutral and external rotation), Gagey test.[2,3]

Positioning

- The patient is positioned in the lateral decubitus position.
- All bony prominences and at-risk neurovascular structures are padded, including peroneal nerve, radial nerve, and greater trochanter.
- An axillary roll and foam headrest are used, and a deflatable beanbag is positioned near the inferior angle of the scapula.
- A dual traction lateral shoulder positioner is used with a sterile arm sleeve, and 5 lb of lateral distraction and distal traction are applied (Fig. 5-1A).
    - A foam roll also can be placed under the axilla for additional distraction.

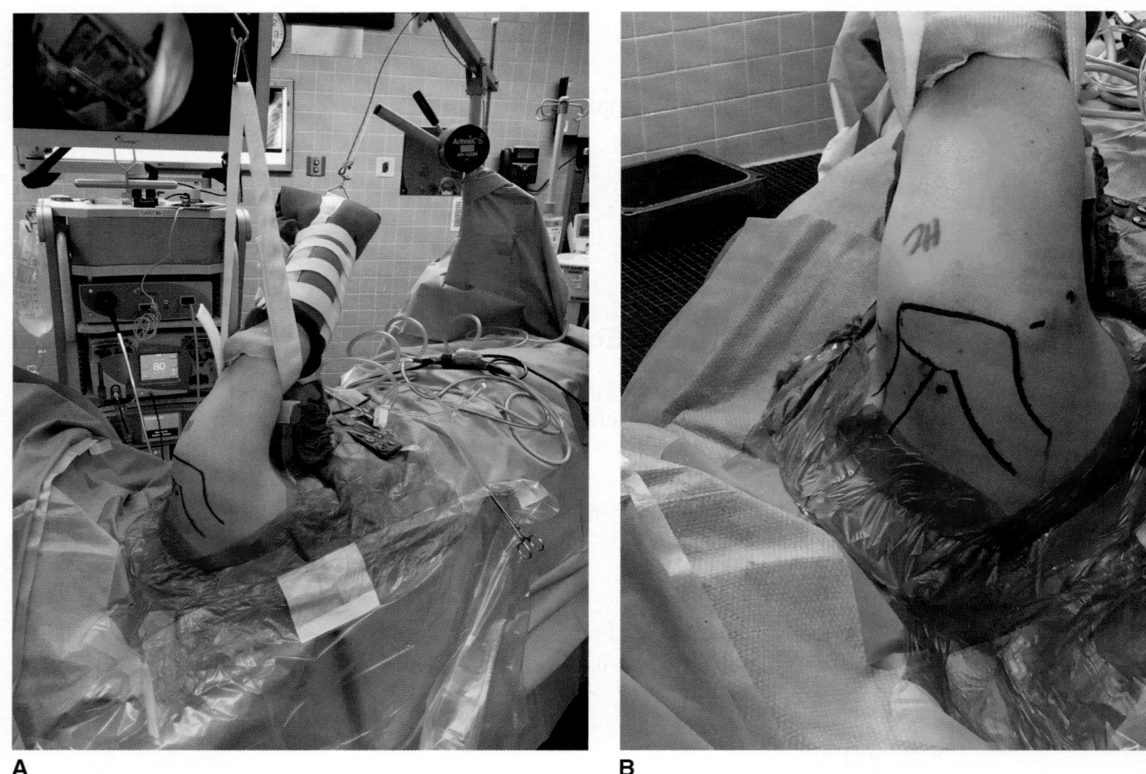

A B

Figure 5-1 | A. Lateral patient positioning. **B.** Demarcated arthroscopic portals.

Arthroscopic Portals (Fig. 5-1B)

- The posterior viewing portal is created in line with the posterolateral margin of the acromion and slightly superior to the standard posterior viewing portal.
- The anterior working portal is placed under needle localization (or inside-out technique) above the superior margin of the subscapularis and in line with the anterolateral margin of the acromion.
- The posteroinferior (7 o'clock) portal is placed under needle localization ~5 cm distal and lateral to the posterior viewing portal.
- The transsubscapularis (5 o'clock) portal is an optional percutaneous portal for anteroinferior anchor placement.
- The anterosuperior portal is an optional viewing portal for posterior and inferior capsular plication.

Diagnostic Arthroscopy

- After establishing the anterior and posterior portals, a thorough 15-point arthroscopic evaluation is conducted (Video 5-1).
- The long head of the biceps is withdrawn intra-articularly to evaluate for hyperemia, synovitis, or other sources of damage.

- The anteroinferior and posteroinferior labrum are inspected for cracking, attenuation, and consistency (Fig. 5-2A and B).
- Laxity and redundancy of the posterior and anterior bands of the inferior glenohumeral complex and axillary pouch are evaluated.
- Competency and volume of the rotator interval are assessed.
- Dynamic examination of glenohumeral translation also can be done under arthroscopic observation for comparison after capsular plication.

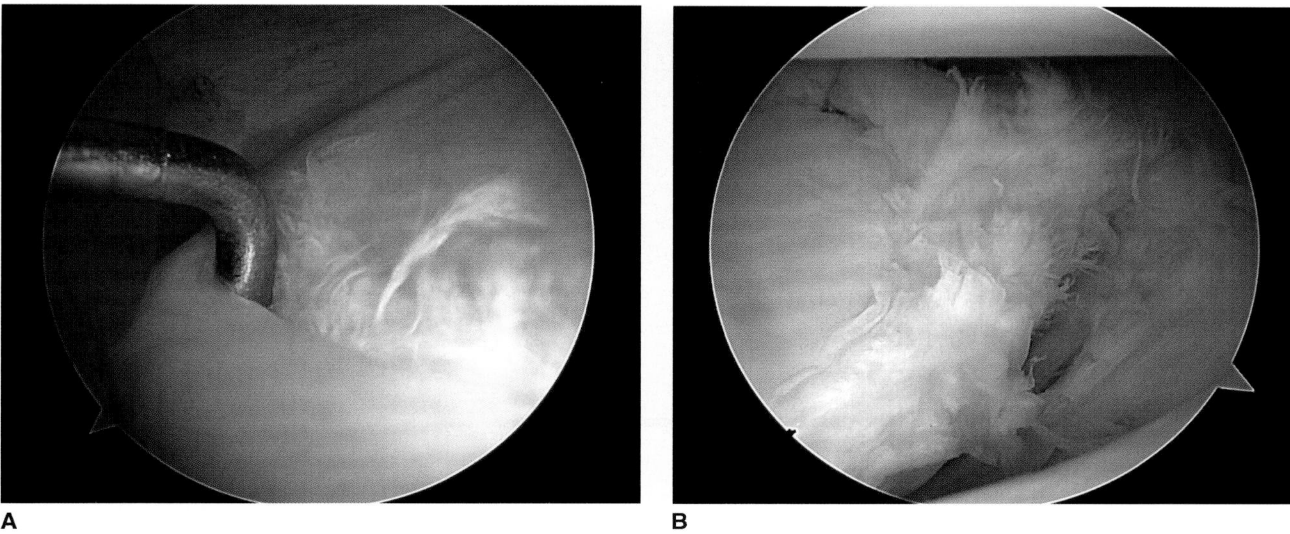

Figure 5-2 | **A.** Posteroinferior labral cracking. **B.** Posteroinferior fraying and capsular injury.

Capsulolabral Preparation

- After arthroscopic confirmation of multidirectional instability, an 8.25-mm cannula is placed in the midanterior portal.
- After needle localization to ensure appropriate trajectory and access for instrumentation of the inferior glenoid, an 8.25-mm cannula also is placed in the posteroinferior portal after tissue dilation (Fig. 5-3A and B).
- An arthroscopic rasp is liberally used for capsular abrasion to generate petechial bleeding.

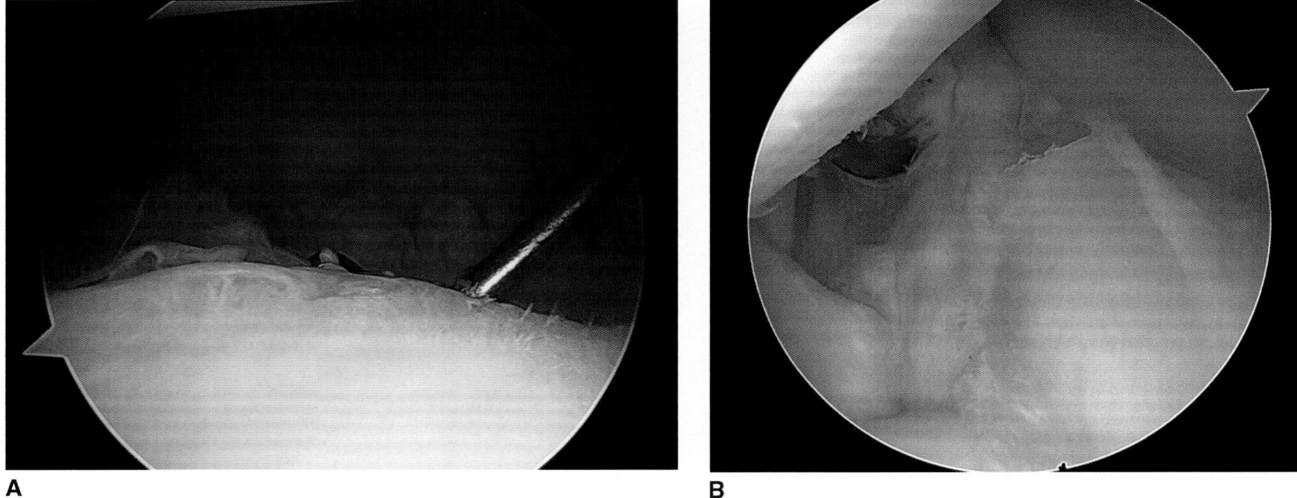

Figure 5-3 | **A.** Posteroinferior portal triangulation. **B.** Posteroinferior portal.

- With labral fissuring or instability, particularly at the chondrolabral junction, a soft tissue elevator can be used to define and mobilize the labrum for subsequent reattachment (Fig. 5-4).[3]
  - Different angled elevators should be used from the anterior and posterior portals.

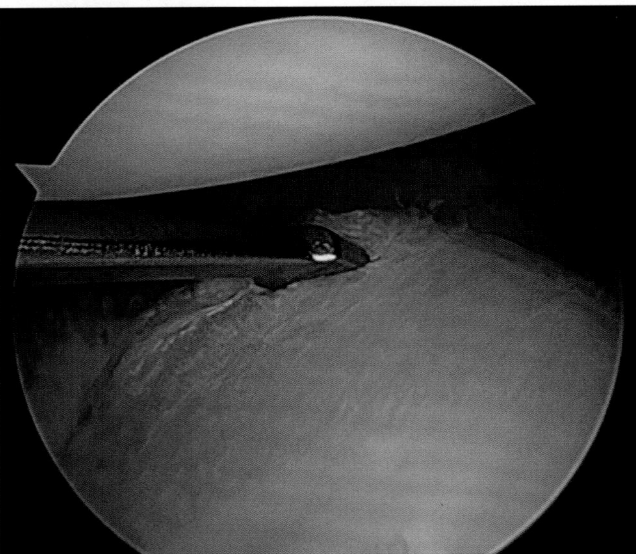

Figure 5-4 | Inferior labral preparation.

  - Care should be exercised to not truncate the labrum or create a segmental or radial split.
  - Mobility of the capsulolabral tissue is evaluated with an arthroscopic grasper.
- Fibrinous and loose labral tissue is debrided from the rim of the glenoid with an arthroscopic shaver.
- A hooded barrel burr is then used to create a bleeding osseous bed on the medial neck of the glenoid.

Capsulolabral Repair (Video 5-2)

- A fish-mouth drill guide is firmly positioned on the glenoid rim at the 6 o'clock position, and drilling is performed until a positive stop (Fig. 5-5).

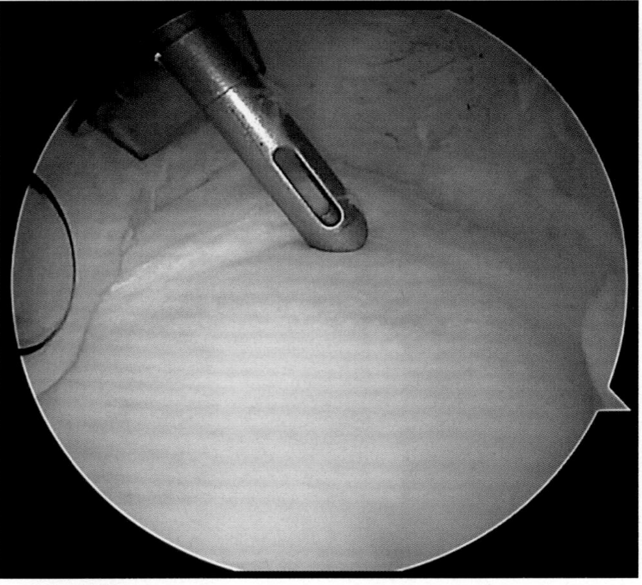

Figure 5-5 | Inferior anchor placement.

- The drill guide is levered up to an angle at or above 50-60 degrees to ensure appropriate bony fixation and avoid skiving into the articular cartilage.
- The drill should be inserted and withdrawn in line with the drill guide to prevent displacing its position on the glenoid.

- The double-loaded 2.4-mm or 3-mm suture anchor is immediately inserted and gently impacted until the anchor is fully seated.
  - The drill sleeve also can be withdrawn slightly to ensure lack of suture anchor prominence.
  - The anchor inserter and drill sleeve are removed together with care to ensure that the suture limbs are not shuttled.
- A ringed suture grasper is used to retrieve three suture limbs through a docking portal, leaving one limb in the posteroinferior portal.
- Angled 45 degrees left (right shoulder) or right (left shoulder), reusable suture-passing devices (Spectrum, ConMed, Largo, FL) are used to penetrate the capsular tissue inferior and posterior to the anchor position (≥1 cm; Fig. 5-6), and a no. 0 Prolene (Johnson & Johnson, Ethicon, Somerville, NJ) shuttling suture is deployed into the joint.[3]

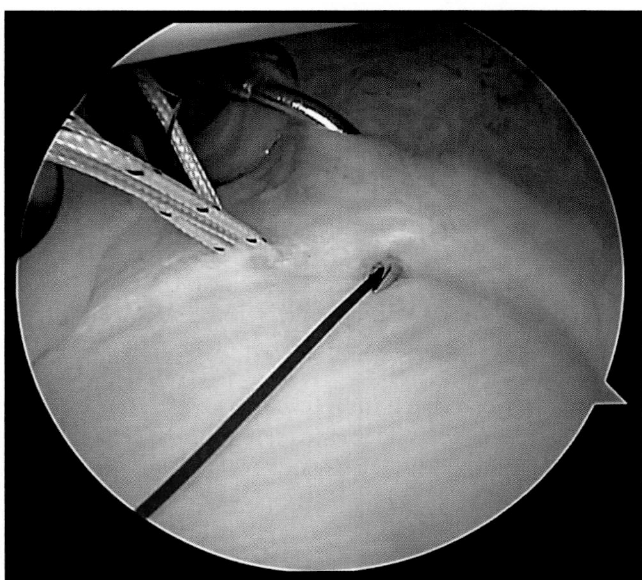

Figure 5-6 | Inferior suture shuttling.

- A ringed grasper is used to retrieve both the Prolene shuttling suture and the isolated anchor suture through the docking portal.
- A half-hitch is created, and the retrieved suture limb is shuttled through the soft tissues and into the posteroinferior portal.
- The suture-passing device is penetrated through the capsule and labrum anterior to the anchor, and the corresponding suture limb is shuttled in similar fashion to create a horizontal mattress configuration.
- Standard arthroscopic knot tying is performed, and the suture tails are cut short.
- The suture shuttling device is passed farther inferiorly (behind the horizontal mattress), and one of the remaining suture limbs is shuttled.
- The other docked suture limb is retrieved through the posteroinferior portal and the sutures are tied, creating a vertical mattress stitch reinforced with the "ripstop" configuration (Fig. 5-7A and B).
- Standard knot tying is done, with the knot directed peripherally to limit prominence.

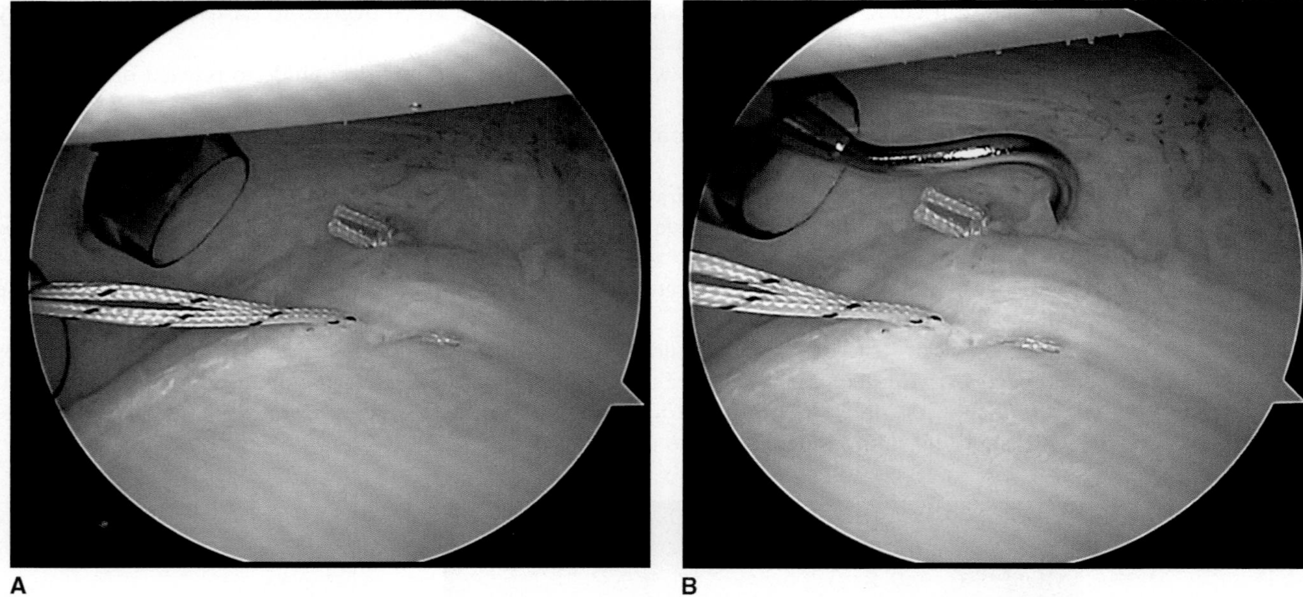

Figure 5-7 | A. Inferior horizontal capsular plication. **B.** Vertical limb suture plication.

- Anterior anchors are placed in similar fashion at 5- to 8-mm increments, at 4:30 and 3 o'clock positions in a right shoulder and 7:30 and 9 o'clock, respectively, in a left shoulder for complete retensioning of the anterior and middle glenohumeral ligament (Fig. 5-8).
  - A tissue grasper can be used through the anterosuperior portal to advance the capsulolabral tissue superiorly and laterally under tension while tissue penetration is achieved with the shuttling device.
- The arthroscopic evaluation is continued from the anterior or anterosuperior portal, and additional points of fixation are obtained with double-loaded suture anchors at 7:30, 9'clock, and 10:30 positions in a right shoulder and 4:30, 3 o'clock, and 1:30 in a left shoulder, with care to advance the tissue and reconstruct the capsulolabral bumper (Fig. 5-9).
  - Alternatively, single-loaded knotless suture anchors with high-tensile suture tape can be used at higher positions on the clockface (ie, above the equator) in either simple or inverted mattress configurations.
- The final repair is inspected and probed; examination under anesthesia is done outside of lateral traction with direct arthroscopic visualization (Video 5-3).

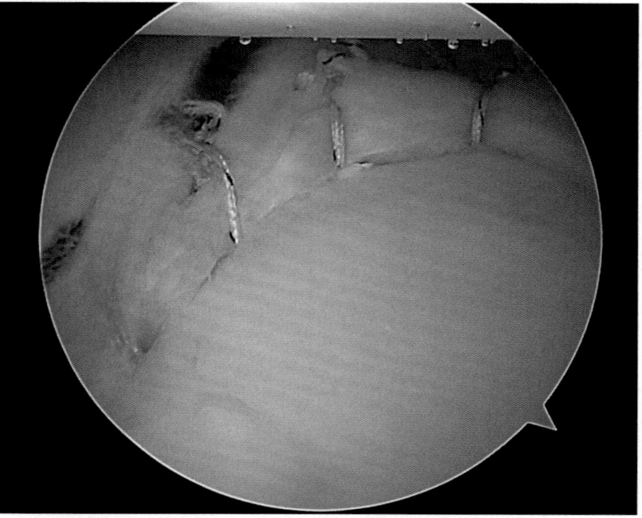

Figure 5-8 | Anterior capsular plication.

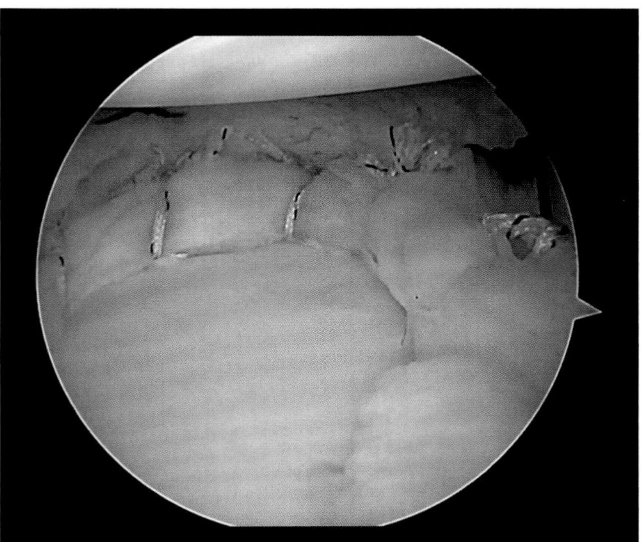

Figure 5-9 | Posterior repair and plication.

Capsular Plication/Rotator Interval Closure (Optional)

- Because of the occasionally tenuous nature of capsular tissue and the high prevalence of systemic laxity conditions, further capsular plication and/or posterior portal closure can be used to augment anchor-based reconstruction.
  - Through the posterior or posteroinferior portal, a curved shuttling device is inserted through the capsule medial and inferiorly, exiting through the labrum, with a "pinch and tuck" technique.
  - A no. 1 PDS suture is deployed into the joint, leaving a lengthy limb of suture intra-articularly.
  - A tissue penetrator is introduced more laterally and superiorly through the capsule, and the free limb of suture is withdrawn into the cannula for intra-articular or extracapsular tying.
- While not routinely part of the senior author's practice, adjunctive rotator interval closure can be considered in high-risk individuals with excessive inferior laxity after 270-degree capsular plication or a sulcus sign that does not diminish with external rotation.[1,3]
  - The anterior cannula is withdrawn beneath the capsular layer of the rotator interval tissue.
  - A crescent suture shuttling device is passed through the rotator interval capsule and superior glenohumeral ligament, and a no. 1 PDS is shuttled, leaving a lengthy suture tail within the joint while the device is removed.
  - A tissue penetrator is introduced through the same anterior portal and passed through the more inferior rotator interval capsule and middle glenohumeral ligament, withdrawing the free suture limb through the anterior portal.
  - With the anterior portal maintained in the extracapsular position, the suture limbs are tensioned under indirect visualization from the intra-articular space (or directly from the lateral portal in the subacromial space).
  - With the arm positioned in 30-45 degrees of external rotation, standard arthroscopic knot tying techniques are used, and the suture limbs are cut short.
  - Alternatively, high-tensile, nonabsorbable suture also can be shuttled in standard fashion at the discretion of the surgeon.

Wound Closure

- Arthroscopic portals are closed with 3-0 Prolene suture and covered with sterile adhesive strips, 4 × 4 gauze dressing, abdominal pads, and adhesive tape.
- A cryotherapy pad and "gunslinger" sling with the shoulder in neutral rotation and slight abduction are worn for 6 weeks.

References

1. Alpert JM, Verma N, Wysocki R, Yanke AB, Romeo AA. Arthroscopic treatment of multidirectional shoulder instability with minimum 270 degrees labral repair: minimum 2-year follow-up. *Arthroscopy*. 2008;24(6):704-711.
2. Forsythe B, Ghodadra N, Romeo AA, Provencher MT. Management of the failed posterior/multidirectional instability patient. *Sports Med Arthrosc Rev*. 2010;18:149-161.
3. Provencher MT, LeClere LE, Romeo AA. Multidirectional and posterior instability of the shoulder: pearls and pitfalls in diagnosis and management. In: Levine W, ed. *Pitfalls in the Management of Common Shoulder Problems*. American Academy of Orthopaedic Surgeons, Rosemont, 2008.

Chapter 6
Open Treatment of Multidirectional Shoulder Instability

THOMAS M. DeBERARDINO
EDUARDO STEWIEN

Introduction

- Neer and Foster[1] described multidirectional instability (MDI) of the shoulder as instability in two or more directions.
- Individuals with generalized joint hypermobility may be at increased risk of sport-related injuries.[2]
- MDI often affects athletic individuals who participate in repetitive overhead movement sports.[3]
- The most frequent complaint is generalized shoulder pain with worsened activity performance and loss of strength.[4]
- The surgical treatment options are open and arthroscopic procedures.[3,5,6]

Sterile Instruments/Equipment

- Arthroscope, 30-degree
- Trimano arm holder (Arthrex, Naples, FL)
- Scorpion suture passer (Arthrex, Naples, FL)
- Lasso suture passer (Arthrex, Naples, FL)
- Knotless SutureTak anchors (Arthrex, Naples, FL)
- SwiveLock anchors (Arthrex, Naples, FL)
- FiberTape + FiberWire sutures (Arthrex, Naples, FL)

Positioning

- The patient is positioned in a beach-chair position with the Trimano arm holder holding the arm (Fig. 6-1).

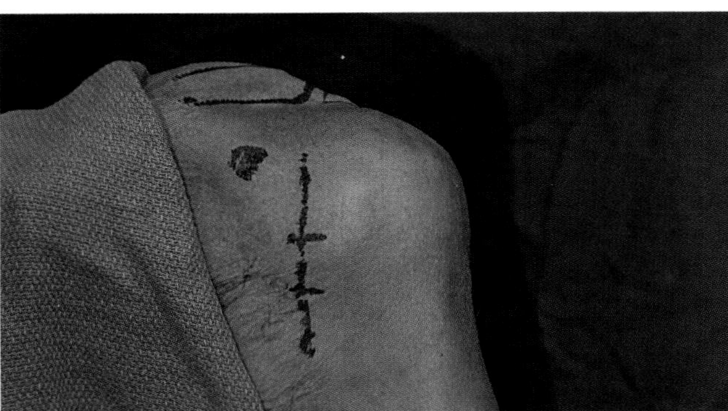

Figure 6-1 | Anterior approach (left shoulder).

Surgical Approach

- A deltopectoral approach is made. (For cosmetic reasons, an axillary approach can be used.)
- The cephalic vein is exposed and retracted laterally with the deltoid; the pectoralis major is medialized.
- The axillary nerve is palpated inferiorly, and a retractor is placed below the conjoint tendon to expose the subscapularis muscle (Figs. 6-2 and 6-3).

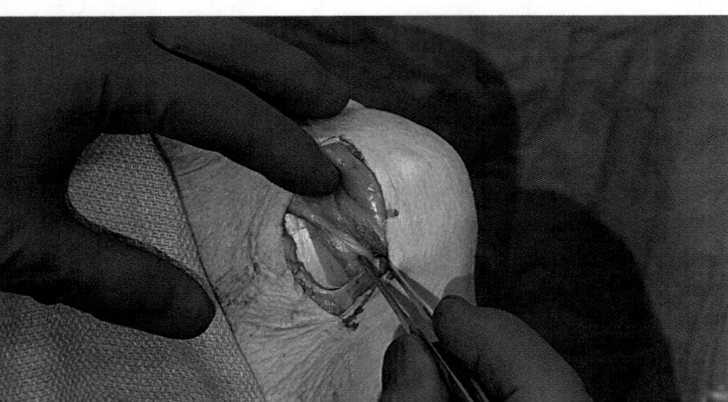

Figure 6-2 | Deltopectoral interval (left shoulder).

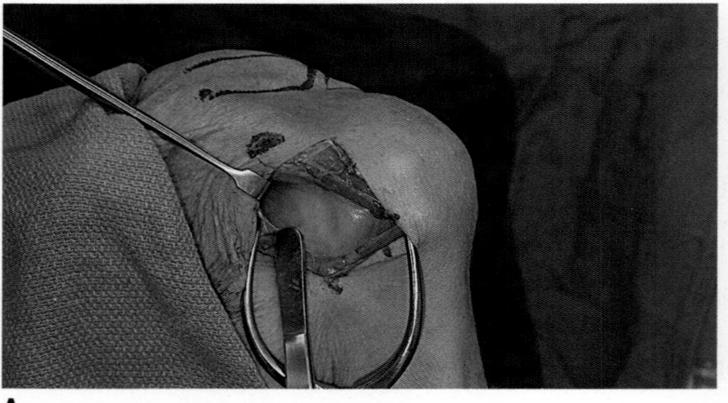

A

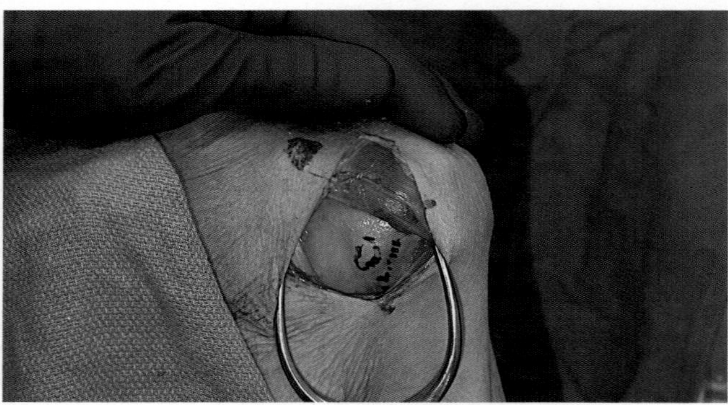

B

Figure 6-3 | A. Exposure of the subscapularis. **B.** Lesser tuberosity identified (left shoulder).

- The "three sisters" (anterior humeral circumflex vessels along the inferior third of the subscapularis) are ligated or cauterized, and the biceps tendon long head is dissected to provide a landmark. Dissection with scissors is carried under the subscapularis from inferior to superior to expose the rotator interval.
- A vertical incision is made 1 cm medial to the biceps tendon to identify the subscapularis and the capsule.
- Sutures passed by the Scorpion suture passer are used to retract the subscapularis and expose the capsule, where a midline incision is made and superior and inferior flaps are created.
- Dissection is carried under the inferior flap until the inferior pouch is seen and the redundant capsule is identified.
- A Fukuda retractor is used to expose the anterior labrum and evaluate the anteroinferior joint area for a Bankart lesion (Fig. 6-4).
- The knotless SutureTak anchors are placed at the 6, 4, and 2 o'clock positions. This can be done in three different ways.
  - A 90-degree Lasso suture passer can be used to pass the sutures through the Bankart lesion and redundant capsule if needed. Then, FiberTape is used to wrap the Bankart lesion, and it is stabilized with a knotless PushLock anchor (Fig. 6-5).
  - The Scorpion suture passer can be used to grab the Bankart lesion and pass a FiberSnare (Arthrex, Naples, FL) to form a cinch stitch. It is quick and easy to hold the lesion inside the loop. The final step is to stabilize the lesion with a 3.5-mm SwiveLock screw-in anchor (Figs. 6-6 and 6-7).

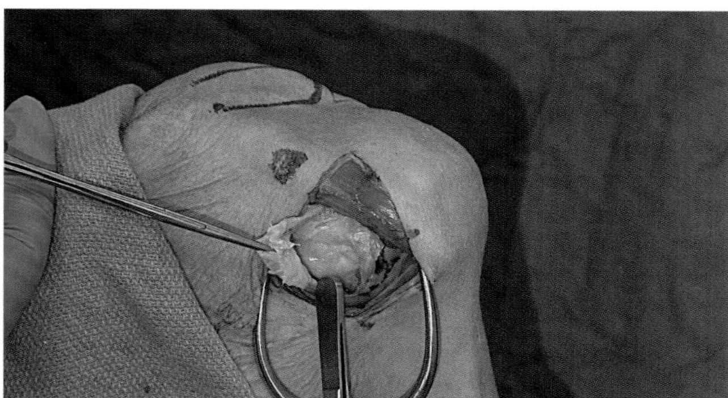

Figure 6-4 | Subscapularis released from underlying capsule.

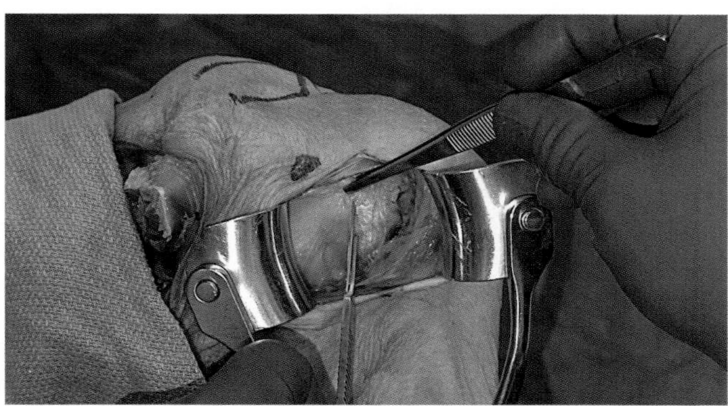

Figure 6-5 | Shoulder prepared for capsulotomy.

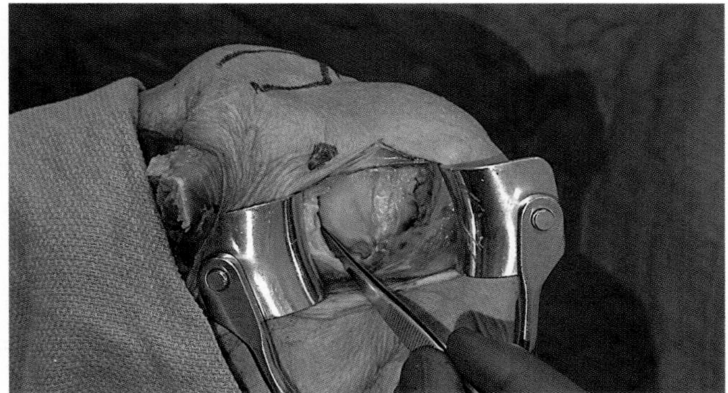

Figure 6-6 | Assessment of capsulolabral complex laxity.

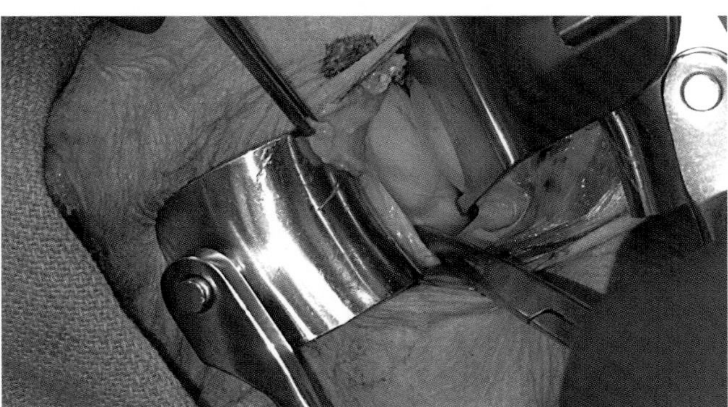

Figure 6-7 | Ready for preparation of the detached labral area with a shaver and/or burr to augment capsulolabral tissue healing to the bone.

- A Lasso suture-passing device is used to pass a hardened FiberStick (Arthrex, Naples, FL) suture directly through the capsulolabral tissue. The suture tails are passed through the anchor eyelet, and the anchor and sutures at the desired tension are passed into a drilled hole (Fig. 6-8).

  Based on surgeon preference or degree of laxity, after the robust inferior flap is properly mobilized, a base-stabilizing closure of the superior interval is completed with the Scorpion suture passer or similar instrument.

- The inferior flap is mobilized underneath the superior flap, and the Scorpion is used to pass the sutures, which are held with knotless SutureTak anchors superiorly and inferiorly to create a stable complex without the redundant capsule. The knotless SutureTak anchors can be used instead of stitches to construct a safer and stronger capsular shift (Figs. 6-9 to 6-11).

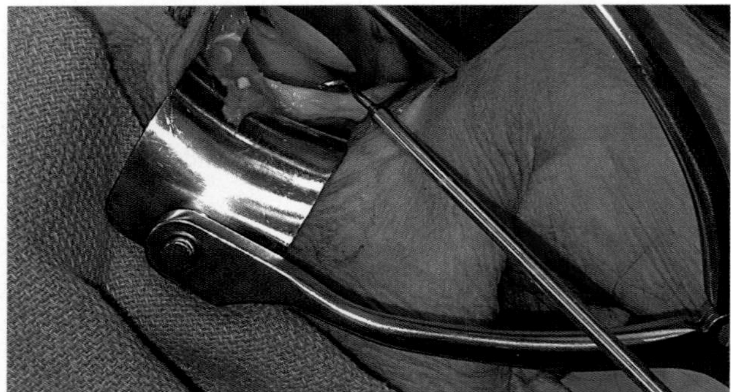

A1

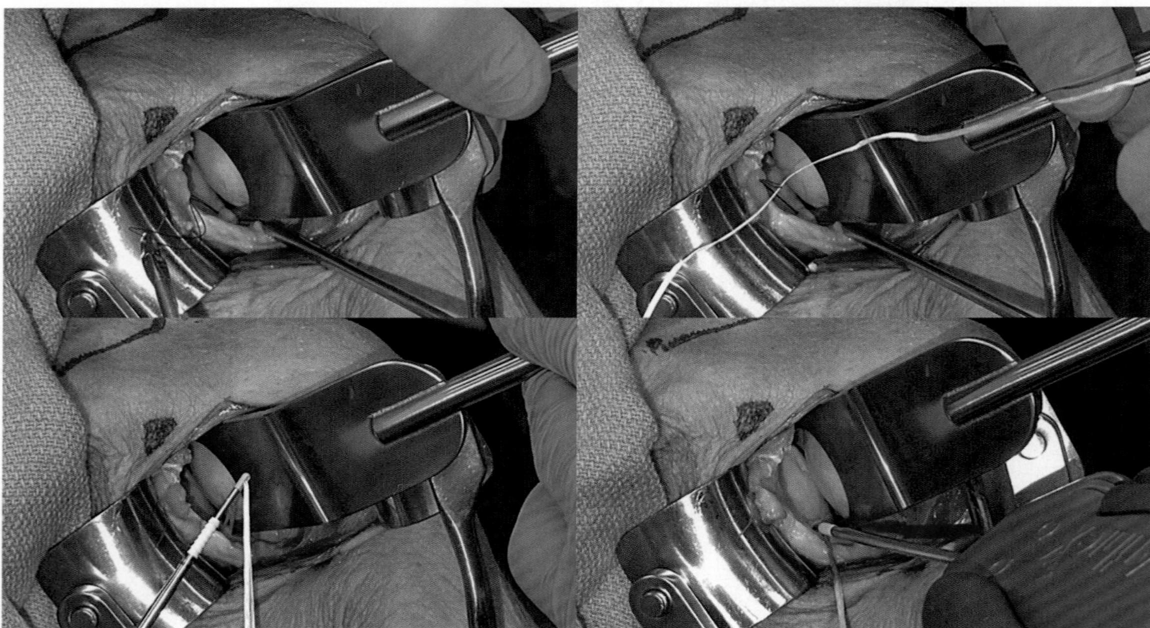

A2

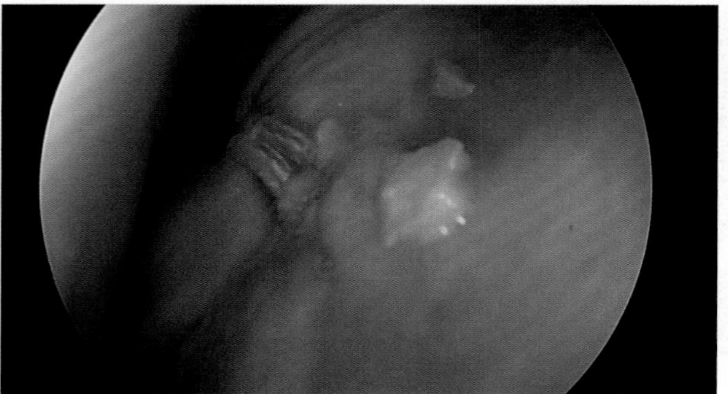

A3

Figure 6-8 | **A1.** Placement of inferior capsulolabral suture. **A2.** Anchor placement. **A3.** Posterior arthroscopic view of open repair appears as if it were completed with the arthroscopic technique.

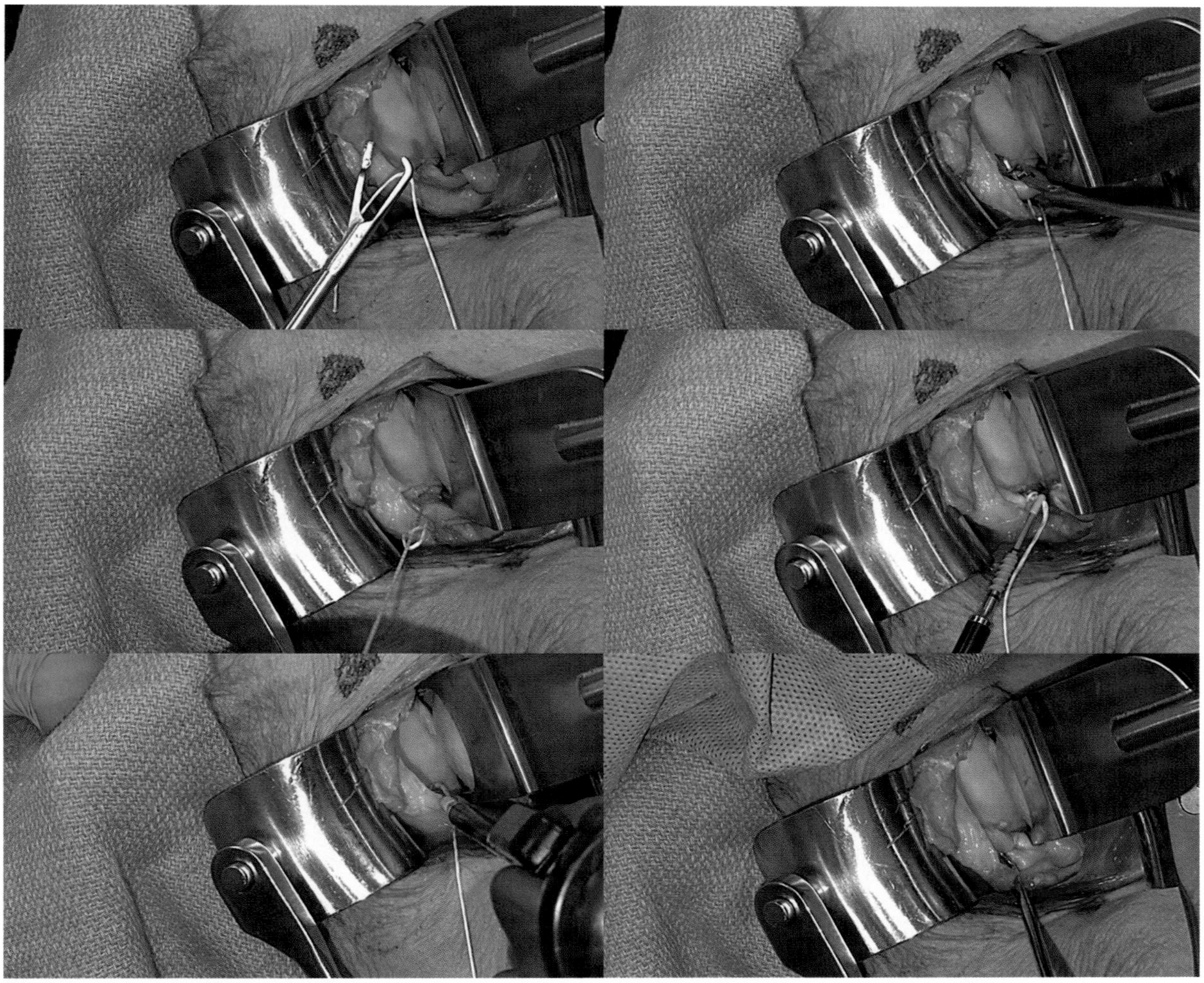

B

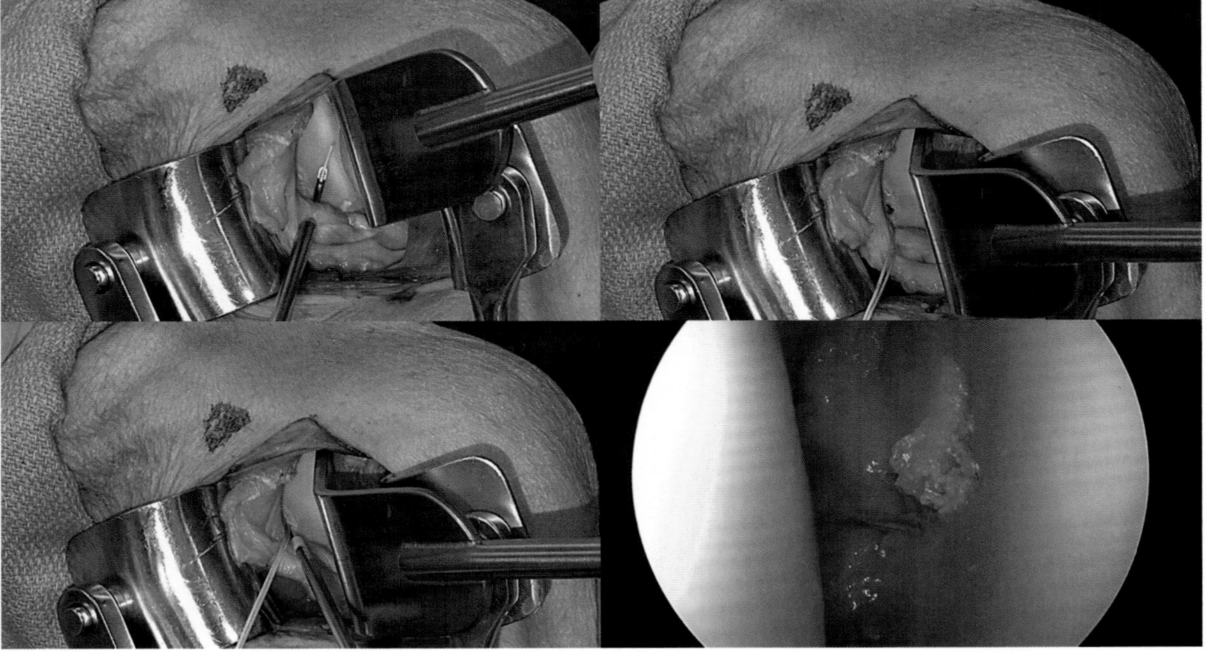

C

Figure 6-8 | (*Continued*) **B.** Placement of second suture anchor. **C.** Final suture anchor placement; posterior arthroscopic view after anchor placement reveals striking similarity in appearance to arthroscopic capsulolabral repair.

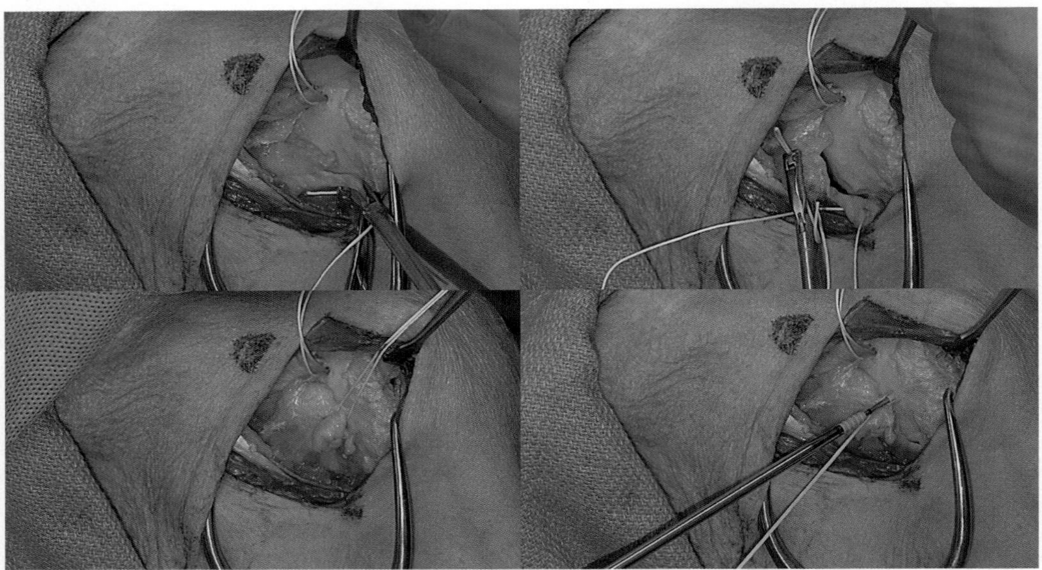

Figure 6-9 | Capsular closure.

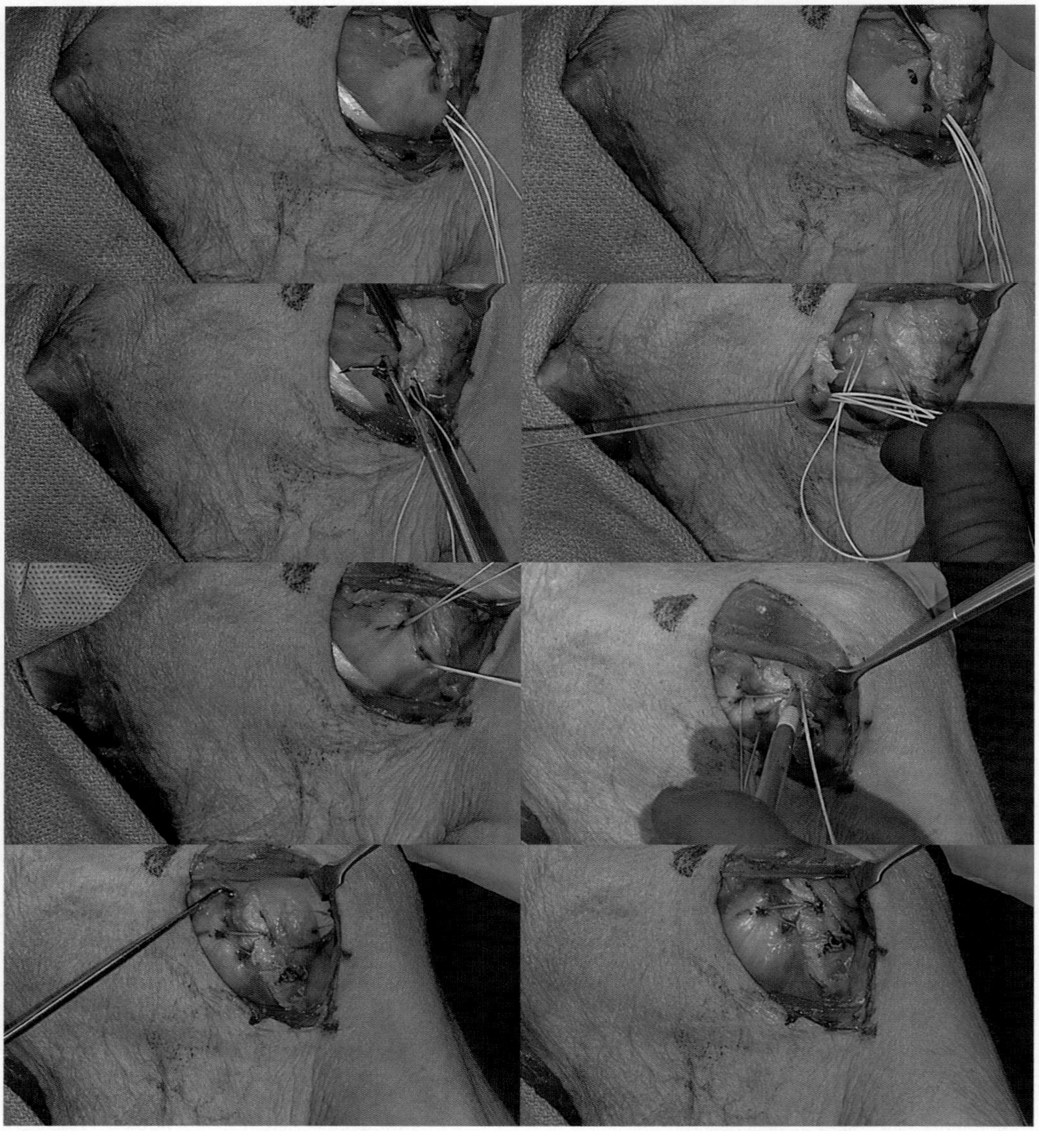

Figure 6-10 | Final closure of subscapularis.

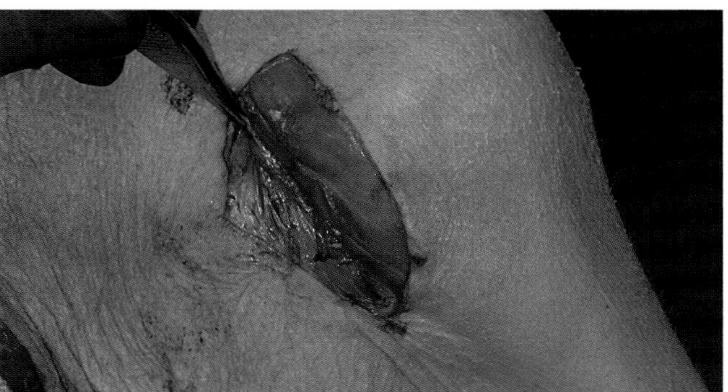

Figure 6-11 | Wound closure.

- The Scorpion is used to pass the sutures to reattach the subscapularis. The lateral flap is mobilized, and the closure over the subscapularis is competed with SwiveLock anchors.
- The wound is closed with the surgeon's standard technique.

References

1. Neer CS, Foster CR. Inferior capsular shift for involuntary inferior and multidirectional instability of the shoulder. A preliminary report. *J Bone Joint Surg Am*. 1980;62(6):897-908.
2. Cameron KL, Duffey ML, DeBerardino TM, Stoneman PD, Jones CJ, Owens BD. Association of generalized joint hypermobility with a history of glenohumeral joint instability. *J Athl Train*. 2010;45(3):253-258.
3. Longo UG, Rizzello G, Loppini M, et al. Multidirectional instability of the shoulder: a systematic review. *Arthroscopy*. 2015;31(12):2431-2443.
4. Forsythe B, Ghodadra N, Romeo AA, Provencher MT. Management of the failed posterior/multidirectional instability patient. *Sports Med Arthrosc*. 2010;18(3):149-161.
5. Bois AJ, Wirth MA. Revision open capsular shift for atraumatic and multidirectional instability of the shoulder. *Instr Course Lect*. 2013;62:95-103.
6. Gaskill TR, Taylor DC, Millett PJ. Management of multidirectional instability of the shoulder. *J Am Acad Orthop Surg*. 2011;19(12):758-767.

Chapter 7
Arthroscopic Treatment of SLAP Lesions

NIKOLAOS K. PASCHOS
KIMBERLY V. TUCKER
JOHN D. A. KELLY IV

Overview

- Superior labrum anterior and posterior (SLAP) lesions are a major cause of a dysfunctional throwing shoulder.
- Both indications and surgical techniques for SLAP lesions have evolved over the years.
- There is no clear consensus for the management of SLAP lesions.
- The type of the SLAP lesion (Fig. 7-1) should be determined, with normal anatomic variants kept in mind (Fig. 7-2).

Indications

- Complete detachment of superior labrum, especially posterior with positive peel-back.
- Tear associated with clear laxity of biceps insertion as examined with probe.
- Elevation of labrum at least 5 mm with associated signs of inflammation, fraying, erythema, fissuring, and granulation.
- Separation of bone-labrum junction, with associated erythema at the respective labrum insertion, with or without excursion of at least 5 mm.
- Age is a determining factor: ≤30 years, SLAP repair; 30-60 years, tenodesis; >60 years, tenotomy.

Preparation for the Repair

- The side of the glenoid is prepared with a shaver or burr to obtain bleeding bone before anchor placement to promote labral healing (Fig. 7-3). This is best accomplished from a contralateral portal.
- Because anchor placement needs to be somewhat perpendicular to the glenoid to avoid injury to the glenoid cartilage and potential anchor failure, portal placement must be selected meticulously and a new portal created when necessary for ideal anchor placement (Fig. 7-4). A percutaneous anchor placement is necessary to obtain the correct trajectory (Fig. 7-5).
- The Port of Wilmington is ideal for posterosuperior tears, while the "7 o'clock" portal is helpful for posteroinferior lesions.
- Iatrogenic chondrolysis (rapid degeneration of articular cartilage) can be avoided by not using thermal radiofrequency devices or administering anesthetics intra-articularly or by infusion.[1-4]

Evolution of Techniques

The different techniques initially used for arthroscopic repair of SLAP tears had inconsistent results, especially in young athletes. The rate of successful outcomes ranged significantly from 40% to 94% of patients.[5-9] This wide range was attributed to the huge variability among different techniques and

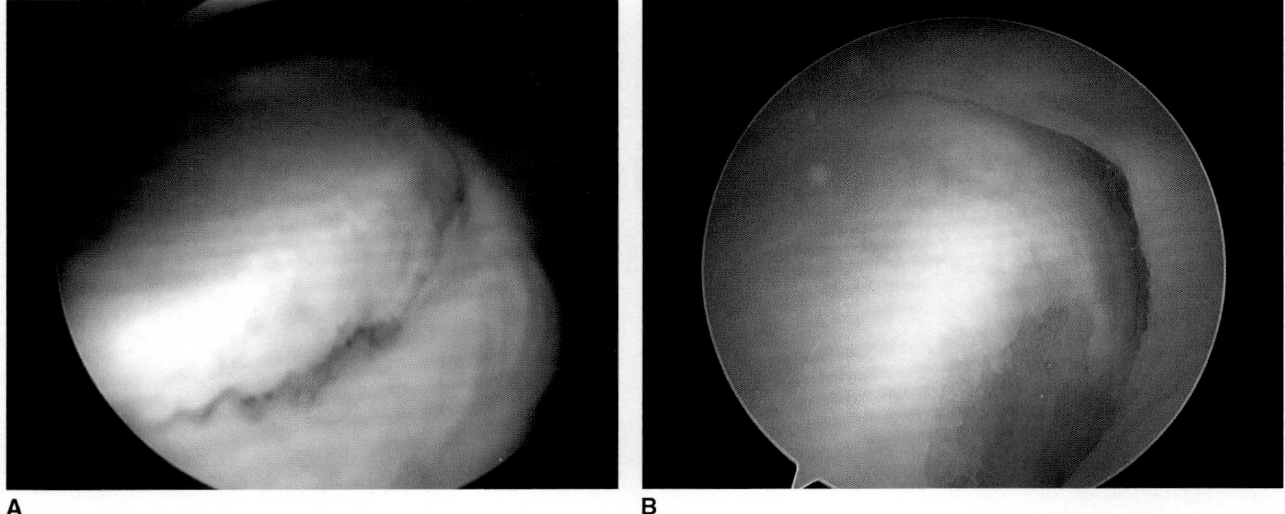

Figure 7-1 | **A.** A good SLAP lesion has stretched tissue that enables thrower to "bring it." **B.** A bad SLAP lesion has significant displacement with adverse mechanical consequences.

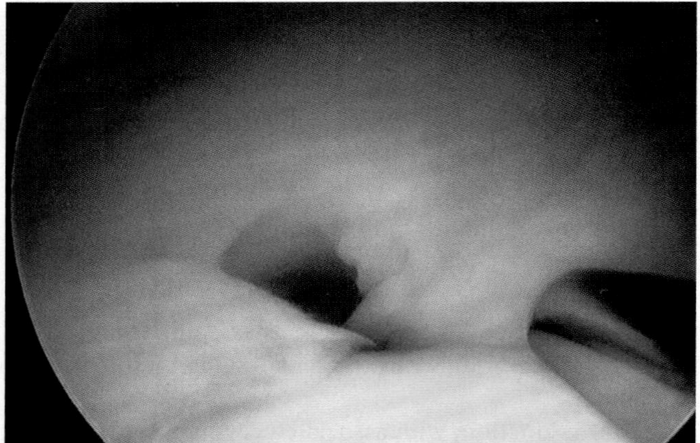

Figure 7-2 | An example of a sublabral foramen, an unattached anterosuperior labrum seen in ~11% of individuals.

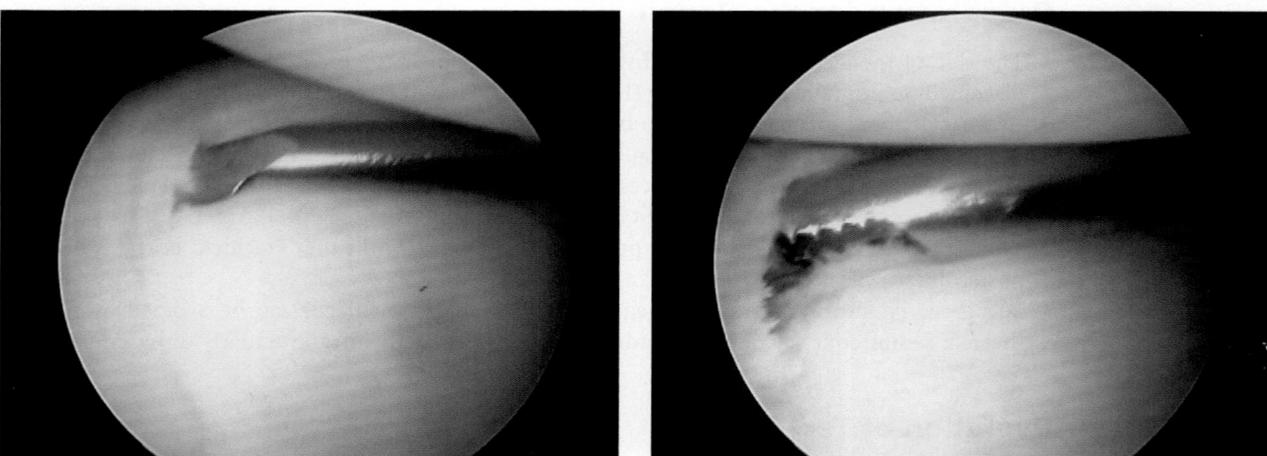

Figure 7-3 | Preparation of the tear from the contralateral portal.

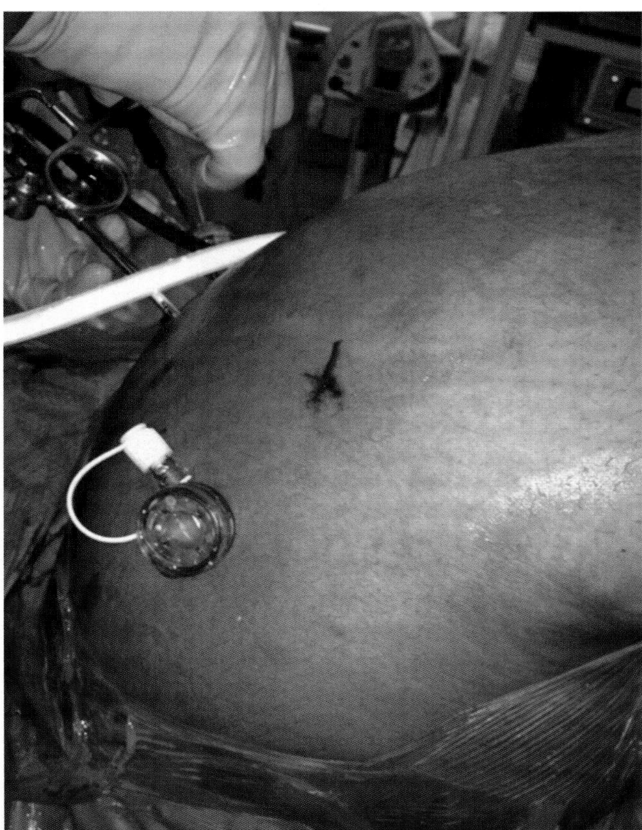

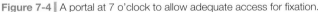

Figure 7-4 | A portal at 7 o'clock to allow adequate access for fixation.

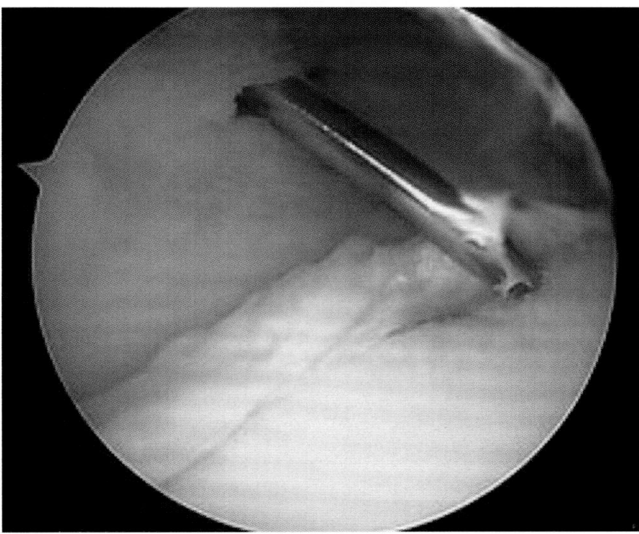

Figure 7-5 | Percutaneous portal creation.

preferences for SLAP repair. Indeed, a high degree of variability was recorded in numerous issues concerning the repair technique.[10] For example, in one study, the number of anchors used for similarly sized SLAP lesions varied significantly with half of the surgeons using from 1 to 2 anchors vs the other half that used 3-4 anchors. A high degree of variability exists in the use of absorbable suture anchors vs metallic anchors, in the position of the anchors, and in the type and configuration of the knot.[10] As techniques evolved, it was realized that these conflicting data might be due to the fact that early techniques overlooked some basic principles of normal superior labrum anatomy restoration. It was also realized that certain risk factors might contribute to increased failure rate. For example, polylactic acid absorbable suture anchors were associated with an increased risk of failure and reoperation (odds ratio 12.7). Smoking status was also found to be linked with increased failure rate, while age, gender, the presence of rotator cuff pathology, the number of anchors, and the duration of symptoms were not found to be associated with increased failure risk of SLAP tear repair.[11]

Technical Tips and Tricks for SLAP Repair

- **Avoidance of overtightening of SLAP repairs.** Rigid suture constructs (tape, fibers) may overconstrain the proximal labrum and impair motion. Loss of external rotation may occur when the capsule is advanced to the glenoid along with the labrum. Some reports suggest tightening of the knots with the arm in external rotation.[12]
- **Recreation of the native anatomy of the labrum's meniscoid appearance**. Advocates of horizontal mattress technique for labral repair highlight the importance of the "bumper effect" for functional

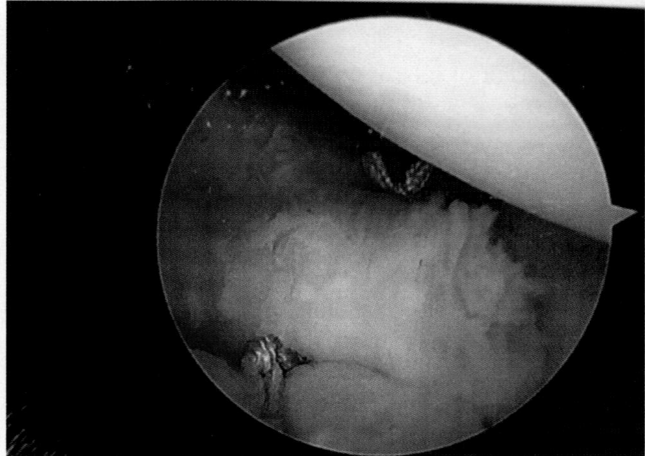

Figure 7-6 | Horizontal mattress technique ensures the recreation of the native bumper effect of the labrum.

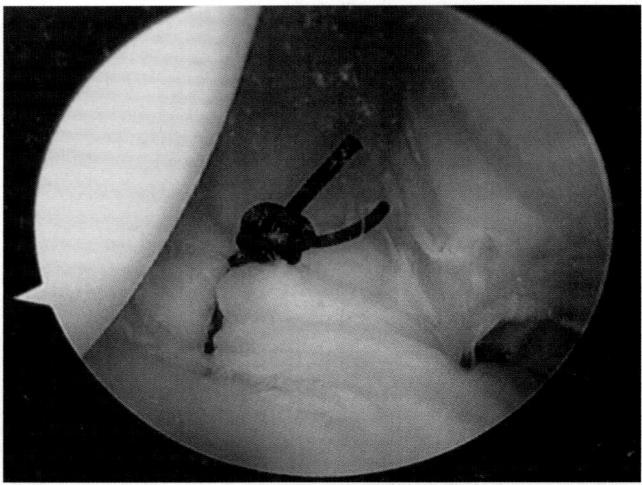

Figure 7-7 | PDS suture used for SLAP repair.

stability of the shoulder that can only be recreated with this technique[13,14] (Fig. 7-6). Furthermore horizontal mattress configuration avoids the threat of "knot abrasion," which can induce appreciable chondral wear (Figs. 7-7 to 7-9). Despite concerns of poor biomechanical strength with horizontal mattress,[15] similar biomechanical studies demonstrated parity or superiority of the fixation strength.[16,17] No significant differences were shown in functional outcomes between the vertical knot and horizontal mattress knot configurations[18,19]; however, some benefit in range of motion and

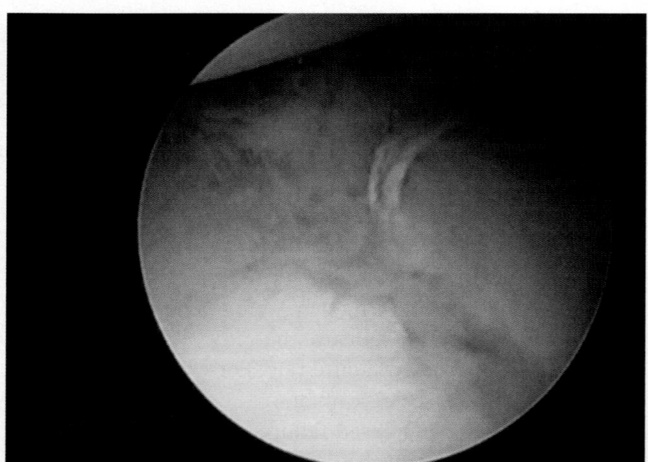

Figure 7-8 | Chondral wear and poor bumper from "tape."

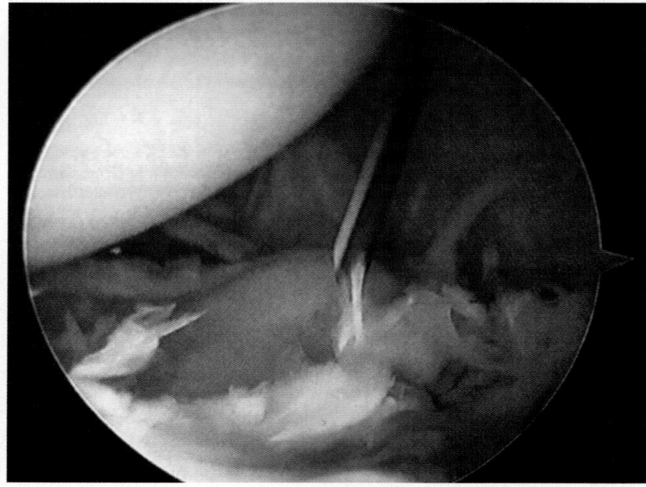

Figure 7-9 | An example of damage caused by a prominent knot.

in early pain relief was recently recorded with horizontal mattress knot configurations.[18] Finally, anchors must not be placed too close to the biceps root, which would in effect "hog-tie" the biceps and prevent bicipital excursion needed to full external rotation (Fig. 7-10).

- **The use of knotless anchors** may reduce the volume of the suture repair in a narrow interval, thus preventing complications from suture-related glenoid erosion,[20] as well as minimizing postoperative pain due to knot impingement during motion.[13] However, the senior author discourages their use due to overconstraint and loss of bumper effect.
- **Avoidance of biceps "sacrifice," unless absolutely necessary.** It is important not to cause additional injury and functional impairment unless clearly indicated from the pathology. The biceps tendon serves an important functional role and, even though the trend recently favors more biceps tenodesis and less SLAP repair, "sacrifice" of the biceps should be considered carefully. The biceps tendon serves as a tension band to the shoulder and confers stability and minimizes shear stress across the joint.

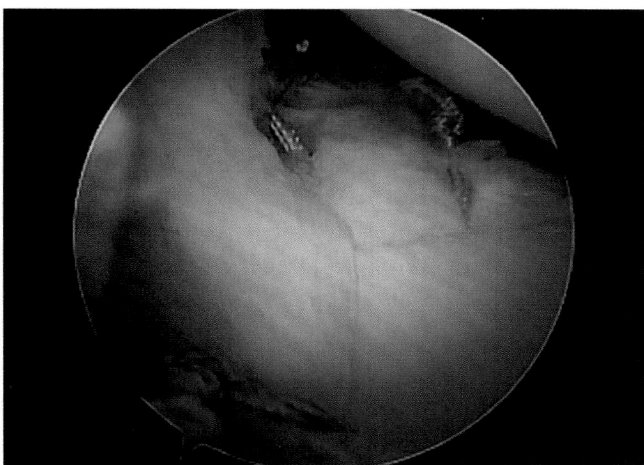

Figure 7-10 | Overconstraint of the biceps by the repair (hog-tied biceps).

- **Prevention of recurrent instability.** Rotator interval closure should be done when indicated to prevent recurrent instability in patients with excessive interval laxity and when the biceps sling is capacious due to coracohumeral ligament laxity.[21] Tightening of the sutures should be done with the shoulder external rotation to avoid loss of motion.
- **Treatment of associated pathology** (eg, rotator cuff tears, posterior capsular contracture, and/or anterior instability). The remplissage technique can be done when a large Hills-Sachs lesion is recognized. Spinoglenoid cysts with suprascapular nerve disorders are frequent with SLAP lesions; cysts should be decompressed if possible in conjunction with arthroscopic SLAP repair.[22] Kinetic chain abnormalities need to be corrected before a return to throwing is begun; otherwise, uncorrected mechanical flaws present preoperatively will increase the risk for recurrence or poor performance.

Equipment

- Large joint arthroscopy equipment (30/70 degree arthroscope)
- Arthroscopic shoulder tray with the following additions:
  - Cannula insertion/dilation instruments
  - 6.0-/7.0-mm or 8.25-mm working cannulas
  - Suture-passing devices (ReelPass Suture Lasso [Arthrex, Naples, FL] or Spectrum [Linvatec, Edison, NJ])
  - Arthroscopic periosteal/labrum elevator/spatula
  - 3.5-/4.5-mm arthroscopic shaver
  - 4.0-/4.5-mm hooded burr
  - No. 1 or no. 0 polypropylene suture
  - No. 1 polydioxanone (PDS) suture
  - 2.4-mm biocomposite short PushLock anchors (Arthrex, Naples, FL)
  - 1.3-mm SutureTape (Arthrex, Naples, FL)
  - Anchor drill with guide and trocar

Patient Positioning and Preparation

- The patient is positioned in the lateral decubitus position on a beanbag.
- Interscalene nerve block typically is used, with or without general anesthesia.
- Bony prominences are padded (fibular head/peroneal nerve, lateral malleolus, axillary roll, pillow between the legs to alleviate low back pressure).
- Five to ten pounds of traction is applied to the operative arm.

Surgical Technique

- Standard posterior (viewing) and anterior (working) rotator interval portals are established for arthroscopic evaluation of all aspects of the labrum.

- The glenoid surface area of labral detachment is prepared with a motorized shaver through the anterior working portal.
- A spinal needle is positioned percutaneously at the lateral edge of the acromion at its posterior one-third and directed to the desired anchor placement.
- A 3-mm percutaneous incision is made, through which the drill guide with a blunt obturator is inserted to penetrate the supraspinatus at its musculotendinous border and enter the glenoid.
- With the guide angled 45 degrees to the articular margin, the tunnel is drilled and the anchor inserted through the guide.
- The suture limb passed through the labrum is retrieved out the anterior cannula.
- A 90-degree suture passer (SutureLasso, Arthrex, Naples, FL) is inserted through the same percutaneous incision, through the supraspinatus, and through the labrum. The suture is shuttled through the labrum, and both suture limbs are retrieved out the anterior cannula with the cannula placed posterior to the biceps tendon.
- The knots are tied with five alternating half-hitches. For a meniscoid-type labrum, the two limbs from each suture were placed in a vertical fashion with 4 mm of tissue bridge between them to achieve a more anatomic repair. The goal during knot tying is to keep the knots on the medial aspect of the labrum and away from the glenohumeral articulation.
- The first anchor is placed posterior to the biceps anchor, with subsequent anchors placed 5 mm more posterior on the glenoid as necessary to achieve complete fixation posteriorly.
- If the anterior aspect of the biceps insertion and labrum is detached, the drill guide is placed percutaneously through the rotator interval just lateral to the anterior working cannula. Anchor placement, suture shuttling, and knot tying are done as for the posterior repair.
- The repair is inspected with a probe and the portals are closed in routine fashion.

Postoperative Management

- A protective sling is worn for 6 weeks.
- Elbow, wrist, and hand exercises are begun immediately after surgery.
- Passive and active assisted range-of-motion exercises are begun at 2 weeks.
- Strengthening exercises for the rotator cuff, scapular stabilizers, and deltoid are begun at 6 weeks, and biceps strengthening at 8 weeks.
- Aggressive strengthening activities are allowed at 3 months, and at 4 months, throwing athletes begin an interval throwing program.
- At 6 months, contact and collision athletes return to sport, and at 7 months, pitchers are allowed maximal throwing effort from the mound.

References

1. Good CR, Shindle MK, Kelly BT, Wanich T, Warren RF. Glenohumeral chondrolysis after shoulder arthroscopy with thermal capsulorrhaphy. *Arthroscopy*. 2007;23:797.e1-797.e5.
2. Levine WN, Clark AM Jr, D'Alessandro DF, Yamaguchi K. Chondrolysis following arthroscopic thermal capsulorrhaphy to treat shoulder instability. A report of two cases. *J Bone Joint Surg Am*. 2005;87:616-621.
3. Scheffel PT, Clinton J, Lynch JR, Warme WJ, Bertelsen AL, Matsen FA III. Glenohumeral chondrolysis: a systematic review of 100 cases from the English language literature. *J Shoulder Elbow Surg*. 2010;19:944-949.
4. Matsen FA III, Papadonikolakis A. Published evidence demonstrating the causation of glenohumeral chondrolysis by post-operative infusion of local anesthetic via a pain pump. *J Bone Joint Surg Am*. 2013;95:1126-1134.
5. Boileau P, Parratte S, Chuinard C, Roussanne Y, Shia D, Bicknell R. Arthroscopic treatment of isolated type II SLAP lesions: biceps tenodesis as an alternative to reinsertion. *Am J Sports Med*. 2009;37:929-936.
6. Ide J, Maeda S, Takagi K. Sports activity after arthroscopic superior labral repair using suture anchors in overhead-throwing athletes. *Am J Sports Med*. 2005;33:507-514.
7. Kim SH, Ha KI, Kim SH, Choi HJ. Results of arthroscopic treatment of superior labral lesions. *J Bone Joint Surg Am*. 2002;84-A:981-985.
8. Yung PS, Fong DT, Kong MF, et al. Arthroscopic repair of isolated type II superior labrum anterior-posterior lesion. *Knee Surg Sports Traumatol Arthrosc*. 2008;16:1151-1157.
9. Rhee YG, Lee DH, Lim CT. Unstable isolated SLAP lesion: clinical presentation and outcome of arthroscopic fixation. *Arthroscopy*. 2005;21:1099.
10. Kibler WB, Sciascia A. Current practice for the surgical treatment of SLAP lesions: a systematic review. *Arthroscopy*. 2016;32:669-683.
11. Park MJ, Hsu JE, Harper C, Sennett BJ, Huffman GR. Poly-L/D-lactic acid anchors are associated with reoperation and failure of SLAP repairs. *Arthroscopy*. 2011;27:1335-1340.
12. Matsuki K, Sugaya H. Complications after arthroscopic labral repair for shoulder instability. *Curr Rev Musculoskelet Med*. 2015;8:53-58.

13. Dines JS, Elattrache NS. Horizontal mattress with a knotless anchor to better recreate the normal superior labrum anatomy. *Arthroscopy*. 2008;24:1422-1425.
14. Chia MR, Hatrick C. Simplified knotless mattress repair of Type II SLAP lesions. *Arthrosc Tech*. 2015;4:e763-e767.
15. Domb BG, Ehteshami JR, Shindle MK, et al. Biomechanical comparison of 3 suture anchor configurations for repair of type II SLAP lesions. *Arthroscopy*. 2007;23:135-140.
16. Morgan RJ, Kuremsky MA, Peindl RD, Fleischli JE. A biomechanical comparison of two suture anchor configurations for the repair of type II SLAP lesions subjected to a peel-back mechanism of failure. *Arthroscopy*. 2008;24:383-388.
17. Yoo JC, Ahn JH, Lee SH, et al. A biomechanical comparison of repair techniques in posterior type II superior labral anterior and posterior (SLAP) lesions. *J Shoulder Elbow Surg*. 2008;17:144-149.
18. Yang HJ, Yoon K, Jin H, Song HS. Clinical outcome of arthroscopic SLAP repair: conventional vertical knot versus knotless horizontal mattress sutures. *Knee Surg Sports Traumatol Arthrosc*. 2016;24:464-469.
19. Silberberg JM, Moya-Angeler J, Martin E, Leyes M, Forriol F. Vertical versus horizontal suture configuration for the repair of isolated type II SLAP lesion through a single anterior portal: a randomized controlled trial. *Arthroscopy*. 2011;27:1605-1613.
20. Rhee YG, Ha JH. Knot-induced glenoid erosion after arthroscopic fixation for unstable superior labrum anterior-posterior lesion: case report. *J Shoulder Elbow Surg*. 2006;15:391-393.
21. Durban CM, Kim JK, Kim SH, Oh JH. Anterior shoulder instability with concomitant superior labrum from anterior to posterior (SLAP) lesion compared to anterior instability without SLAP lesion. *Clin Orthop Surg*. 2016;8:168-174.
22. Hashiguchi H, Iwashita S, Ohkubo A, Takai S. SLAP repair with arthroscopic decompression of spinoglenoid cyst. *SICOT J*. 2016;2:1.

Chapter 8

Arthroscopic Treatment of Internal Impingement

CHRISTOPHER A. LOOZE
JEFFREY R. DUGAS

Positioning

- An examination is performed under anesthesia with the patient supine before he or she is turned to the lateral decubitus position.
  - Particular attention should be paid for evidence of internal rotation deficit and/or anterior or posterior instability.
- We prefer the lateral decubitus position, but the procedure also can be done with the patient in the beach-chair position.
  - All bony prominences are carefully padded, including the greater trochanter, fibular head, and elbow. An axillary roll is placed under the down axilla.
- Approximately 10 lb of traction is applied to the operative limb.
  - The arm should be in ~15 degrees of forward flexion and 45 degrees of abduction.

Portal Placement

- The glenohumeral joint is insufflated with 60 cc of normal saline.
  - If performed appropriately, the shoulder should internally rotate.
- A posterior portal is created ~2 cm inferior and medial to the posterolateral corner of the acromion.
  - If a posterior release is planned, this portal can be shifted laterally to give a better approach to the posterior capsule.
- The anterior portal is placed just lateral to the coracoacromial (CA) ligament, which should be marked as a line connecting the coracoid to the anterolateral corner of the acromion.
- Accessory portals can be used depending on individual pathology.

Defining Pathology

- An intra-articular diagnostic arthroscopy is performed. It is important to evaluate the shoulder from both the posterior and anterior portals.
- Commonly seen pathologies with internal impingement
  - Glenohumeral internal rotation deficit
  - Bennett lesion
  - Posterior, partial-thickness rotator cuff tears
  - Superior labrum anterior and posterior (SLAP) tears
  - Posterosuperior labral tears

Glenohumeral Internal Rotation Deficit (GIRD)

- If an internal rotation deficit exists and has been refractory to physical therapy, a posterior capsular release is performed.
- The release is done with the arthroscope in the anterior portal, using the posterior portal as the working portal.
- If there is difficulty obtaining an appropriate angle for the capsulotomy, a second accessory posterior portal can be made.
  - The surface landmark for this portal usually is lateral to the standard posterior portal and should provide a steeper angle to the glenoid/capsule.
- The capsulotomy is largely posteroinferior and should start at the 10 o'clock position and extend down to the 6:30 o'clock position. The capsulotomy should be adjacent to the margin of the labral tissue with a small cuff of capsular tissue intervening. The posterior band of the inferior glenohumeral ligament (IGHL) should be released and marks the inferiormost extent of the release (Fig. 8-1A and B).
- We typically begin the capsulotomy with a shaver and proceed until we see muscular fibers. The inferior capsulotomy can be performed with a meniscal biter to avoid injury to deeper structures, including the axillary nerve.

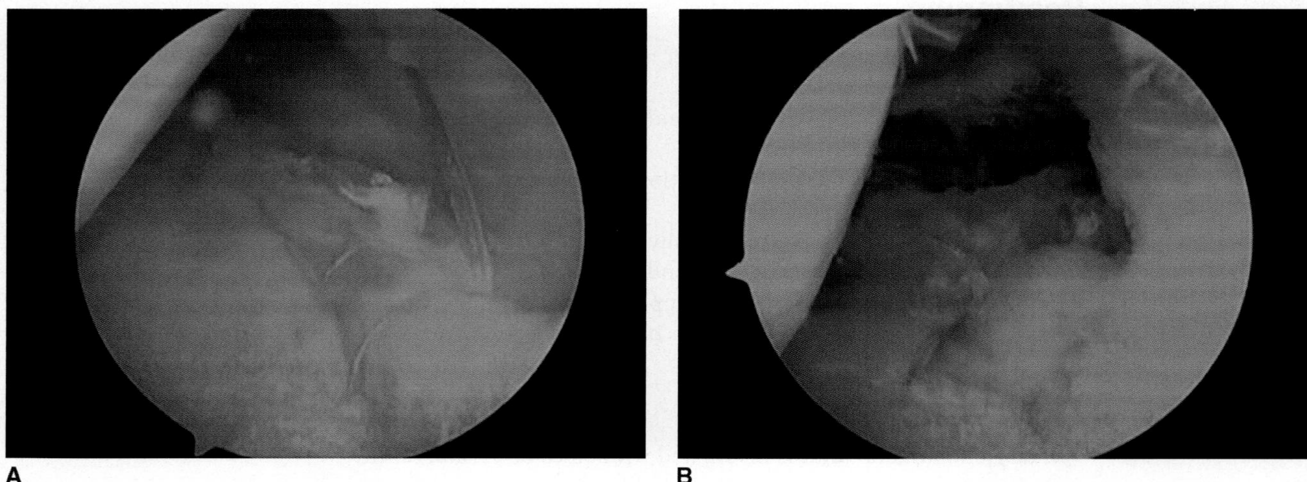

Figure 8-1 | Combination of a posterior labral repair with capsular release (right shoulder). **A.** Appearance of the capsule after labral repair. **B.** Muscular fibers after capsular release.

Bennett Lesion

- Bennett lesions often can be identified on plain radiographs (Fig. 8-2A).
- It is controversial as to whether this represents a traction osteophyte from the posteroinferior capsule or the triceps attachment.
- Excision is performed when the patient has posterior symptoms or evidence of an internal rotation deficit for which nonoperative management has failed.
- A capsular release is performed as described above.
- The lesion often can be palpated with a probe or shaver through the capsule and typically is located adjacent to the posteroinferior margin of the glenoid (Fig. 8-2B).
- Excision is done with the arthroscope in the anterior portal. If there is difficulty visualizing the lesion, a 70-degree scope can be used or an accessory portal can be made (Fig. 8-2C). If the accessory portal is created, the arthroscope can be introduced through the standard posterior portal with the accessory portal as the working portal.
- The bony prominence is excised, and a smooth margin is created at with the remainder of the glenoid. We typically perform this with a shaver. The inferior margin often is confluent with the inferior scapular neck. Care must be taken not to create a divot in the neck. The triceps attachment may need to be elevated to determine the true extent of the lesion and to fully excise it.

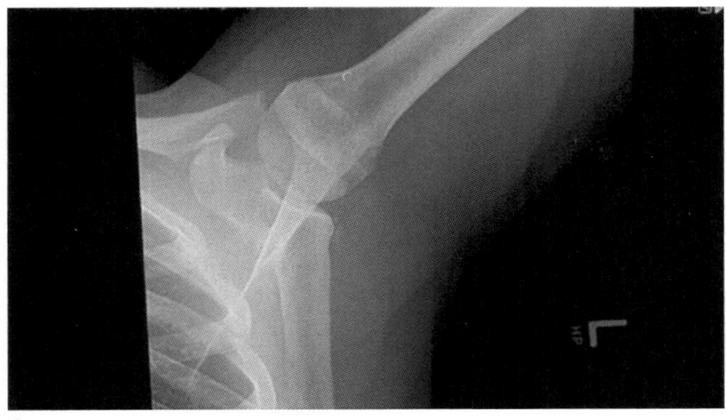

A

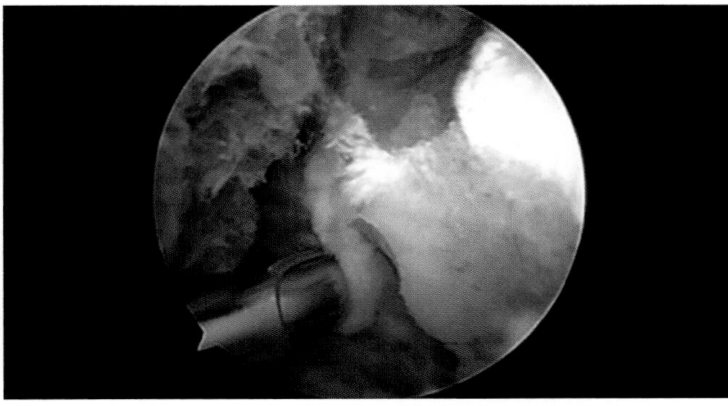

B

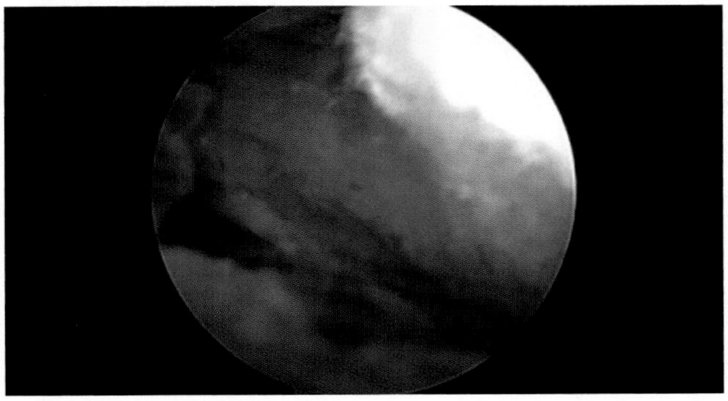

C

Figure 8-2 | A. Radiograph of the shoulder demonstrating a Bennett lesion with surrounding calcification. **B.** The Bennett lesion viewed from the posterior portal with an accessory portal made as a working portal. **C.** The burred-down Bennett lesion with a smooth, confluent surface with the scapular neck.

Partial-Thickness Rotator Cuff Tears

- Typically, these are articular-sided and found in the posterior aspect of the rotator cuff.
- If the tear is <75% thickness, we debride it with care not to violate any healthy-appearing rotator cuff tissue (Fig. 8-3A and B).
- If the tear is >75% thickness, we repair it (Fig. 8-4A).
  - The arthroscope is introduced into the subacromial space, and a lateral portal is created.
  - The bursa is excised to expose the rotator cuff.
    - For overhead athletes, we leave the CA ligament intact and do not perform an acromioplasty unless symptoms of subacromial impingement are present or acromioplasty is required for visualization.
  - We prefer to prepare the bone bed and place anchors intra-articularly through the standard anterior or posterior portal. This often can be achieved with the use of curved drill guides and all-suture anchors (Fig. 8-4B).

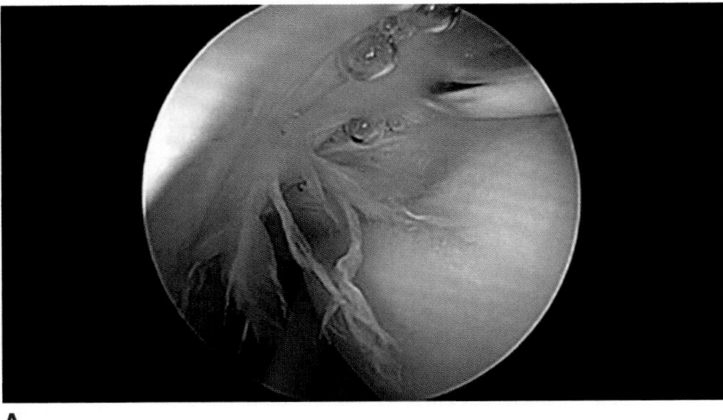

A

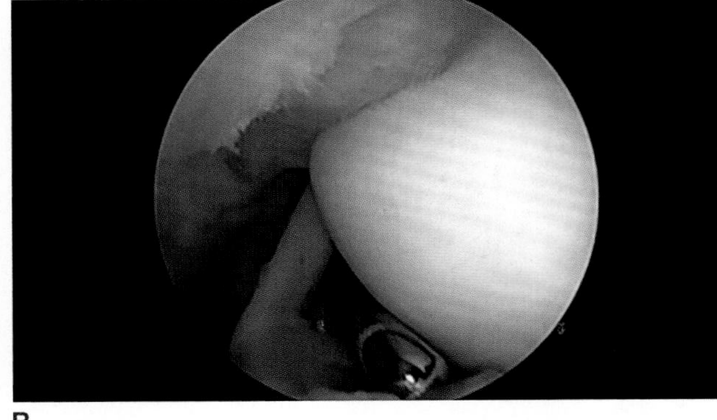

B

Figure 8-3 | Common appearance of the posterior partial-thickness rotator cuff tear with internal impingement **(A)** before and **(B)** after debridement.

- If adequate debridement and anchor placement are not possible from the standard portals, an accessory portal can be created just off the acromion. A small split is made in the partial-thickness tear in line with the rotator cuff fibers.
- The surface is prepared for repair to a bleeding bone bed, devoid of soft tissue.
  - Care is taken not to decorticate the bone, which would decrease the pullout strength of the anchors.
- A row of anchors is placed adjacent to the articular surface.
- The sutures are passed with an 18-gauge spinal needle and a wire suture shuttle to minimize trauma to the intact rotator cuff (Fig. 8-4C).
  - A bird beak or a suture passer also can be used but will induce more trauma to the intact cuff.

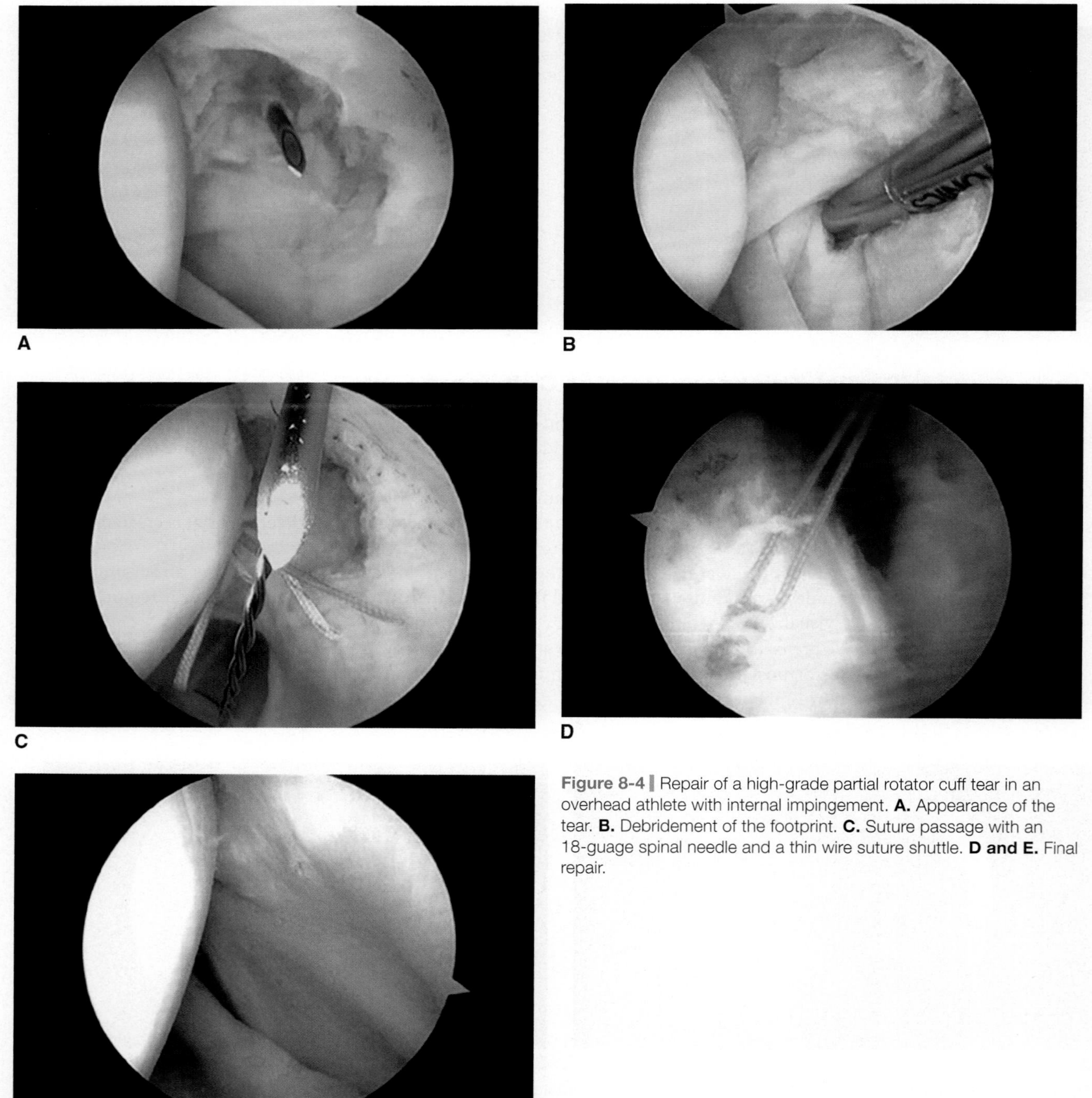

Figure 8-4 | Repair of a high-grade partial rotator cuff tear in an overhead athlete with internal impingement. **A.** Appearance of the tear. **B.** Debridement of the footprint. **C.** Suture passage with an 18-guage spinal needle and a thin wire suture shuttle. **D and E.** Final repair.

- The sutures are tied in a mattress fashion from the subacromial space (Fig. 8-4D and E).
- In throwers with partial-thickness tears, we do not place a lateral row to avoid overtensioning of the rotator cuff. If a full-thickness tear is present, we place a lateral row with SwiveLock anchors (Arthrex, Naples, FL) in a 2 × 2 or a 1 × 1 fashion.

Labral Tears

- **SLAP Tears/Posterior-Superior Labral Tear**
  - If the patient has a detachment of the anchor without evidence of bicipital groove pain or biceps tendinosis along the course of the tendon, we perform a SLAP repair (Fig. 8-5A).
  - Posterosuperior labral tears also are common, in isolation or in combination with a SLAP tear. These are repaired if there is a detachment and debrided if fraying is present.
    - This typically can be done through standard anterior and posterior portals.
    - The bone bed is prepared with a shaver, with care taken to obtain an adequate bone bed devoid of soft tissue. Usually, this is best performed with the anterior portal as the working portal.
    - Anchors are placed ~1 hour apart along the course of the tear, starting with the most posterior anchors (Fig. 8-1A).
      - We use all-suture anchors to allow smaller drill holes and the use of curved drill guides.
      - The anchors are loaded with FiberTape (Arthrex, Naples, FL) to allow low-profile knots to avoid abrasion of the superior rotator cuff. Alternatively, knotless anchors can be used to avoid abrasion of the undersurface of the rotator cuff.
      - Anchors should be placed at the articular margin.

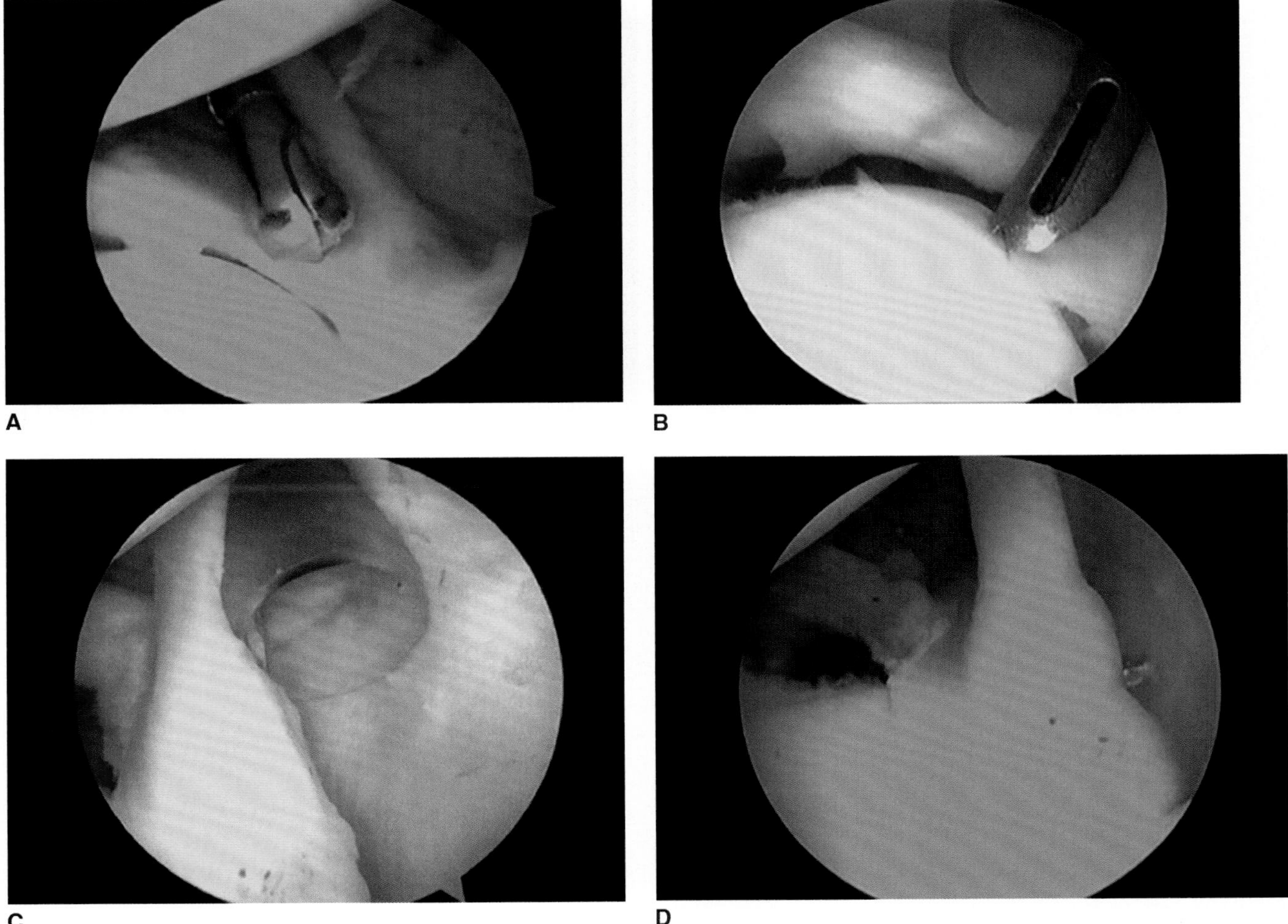

Figure 8-5 | A. Type II SLAP tear (left shoulder). **B.** Anchor placement to reattach the biceps anchor. **C.** Suture passage behind the biceps in a mattress fashion. **D.** The completed repair.

- The limbs of the suture are passed through the labral tissue with a 70-degree suture passer in a simple fashion.
- The sutures are tied down on the nonarticular surface.
- The superior anchor designed to reattach the biceps anchor is placed just underneath the biceps anchor (Fig. 8-5B). This can be done with a curved drill guide placed through the anterior portal. Alternatively, if an adequate angle cannot be obtained, a Port of Wilmington or Neviaser accessory portal can be made.
- These sutures are passed in a horizontal mattress fashion behind the biceps anchor and tied down (Fig. 8-5C).
- If the tear propagates anteriorly, we place an anterior anchor. Care is taken to provide adequate spacing between the biceps anchor and the adjacent suture anchors to avoid strangulating the biceps tendon.
- The anchor is probed to ensure that it is stable but allows normal biceps mobility (Fig. 8-5D).

- If the patient has undergone previous SLAP repair and has a recurrent tear or has a predominance of bicipital groove pain with MRI and arthroscopic evidence of biceps tendonitis/tendinosis, we perform a open, subpectoral biceps tenodesis (Fig. 8-6A).
  - The biceps is cut at its base with a meniscal biter (Fig. 8-6B).
  - The stump is excised with an arthroscopic shaver (Fig. 8-6C).
  - If the labral tissue is relatively stable to probing and there is minimal propagation of the tear into the posterior labrum, we do not perform a labral repair.
  - The biceps tenodesis is performed through an open subpectoralis approach.

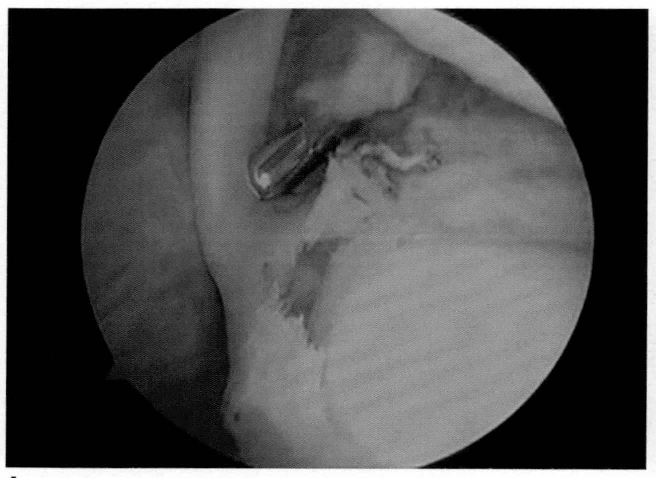
A

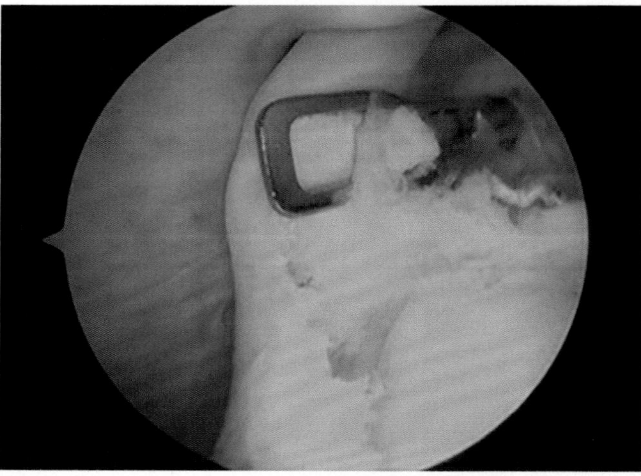
B

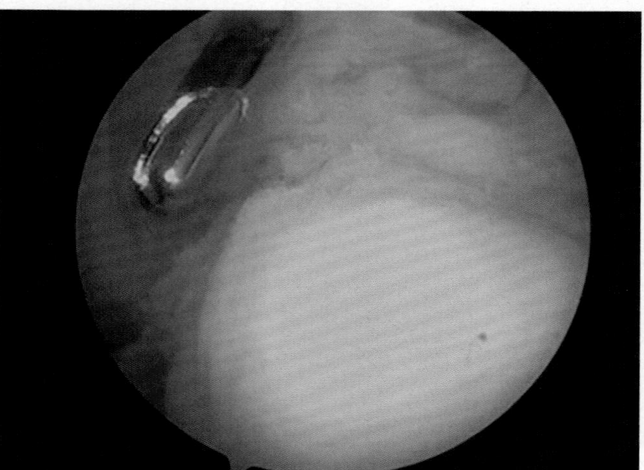
C

Figure 8-6 | **A.** Thrower with a failed SLAP repair. **B.** Biceps cut at its base. **C.** Debridement of the remaining stump.

- An ~3-cm longitudinal incision is made in line with the biceps tendon, with one-third of the incision above the pectoralis tendon and two-thirds below.
- Subcutaneous tissue is dissected to the level of the pectoralis fascia, which is then opened with electrocautery.
- The undersurface of the pectoralis tendon can be traced to the bicipital groove. The correct plane is above the short head of the biceps and coracobrachialis and underneath the pectoralis major.
- The pectoralis major is retracted with an Army-Navy retractor. Care should be taken to retract the medial structures gently to avoid neurovascular injury. We prefer to use digital retraction, but a second Army-Navy retractor also can be used.
- The biceps tendon is identified and delivered through the wound.
  - The groove often needs to be opened with electrocautery before identification and delivery of the tendon.
- The tendon is whipstitched from the myotendinous junction to ~4 cm proximal. Excess tendon is cut.
- The tendon is then loaded onto the SwiveLock anchor.
- An Army-Navy retractor is again used to retract the pectoralis tendon. The pallium pectoralis is identified at the top of the bicipital groove.
  - This is a fold of fascia that can be palpated at the top of the attachment of the pectoralis and creates a roof over the bicipital groove.
- Tissue is cleared from this area with electrocautery to expose the location for the drill hole.
- The goal is to place the drill hole at the metaphyseal-diaphyseal junction. Low placement will result in a stress riser.
- The reamer is used to create a unicortical drill hole for a 5.5-mm SwiveLock anchor.
- The SwiveLock is docked with the tendon and screwed into position.
- The sutures are tied over the top of the tenodesis.
- The tendon is checked for appropriate placement and tension.

Chapter 9

Open and Arthroscopic Treatment of Humeral Avulsions of the Glenohumeral Ligament (HAGL)

TIM WANG
MICHAEL H. MCGRAW
ANSWORTH A. ALLEN

Background, Diagnosis, and Interpretation

- Injuries to the inferior glenohumeral ligament (IGHL) and capsulolabral complex may occur at the glenoid origin (40%) or present as an intrasubstance tear (35%) or tear at the humeral insertion (25%).
- The incidence of humeral avulsion of the glenohumeral ligament (HAGL) is 1%-9% in patients presenting with glenohumeral instability (Fig. 9-1).
- Special attention should be paid to intrasubstance tears of the IGHL and capsule, which appear parallel to its fibers. This may present similarly to an HAGL but without frank capsular detachment at the humeral insertion and can be repaired with side-to-side sutures passed and tied arthroscopically. In these cases, imaging is consistent with escape of fluid from the capsule and a positive "J sign" on MRI, but an intact humeral attachment is seen arthroscopically.[1,2]
- Biomechanical studies show that large anterior HAGL lesions increase glenohumeral rotation and translation. Repair of these large HAGL lesions restores range of motion (ROM) and translational stability similar to native condition.[3,4]

Open Repair

- Positioning
  - Beach chair, with patient elevated 45 degrees
  - Arm holder as preferred
- Approach
  - The arm is positioned so that it is forward-flexed in line with the body and in neutral rotation to assist with the surgical approach.
  - An incision is made over the deltopectoral interval, slightly more vertically than otherwise would be used for shoulder arthroplasty or proximal humeral work. The incision should extend from superior border of the coracoid to just above the axillary fold, ~7 cm.
  - Dissection with cautery is carried through fat until deep muscular fascia is reached. The cephalic vein (typically found proximally and medially in the wound) is identified, the plane medial to the vein is dissected, and the vein is retracted laterally. Crossing veins are ligated with cautery.

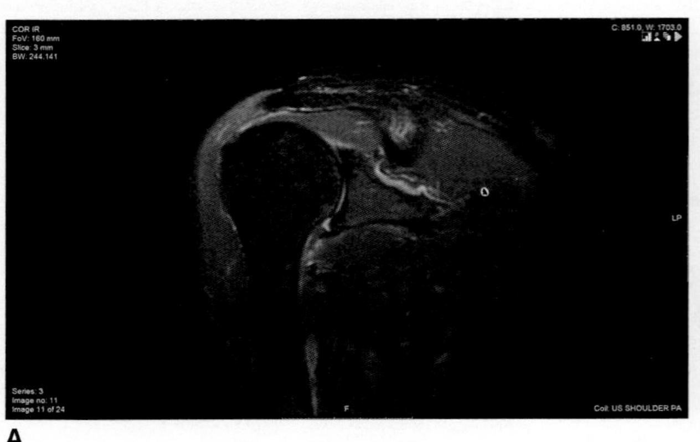
A

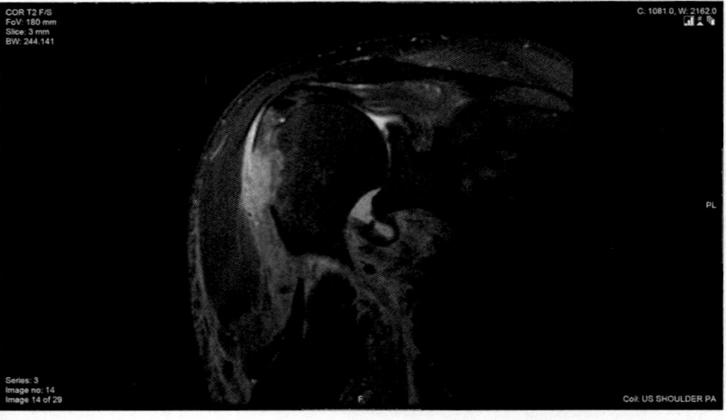
B

Figure 9-1 | Coronal T2-weighted MRI images of a right shoulder demonstrating normal-appearing inferior capsular attachment on the anatomic neck of the humerus as a normal "U"-shaped structure **(A)**. An example of a right shoulder with HAGL lesion is presented **(B)**, as demonstrated by an abnormal "J"-shaped axillary pouch and associated signal intensity of the inferior capsule indicating soft tissue edema. Also noted is a displaced fracture to the greater tuberosity.

  - The deep deltopectoral interval is developed and retracted with a self-retaining retractor (Kolbel retractor, George Tiemann & Co., Hauppauge, NY).
  - The clavipectoral fascia is incised with Metzenbaum scissors lateral to the muscular component of the conjoint tendon.
  - The Kolbel retractor is adjusted to retract the proximal conjoint tendon medially, with care not to place excessive tension on the musculocutaneous nerve.
  - The arm is externally rotated to place tension on the subscapularis tendon.
  - Landmarks include the long head of the biceps tendon and the bicipital groove laterally and the upper border of the subscapularis tendon and rotator interval proximally.
- Tenotomy and release
  - An L-shaped subscapularis tenotomy is made with a vertical limb 1 cm medial to the insertion on the lesser tuberosity at the superolateral corner of the subscapularis and the transverse limb inferiorly (Fig. 9-2). This maintains a 1-cm cuff of subscapularis tendon insertion laterally for repair. We begin this tenotomy inferiorly.

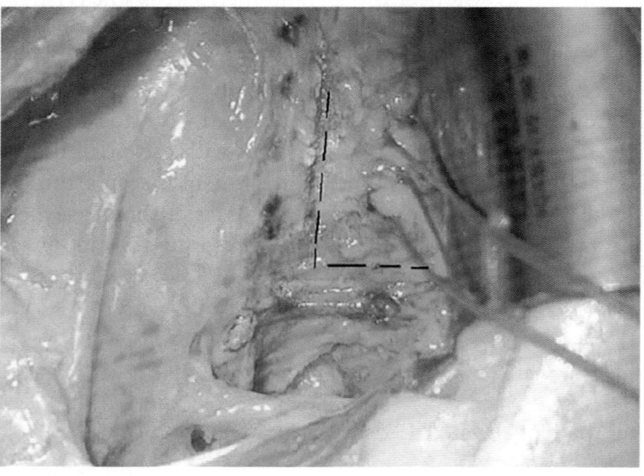

Figure 9-2 | The L-shaped incision made in the inferior portion of subscapularis insertion 1.5 cm medial to the lesser tuberosity. (Arciero RA, Mazzocca AD. Mini-open repair technique of HAGL (humeral avulsion of the glenohumeral ligament) lesion. *Arthroscopy*. 2005;21(9):1152.)

  - The upper two-thirds of the subscapularis typically appear more tendinous, while the lower one-third typically appears more muscular. At this junction, a transverse plane is developed parallel to the fibers of the subscapularis with two small Freer elevators.
  - The plane between the upper two-thirds of the subscapularis (superficial) and the anterior capsule (deep) is developed with a small periosteal elevator, which is left in place to place tension on the subscapularis tendon.

- With the subscapularis insertion still attached but retracted, the inferior capsule is examined to confirm that the capsule is completely avulsed from the humerus, because sometimes only a portion of the capsule is avulsed. In cases of incomplete capsular detachment, we detach only a portion of the subscapularis, instead of its entirety.
- Further release of the subscapularis tendon progresses from inferior to superior, medial to its insertion. We find needlepoint cautery helpful to start with a partial-thickness release of the subscapularis tendon to prevent injury to the anterior capsule, deep to the tendon.
- Tagging sutures are placed (we prefer a Mason-Allen type stitch) from inferior to superior as the release progresses.
- Once the tendon is fully released, the plane between the subscapularis and the anterior glenoid medially is bluntly developed, and the subscapularis is retracted medially.

- Alternatively, the upper half of the subscapularis can be preserved.
  - An L-shaped tenotomy is made with the transverse limb at the inferior border of the subscapularis, splitting muscle fibers, and the vertical limb is 1.5 cm medial to lesser tuberosity traversing the inferior half of tendon, leaving the superior half of subscapularis tendon undisturbed.[9]
- The axillary nerve is palpated inferiorly.
- The subscapularis is tagged and retracted medially and superiorly.
- As the interval between the capsule and subscapularis is dissected, the HAGL lesion will become visible at the anteroinferior aspect of the glenohumeral neck.
- The remaining anterior capsule is released off the humeral neck and mobilized for repair.
  - This is done as an inverse L-shaped capsulotomy, with the transverse limb along the rotator interval and the vertical limb on the border of the anatomic neck/articular margin of the humerus.
  - The release of the anterior capsule is continued from superior to inferior.
  - At the anteroinferior quadrant of the glenohumeral joint (5-6 o'clock on a right shoulder), the avulsion of the capsule from the humeral neck will be visible extending posteroinferiorly (Fig. 9-3).

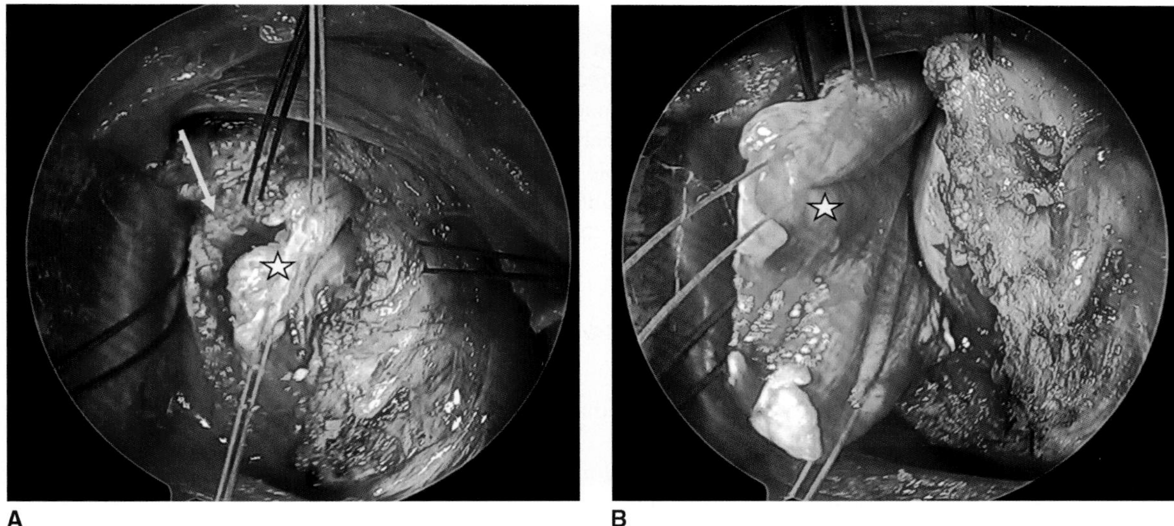

Figure 9-3 | Anterior view of dissection left shoulder. **A.** The plane between the subscapularis (*yellow arrow*) and anterior capsule (*star*) has been developed. With medial retraction **(B)** of these structures, the anatomic neck and capsular attachment on the humerus can be visualized.

Arthroscopic Repair

Positioning Pearls: Lateral Decubitus Position

- Lateral positioning can be used with the arm suspended or in traction, with the benefit of glenohumeral joint distraction to increase working space; however, this position may make it more difficult if intraoperative findings suggest a need to convert to an open procedure.
- General anesthesia is administered while the patient is on a padded beanbag.
- The patient is then positioned in the lateral decubitus position on the beanbag, taking care to place an axillary roll two fingerbreadths below the axillary fold.

- Hip and knee flexion is ensured, and adequate padding is placed for the "down side" elbow and wrist, greater trochanter, fibular head, and lateral malleolus, with pillows placed between the legs.
- The operative arm should be placed in 40-50 degrees of abduction and 15 degrees of forward flexion, with 5-10 lb of balanced suspension.

Positioning Pearls: Beach Chair

- Advantages of beach chair positioning include improved orientation of anatomy and the ease to convert to open stabilization if needed.
- General anesthetic is preferred for maximal muscular relaxation.
- Before sitting the patient up, he or she is moved both proximally and toward the operative side to ensure that the buttocks will be centered at the break of the bed. Moving the patient to the operative side will maximize posterior exposure of the shoulder and allow space for manipulation of the arthroscopic instruments.
- The back of bed is elevated to 70 degrees, and the hips and knees are flexed to minimize pressure sores and nerve injuries in the lower extremities. A kidney post positioner can be used along the greater trochanter and iliac crest to protect the patient from excessive lateral translation. The nonoperative arm is placed on a well-padded arm holder or pillows.
- Ideally, exposure should extend to the medial border of the scapula posteriorly and medial to the coracoid anteriorly.
- An arm positioner such as SPIDER2 (Smith & Nephew, Memphis, TN) or Trimano (Arthrex, Naples, FL) is used to maintain arm position.
- The head and neck should be in neutral position in both the coronal and sagittal planes.
- A large bump (three folded sheets wrapped in an elastic bandage) can be placed in the axilla with the arm maximally adducted to provide distraction of the glenohumeral joint.

Examination Under Anesthesia

- Passive ROM: forward flexion, abduction, external rotation with arm at the side, and external and internal rotation with 90 degrees of abduction
- Anterior, posterior, inferior load, and shift
  - Grade 1+ humeral head unable to be translated over rim
  - Grade 2+ humeral head able to translate over rim but spontaneously reduces
  - Grade 3+ humeral head able to translate over rim and remains dislocated, requiring manual maneuver to reduce
- Sulcus sign

Common Portals Used for HAGL Repair

- Standard posterior
  - 2 cm inferior and 2 cm medial to posterolateral border of the acromion
- Anterior rotator interval
  - Created just above the tendon of the subscapularis, can be created "inside out" or "outside in" with spinal needle localization.
  - Trajectory is planned for placement of humeral anchor for HAGL repair, as well as possible glenoid anchor if needed for treatment of concurrent labral tear.
- Anterolateral superior
  - Made with spinal needle localization in the lateralmost extent of the rotator interval
  - Skin incision is just off the anterolateral border of the acromion; entry into the joint should be adjacent to the biceps tendon laterally and just anterior to the anterior margin of the supraspinatus tendon.
- Anteroinferior "5 o'clock portal"
  - Made with spinal needle localization through the subscapularis muscle, ~2 cm inferior to the lateral border of the coracoid; entry into the joint should be visualized 1 cm inferior to the upper border of the subscapularis and as lateral as possible.[5] Follow with dilation using a blunt trocar, which is exchanged for a 5-mm cannula.
  - The portal is created with the arm in neutral rotation and adduction to increase the distance from musculocutaneous nerve.
- Posteroinferior "7 o'clock portal"

- This portal is made with spinal needle localization while viewing from the anterolateral superior portal.
- A skin incision is made 3-4 cm lateral to the posterolateral border of the acromion, angled 30 degrees medially and slightly inferior.
- Placing a cannula through this portal is avoided to prevent damage to the posterior capsule, which would preclude repair.
- The suprascapular nerve is 28 mm away and the axillary nerve is 39 mm away (Davidson and Rivenburgh).

- Posterior axillary pouch portal
  - This portal is made with spinal needle localization while viewing from the anterolateral superior portal.
  - A skin incision is made 2 cm directly inferior to the posterolateral border of the acromion and 2 cm lateral to the standard posterior viewing portal.

Diagnostic Arthroscopy

- Standard diagnostic shoulder arthroscopy is done viewing from the posterior portal.
- For optimal viewing of an HAGL lesion, the shoulder is placed in abduction and external rotation for an optimal angle toward the humeral neck directly inferior to the articular surface.
  - The typical HAGL lesion can be viewed through a standard posterior portal with a 30-degree arthroscope viewing toward the axillary pouch.[6] The IGHL fibers are seen traversing from the humeral neck to the glenoid neck. Disruptions in the fibers are seen as a capsular tear, and underlying fibers of subscapularis are seen through the defect. Internal and external rotation of the arm exposes the different portions of the ligaments (Fig. 9-4).

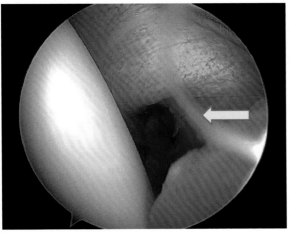

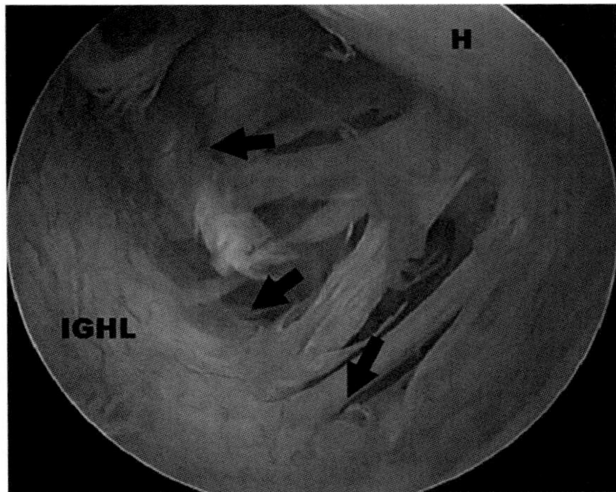

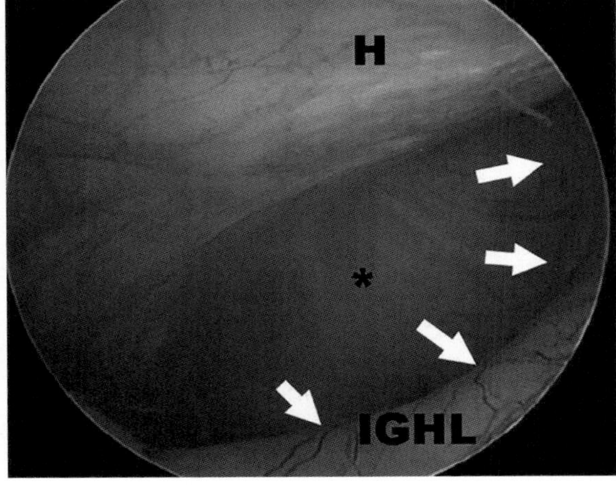

C

Figure 9-4 | A and B. Examples of HAGL lesions as viewed arthroscopically. *Arrows*: torn edge of IGHL; *asterisk*: bridging fibrous adhesions. H, humeral head; IGHL, inferior glenohumeral ligament. (Page RS, Bhatia DN. Arthroscopic repair of humeral avulsion of glenohumeral ligament lesion: anterior and posterior techniques. *Tech Hand Up Extrem Surg*. 2009;13(2):98-103.) **C.** Arthroscopic view from posterior portal of a left shoulder. Humeral head on right; HAGL lesion is seen with detachment of the inferior capsule from the anatomic neck of the humerus (*arrow*).

- Working portals
  - Using the standard posterior portal as the primary viewing portal, either a 30- or 70-degree arthroscope is used.[7]
    - Working portal option 1: Anterosuperior lateral portal with an 8.5-mm cannula (working) and an anteroinferior 5 o'clock portal with a 6-mm cannula (suture shuttle)
    - Working portal option 2: Anterior rotator interval portal with an 8.5-mm cannula (working) and a posteroinferior 7 o'clock portal with a 6-mm cannula (suture shuttle)
  - Anterior viewing through the anterolateral superior viewing portal
    - Anterior HAGL lesions also can be viewed from the anterolateral superior portal, with the arthroscope anterior to the humeral head and looking laterally at the humeral capsular insertion.
    - Posterior HAGL ("reverse HAGL") lesions can be viewed from the anterolateral superior portal, posterior to the humeral head, with the lens looking lateral at the humeral capsular insertion.
  - Placement of a large bump (rolled sheets or drapes) high in the axilla, followed by adduction of the arm, can aid in distraction of the glenohumeral joint to increase the working space.
    - Alternatively, rolled gauze can be wrapped around the proximal humerus, with a loop made and then wrapped around an assistant (tied by the circulating nurse posteriorly) to provide a distractive force on the joint when the assistant "water-skis" on the gauze.

Preparation and Fixation Techniques[8]

- An arthroscopic shaver and ablation device (anteroinferior 5 o'clock portal is ideal) are used to debride adhesions and perform synovectomy until the free lateral edge of the IGHL is identified.
- The avulsed capsular tissue is identified, and a grasper is used to assess tissue quality and mobility.
  - If a concurrent labral tear is identified, treating the HAGL lesion before the labral repair helps avoid overtensioning of the medial aspect of the glenohumeral joint.
- An arthroscopic shaver, burr, or rasp is used to prepare a bony bed for reduction along the humeral neck.
- The trajectory for suture anchor placement in the inferior humeral neck is confirmed with a spinal needle.
  - The arm is rotated as needed to get the appropriate angle.
  - An anchor is inserted percutaneously, with the entry site on the skin between the standard posterior portal and the accessory posterior-lateral portal.
- Two or three suture anchors (we use 3.0-mm PEEK SutureTak suture anchors with no. 2 FiberWire, Arthrex, Naples, FL) are placed along the humeral neck, spaced 5-10 mm apart. The humerus is rotated as needed to achieve the proper angle for anchor placement (abduction and external rotation).
- After the suture anchors are placed, a single limb of suture is retrieved through the anterosuperior lateral portal, with the other suture limb remaining out of the percutaneous wound (or coming out of the anteroinferior portal).
- A curved suture passer is passed through the avulsed capsular tissue, and the PDS suture is shuttled through.
  - Suture limbs are passed individually through the IGHL with a curved suture passer.
  - Once it has penetrated the tissue, the PDS passing suture is retrieved with a grasper from the anterolateral superior portal.
  - A single loop is tied in the PDS passing suture and used to snare the limb of suture from the anchor, which was previously retrieved from the anterolateral superior portal.
  - The curved suture passer is removed, and the PDS suture is pulled from the 7 o'clock portal to shuttle the suture through tissue and out the 7 o'clock suture.
  - This process is repeated with the second suture, so that two limbs are coming out of the 7 o'clock portal passed through in a horizontal mattress fashion.
- An arthroscopic knot is tied with the arm in slight abduction and slight external rotation (15 degrees) such that the knot lies intra-articular.
  - Caution is required in passing sutures at the 6 o'clock position, and no more than 1 cm of tissue should be taken to avoid the risk of injury to the axillary nerve.
  - Alternatively, a Viper suture passer (Arthrex, Naples, FL) from the 7 o'clock portal can be used to penetrate the avulsed capsule and retrieve the suture.
- The suture-passing sequence continues from posteroinferiorly to anterosuperiorly.
- As suture passage progresses anteriorly, a 5 o'clock portal, either percutaneous transsubscapularis or through a 5-mm cannula, will achieve the proper angle toward the humeral neck.

- Caution is required when passing sutures to avoid the musculocutaneous nerve (arm in adduction and neutral rotation) and the axillary nerve.

Alternate Single-Portal Technique for Treatment of Anterior HAGL Lesions[7]

- The humeral neck is prepared as above, and a suture anchor is placed along the inferior humeral neck. A single limb of suture is retrieved from the anteroinferior 5 o'clock portal.
- A curved suture shuttle is inserted from the anteroinferior 5 o'clock cannula, grabs a bite through the IGHL 5-10 mm medial, and the PDS passing suture is shuttled. The suture shuttle is removed and the end of the suture exiting the cannula is tagged with a clamp.
- The suture retriever is used to grasp the free end of the PDS passing suture from anteroinferior cannula. A loop is created in the free end of the passing suture and tied around the free suture limb from the previously retrieved anchor.
- The anterior strand is shuttled through the IGHL and out the anteroinferior cannula.
- This is repeated for the second suture. The position of the suture strands determines the magnitude of capsular shift.
- An arthroscopic knot is tied through the anteroinferior cannula with the arm in slight abduction and slight external rotation (15 degrees) such that the knot lies intra-articular.

Arthroscopic Technique for Repair of Posterior HAGL Lesions

- Portals
  - Standard posterior viewing portal with 30- or 70-degree arthroscope
  - An axillary pouch portal is created 2 cm directly inferior to the posterolateral corner of the acromion with spinal needle localization, above the posterior band of the IGHL, and a working cannula is inserted. The angle for suture anchor placement along the inferior humeral neck is confirmed.
  - Standard anterior portal in rotator interval (working)
- A shaver is introduced through the axillary pouch portal to debride adhesions and perform synovectomy. Preparation of the humeral neck is similar to that described above.
- Suture anchors are inserted through the axillary pouch portal, and a single limb is retrieved through the anterior portal.
- A curved suture shuttle from the anterior portal cannula is used to pass the PDS shuttle suture, and sutures are shuttled to pass through the torn edge of the IGHL. Sutures are retrieved through the axillary pouch portal or the 5 o'clock portal.
- This is repeated, and sutures are tied with a mattress stitch.

Repair of HAGL Lesion

- The avulsed capsule from the humeral neck is identified, and the leading edge of the ligament is tagged with suture.
- The capsular insertion on the humeral neck is prepared with a curette, burr, or rasp.
- Two or three suture anchors (G4 Anchor, Mitek Sports Medicine, Raynham, MA or 3-mm PEEK SutureTak, Arthrex, Naples, FL) are placed along the humeral neck at the anatomic insertion of the glenohumeral ligaments.
- The shoulder is positioned in slight abduction, forward flexion, and external rotation for optimal tensioning.
  - The position of repair is determined by examination of the contralateral extremity to determine how tight to make it. Usually, forward flexion allows reduction of the humeral head and about 30 degrees of abduction and external rotation.
  - If the tear extends into the rotator interval, we repair it with the arm in maximal adduction and 30 degrees of external rotation.
- Sutures are passed through the capsule and glenohumeral ligaments in a horizontal mattress configuration and are tagged together. Once all sutures are passed, they are tied sequentially from inferior to superior.
- We routinely close the rotator interval with one or two sutures.
- The arm is maximally internally rotated, and the subscapularis tenotomy is reapproximated with heavy suture.

- The shoulder is gently moved through an ROM to ensure that the subscapularis repair remains intact and moves as a unit.
- The deltopectoral fascia is closed with interrupted suture (no. 2 Orthocord, DePuy Synthes Mitek Sports Medicine, Raynham, MA) in case further surgery is necessary; colored suture assists in locating the rotator interval.
- The deep dermal tissue is closed with deep buried 2-0 Vicryl.
- The skin is closed with no. 2-0 Prolene in a running subcuticular fashion, with an escape stitch.
- Sterile dressings are placed and the patient is placed in a shoulder immobilizer.

Postoperative Care

0-2 wk	The shoulder is maintained in a sling. Distal ROM of the elbow, wrist, and hand is allowed. External rotation is limited to neutral.
2-4 wk	Passive abduction and forward flexion in the scapular plane to 60 degrees are allowed. External rotation is limited to neutral.
4-6 wk	Passive abduction and forward flexion in the scapular plane to 90 degrees are allowed. External rotation is limited to 30 degrees.
6-9 wk	Passive abduction and forward flexion in the scapular plane progress to full. External rotation to 60 degrees is allowed.
9-12 wk	External rotation in 45 degrees of abduction is allowed.
12 wk+	External rotation in 90 degrees of abduction is allowed, and strengthening is begun.

Return to sport is allowed at 6 months postoperatively.

References

1. Melvin JS, Mackenzie JD, Nacke E, Sennett BJ, Wells L. MRI of HAGL lesions: four arthroscopically confirmed cases of false-positive diagnosis. *AJR Am J Roentgenol.* 2008;191(3):730-734.
2. Mizuno N, Yoneda M, Hayashida K, Nakagawa S, Mae T, Izawa K. Recurrent anterior shoulder dislocation caused by a mid-substance complete capsular tear. *J Bone Joint Surg Am.* 2005;87(12):2717-2723.
3. Park KJ, Tamboli M, Nguyen LY, McGarry MH, Lee TQ. A large humeral avulsion of the glenohumeral ligaments decreases stability that can be restored with repair. *Clin Orthop Relat Res.* 2014;472(8):2372-2379.
4. Southgate DF, Bokor DJ, Longo UG, Wallace AL, Bull AM. The effect of humeral avulsion of the glenohumeral ligaments and humeral repair site on joint laxity: a biomechanical study. *Arthroscopy.* 2013;29(6):990-997.
5. Kon Y, Shiozaki H, Sugaya H. Arthroscopic repair of a humeral avulsion of the glenohumeral ligament lesion. *Arthroscopy.* 2005;21(5):632.
6. Parameswaran AD, Provencher MT, Bach BR, Verma N, Romeo AA. Humeral avulsion of the glenohumeral ligament: injury pattern and arthroscopic repair techniques. *Orthopedics.* 2008;31(8):773-779.
7. Page RS, Bhatia DN. Arthroscopic repair of humeral avulsion of glenohumeral ligament lesion: anterior and posterior techniques. *Tech Hand Up Extrem Surg.* 2009;13(2):98-103.
8. George MS, Khazzam M, Kuhn JE. Humeral avulsion of glenohumeral ligaments. *J Am Acad Orthop Surg.* 2011;19(3):127-133.
9. Arciero RA, Mazzocca AD. Mini-open repair technique of HAGL (humeral avulsion of the glenohumeral ligament) lesion. *Arthroscopy.* 2005;21(9):1152.

Chapter 10

Arthroscopic Treatment of Humeral Avulsions of the Glenohumeral Ligament (HAGL)

WILLIAM H. ROSSY
JEFFREY S. ABRAMS

Anesthesia

- Interscalene nerve block followed by general anesthesia

Instruments/Equipment/Implants

- Arthroscopic tower with 30-degree and 70-degree arthroscope
- Curved suture hook for suture shuttling
- 4.5-mm double-loaded suture anchor
- Arthroscopic cannulas in varying sizes (5.5 mm and 7.0 mm)

Positioning

- The patient can be positioned in the lateral decubitus position using a beanbag or in the beach-chair position. We prefer the lateral decubitus position.
  - Care is taken to pad all bony prominences.
  - An axillary roll is placed to minimize the risk of contralateral brachial plexus injury.
- The patient is leaned posteriorly 15 degrees to ensure that the glenoid is parallel to the floor.
- The operative extremity is placed in a balanced suspension system, and depending on patient's size, 10-15 lb of traction are hung to obtain the desired distraction.
- Adjustments to the suspension system are made to place the arm in 20 degrees of forward flexion and ~50 degrees of abduction.
  - A sterile bump can then be placed in the axilla to improve visualization and access to the axillary recess during the surgery.

Portal Placement (Fig. 10-1)

- *Standard Posterior Portal*
  - A longitudinal skin incision is made ~2 cm distal and 1 cm medial to the posterolateral tip of the acromion.
  - Care should be taken not to make the portal too lateral, as this may lead to a less than optimal trajectory for viewing or gaining access to the site of avulsion of the inferior glenohumeral ligament (IGHL).

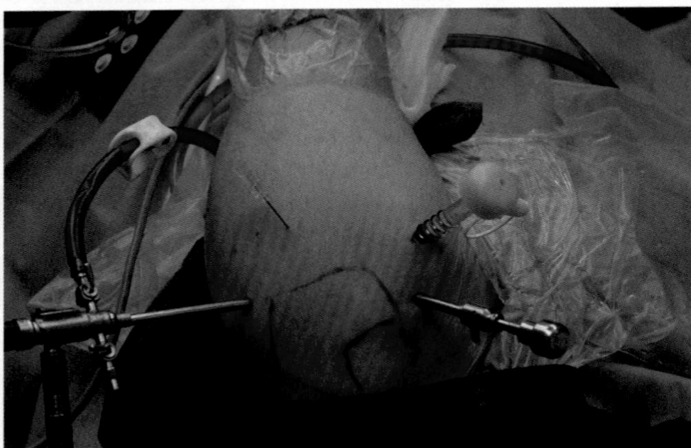

Figure 10-1 | Portals for HAGL repairs: arthroscope is in posterior viewing portal. Spinal needle marks the accessory posterior portal. Cannula is in the anterior working portal. Metal trocar is in the anterosuperior portal.

- *Standard Anterior Portal*
  - This portal is created under direct vision through the center of the rotator interval.
  - A smooth, 5.5-mm cannula is placed through a small skin incision into the interval.
  - For anterior humeral avulsion of the glenohumeral ligament (HAGL) lesions, a second anterior portal (low anterior portal) may be desired for suture management. In this instance, the standard anterior portal should be shifted to the superior aspect of the rotator interval to ensure room for a second cannula.
- *Low Anterior Portal (optional)*
  - While viewing from the posterior portal, a spinal needle is placed between the coracoid and anterior corner of the acromion, ~1 cm distal to the standard anterior portal.
  - The spinal needle should enter the joint through the inferior aspect of the rotator interval.
  - Once location is confirmed, a small skin incision is made and a Wissinger rod is placed along the same trajectory as the needle.
  - A 5.5-mm cannula is then passed over the rod.
- *7 O'Clock Portal (optional)*
  - This portal is optional for anterior HAGL lesions; however, it can be used for suture management with these lesions.
  - It facilitates visualization as well as instrumentation in reverse HAGL (rHAGL) lesions involving avulsion of the posteroinferior glenohumeral ligament.
  - With the arthroscope in the anterior portal, an 18-gauge spinal needle is used to identify optimal portal placement.
  - The spinal needle should enter the skin ~4 cm lateral to the posterolateral tip of the acromion.
    - Analysis of the needle trajectory is crucial to ensure proper position of the portal.
    - The needle trajectory should be perpendicular to the floor.
  - Once trajectory is confirmed, a small skin incision is made and a Wissinger rod is placed along the same trajectory as the needle into the joint.
  - A 7-mm cannula is then passed over the Wissinger rod into the joint.

Diagnostic Arthroscopy/Identification of Injury

- While viewing through the posterior portal, the anteroinferior quadrant of the glenohumeral joint is inspected.
- A full assessment of the anteroinferior labrum should be made because labral tears have been found to occur concomitantly in these patients.
- The leading edge of the IGHL can be seen medially, often scarred down to the medial interval tissue.
- The underlying subscapularis muscle fibers are easily visualized, a finding pathognomonic for HAGL lesions.
  - At this point, the arthroscope can be switched into the anterior portal to better visualize the IGHL's footprint on the anterior humeral neck or a 70-degree arthroscope can be used to better visualize the footprint from the posterior viewing portal (Fig. 10-2).

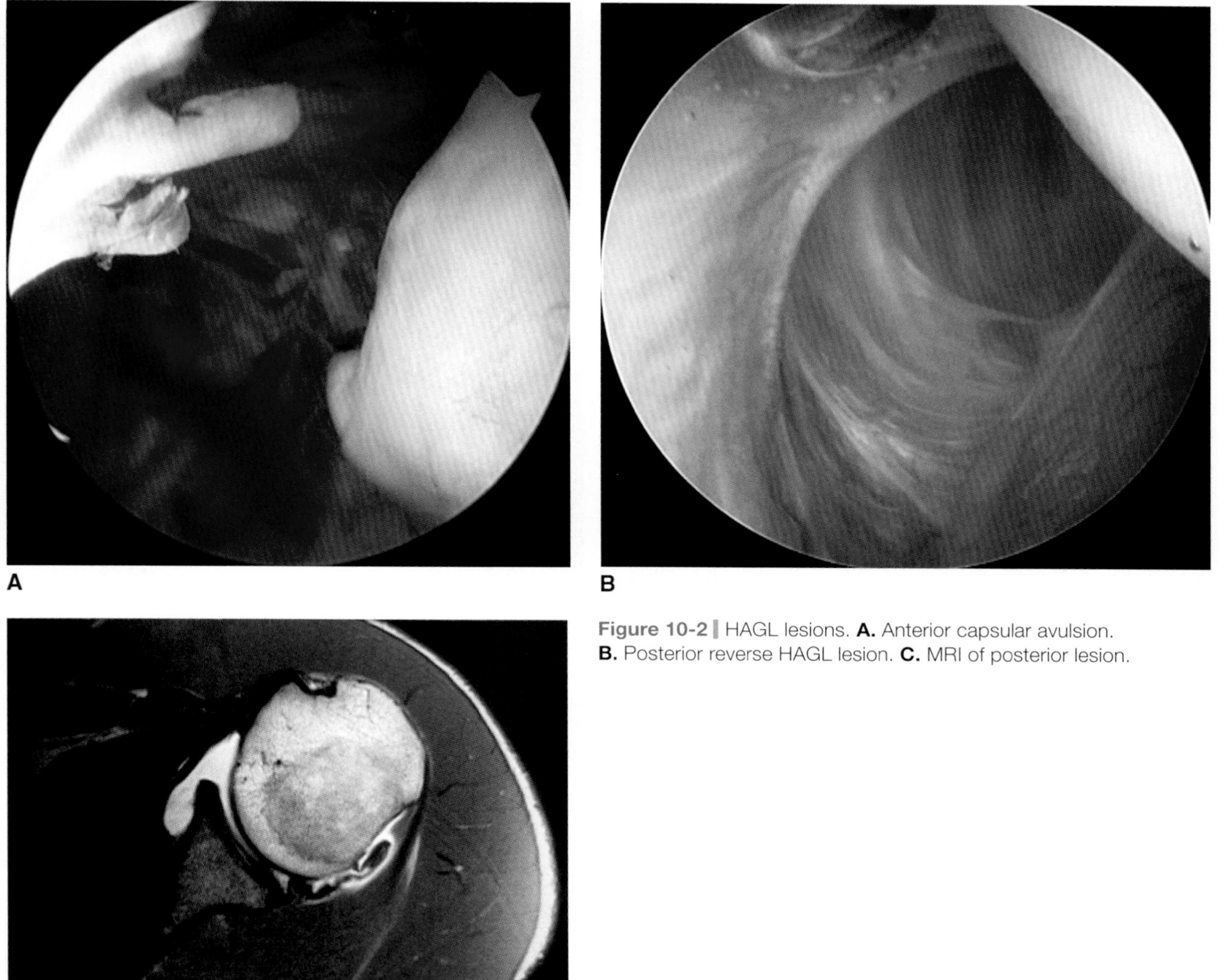

Figure 10-2 | HAGL lesions. **A.** Anterior capsular avulsion. **B.** Posterior reverse HAGL lesion. **C.** MRI of posterior lesion.

Soft Tissue Mobilization/Traction Stitch

- Anterior lesions:
  - With the arthroscope in the posterior portal, an atraumatic grasping instrument is passed through the anterior portal and the leading edge of the IGHL is freed and mobilized back to its origin on the humeral neck (Fig. 10-3).
  - A suture hook can be used to shuttle a suture through the ligament to serve as a traction stitch to aid mobilization back to the footprint (Fig. 10-4).
- Posterior lesions:
  - With the arthroscope in the anterior portal, an atraumatic grasping instrument is passed through the 7 o'clock portal.
  - The leading edge of the posterior IGHL is grasped and freed (Fig. 10-5).
  - Soft tissue mobilization is performed to ensure reduction of the posterior IGHL back to the humeral neck footprint.

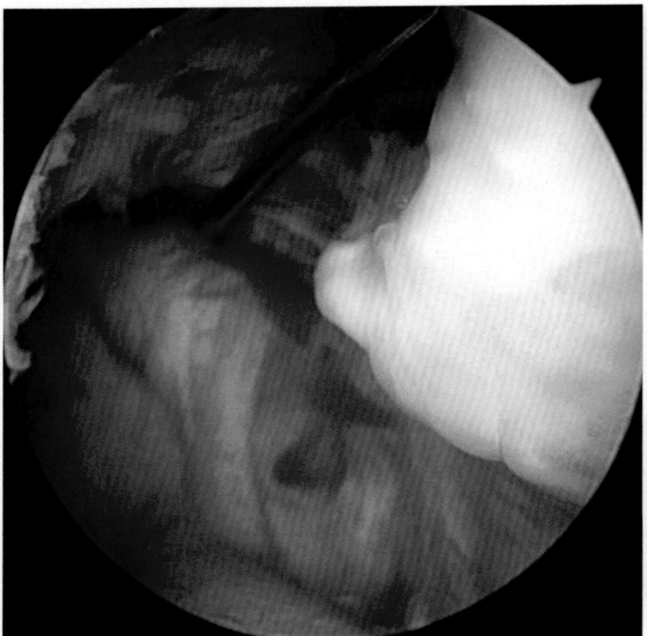

Figure 10-3 | A grasper is used to mobilize the free edges of the tear.

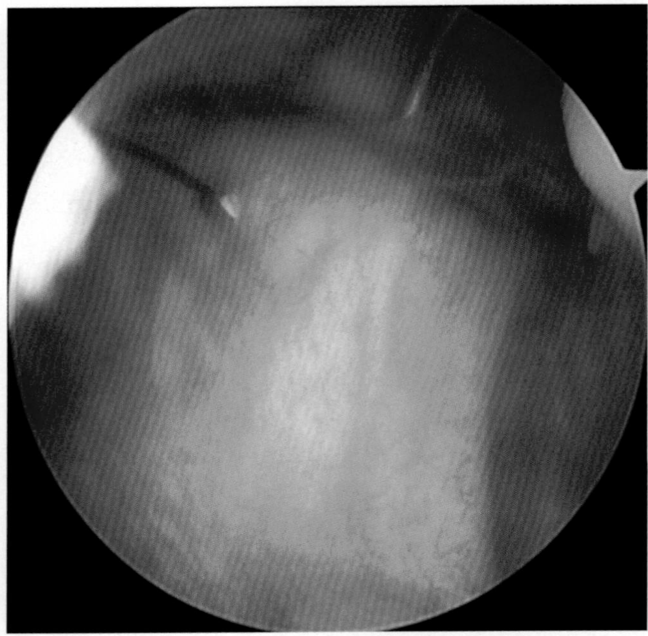

Figure 10-4 | A traction stitch can be placed in the margin of the anteroinferior tear.

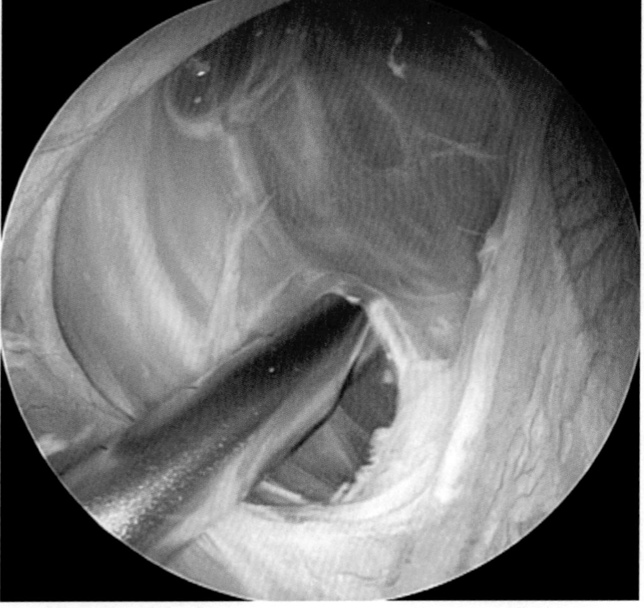

Figure 10-5 | Margins of the reverse HAGL can be mobilized.

Fixation/Repair

- A combination of humeral internal and external rotation, as well as periodically changing the arthroscope to view from anteriorly and posteriorly, will optimize visualization of the site of avulsion from the humerus.[1]
- Once identified, an arthroscopic shaver is used to decorticate the bone to a bleeding bed to optimize ligament healing (Fig. 10-6).
- A spinal needle is used to localize the lesion on the humerus. Careful attention must be paid to ensure that the spinal needle is directed perpendicular to the bone (Fig. 10-7).
- Once appropriate orientation of the needle is confirmed, a separate, percutaneous incision is made and a double-loaded 4.5-mm anchor is percutaneously placed in the center of the lesion (Fig. 10-8).

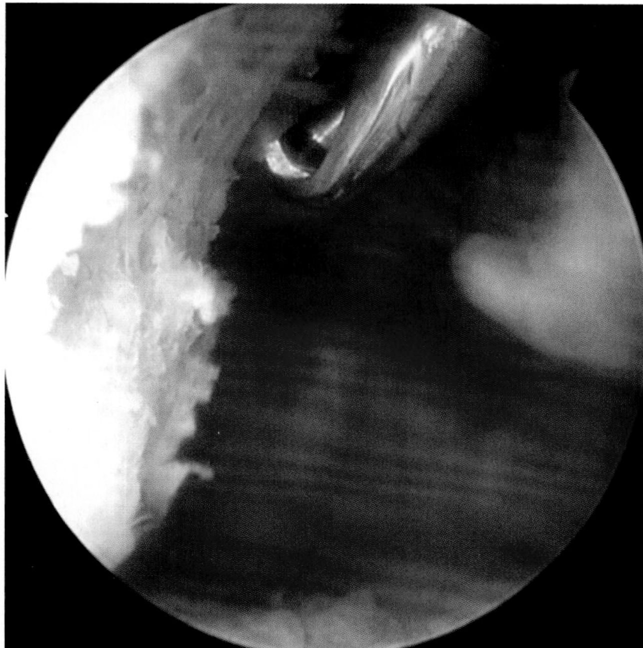

Figure 10-6 | Debridement and abrasion of the humeral attachment site.

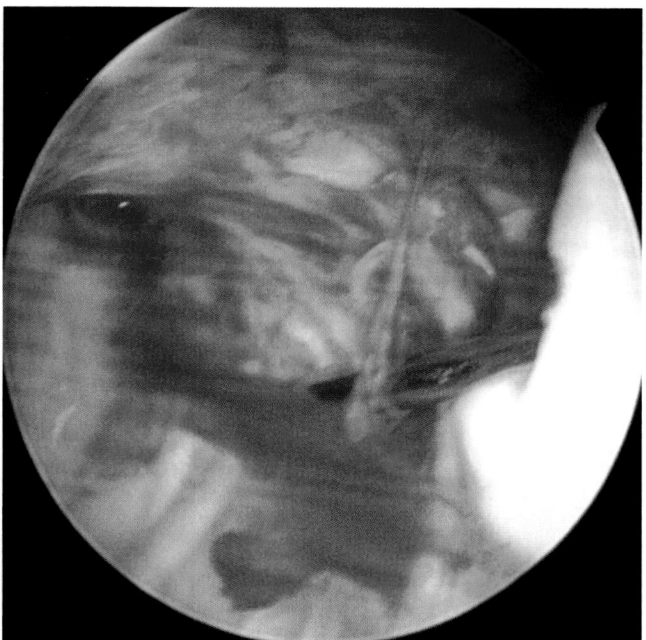

Figure 10-7 | Spinal needle localization for cannula placement through the defect.

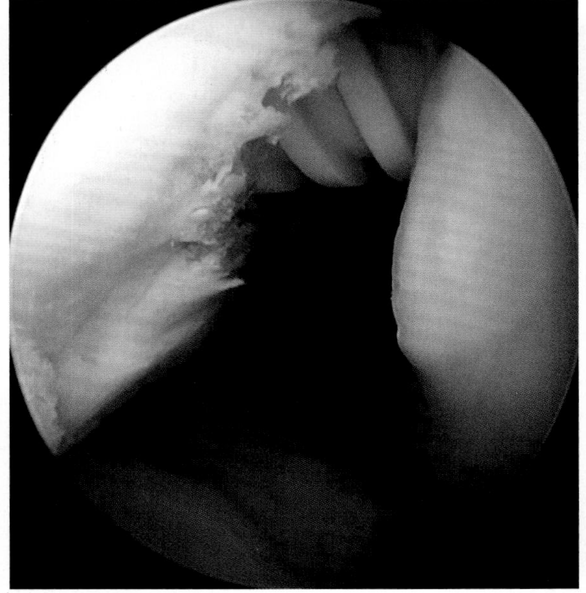

A

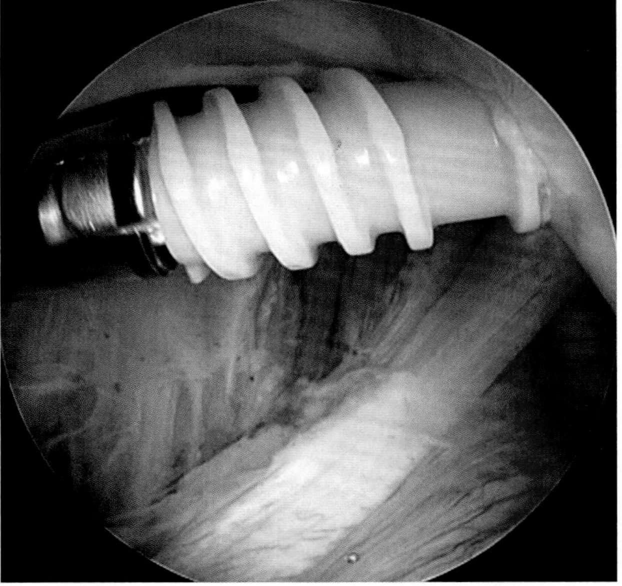

B

Figure 10-8 | Suture anchor insertion. **A.** Anterior suture anchor placement for repair of HAGL lesion. **B.** Posterior suture anchor placement for repair of reverse HAGL lesion (rHAGL).

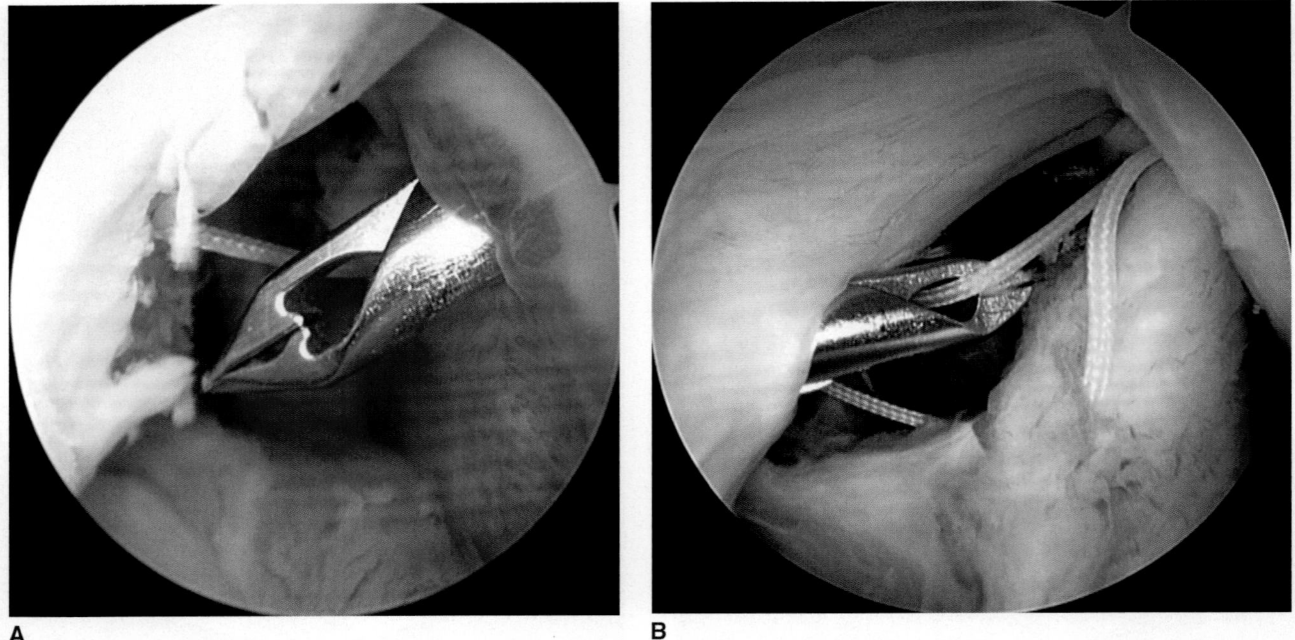

Figure 10-9 | A penetrator instrument pierces the detached capsule to retrieve sutures from anchors. **A.** Anterior capsule suture retrieval. **B.** Posterior capsule suture retrieval.

- A curved soft tissue penetrator is passed through the freed ligament and used to retrieve the sutures and pull them through the tissue to be repaired (Fig. 10-9A and B).
- Once all sutures are passed, an arthroscopic sliding knot is used to reduce the avulsed glenohumeral ligament back to its anatomic footprint on the humerus (Fig. 10-10A and B).

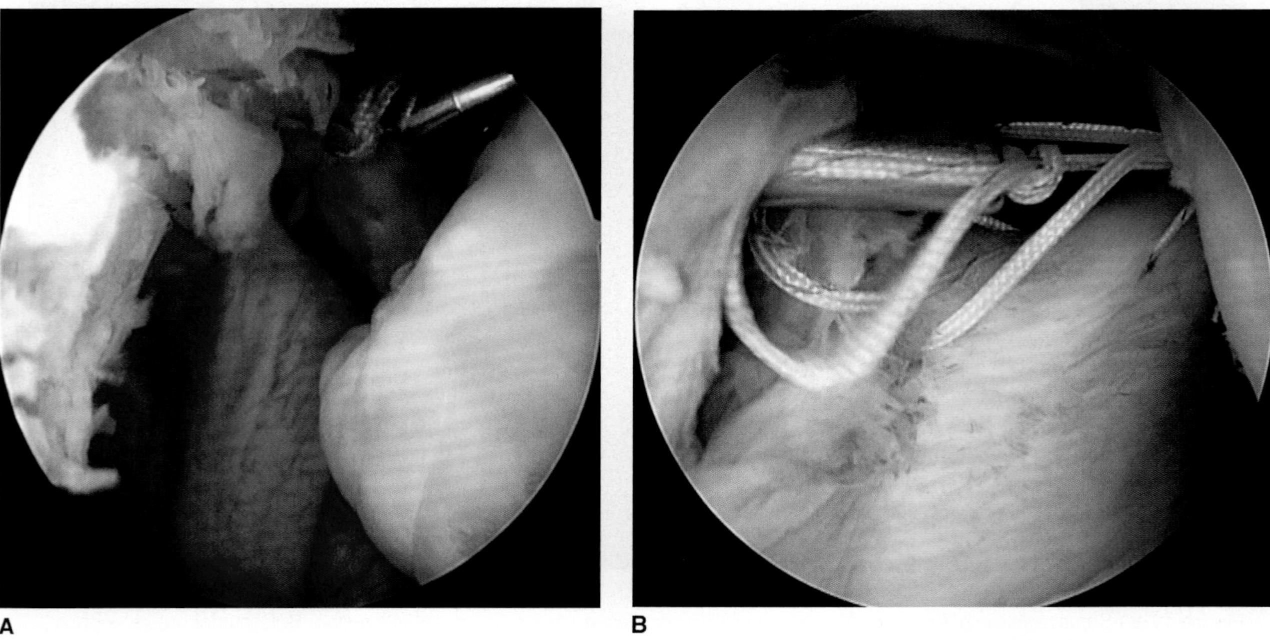

Figure 10-10 | Curved suture hooks are used to repair inferior suture margins. **A.** Anterior HAGL. **B.** Posterior rHAGL.

- With anterior lesions, once the repair is completed, the muscle belly of the subscapularis is no longer exposed (Fig. 10-11).
- With posterior lesions, side-to-side sutures reinforce the capsular repair (Fig. 10-12).

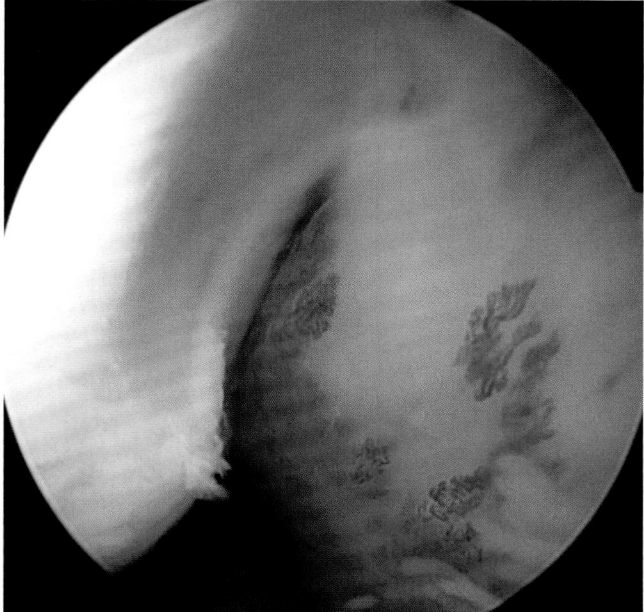

Figure 10-11 | Repaired anterior HAGL lesion.

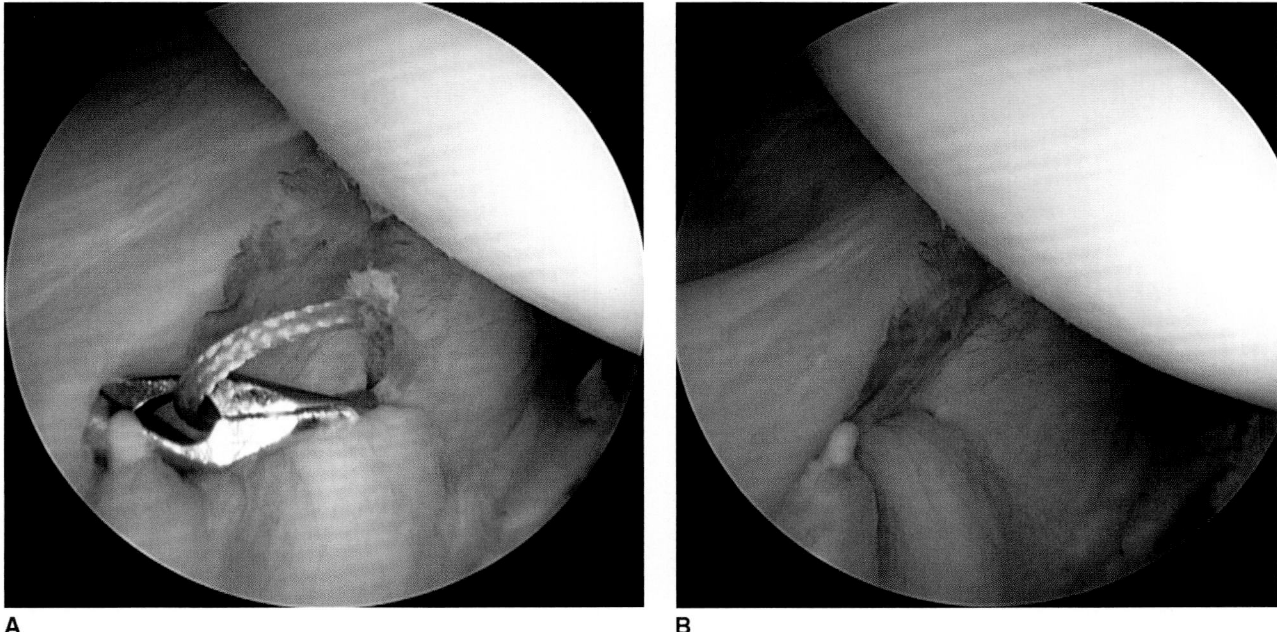

Figure 10-12 | Repaired posterior rHAGL lesion. **A.** Side-to-side sutures placed and tied to close the medial defect. **B.** Completed rHAGL repair.

Postoperative Rehabilitation

- Patients are placed in a sling with an abduction pillow; these are used for a total of 6 weeks.
- Formal physical therapy can start as soon as 1 week postoperatively for passive and active-assisted range of motion only.
  - Forward elevation is restricted to 90 degrees in the plane of the scapula.
  - No internal or external rotation is permitted until the patient is out of the sling at 6 weeks.
- Once the sling is discontinued, range of motion is progressed as tolerated.

- Isometrics, light-band strengthening, and scapular stabilization exercises are begun 6 weeks postoperatively.
- If the patient is pain free at 8 weeks, he or she may begin strengthening with light weights (<5 lb).
- More aggressive strengthening is gradually started at 3 months, with a planned return to sport or activity, without restriction, at 6 months.

Reference

1. Abrams JS. Arthroscopic repair of posterior instability and reverse humeral glenohumeral ligament avulsion lesions. *Orthop Clin North Am.* 2003;34(4):475-483.

Chapter 11

Arthroscopic Subacromial Decompression

DAYNE T. MICKELSON
DEAN C. TAYLOR

Background and Preoperative Planning

- Acromion anatomy (Fig. 11-1)

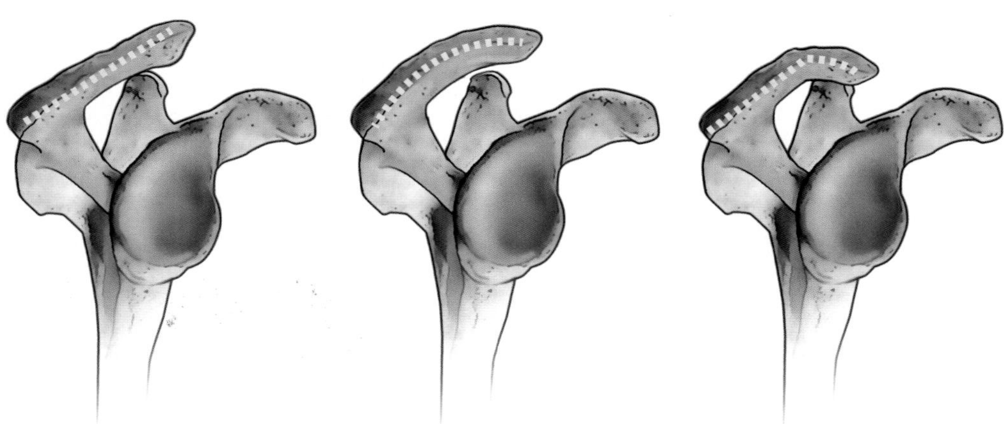

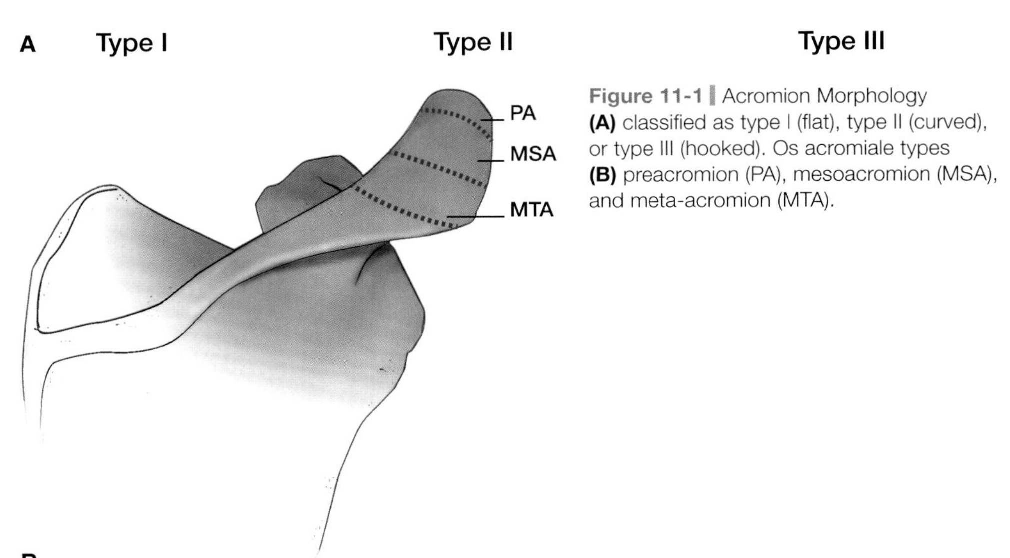

Figure 11-1 | Acromion Morphology **(A)** classified as type I (flat), type II (curved), or type III (hooked). Os acromiale types **(B)** preacromion (PA), mesoacromion (MSA), and meta-acromion (MTA).

- Acromion morphology[1]
- Os acromiale
  - Acromioplasty as a treatment for os acromiale should be used with caution because it may destabilize the acromion.
  - Excision of a symptomatic unstable os acromiale is effective and safe if the deltotrapezial fascia is not disrupted.
- The subacromial bursa vascular supply encountered during bursectomy[2]:
  - Anterior bursa: Superficial to the coracoacromial (CA) ligament is the acromial branch of the thoracoacromial artery (Fig. 11-2).

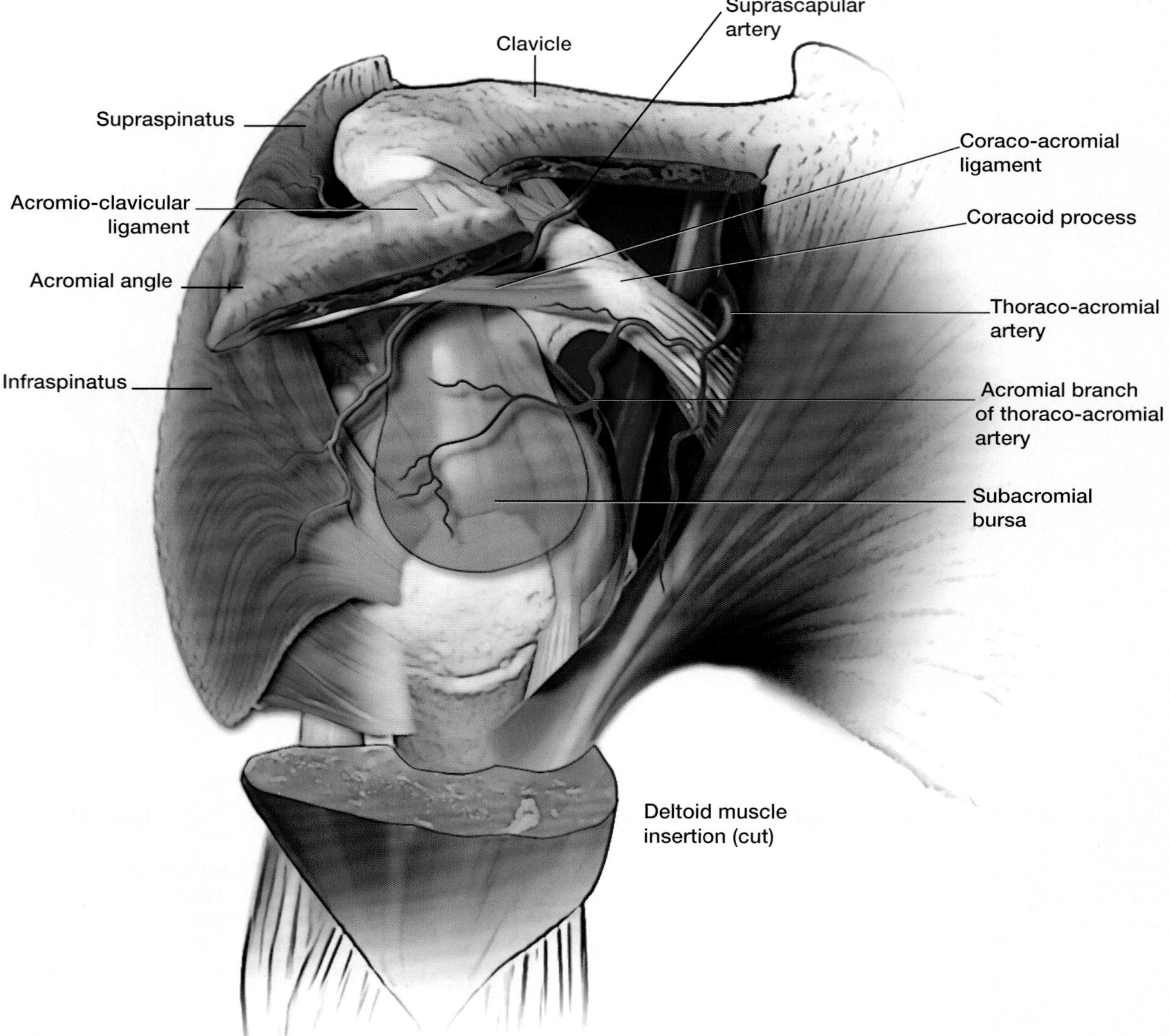

Figure 11-2 | Shoulder and subacromial bursa location as viewed from superolateral. The veil is posteriormost aspect of the bursa. Coracoacromial ligament with acromial branch of the thoracoacromial artery superficial to it.

  - Posterior bursa: posteromedial acromial branch of the suprascapular artery.
  - Medial bursa: Fat in this area is vascularized from the anterior and posterior arteries of the acromioclavicular joint.
- Pathology
  - Neer initially described acromioplasty and extrinsic impingement of the rotator cuff from the CA ligament and anterior inferior edge of the acromion.[3]

- When the arm is elevated, the subacromial bursa helps decrease contact between the CA arch and the rotator cuff. However the bursa can become irritated and inflamed (Fig. 11-2).
  - Pathologic changes to the rotator cuff are thought to arise from both intrinsic and extrinsic processes.
    - Tears caused by intrinsic degenerative changes of the cuff
    - Tears caused by extrinsic impingement from a hooked acromion or anteroinferior undersurface CA enthesophyte
- Indications—Failure of satisfactory nonoperative management (3-6 months) trial
  - Consistent physical examination findings
    - Neer impingement sign and Hawkins test are sensitive but not specific.[4]
  - Physical therapy with emphasis on scapular stabilization and periscapular strengthening
  - Response to diagnostic/therapeutic subacromial steroid and anesthetic injection.
  - Continued significant pain affecting quality of life
- Anesthesia—regional block with monitored anesthesia care sedation

Sterile Instruments/Equipment

- Thirty-degree arthroscope, light source, and pump
- Fluid with epinephrine 1:1000 in each 3 L bag of lactated Ringer solution
- 10 cc 1% lidocaine with epinephrine (1:100 000)
- Instruments
  - Spinal needle
  - Probe
  - Arthroscopic ablation wand
  - Shaver 5.5 mm (4.0-mm shaver if small shoulder) or optional burr
  - Two 5.5 mm × 70 mm cannulas without fenestrations
  - Possible instruments for rotator cuff repair (Tip—see Table 11-1)

Table 11-1 | Subacromial decompression tips and tricks

Timing of Operation	Tip or Trick
Preoperatively	Always be prepared to do a rotator cuff repair. Have the necessary instruments available.
Before Prepping and Draping	Remember to complete a full shoulder examination under anesthesia once the patient is relaxed.
Prepping and Draping	A pneumatic limb positioner helps provide inferior traction on the humeral head during subacromial decompression to enlarge the space.
Diagnostic Arthroscopy	Verify you are in the glenohumeral joint by sweeping the trocar inferior and superior to feel the camera slide between the humeral head and glenoid.
Subacromial Bursoscopy	Avoid sweeping medial and lateral in the subacromial space, which can create unnecessary bleeding.
Subacromial Decompression	When entering the subacromial bursa, aim for the bursal space located under the anterolateral portion of the acromion (Fig. 11-5A)
Subacromial Decompression	Visualization may be difficult during initial bursectomy. Run shaver facing up (away from rotator cuff) and toward the camera to clear space for viewing.
Subacromial Decompression	Avoid the fat in the posteromedial aspect of the subacromial space—this area will bleed significantly.
Subacromial Decompression	Be prepared for bleeding from the acromial branch of the thoracoacromial artery when dissecting around the CA ligament.
Acromioplasty	If the anterior overhang is too large (and shaver/burr cannot advanced in an anterior direction), then move inferior to bone overhang and resect it from directly underneath.
Acromioplasty	Before closing, return the camera to the posterior portal and verify resection. Best view is a horizon tangential view: 30-degree scope rotated to view toward 6 o'clock while dropping hand to keep the tip of the scope on the undersurface of the acromion.

Positioning and Operative Preparation

- Sitting (beach chair) position (Fig. 11-3)
  - Legs flexed at hips and knees.
  - Head in neutral position in both coronal and sagittal plane.
  - All bony prominences padded, including nonoperative arm on arm holder.
  - Operative arm positioning device can be used (optional).

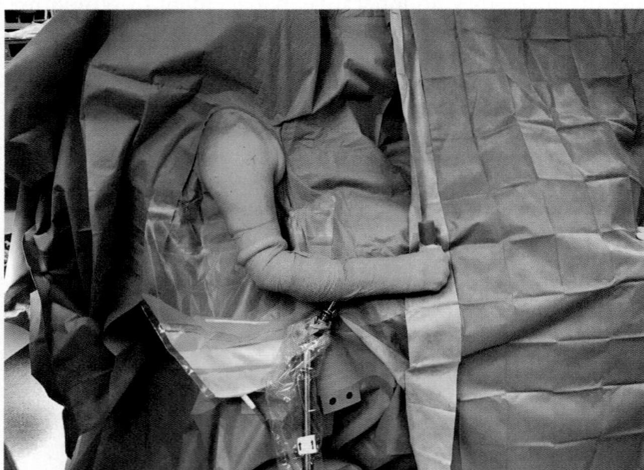

Figure 11-3 | Beach chair position and draping. Operative arm in pneumatic limb positioner. Extremity drape and additional sheets placed over bar located across anesthesia IV poles. Sterile Mayo table will be brought in over legs for instrument management.

- Preoperative physical examination (Tip—see Table 11-1)
  - Forward elevation
  - External rotation at 0 degrees of abduction
  - Internal rotation at 90 degrees of abduction
  - External rotation at 90 degrees of abduction
  - Cross-body adduction
  - Anterior and posterior load and shift
  - Inferior humeral head translation
- Preparation and draping (Fig. 11-3)
  - Operative arm in pneumatic limb positioner
    - Assists in providing inferior traction of humerus during bursoscopy
  - Draping up over bar located across anesthesia IV poles
  - Sterile Mayo table over legs for arthroscopic instrument setup and cord management

Subacromial Decompression

- **Surface Anatomy and Portals (Fig. 11-4)**
- **Diagnostic Arthroscopy**

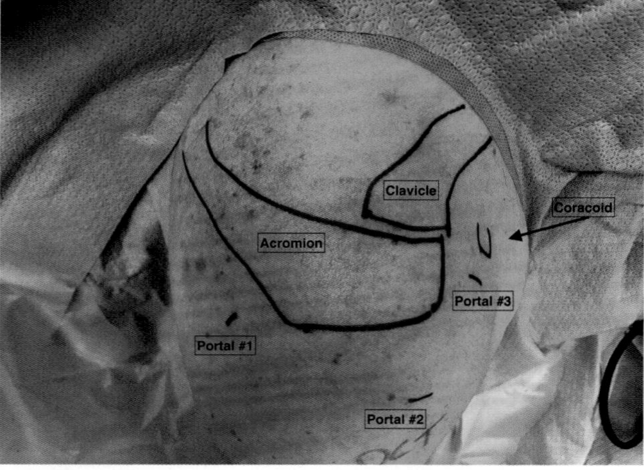

Figure 11-4 | The patient's right shoulder viewing from lateral demonstrating portal positions and surface anatomy. Superficial anatomy drawn out includes the coracoid, acromion, clavicle, and acromioclavicular joint. Portal no. 1 (vertical posterior portal): made in the soft spot of posterior shoulder inferomedial to the posterolateral corner of the acromion. Portal no. 2 (horizontal anterolateral portal): made 3 cm lateral to the anterolateral corner of the acromion. Portal no. 3 (vertical anterior portal): made half way between the coracoid and the anterolateral corner of the acromion. This portal is made during diagnostic arthroscopy through the rotator interval under direct visualization.

- Portals are injected with 1% lidocaine with epinephrine for hemostasis.
- Posterior portal incision is made with no. 11 blade.
- The glenohumeral joint is entered with trocar and cannula by aiming toward coracoid between glenoid and humeral head (Tip—see Table 11-1).
- The cannula is placed through the anterior portal into the joint for outflow and probing.
  - Spinal needle localization into the rotator interval
- Standard diagnostic arthroscopy is completed.

- **Bursoscopy Entry and Preparation**
  - The arthroscope is moved into the subacromial bursa located in the anterior portion of the subacromial space inferior and posterior to the CA arch (Fig. 11-5A).

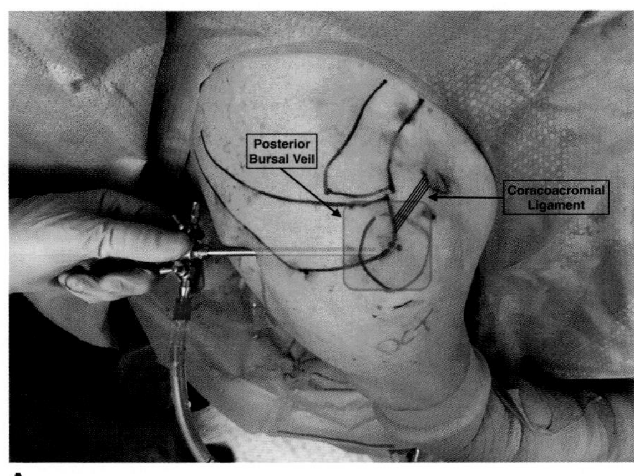

A

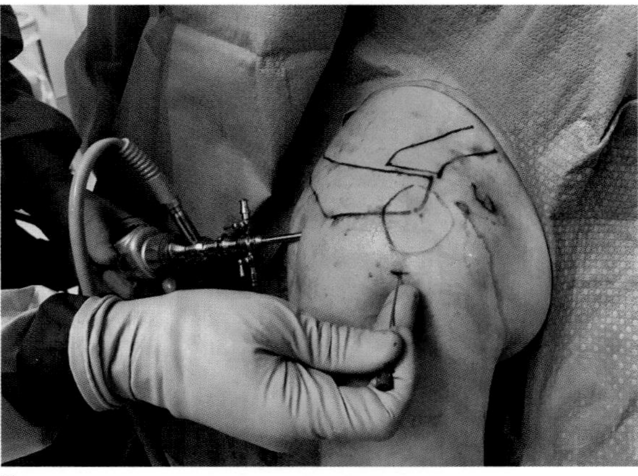

B

Figure 11-5 | The patient's right shoulder viewing from lateral demonstrating arthroscope entry into the subacromial bursa **(A)**. The subacromial bursa (*red rectangle*) is located in the anterior portion of the subacromial space and under and posterior to the coracoacromial arch. The posterior bursal veil can obscure entry into the bursa. Arthroscope viewing from posterior and needle localization into subacromial space from anterolateral portal **(B)**.

  - The glenohumeral is exited, and a trocar from the posterior portal is used to feel the posterior edge of the acromion and joint slide just underneath.
  - The trocar is advanced anteriorly to enter the bursa. The trocar must get past the posterior bursal veil, which can obscure view (Figs. 11-5A and 11-6A).
    - Sweeping medial and lateral in the subacromial space can create unnecessary bleeding (Tip—see Table 11-1).
    - Positioning the arm in adduction with neutral rotation and inferior traction using arm positioner or manual traction can help improve entry into the space (Tip—see Table 11-1).
- Initial visualization within the space can be difficult because of inflamed bursa and adhesions
  - If a full-thickness rotator cuff tear is present, the bursa may be open and inflated, aiding visualization, due to fluid extravasation from the glenohumeral joint into the subacromial space during diagnostic arthroscopy.
  - Undersurface fraying of the CA ligament can identify site of impingement (Fig. 11-6B).
- A spinal needle from the anterolateral portal (Fig. 11-5B) is used to localize within the bursa and verify that the trajectory of the needle is parallel to the undersurface of the acromion (Fig. 11-6C).
  - Once verified, a horizontal lateral incision is made (Fig. 11-4), followed by a hemostat to enlarge the incision.
- A shaver is placed through the anterolateral portal to begin bursectomy and improve visualization.
  - The shaver blade should be kept facing up to prevent damage to rotator cuff (Fig. 11-6D) and allow bursal tissue and adhesions to be sucked into the shaver.
- The cannula is repositioned from the anterior portal into the subacromial space medial to the CA ligament to function as outflow (Fig. 11-6D).

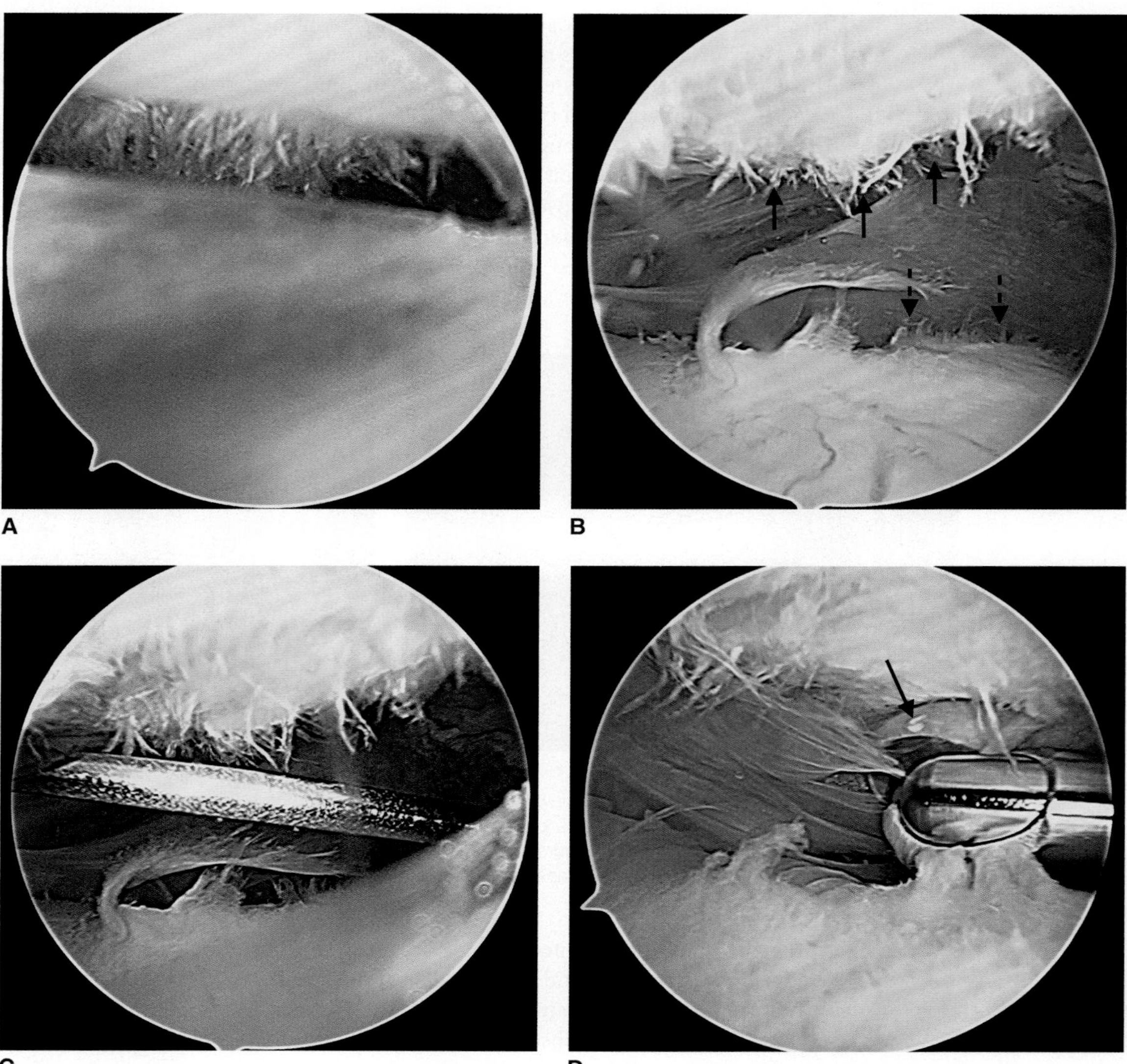

Figure 11-6 | Arthroscopic view of the patient's right shoulder viewing from posterior portal. The posterior bursa veil obscures view into the subacromial space **(A)**. Advancing into the bursa provides view of the subacromial space and site of impingement—fraying of the undersurface of the coracoacromial ligament (*solid arrows*) and bursal side of the supraspinatus (*dashed arrows*) **(B)**. Spinal needle localization through the anterolateral portal (**C**). Bursal debridement using shaver working through the anterolateral portal with outflow cannula (*arrow*) from anterior portal repositioned into subacromial space behind **(D)**.

- **Subacromial Bursectomy**
  - Bursa, adhesions, and inflamed tissue within field of view.
    - Debridement progresses from anterior to posterior and medial to lateral to enlarge visual space.
  - Viewing and working portals.
    - Switching sticks are placed in the posterior and anterolateral portals.
      - The camera is moved to anterolateral viewing portal (Fig. 11-7A).
      - A second cannula is placed from posterior to become a working portal.
  - A shaver is used to remove the posterior veil and work anterior to define acromion.
  - An ablation device is used for hemostasis and to clear off the undersurface of acromion (Figs. 11-7B and 11-8A).
    - Starting posteriorly and moving anteriorly sweeping medial and lateral.
      - The anterior extent of the acromion to the CA ligament is identified (Fig. 11-8A).
      - Laterally, the anterolateral corner and lateral border of acromion are identified.
      - Continue to clear off anterior acromion moving medially until defined the acromioclavicular joint.

Chapter 12
Arthroscopic Treatment of Partial-Thickness Rotator Cuff Tears

CORY M. STEWART
TYLER J. HUNT
LAURENCE D. HIGGINS

Sterile Instruments/Equipment

- Beach chair, ensuring that maximal weight tolerance is not exceeded based on individual beach-chair specifications
- Arm holder (pneumatic, mechanical, or battery powered); if not available, a Mayo stand or a surgical assistant can be used to hold and manipulate the arm
- Thirty-degree arthroscope, possible 70 degrees
- Arthroscopic burr
- Arthroscopic shaver
- Arthroscopic radiofrequency device
- No. 11 blade, both for skin incisions and for making a portal through the rotator cuff
- Arthroscopic biting instruments, both straight and angled
- Implants
  - Anchor(s): either all suture, or absorbable or nonabsorbable nonmetallic anchors depending on preference. Metal anchors are generally avoided due to distortion of future magnetic resonance imaging (MRI) studies
- Smooth and threaded cannulas
- Arthroscopic suture passer, both straight and curved depending on tear configuration.
- Beanbag, or other lateral positioner (pegboard, lateral positioning arms) if lateral positioning is preferred

Positioning

- The authors prefer beach-chair positioning for partial-thickness rotator cuff tears; lateral decubitus positioning is an option for those who exclusively use this position for shoulder arthroscopy.
  - All bony prominences must be adequately padded if using a lateral decubitus position—both the elbow of the upper extremity and the fibular head of the lower extremity.
  - Case reports also exist of partial-thickness ulcers at bony prominences about the pelvis due to inadequate padding of the beach chair. The authors typically add additional gel padding in the lumbosacral area (Fig. 12-1).

Surgical Approach

- Bony landmarks including coracoid, acromion, scapular spine, and clavicle are marked with a skin marker.
- A standard posterolateral portal is established first, roughly 2 cm inferior and 2 cm medial to posterolateralmost aspect of acromion.

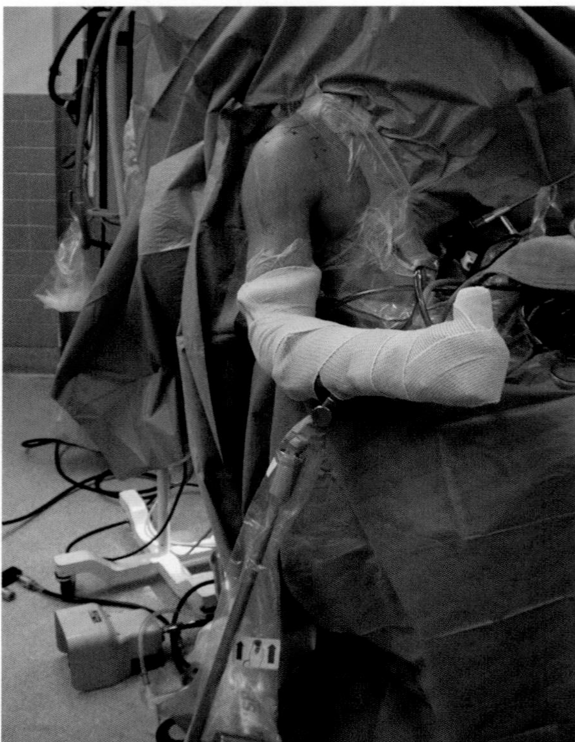

Figure 12-1 | Patient seated in the beach-chair position. Arm is held with a pneumatic arm holder secured to the back of the operative table. Edges of drapes are sealed with either clear or iodine-impregnated adhesives.

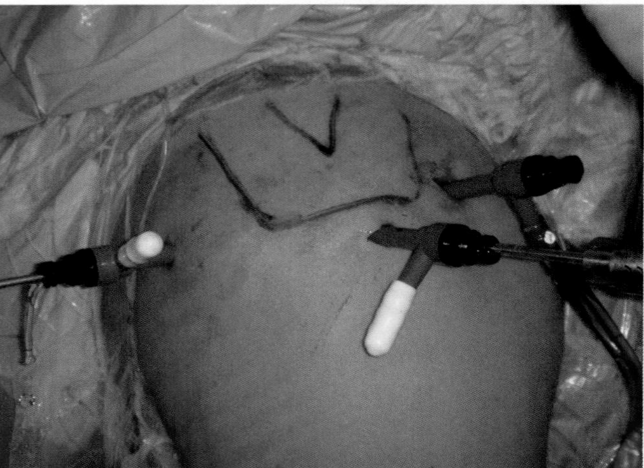

Figure 12-2 | Traditional anterior, posterior, and lateral portals with corresponding cannulas. The clavicle, acromion, and scapular spine are identified with a skin marker.

- The anterior portal is established under direct visualization using outside-in technique, though inside-out technique can also be utilized (Fig. 12-2).
- Diagnostic intra-articular arthroscopy is performed at the outset of the procedure to evaluate for concomitant pathology, ensuring that the biceps tendon, labrum, articular surfaces, axillary recess, subscapularis insertion, and remainder of rotator cuff are completely visualized and free of lesions.
- Particular care is paid to the articular side of rotator cuff insertion if exam or imaging studies are concerning for rotator cuff pathology.
- Arthroscope is then passed into the subacromial space.
- Bony or soft tissue decompression is performed depending on preoperative symptoms and extent of pathology/spur formation.
- Complete bursectomy is performed to ensure adequate visualization of rotator cuff.
- Depending on extent and location of the partial-thickness tear, a repair is performed. Significant bursal-sided tears are generally completed and repaired in standard fashion. Repair of an articular-sided tear is generally more complicated and is accomplished via the methods described in the "Tips and Tricks" section below.

Bursal-Sided Partial-Thickness Rotator Cuff Tears

Treatment of bursal-sided, partial-thickness rotator cuff repairs remains a controversial subject with regard to determining if a debridement or a repair should be performed. Previous authors have attempted to quantify tendon quality and tear thickness to set thresholds that necessitate surgical repair. Generally, the authors surgically repair bursal-sided tears that involve in excess of 50% of the normal tendon thickness (Fig. 12-3).[1,2]

Arthroscopic examples of bursal-sided rotator cuff tears (Figs. 12-4 and 12-5).

Articular-Sided Partial-Thickness Rotator Cuff Tears

Similar to bursal-sided tears, articular-sided tears have been an area of discussion and debate. Many surgeons use 50% tear thickness when compared to healthy tendon tissue as a threshold above which tendon repair is indicated. Techniques used to repair articular-sided tears vary but broadly fall into two

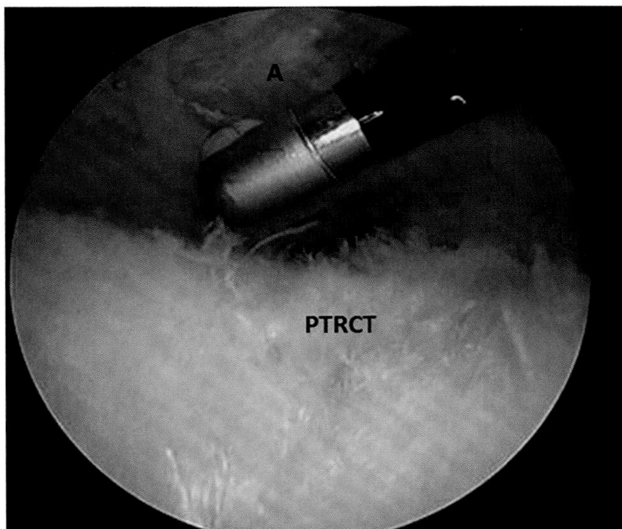

Figure 12-3 | View from the posterior portal of subacromial space looking down at a frayed and partially torn rotator cuff. A subacromial decompression is being performed using a radiofrequency device (pictured). PTRCT, partial-thickness rotator cuff tear; A, acromion.

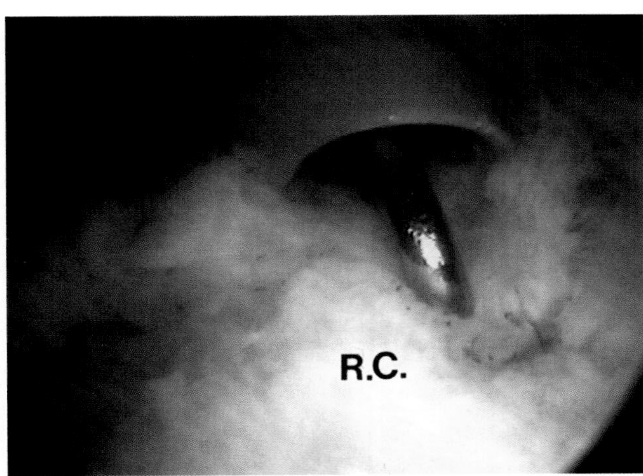

Figure 12-4 | View from the posterior portal looking down at the rotator cuff from the subacromial space. Note the thinned tendon tissue as evidenced by the probe easily penetrating the rotator cuff. R.C., rotator cuff.

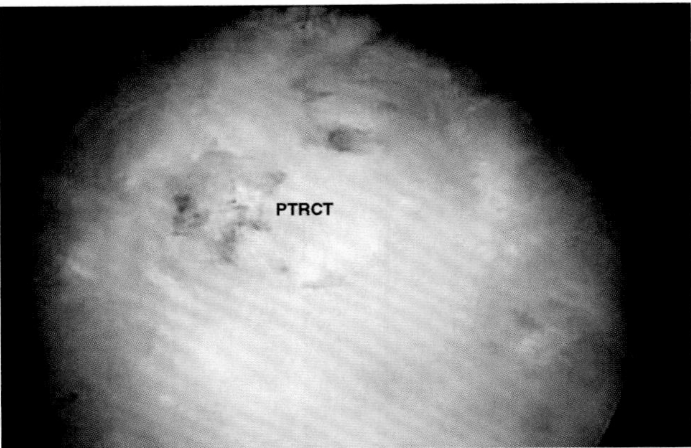

Figure 12-5 | Partial-thickness, bursal-sided rotator cuff tear after debridement as viewed from the posterior portal looking down from the subacromial space. PTRCT, partial-thickness rotator cuff tear.

main groups. One technique involves an in situ repair of the partial-thickness tear through an intact tendon, while the other technique consists of completion and debridement of a partial-thickness tear with subsequent repair. Though prior studies have demonstrated little difference in long-term outcome, a 2012 study by Shin demonstrated two key differences in outcomes between the techniques.[3-6] The completion and repair group demonstrated a higher incompetent cuff rate, while the group that had in situ fixation had a slower restoration of function and more stiffness.[5]

- Normal appearance of the rotator cuff when viewed intra-articularly (Fig. 12-6)
- MRI appearance of a partial-thickness, articular-sided rotator cuff tear (Figs. 12-7 and 12-8)
- Intra-articular appearance of several articular-sided rotator cuff tears (Figs. 12-9 and 12-10)

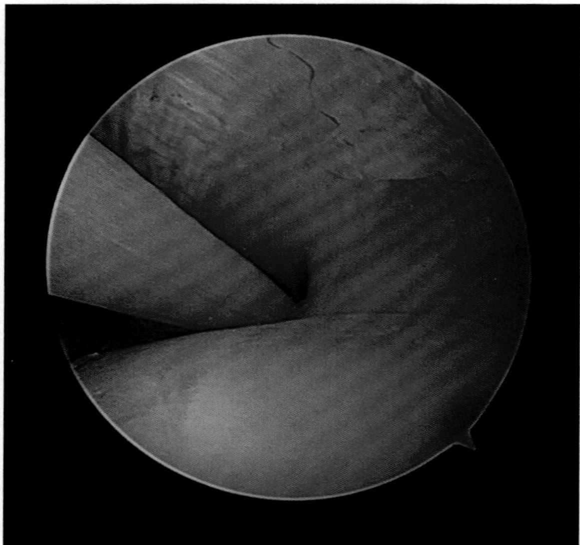

Figure 12-6 | View from the posterior portal demonstrating normal appearance of rotator cuff insertion when viewed from within the glenohumeral joint.

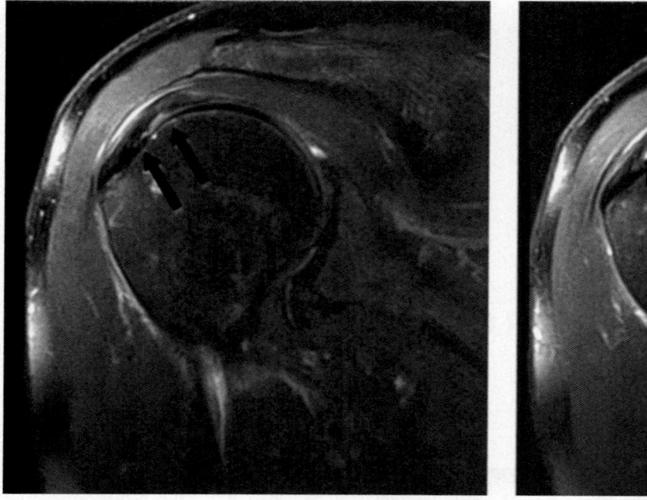

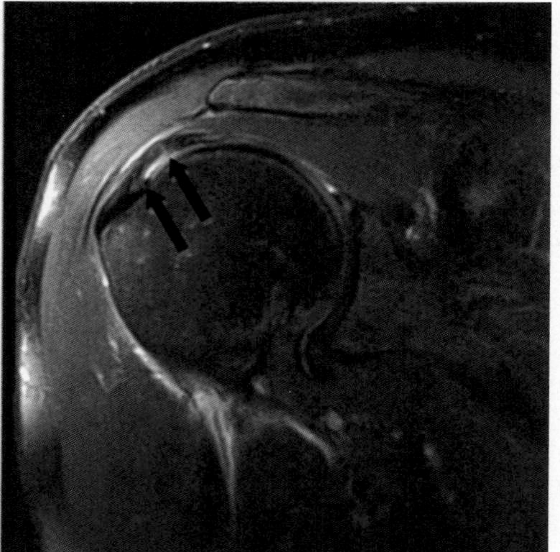

Figure 12-7 | Coronal T2-weighted images demonstrating a partial-thickness, mostly articular-sided tear of the supraspinatus tendon. Arrows denote partial-thickness, articular sided tearing of the supraspinatus with uncovering of the normal anatomic footprint.

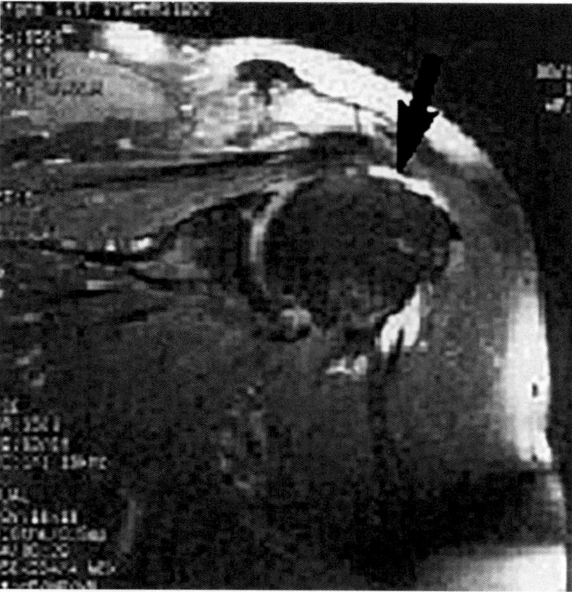

Figure 12-8 | Fat-suppressed, T2 imaging of an articular-sided rotator cuff tear with *arrow* indicating passage of fluid in area of normal rotator cuff insertion.

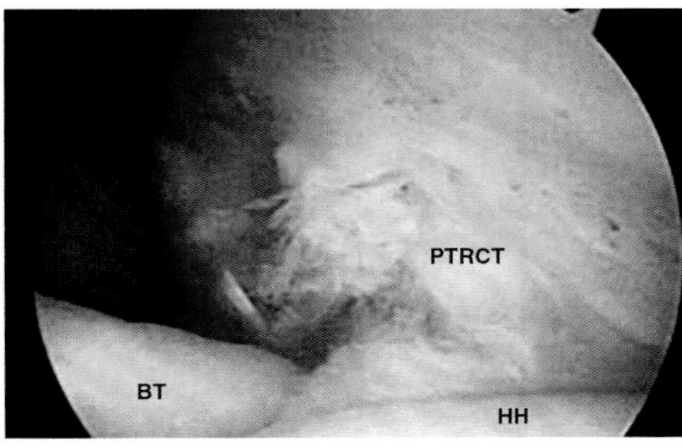

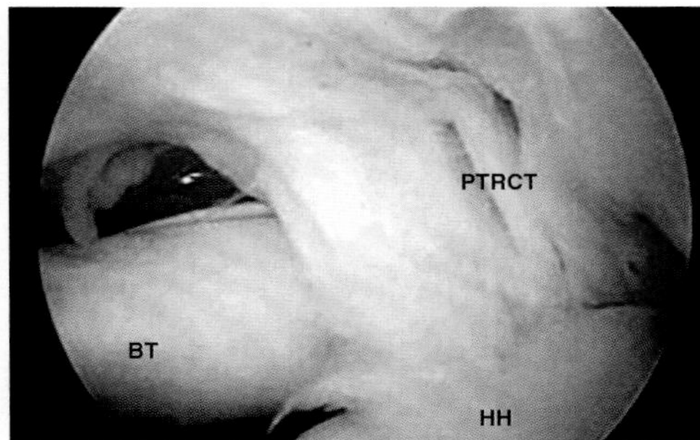

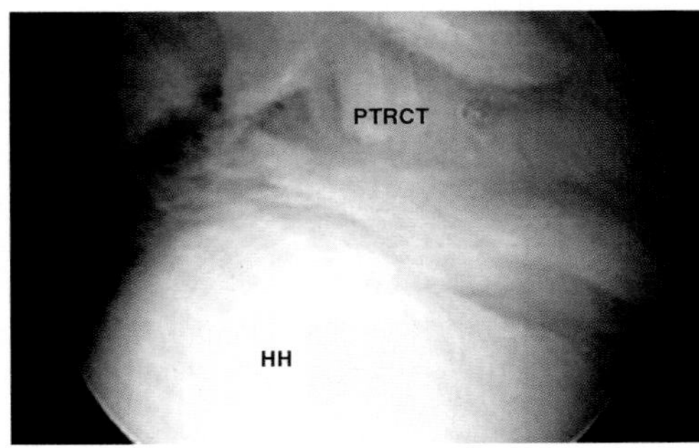

Figure 12-9 | Intra-articular view from posterior portal of three different articular-sided rotator cuff tears with varying degrees of severity. All images demonstrate uncovering of the attachment at the greater tuberosity with associated fraying of the rotator cuff tendon. PTRCT, partial tear of the rotator cuff tendon; HH, humeral head; BT, biceps tendon.

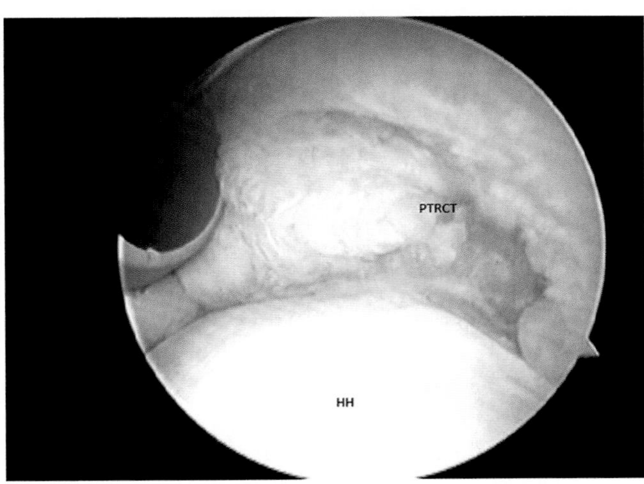

Figure 12-10 | Partial-thickness rotator cuff tear after debridement demonstrating a near full-thickness articular-sided tear. PTRCT, partial-thickness rotator cuff tear; HH, humeral head.

Tips and Tricks

Partial Articular-Sided Supraspinatus Tear (PASTA) Repair Technique

- Articular-sided tears can present a difficult problem for both the general orthopedic surgeon and the shoulder specialist.
- Incomplete tears force the surgeon to either complete the rotator cuff tear and repair from the subacromial space or to repair the tear in situ.
- An in situ repair preserves intact rotator cuff tissue but is more technically challenging.
- A variety of arthroscopic tools can be used for passing suture; in general, the authors prefer straight, penetrating suture retrievers but use gently curved suture passing devices in certain circumstances.
- In the images below and in an associated video 12-1, the authors demonstrate an in situ PASTA repair using a transcuff portal (Figs. 12-11 to 12-15).

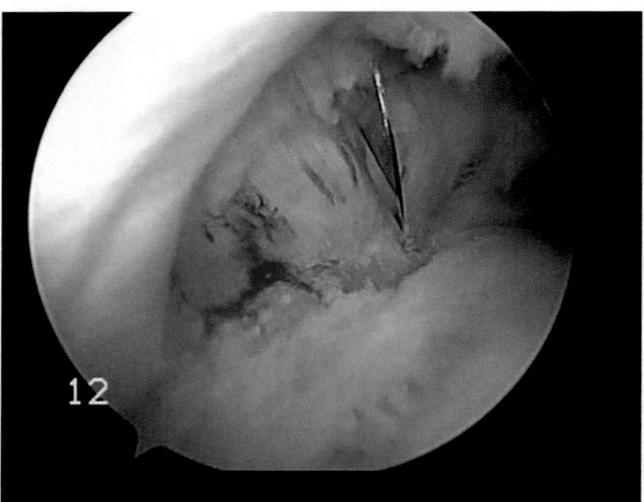

Figure 12-11 | Looking up from an intra-articular position at a PASTA lesion—viewing from a posterior portal, a no. 11 blade is passed from a lateral skin incision to make a small opening in the supraspinatus tendon.

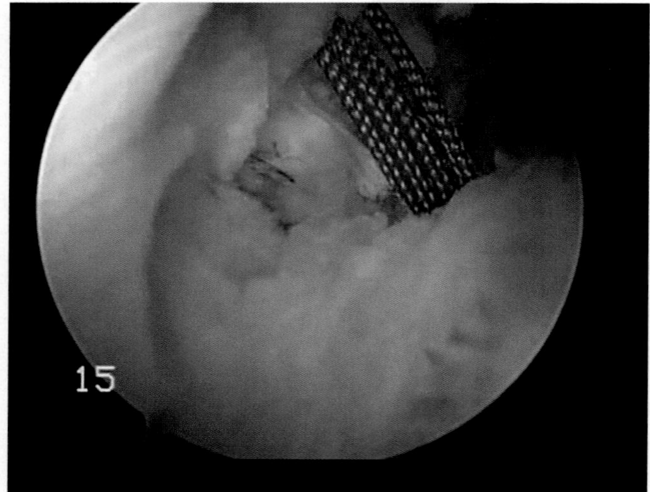

Figure 12-12 | An anchor is passed along the same trajectory.

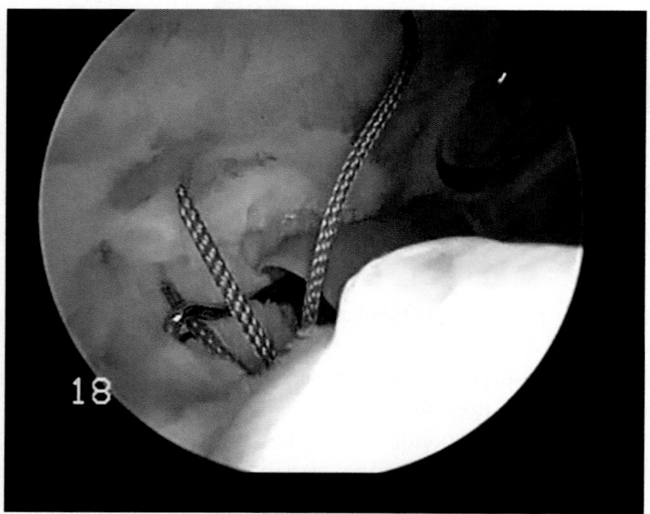

Figure 12-13 | Sutures are removed via the anterior portal.

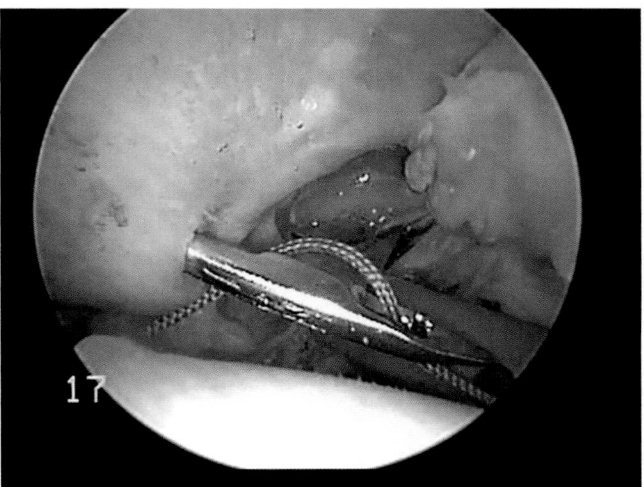

Figure 12-14 | A penetrating suture retrieval device is passed through the intact cuff in the area of the rotator cuff footprint.

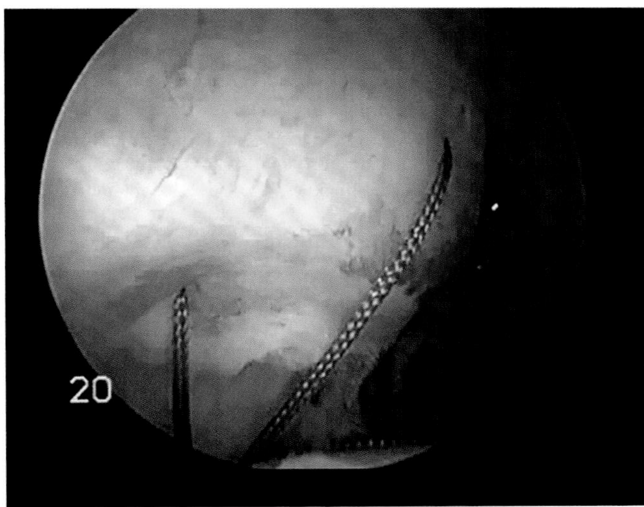

Figure 12-15 | Four separate passes are made through the rotator cuff while viewing from an intra-articular position.

- The arthroscope is then moved to the subacromial space, and a complete bursectomy is performed.
- Depending on symptoms and the patient's anatomy at the time of surgery, a bony subacromial decompression is performed (Figs. 12-16 and 12-17).

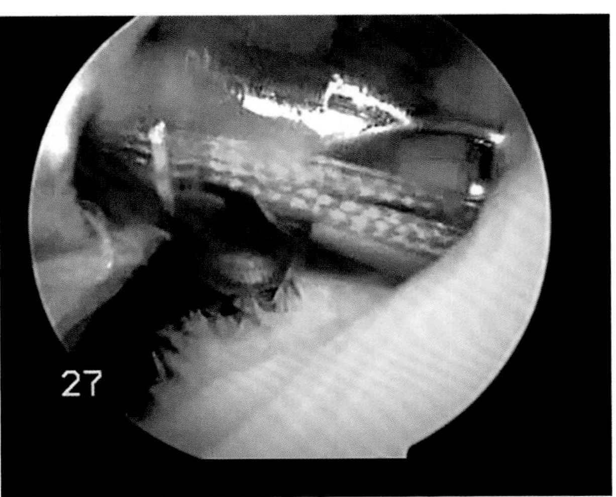

Figure 12-16 | Viewing the subacromial space, the rotator cuff is to the right. Sutures are removed via a cannula in the lateral portal and tied.

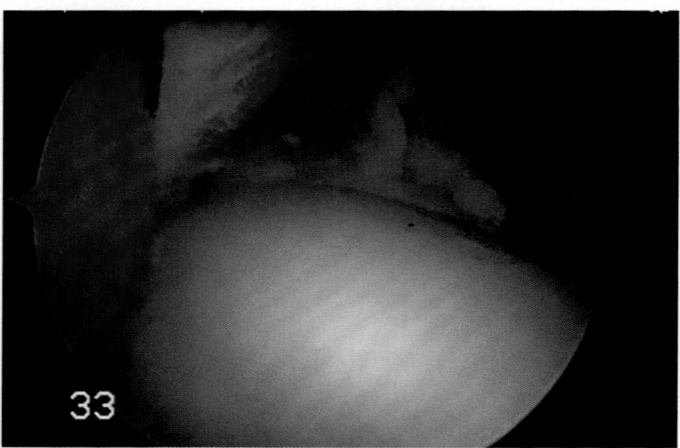

Figure 12-17 | The arthroscope is then brought back into an intra-articular position and the repaired rotator cuff is visualized. Note that the footprint has been reapproximated to its normal location on the greater tuberosity.

References

1. Wolff AB, Magit DP, Miller SR, Wyman J, Sethi PM. Arthroscopic fixation of bursal-sided rotator cuff tears. *Arthroscopy*. 2006;22(11):1247.e1-1247.e4. doi:10.1016/j.arthro.2006.05.026.
2. Yang S, Park H-S, Flores S, et al. Biomechanical analysis of bursal-sided partial thickness rotator cuff tears. *J Shoulder Elbow Surg*. 2009;18(3):379-385. doi:10.1016/j.jse.2008.12.011.
3. Franceschi F, Papalia R, Del Buono A, et al. Articular-sided rotator cuff tears: which is the best repair? A three-year prospective randomised controlled trial. *Int Orthop*. 2013;37(8):1487-1493. doi:10.1007/s00264-013-1882-9.
4. Sethi PM, Rajaram A, Obopilwe E, Mazzocca AD. Partial articular-sided rotator cuff tears: in situ repair versus tear completion prior to repair. *Orthopedics*. 2013;36(6):771-777. doi:10.3928/01477447-20130523-23.
5. Shin SJ. A comparison of 2 repair techniques for partial-thickness articular sided rotator cuff tears. *Arthroscopy*. 2012;28(1):25-33. doi:10.1016/j.arthro.2011.07.005.
6. Sun L, Zhang Q, Ge H, Sun Y, Cheng B. Which is the best repair of articular-sided rotator cuff tears: a meta-analysis. *J Orthop Surg Res*. 2015;10(1):84. doi:10.1186/s13018-015-0224-6.

Chapter 13
Arthroscopic Single-Row Rotator Cuff Repair

BRENDAN M. PATTERSON
NATHAN D. ORVETS
KEN YAMAGUCHI

Sterile Instruments/Equipment

- Standard 30-degree arthroscope
- Self-passing suture passing instrument
- No. 2 braided nonabsorbable sutures
- 4.75-mm self-punching BioComposite suture anchors (Arthrex, Naples, FL).

Positioning

- The patient is positioned in the beach-chair position. Lateral decubitus positioning also can be used depending on surgeon preference.[1]
- Care is taken to keep cervical spine alignment in neutral and to protect the ulnar nerve of the nonoperative extremity.
- Before preparing and draping, the subacromial space is injected with local anesthetic mixed with epinephrine. This provides improved hemostasis during subacromial bursectomy, which is critical for optimal visualization during rotator cuff repair.
- The operative extremity is draped free and placed into an articulating arm holder.

Surgical Approach

Portal Placement and Diagnostic Arthroscopy

- Bony landmarks are identified and marked to allow accurate portal placement.
- The posterior portal is positioned ~2 cm inferior to the scapular spine in line with the posterolateral corner of the acromion (Fig. 13-1).
- The posterior portal, positioned slightly more lateral than the traditional soft-spot portal, allows improved viewing of the greater tuberosity and rotator cuff tear.
- A lateral working portal is positioned ~2 to 3 cm distal to the lateral border of the acromion. This portal is created with spinal needle localization and is placed at the center of the tear (Fig. 13-2).
- An additional posterolateral working portal can be made in the case of larger tears that necessitate more working space.
- Care is taken to ensure that the lateral portals are placed in an inferior position in relation to the lateral border of the acromion. This serves two important purposes.
  - Low portal placement allows instruments to be passed parallel to the rotator cuff during repair.
  - The portals also tend to migrate superiorly relative to the rotator cuff as swelling occurs during arthroscopic shoulder surgery.
- The anterior portal is located ~2 cm inferomedial to the anterolateral corner of the acromion and lateral to the coracoid (Fig. 13-3).[2]

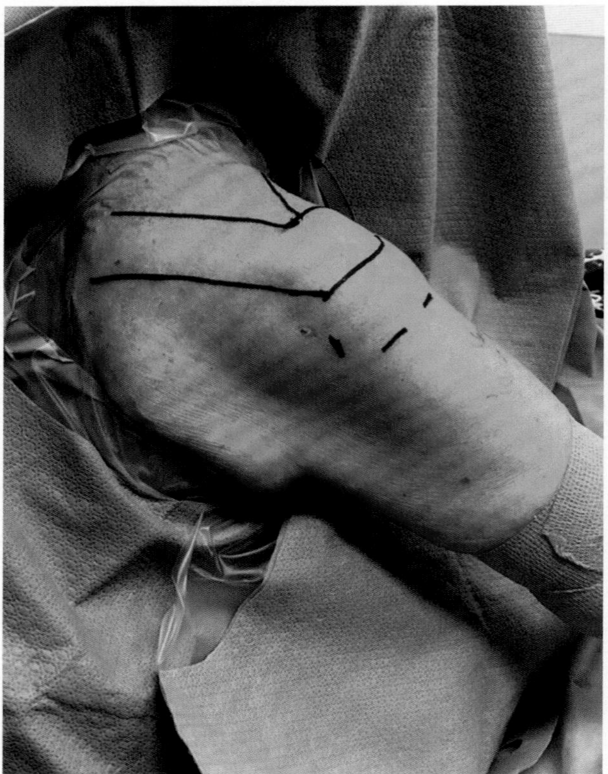

Figure 13-1 | A posterior portal in line with the posterolateral corner of the acromion is preferred.

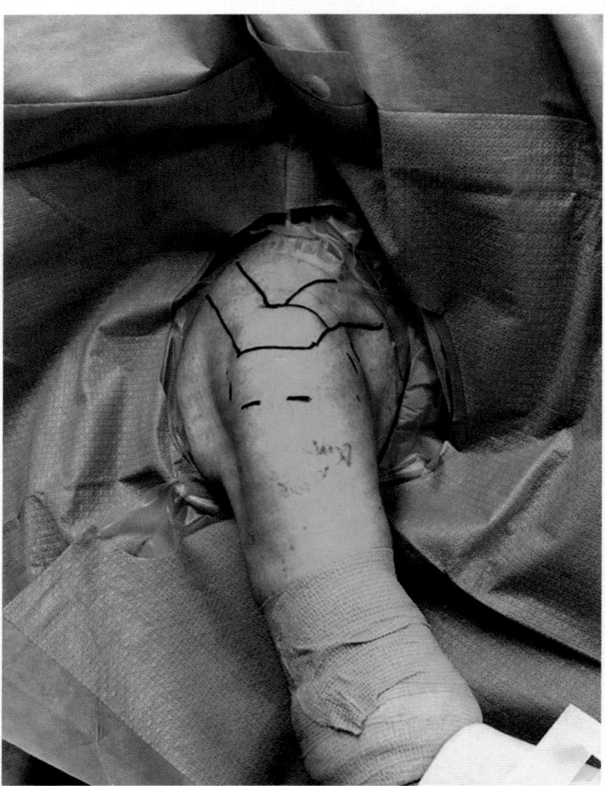

Figure 13-2 | Lateral portals are marked 2-3 cm distal to the lateral border of the acromion.

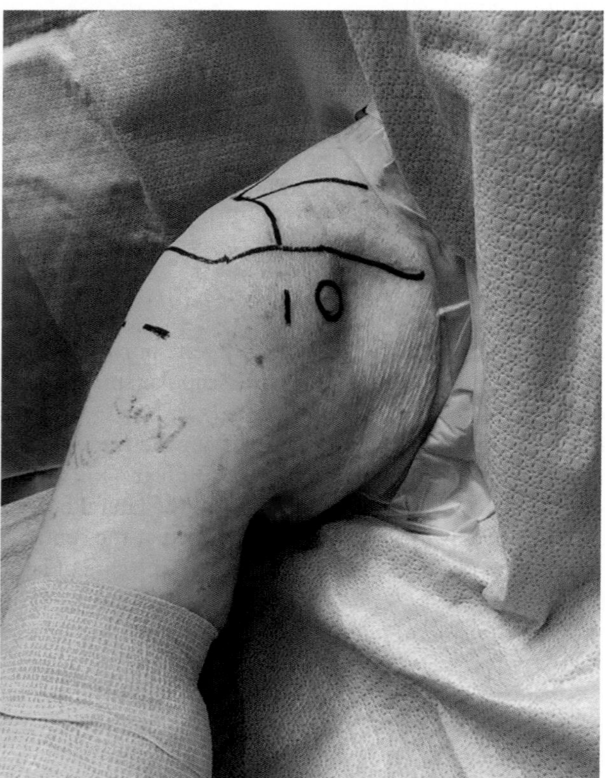

Figure 13-3 | A standard anterior portal is marked lateral to the coracoid.

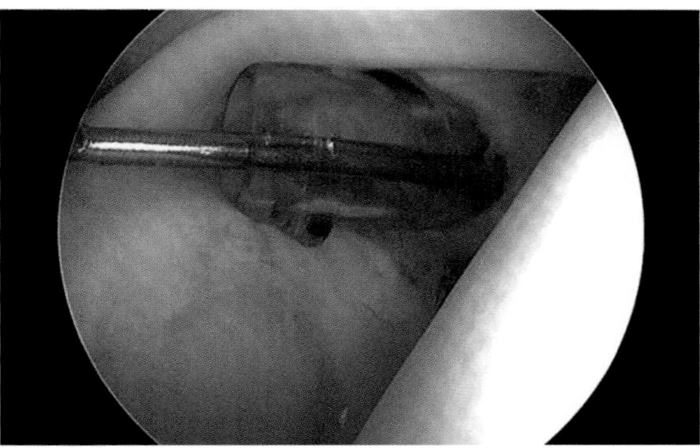

Figure 13-4 | The anterior portal is made under direct vision within the rotator interval.

- Once the posterior portal is established, a cannula is placed anteriorly within the rotator interval with spinal needle localization (Fig. 13-4).
- A complete diagnostic arthroscopy of the glenohumeral joint is performed.
- A rotator interval release is commonly performed. Visualization of the coracoacromial ligament indicates complete rotator interval release.

Repair Technique

- Following diagnostic arthroscopy, the arthroscope is removed from the glenohumeral joint and placed in the subacromial space. A sweep of the subacromial space is performed from the posterior portal with the blunt trocar in the camera sheath to clear any adhesions and improve viewing.
- The rotator cuff tear is viewed from the subacromial space, and the lateral working portal is made with spinal needle localization in line with the apex of the rotator cuff tear (Fig. 13-5).
- The arthroscopic shaver is used to clear the bursa from the subacromial space to allow adequate visualization of the rotator cuff tear.
- A fully threaded large cannula is placed in the lateral working portal.
- A soft-tissue ablation device can be used to facilitate bursectomy from the undersurface of the acromion and to achieve hemostasis, which is critical for appropriate visualization during rotator cuff repair.
- An arthroscopic shaver is used to debride any remaining soft tissue from the greater tuberosity at the insertion point of the rotator cuff.
- The greater tuberosity should be decorticated to facilitate tendon to bone healing. Because bony integrity is not required for suture anchor fixation, a burr can be used to expose bleeding bone (Fig. 13-6).
- The lateralmost portion of the rotator cuff tendon should be carefully debrided if there is degenerative tissue present that may impede healing.

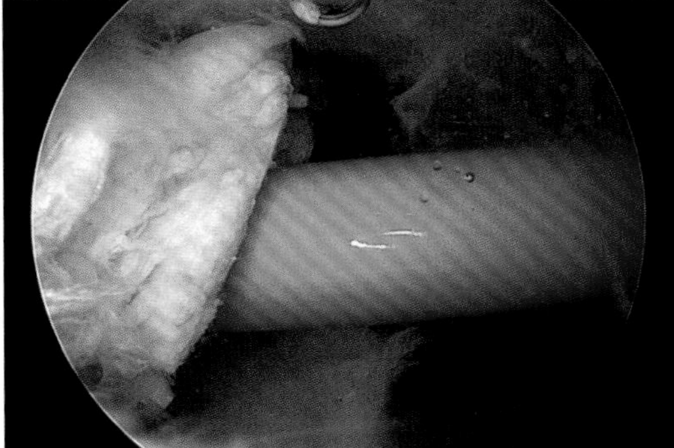

Figure 13-5 | The lateral portal is centered at the midpoint of the rotator cuff tear.

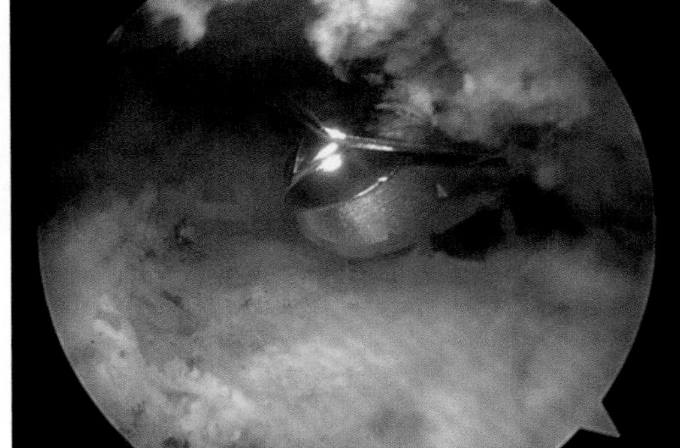

Figure 13-6 | A burr allows decortication of the greater tuberosity.

Suture Configuration and Anchor Placement

- Using the lateral portal as the working portal, a no. 2 nonabsorbable suture is passed through the anterior portion of the torn rotator cuff tendon with a suture passing instrument. The other limb of this same suture is passed ~1 cm posterior to the first limb in a horizontal mattress configuration (Fig. 13-7).

- Suture limbs are shuttled through the anterolateral portal to facilitate efficient suture management.
- The number of sutures required varies according to the spacing of suture passes and size of the tear; because a horizontal mattress configuration is used, an even number of passes is required.
- Because a medial row is not required to lock tendon fixation, a maximal tissue depth of the suture passer "bite" can be used.[3] The most anterior and posterior suture limbs can be pulled slightly more lateral than central sutures to prevent dog ears in the repair construct (Fig. 13-7).
- A soft-tissue ablation device is used to clear the bursal tissue from the lateral cortex of the greater tuberosity to localize the proper insertion site for the lateral row anchors.
- The suture limbs that will be passed through each anchor are then retrieved through the lateral cannula.
- These suture limbs are shuttled through a 4.75-mm self-punching BioComposite suture anchor. This anchor secures the free suture ends in bone without the necessity of a knot.
- The suture anchor is placed through the lateral portal and impacted to the desired insertion site (Fig. 13-8).

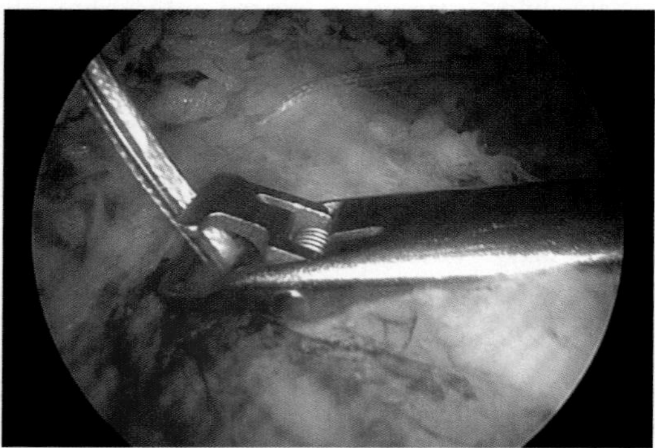

Figure 13-7 | Sutures are passed with a self-passing suture passing instrument from anterior to posterior with a horizontal mattress configuration.

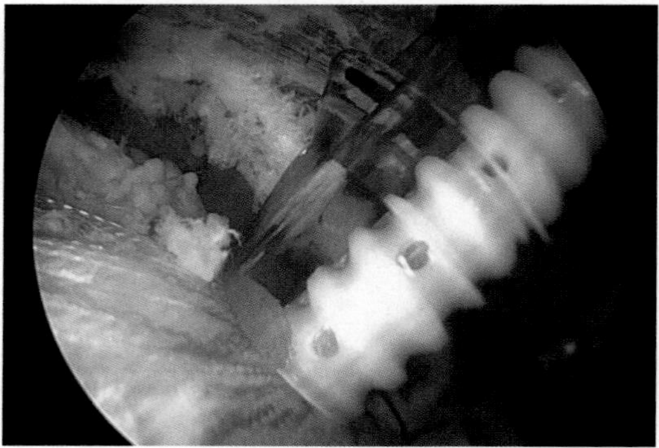

Figure 13-8 | A self-punching suture anchor allows secure fixation of the repair construct.

- Before final suture anchor fixation, the suture limbs are carefully tensioned to restore contact with the rotator cuff footprint. This should be done carefully to avoid overtensioning the rotator cuff.
- The suture limbs are cut once the anchor has been placed (Fig. 13-9).

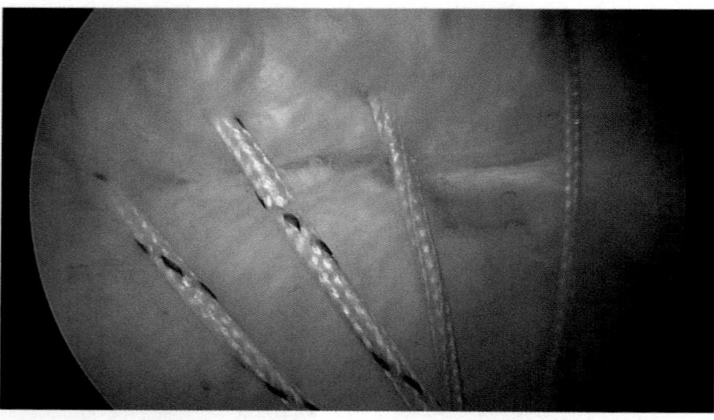

Figure 13-9 | The single-row tension band repair construct viewed from the lateral portal.

- Because most tears are crescent-shaped, a second suture anchor rarely is required and is not optimal. Eight suture limbs can be fitted to one anchor with the system we use.
- An acromioplasty is performed according to surgeon preference, generally before repair.

References

1. Peruto CM, Ciccotti MG, Cohen SB. Shoulder arthroscopy positioning: lateral decubitus versus beach chair. *Arthroscopy.* 2009;25(8):891-896.
2. Paxton ES, Backus J, Keener J, Brophy RH. Shoulder arthroscopy: basic principles of positioning, anesthesia, and portal anatomy. *J Am Acad Orthop Surg.* 2013;21(6):332-342.
3. Boileau P, Brassart N, Watkinson DJ, Carles M, Hatzidakis AM, Krishnan SG. Arthroscopic repair of full-thickness tears of the supraspinatus: does the tendon really heal? *J Bone Joint Surg Am.* 2005;87(6):1229-1240.

Chapter 14
Arthroscopic Double-Row Rotator Cuff Repair

ANDREW E. APPLE
MICHAEL J. O'BRIEN
FELIX H. SAVOIE

Introduction

- Double-row, transosseous equivalent rotator cuff repair has been shown to be biomechanically stronger than single-row repairs, but until recently, functional outcomes were equivalent.[1-3]
- Recent clinical studies demonstrate improved strength and decreased re-tear rates in rotator cuff tears larger than 3 cm with adequate tendon mobility.[4,5]
- Advantages of double-row repair[1]:
  - Better footprint coverage
  - Greater surface area contact
  - Decreased motion at footprint bone-tendon junction
  - Pressurized contact area

History

- The patient may have an inciting injury, but gradual onset is more common.
- Common symptoms
  - Anterolateral shoulder pain exacerbated by overhead reaching
  - Difficulty or weakness with overhead activities
  - Pain at night, especially while sleeping on the affected shoulder

Physical Examination

- Overall posture and position of the shoulder (protraction vs retraction) are evaluated.
- The shoulder is inspected for atrophy of the supraspinatus and infraspinatus fossa and for deltoid atrophy.
- Tenderness to palpation is tested over the greater tuberosity.
  - By extending the elbow behind the body, and palpating the greater tuberosity while internally and externally rotating the arm, the examiner can feel for any palpable defects in the rotator cuff tendons.
- Active and passive range of motion is compared to the contralateral shoulder.
- Manual strength testing is graded on a five-point scale.[6]
- Supraspinatus
  - Jobe empty-can test: weakness and/or pain with resisted forward elevation with the shoulder internally rotated in the scapular plane.
  - Supraspinatus isolation test: weakness and/or pain with resisted forward elevation with the arm in neutral, thumb up (full can test), in the plane of the scapula.

- Whipple test: weakness and/or pain with resisted forward flexion with the arm in neutral in front of the contralateral shoulder indicates scapular dyskinesis or partial-thickness supraspinatus tear.
- Drop arm test: the patient is unable to slowly and smoothly lower the arm from 90 degrees of abduction to his or her side.

- Infraspinatus
  - Weakness with external rotation.
    - With the arm adducted and in 30-40 degrees of external rotation, external rotation strength is checked against resistance.
    - In the 90/90 position for partial upper infraspinatus tears.
  - External rotation lag sign: with the shoulder adducted, the arm is passively externally rotated as far as possible, and the patient is unable to maintain this position once the examiner releases the arm.
- Teres minor
  - With the elbow supported and the arm abducted to 90 degrees, external rotation strength is checked against resistance.
  - Hornblower's sign: while the arm is supported in 90 degrees of shoulder abduction, 90 degrees of elbow flexion, and 90 degrees of external rotation, the patient is unable to maintain the arm in maximal shoulder external rotation, and the arm drops forward.
- Subscapularis
  - Lift-off test: the patient, positioned with the dorsum of the hand against the lumbar spine, is unable to lift off away from the back.[7]
    - For partial tears, strength is compared to the contralateral side.
  - Belly press test: with patient's palm on the abdomen, he or she is unable to bring the elbow forward, anterior to the plane of the body, or more subtly is unable to keep the hand on the belly when the examiner manually holds elbow forward.
  - Bear hug test: patient places hand of the affected shoulder on the contralateral shoulder and experiences pain and/or weakness when the examiner attempts to lift the hand superiorly off the shoulder while pushing down on the elbow.[8]

Imaging

- Radiographs
  - Standard shoulder series including Grashey and axillary lateral views
    - Evaluate for proximal humeral migration, degenerative changes, any abnormal bony morphology, calcific tendinosis.
    - Evaluate the lateral acromion for overhand and acromial index.
- Ultrasound
  - Can detect partial-thickness tears, full-thickness tears, and biceps tendonitis
  - Inexpensive, high sensitivity/specificity
  - Operator dependent
- Magnetic resonance imaging (MRI)
  - Can detect partial-thickness tears, full-thickness tears, and biceps tendonitis
    - Magnetic resonance arthrography (MRA) is the most sensitive and specific for full-thickness rotator cuff tears.
  - Also evaluates muscle atrophy, fatty infiltration, specific tendon involvement, and degree of rotator cuff retraction
  - Can evaluate acromion morphology, acromiohumeral distance, acromioclavicular joint, and suprascapular nerve

Surgical Indications

- Indications for rotator cuff repair:
  - Pain and functional impairment despite appropriate nonoperative management
  - Complete tear in young active individual
- Indications for double-row rotator cuff repair
  - Full-thickness tears, 2.5 cm or larger
  - Good tendon thickness and quality.
  - Tendons are easily reducible to the lateral border of the greater tuberosity, to ensure repair under minimal tension.

- Full passive range of motion.
- High activity level.
- Failed nonoperative treatment.

Positioning

- Beach-chair or lateral decubitus position is acceptable, depending on surgeon preference.

Portal Placement

- Standard posterior viewing portal
- Anterior portal in rotator interval
  - For any necessary intra-articular work
- Anterolateral portal 3 cm lateral to the anterior corner of the acromion
  - To accomplish work in the subacromial space.
  - We prefer to view from the lateral portal, to better evaluate tear configuration, and pass sutures through the anterior and posterior portals.
- Accessory portals
  - Anterolateral portal, posterolateral portal, Neviaser portal

Double-Row Rotator Cuff Repair: Surgical Technique

- Diagnostic arthroscopy is done to evaluate intra-articular pathology; integrity of the labrum, biceps tendon, and biceps anchor; articular cartilage lesions of the glenohumeral joint; presence of loose bodies and to confirm the presence of a rotator cuff tear.
- The rotator cuff tear pattern is evaluated.
  - After the intra-articular diagnostic arthroscopy, the arthroscope is redirected into the subacromial space. A medial-to-lateral sweeping motion is performed to confirm appropriate placement of the arthroscope, gain access anterior to the subacromial bursa, and release subacromial adhesions.
  - Next, a lateral portal is established using an outside-in technique with a spinal needle. The spinal needle should be parallel with the undersurface of the acromion and in line with the supraspinatus tendon tear.
  - A shaver is used to perform a partial lateral bursectomy. Bursectomy is crucial to obtaining a full view of the rotator cuff for tear pattern recognition and appropriate anchor placement.
  - Finally, the arthroscope is repositioned to the lateral portal for in-line viewing of the rotator cuff to determine tear size, retraction, and pattern recognition (eg, U-shaped, L-shaped, crescent-shaped, delaminated) (Fig. 14-1).

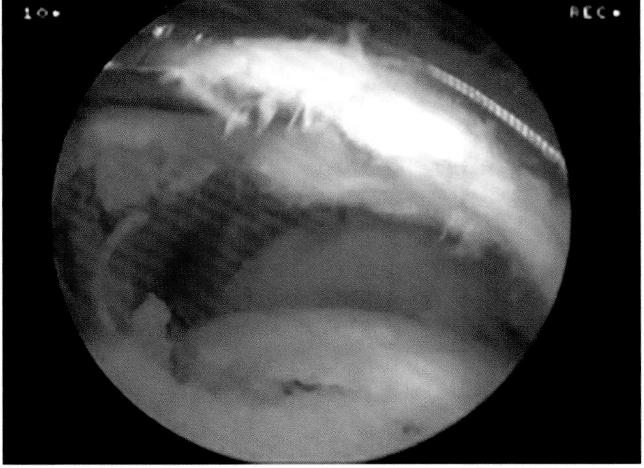

Figure 14-1 | An arthroscopic view from the lateral portal. A grasper is used to determine tear pattern and mobility.

- Assessment and mobilization of the tear
  - A grasper can be used to pull the free edge of the tear laterally to determine the shape and configuration of the tear, tendon tension, and mobility.
    - The corner of an L-shaped tear should be located so that it can be appropriately reduced to the tuberosity for anatomic repair.

- To perform a double-row repair, the tendon must have enough lateral excursion to reach the lateral edge of the greater tuberosity footprint.
- Any necessary releases are performed.
  - If the tear is difficult to reduce back to the tuberosity, releases may be necessary: this is one of the major keys to successful repair surgery.
  - Releases can be performed inferiorly, between the rotator cuff and glenoid labrum, and superiorly, between the rotator cuff and acromion, spine of scapula, and deltoid.
  - The coracohumeral ligament should be released between the supraspinatus tendon and coracoid in the subacromial space.
  - In cases of tendon retraction medial to the level of the glenoid, release of the suprascapular nerve at the suprascapular notch should be considered.[9]
- Preparing the footprint
  - The cortical bone at the footprint is abraded to stimulate healing.
    - Care should be taken not to remove cortical bone at the footprint, which may decrease the strength of the suture anchor construct.
  - Microfracture of the tuberosity also can be done to release marrow elements to facilitate healing.[10]
    - Osteopenic bone and greater tuberosity cysts may compromise anchor fixation.
- Margin convergence
  - If the tear pattern permits, placement of margin convergence sutures can approximate the tendon edges and decrease the volume of the tear to allow attachment of the tendon to the greater tuberosity bone with fewer suture anchors.
  - Sutures typically are placed in mattress fashion from posteromedial to anterolateral, in the line of pull of the infraspinatus. Typically, 2-4 sutures are used.
  - The lateral margin convergence suture can be left untied until the end of the procedure, because tying this suture will close the tendon over the optimal placement site for the medial row anchor.
- Medial-row suture anchors
  - The medial-row suture anchors are placed as far medially as possible, just lateral to the edge of the humeral head articular cartilage.
    - If more than one anchor is used, they should be spaced evenly from anterior to posterior.
    - Care must be taken to avoid overlapping anchor tunnels.
  - Anchors are inserted at a 45-degree angle (dead man's angle) to maximize pullout strength.
  - Figure 14-2 demonstrates appropriate placement of the medial-row anchor, just lateral to the articular cartilage margin. Trephination holes have been made in the greater tuberosity to deliver marrow contents to the repair site and facilitate healing.
  - Medial-row sutures should be placed through the tendon in horizontal mattress suture configuration. Both limbs of each suture are passed through the tendon, 5-8 mm lateral to the muscle-tendon junction as viewed from the bursal surface (Fig. 14-3).

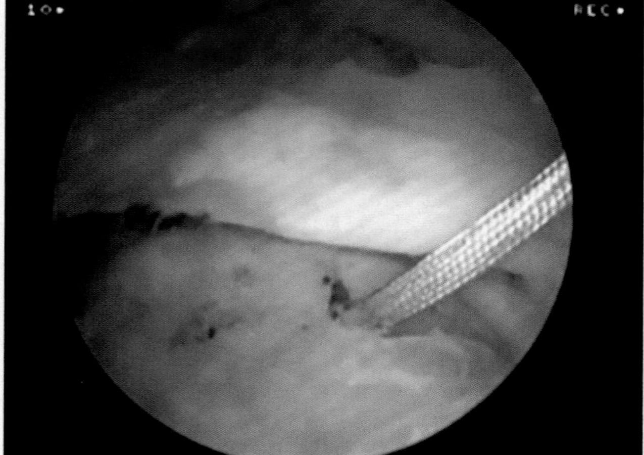

Figure 14-2 | An appropriate placement of the medial-row anchor, just lateral to the articular cartilage margin. Trephination holes have been made in the greater tuberosity to deliver marrow contents to the repair site and facilitate healing.

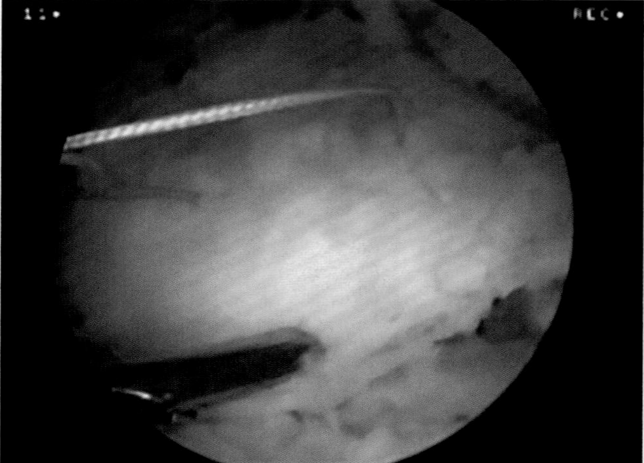

Figure 14-3 | Medial-row sutures should be placed through the tendon in horizontal mattress suture configuration. Both limbs of each suture are passed through the tendon, 5-8 mm lateral to the muscle-tendon junction as viewed from the bursal surface.

  - The sutures should not be placed too medial, which may overtighten the repair and risk recurrent type 2 failure and retear.
  - A small-diameter retrograde retriever can be used to minimize tendon damage and allow precise suture placement.
  - With the arthroscope viewing from the lateral portal, the retrograde retriever is placed through the anterior and posterior portals to accurately pass sutures through the tendon (Fig. 14-4).
- Once the medial-row anchors have been placed and sutures are passed, the previously placed margin convergence sutures are tied in place.
- Next, the medial-row sutures are tied, with the knot resting on the superior aspect of the tendon. The sutures are not cut but are left intact for incorporation into the lateral row of fixation.
- Figure 14-5 shows the medial-row sutures tied, with tails intact for incorporation into the lateral row.

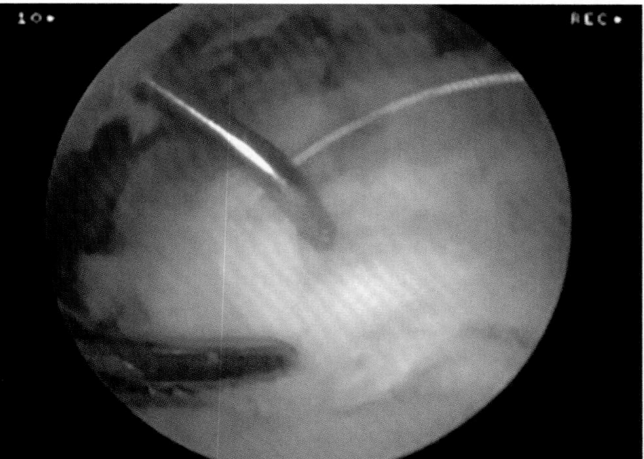

Figure 14-4 | With the arthroscope viewing from the lateral portal, the retrograde retriever is placed through the anterior and posterior portals to accurately pass sutures through the tendon.

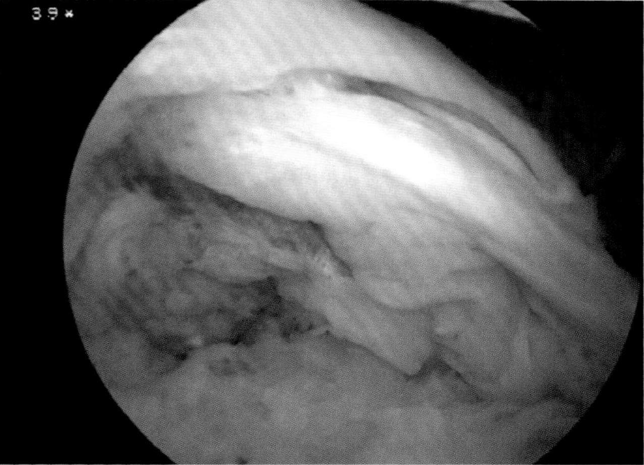

Figure 14-5 | Medial-row sutures tied, with tails intact for incorporation into the lateral row.

- Knotless constructs also are an option, with medial-row sutures or tapes that are passed, not tied, and incorporated directly into lateral-row fixation.
- Lateral-row suture anchors
  - One limb of each medial row knot is retrieved through the lateral portal.
  - These sutures are threaded through the eyelet of the lateral row anchor and the sutures are tensioned; 2-4 sutures can be placed through each lateral row anchor.
  - The rotator cuff tear is reduced and assessed. The pilot hole for the lateral anchor is tapped, just lateral to the lateral edge of the reduced tendon.
    - This placement maximizes tendon to bone surface area coverage
  - Maintaining tension on the sutures, the lateral row anchor is inserted and impacted into the bone. The sutures are tensioned, and the anchor is secured and deployed. The sutures are cut flush with the anchor.
  - For placement of a second lateral row anchor, the procedure is repeated.
  - The final construct may consist of 1 or 2 medial row anchors, a cruciform suture pattern, and 1 or 2 lateral row anchors.
  - Figure 14-6 demonstrates the final construct with 1 triple-loaded medial anchor and 1 lateral-row anchor.

Postoperative Protocol

- Postoperatively, an abduction pillow sling is worn for 6-8 weeks, depending on tear size and chronicity.
- During the first 6 weeks, patients are instructed to work on scapular retraction and passive range of motion, using the opposite extremity to assist the operative one.

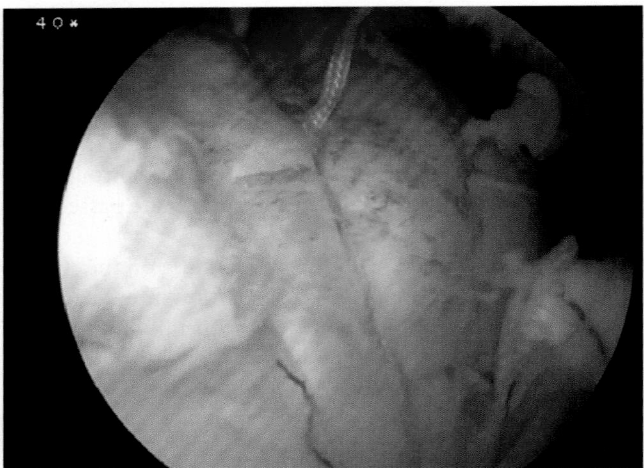

Figure 14-6 | The final construct with 1 triple-loaded medial anchor and 1 lateral-row anchor.

- At 6 weeks, an ultrasound evaluation of the rotator cuff is performed, and therapy for passive, active-assisted, and active range of motion is initiated while monitoring the scapula to maintain a retracted shoulder position during all exercises.
- At 12 weeks, a second ultrasound to confirm repair integrity and also evaluate the healing process and tendon quality allows patient-specific increase in activity and therapy.
- At 16 weeks, integrated rehabilitation, proprioceptive neuromuscular facilitation patterns, and sport and work conditioning are initiated.

Summary of Key Points

1. Releases: under and over the tendon as well as the coracohumeral ligament to facilitate tension-free repair. If the A-H distance is narrowed, the inferior capsule should be released as well.
2. The medial bursa, which overlies the muscle and is an essential part of the blood supply to the tendon, should be preserved.
3. Greater tuberosity preparation: microfracture and trephination holes are made to improve blood supply and marrow stem cell access.
4. Fewer anchors are better: 1 triple-loaded anchor medial often is sufficient, more rarely 2, and 3 anchors only when 3 or more tendons are involved.
5. Margin convergence sutures can be used to relieve tension and also can function as "rip-stop" stitches in large to massive tears.
6. Lateral-row anchors should remain high and be inserted at Burkhart's dead man's angle for improved repair construct strength.

References

1. Wall LB, Keener JD, Brophy RH. Double-row vs single-row rotator cuff repair: a review of the biomechanical evidence. *J Shoulder Elbow Surg.* 2009;18:933-941.
2. Mascarenhas R, Chalmers PN, Sayegh ET, et al. Is double-row rotator cuff repair clinically superior to single-row rotator cuff repair: a systematic review of overlapping meta-analyses. *Arthroscopy.* 2014;30(9):1156-1165.
3. Ma HL, Chiang ER, Wu HH, et al. Clinical outcome and imaging of arthroscopic single-row and double-row rotator cuff repair: a prospective randomized trial. *Arthroscopy.* 2012;28(1):16-24.
4. Millett PJ, Warth RJ, Dornan GJ, et al. Clinical and structural outcomes after arthroscopic single-row versus double-row rotator cuff repair: a systematic review and meta-analysis of level I randomized clinical trials. *J Shoulder Elbow Surg.* 2014;23:586-597.
5. Denard PJ, Jiwani AZ, Lädermann A, Burkhart SS. Long-term outcome of arthroscopic massive rotator cuff repair: the importance of double-row fixation. *Arthroscopy.* 2012;28(7):909-915.
6. Riff A, Yanke AB, Van Thiel GS, Cole BJ. Arthroscopic rotator cuff repair: double-row techniques. In: Cole BJ, Sekiya JK, eds. *Surgical Techniques of the Shoulder, Elbow, and Knee in Sports Medicine.* 2nd ed. Philadelphia, PA: Saunders; 2013:225-239.
7. Gerber C, Krushell RJ. Isolated rupture of the tendon of the subscapularis muscle. Clinical features in 16 cases. *J Bone Joint Surg Br.* 1991;73(3):389-394.
8. Jain NB, Wilcox NB III, Katz JN, Higgins LD. Clinical examination of the rotator cuff. *PM R.* 2013;5(1):45-56.
9. Savoie FH III, Zunkiewicz M, Field LD, Replogle WH, O'Brien MJ. A comparison of functional outcomes in patients undergoing revision arthroscopic repair of massive rotator cuff tears with and without arthroscopic suprascapular nerve release. *J Sports Med.* 2016;20(7):129-134.
10. Milano G, Saccomanno MF, Careri S, Taccardo G, De Vitis R, Fabbriciani R. Efficacy of marrow-stimulating technique in arthroscopic rotator cuff repair: a prospective randomized study. *Arthroscopy.* 2013;29(5):802-810.

Chapter 15
Open Subscapularis Repair

JOSEPH A. BOSCO III

Indications

- Retracted tear (Fig. 15-1)
  - Difficult to mobilize arthroscopically
- Isolated tear
  - Open approach can be combined with mini-open supraspinatus and/or infraspinatus repairs.

Sterile Instruments/Equipment

- Surgical assistant
  - For deltopectoral approach
    - Difficult to retract deltoid laterally
- No. 2 synthetic, nonabsorbable braided suture on a no. 2 curved Mayo needle
  - Traction sutures
- 4.5-mm suture anchors (2-4) with no. 2 synthetic, nonabsorbable braided suture
- No. 5 curved Mayo needles
- Right-angled retractors
  - Richardson or Army/Navy
- Self-retaining retractors
  - Weitlaner retractor

Positioning and Preparation

- Beach chair
  - Difficult to do in lateral position
- Bony landmarks are marked (Fig. 15-2)
  - Coracoid process
  - Acromion: anterior and lateral borders
  - Anterior clavicle
  - Acromioclavicular joint

Surgical Approach/Technique

- Classic open deltopectoral approach
  - A 4- to 6-cm-long incision is made.
  - The incision begins slightly lateral and inferior to coracoid.
  - The deltopectoral interval is identified.
  - The cephalic vein is identified in the interval and retracted laterally.
  - Richardson retractors are placed under the deltoid and vein, and both are retracted laterally.
  - The clavipectoral fascia is incised, and conjoined tendon is identified medially.
  - The bicipital groove is identified (between the greater and lesser tuberosities) (Fig. 15-3).
  - The long head of the biceps tendon (LHBT) is an excellent landmark for the bicipital groove.

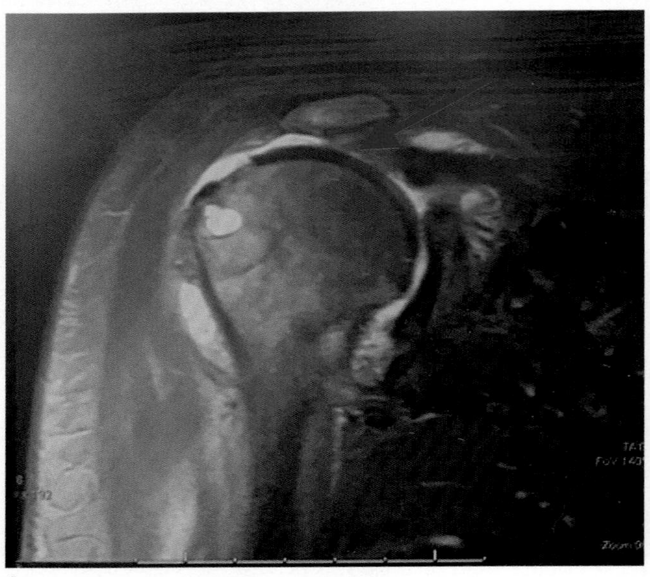
A

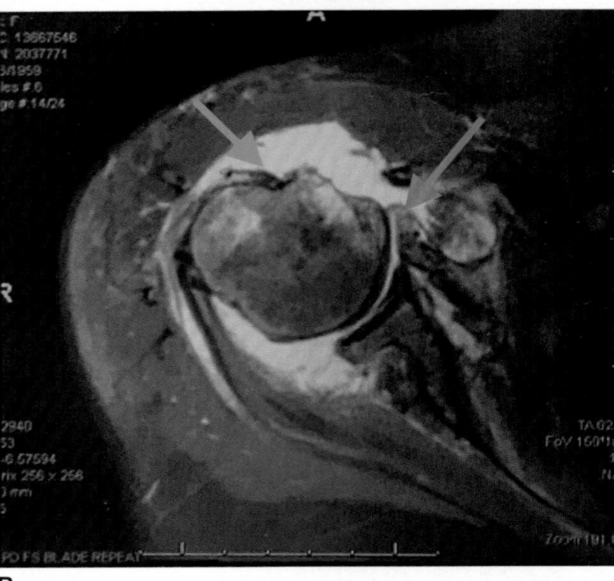
B

Figure 15-1 | A. Coronal T2-weighted MRI indicating an acute, massive, retracted tear of the supraspinatus tendon. The lateral edge (*blue arrow*) is retracted past the apex of the humeral head. **B.** Axial T2 weighted image demonstrating subscapularis tear retracted nearly to the level of the glenoid (*red arrow*). The bicipital groove is empty, indicating a retracted LHBT tear (*green arrow*).

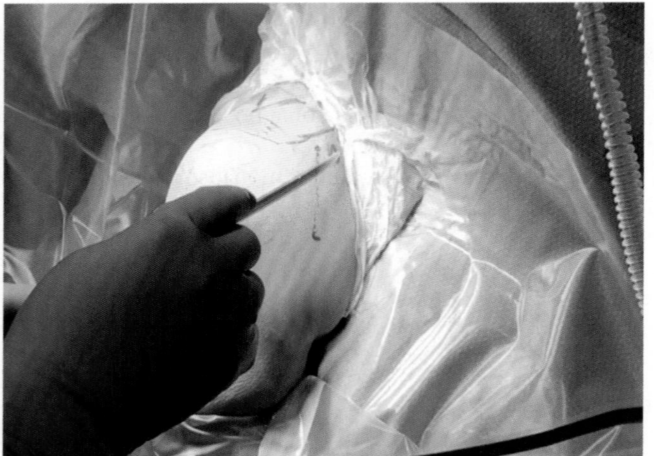

Figure 15-2 | Surgical landmarks and incision. Right shoulder with patient in the beach chair position. The scissors point to the coracoid. The clavicle, acromion, and acromioclavicular joint are marked. The *vertical line* indicates the planned incision.

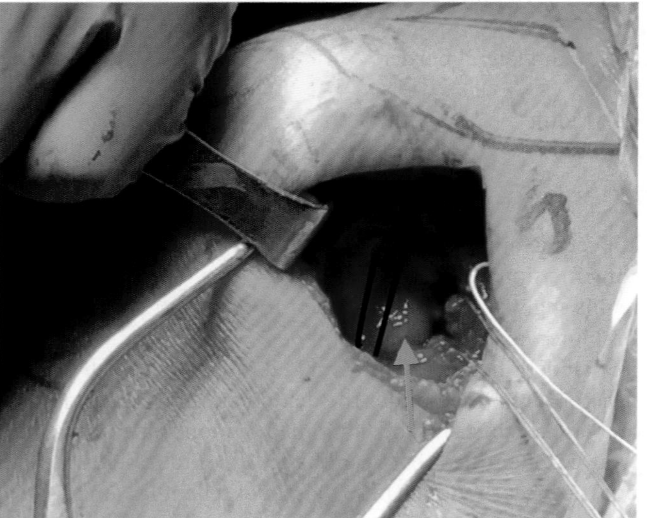

Figure 15-3 | The bicipital groove lies between the *vertical black lines*. The *green arrow* points to the lesser tuberosity.

Box 15.1. Tips for managing the long head of the biceps tendon (LHBT)

- LHBT is in bicipital groove.
  - Perform tenotomy at insertion.
  - Remove excess intra-articular portion (2-3 cm).
  - Perform tenodesis in bicipital groove with 1-2 suture anchors.
- LHBT is medially subluxed or dislocated from groove.
  - Identify tendon.
  - Perform tenotomy at insertion.
  - Remove excess intra-articular portion (2-3 cm).
  - Perform tenodesis in bicipital groove with 1-2 suture anchors.
- LHBT is absent.
  - Either locate LHBT distally (may need to extend incision distally) and tenodese as above, or . . .
  - Do not locate LHBT and leave tendon tenotomized without tenodesis.

- The LHBT, however, frequently is subluxed/dislocated medially because the subscapularis tendon forms the roof of the bicipital groove and is the main soft tissue restraint to medial subluxation of the biceps.[1]
  - The tendon may even be absent.
- See tips for dealing with LHBT (Box 15.1).
- The humerus is externally rotated and the lesser tuberosity is identified.
  - The LHBT forms the medial border of the bicipital groove.
- The conjoined tendon is retracted medially to identify the retracted subscapularis tendon (Fig. 15-4).
  - It should be kept in mind that the musculocutaneous nerve can exit the conjoined tendon as close as 19 mm distal to the coracoid process.[2]
- The lateral border of the subscapularis tendon is grasped with a Kocher clamp and mobilized laterally (Fig. 15-5).

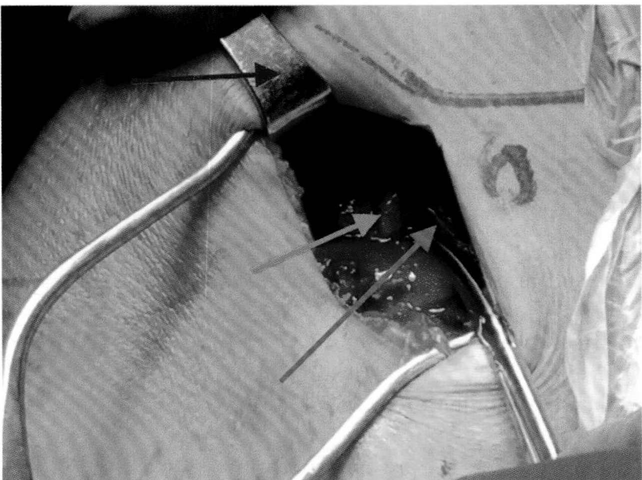

Figure 15-4 | The conjoined tendon (*purple arrow*) is retracted medially to expose the lateral edge of the subscapularis tendon (*green arrow*). Lateral retraction of the anterior deltoid (*blue arrow*) frequently requires a surgical assistant.

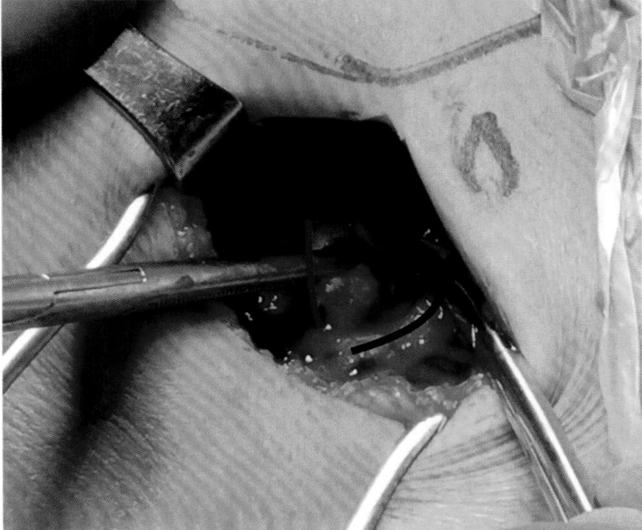

Figure 15-5 | A Kocher clamp is used to grasp and laterally mobilize the subscapularis tendon. The *curved black line* and the *blue line* indicate the lateral borders of the conjoined and subscapularis tendons, respectively.

- Two or three no. 2 horizontal mattress grasping sutures are placed in the tendon (Fig. 15-6).
- The sutures and gentle blunt dissection are used to mobilize the subscapularis laterally.
- Two or three vertically arranged 4.5-mm suture anchors are placed in the lesser tuberosity (Fig. 15-7).

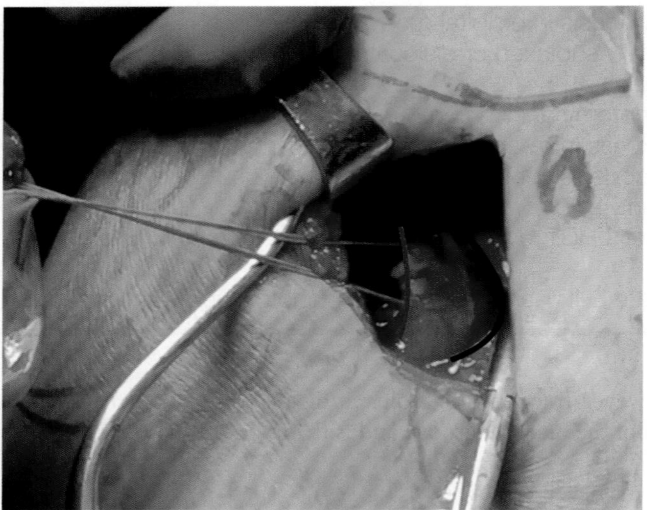

Figure 15-6 | Traction sutures are placed in the tendon to assist in lateral mobilization. The *blue and black lines* represent the lateral borders of the subscapularis and conjoined tendons, respectively.

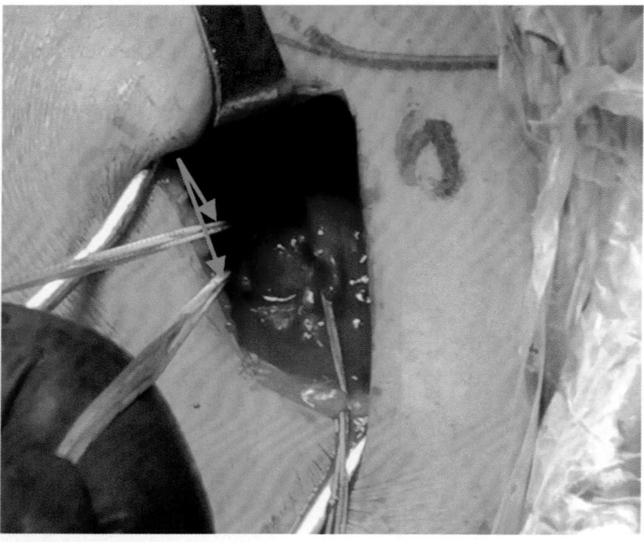

Figure 15-7 | Two double-loaded suture anchors are placed into the lesser tuberosity. The *green arrows* indicate the sutures from each anchor.

  - The humerus is internally rotated, and the sutures from anchors are passed through the subscapularis in horizontal mattress fashion (Fig. 15-8).
  - The subscapularis is reattached by tying the sutures.
  - The humerus is externally rotated to determine tension on the repair (Fig. 15-9).
    - This will be used to guide the postoperative rehabilitation protocol.
- Treatment of concomitant supraspinatus and/or infraspinatus tears
  - The humerus is maximally internally rotated to access the greater tuberosity.
  - The deltoid also can be split between its anterior and middle bellies to gain access to the tendons.
- Posteromedial arthrotomy

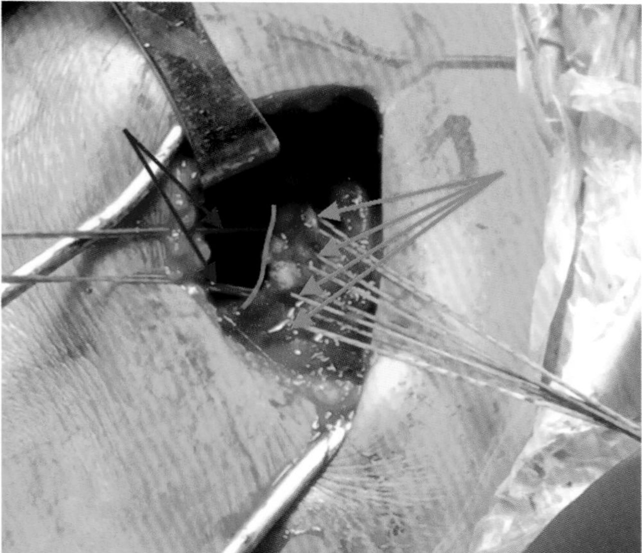

Figure 15-8 | The *green arrows* point to the four sets of horizontal mattress sutures (two sets from each of the double-loaded anchors). The *purple line* marks the lateral border of the subscapularis tendon, which overlies the lesser tuberosity. The *blue arrows* indicate the traction sutures. Note that the mobilized subscapularis tendon reaches the lesser tuberosity.

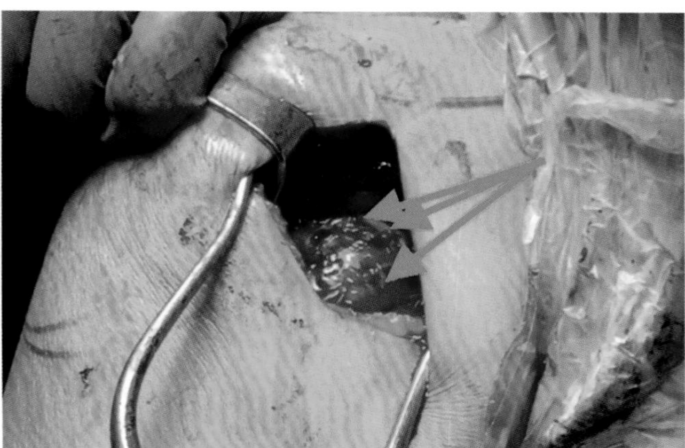

Figure 15-9 | *Green arrows* indicate the suture knots. The proximal humerus is rotated 30 degrees, and there is little tension on the repair. Since this surgery was performed only 2 weeks after the acute tear, the subscapularis was easily mobilized.

Postoperative protocol

- Shoulder sling for 6 weeks
  - Sling is removed for pendulum exercises immediately after surgery.
- Postoperative week 1
  - Active and passive external rotation is begun, limited to degrees noted during interoperative external rotation.
- Postoperative week 6
  - Sling is discontinued.
  - Resistive internal and external rotation rotator cuff strengthening exercises are begun.
  - No limits are placed on range of motion.

References

1. Gleason PD, Beall DP, Sanders TG, et al. The transverse humeral ligament: a separate anatomical structure or a continuation of the osseous attachment of the rotator cuff? *Am J Sports Med.* 2006;34(1):72-77.
2. Bach BR Jr, O'Brien SJ, Warren RF, Leighton M. An unusual neurological complication of the Bristow procedure. A case report. *J Bone Joint Surg Am.* 1988;70(3):458-460.

Chapter 16
Arthroscopic Subscapularis Repair

ROBERT U. HARTZLER
STEPHEN S. BURKHART

Instruments and Equipment

- 30- and 70-degree arthroscopes
- Antegrade and retrograde suture passers
- Suture anchors
- Arthroscopic pump
- Arthroscopic shaver and burr (5 mm) and electrocautery device
- Arthroscopic ring curettes and elevators (15 and 30 degrees)
- Arthroscopic cannulas
- 18-gauge spinal needles

Positioning and Operating Room Setup

- We recommend the lateral position (Fig. 16-1A) with the patient leaning backward 20-30 degrees so that the glenohumeral joint lies horizontal and the working space in front of the shoulder remains open.
  - Goggles should be placed on the patient to protect the eyes, because the angle of approach to the lesser tuberosity often is very close to the face (Fig. 16-1B).
- A skilled surgical tech stands across from the surgeon (Fig. 16-2A) and manipulates the arm to improve visualization and access to critical working spaces.
  - The posterior lever push (Fig. 16-2B) is performed by applying a posteriorly directed force and an anteriorly directed counter force to the proximal and distal humerus, respectively.

Surgical Approach and Intraoperative Diagnostic Techniques

- Subscapularis repair and arthroscopic long head of biceps (LHB) tenodesis should be done first if there is an associated posterosuperior rotator cuff tear, because anterior swelling can compromise the ability to carry out these procedures arthroscopically.
- LHB tenodesis high in the groove[1] (Chapter 17) is almost always indicated with arthroscopic subscapularis tendon repair:
  - Tenodesis protects the subscapularis repair from abrasion by the LHB when the medial sling is incompetent.
  - LHB tendon pathology (medial subluxation, partial tearing) commonly occurs with subscapularis tendon tears (Fig. 16-4B).
- Working anterosuperior-lateral (ASL) and anterior portals are created with an outside-in technique aided by spinal needles:
  - The ASL skin incision usually is located just off the anterolateral corner of the acromion (Fig. 16-3A) and should result in a perpendicular angle of approach to the proximal bicipital

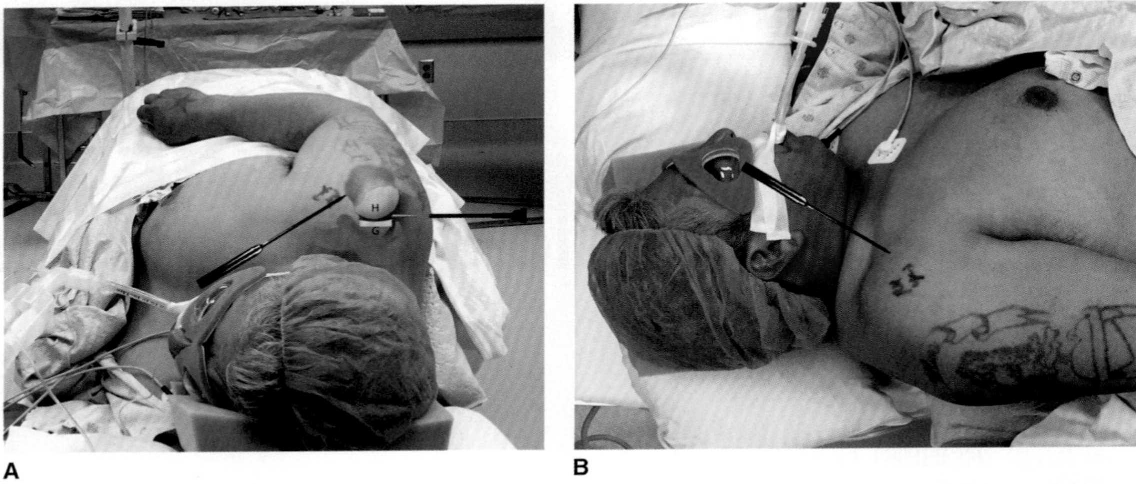

Figure 16-1 | Lateral positioning (right shoulder) shown from the head of the table **(A)** and superior **(B)** with the patient leaning back 20-30 degrees ensures that there is adequate working space anteriorly. Goggles should be placed before draping, because the instruments for placing anchors in the lesser tuberosity will pass very close to the patient's face. G, glenoid; H, humeral head.

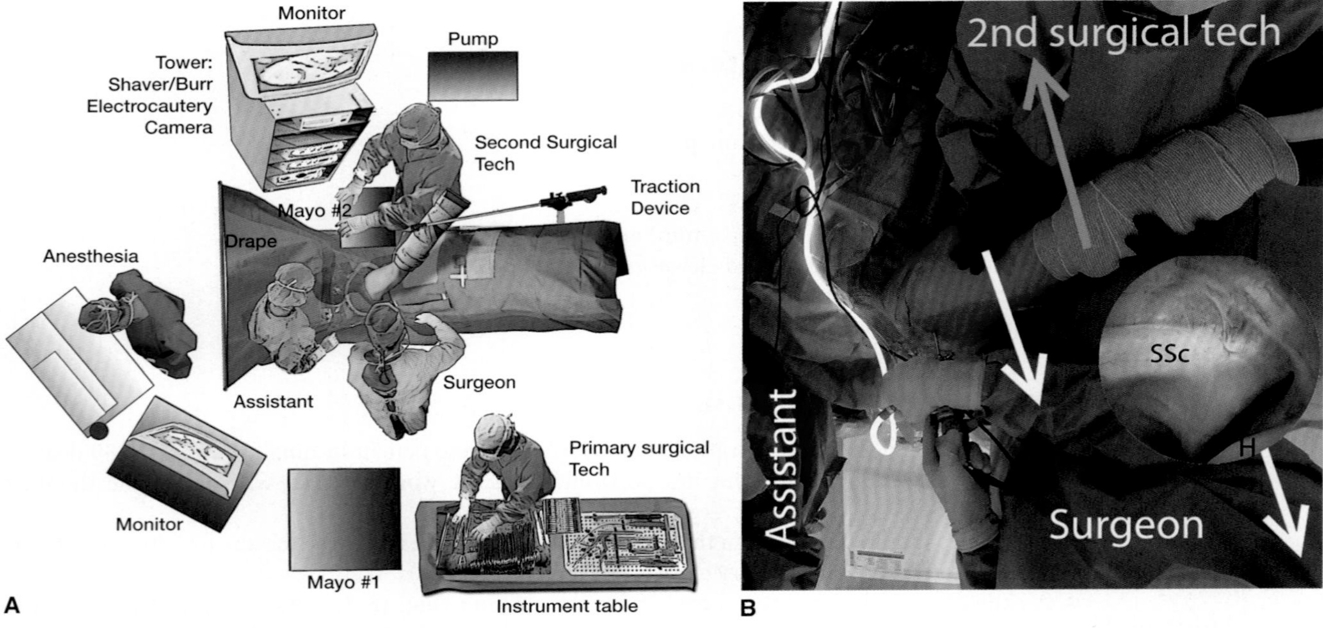

Figure 16-2 | Schematic **(A)** and photo **(B)** of our standard operating room setup (right shoulder) demonstrates how the second surgical technician can apply the posterior lever push to improve the arthroscopic view (**inset**) of the subscapularis (SSc) and lesser tuberosity. A posterior force is applied to the upper arm (*white arrow*), and an anterior counter force is applied to the lower arm (*green arrow*), H, humeral head.

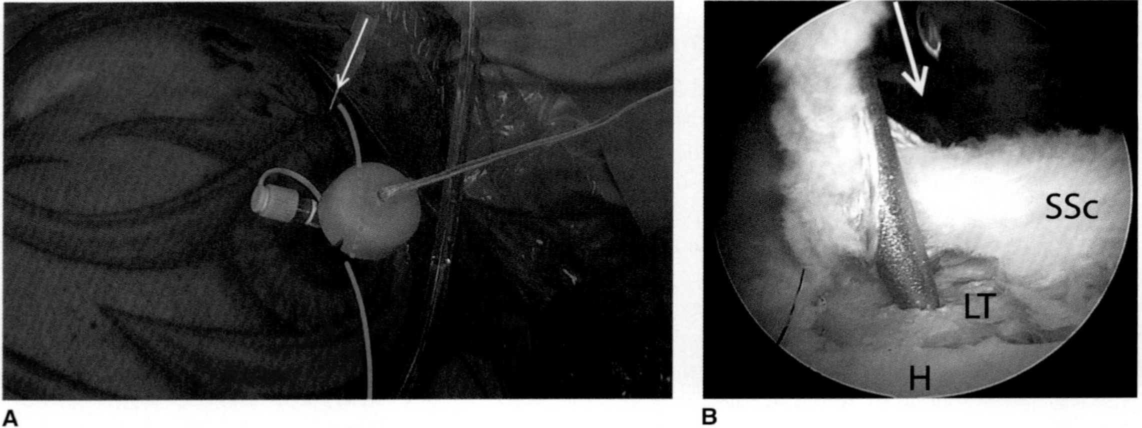

Figure 16-3 | Left shoulder external view **(A)** and 70-degree arthroscopic view **(B)**. The anterosuperior-lateral (ASL) portal (cannulated) is typically located just off the anterolateral corner of the acromion (*blue line*) on the skin. A spinal needle (*white arrow*) shows the location of an accessory anterior portal, which often seems "very medial" but is necessary to gain the correct angle of approach (*white arrow*, **B**) to the lesser tuberosity (LT). H, humeral head; SSc, subscapularis.

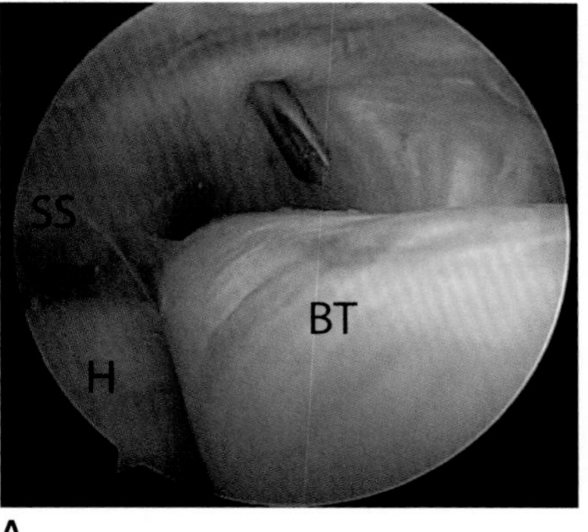

A

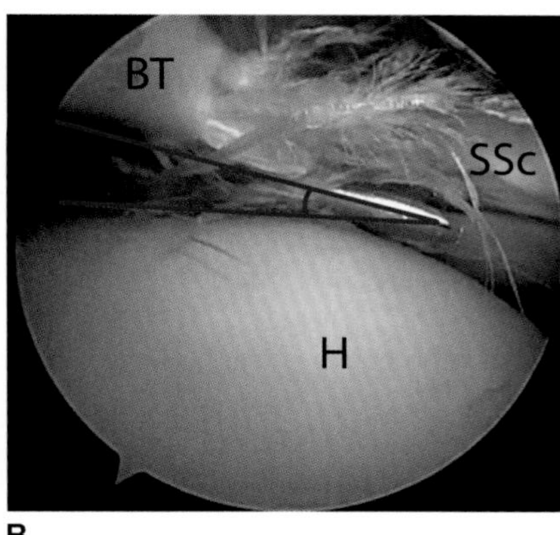

B

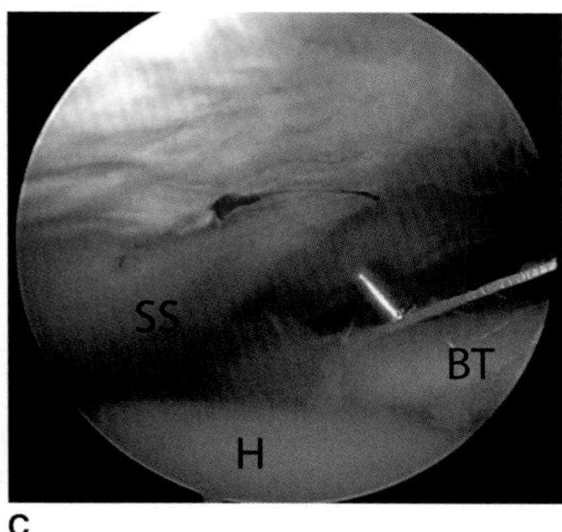

C

Figure 16-4 | Creation of an ASL portal (left shoulder) using an outside-in technique with a spinal needle to ensure the correct working angles from the chosen skin location. **A.** 70-degree view of the top of the bicipital groove shows a good angle for biceps tenodesis. **B.** 70-degree view of the tear shows a good working angle (shallow) to the lesser tuberosity. **C.** 30-degree view shows the portal created through the rotator interval anterior to the supraspinatus tendon (SS). Note the high-grade partial tearing of the medially subluxated BT **(B)**. BT; biceps tendon; H, humeral head; SSc, subscapularis.

groove (for a high tenodesis) (Fig. 16-4A) with a shallow (10 to 15 degrees) angle to the lesser tuberosity (Fig. 16-4B).
    - The ASL portal is made anterior to the supraspinatus through the rotator interval (Fig. 16-4C).
    - A cannula usually is used through the ASL portal.
  - Anterior portal(s) usually are required for anchor placement to improve the angle of approach to the lesser tuberosity (Figs. 16-3B and 16-11)
    - Spinal needle placement often appears to be "very medial" on the skin (Fig. 16-3A).
    - Anterior portals can be used for retrograde suture passage or for suture management and typically are percutaneous (noncannulated).
- Diagnostic techniques
  - Subscapularis tears remain generally underrecognized and undertreated. A high index of suspicion and a systematic examination of the bicipital groove, subcoracoid space, and tendon insertion should be used to avoid a missed diagnosis.
  - Use of a 70-degree arthroscope is critical when assessing these areas, because it greatly expands the surgeon's field of view (Fig. 16-5) and can aid in diagnosing occult tears.[2]
    - The medial side wall of the bicipital groove is examined for tearing (Fig. 16-12A and B), because this can reveal an occult tear.
    - Rarely, takedown of the medial sling is required to demonstrate an occult tear.[3]
  - The posterior lever push with internal rotation often reveals nonretracted (Fig. 16-5C) or occult subscapularis tears.
  - Viewing can be optimized by controlling bleeding through fluid management.

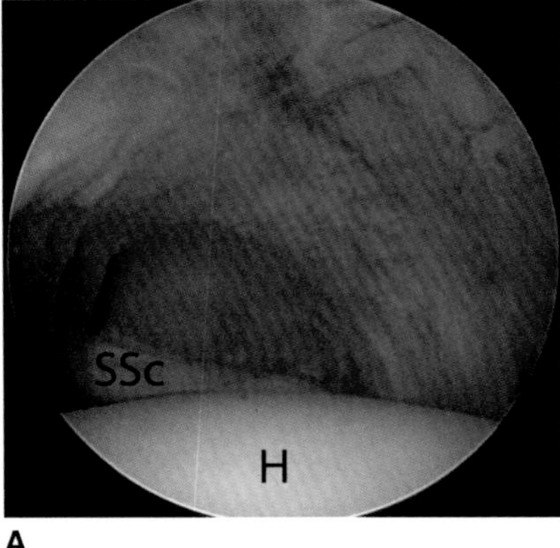

A

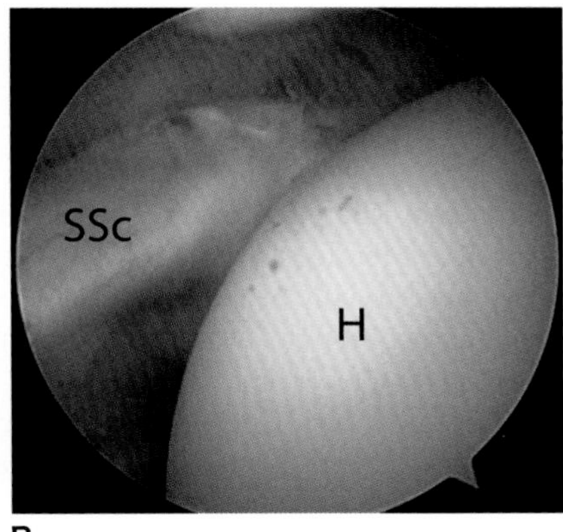

B

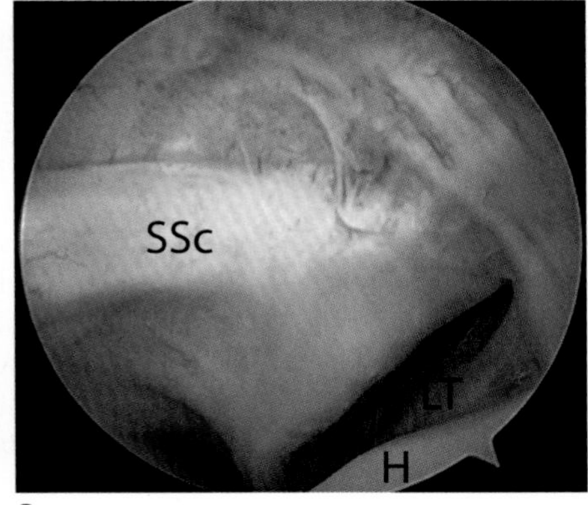

C

Figure 16-5 | The subscapularis (SSc) tendon often looks normal on casual inspection with a 30-degree scope (right shoulder) **(A)**. A 70-degree scope dramatically improves the view of the subscapularis **(B)**; however, the bare lesser tuberosity (LT) is not seen until internal rotation with the posterior lever push is applied **(C)**. H, humeral head.

- The pump is run at an adequate pressure (minimum 60 mm Hg).
- Fluid extravasation from portals is stopped with cannulas or the Dutch boy technique (manual pressure by assistant) to minimize fluctuations in pressure and turbulence.
- Recognition of the "comma sign" is critical when a retracted subscapularis tear is present.[4]
  - The comma tissue is the lateral part of the rotator interval capsule and contains the coracohumeral and superior glenohumeral ligaments.
  - The comma tissue connects the superolateral subscapularis tendon with the supraspinatus tendon.
- In primary, retracted subscapularis tears, the upper tendon border usually lies at the middle of the glenoid.

- Working in the subcoracoid space is essential in treating subscapularis tears.
  - Work in this area is always started by opening the rotator interval medial to the comma with a shaver or cautery from an ASL portal while viewing with a 30-degree arthroscope from a posterior portal (Fig. 16-6A).

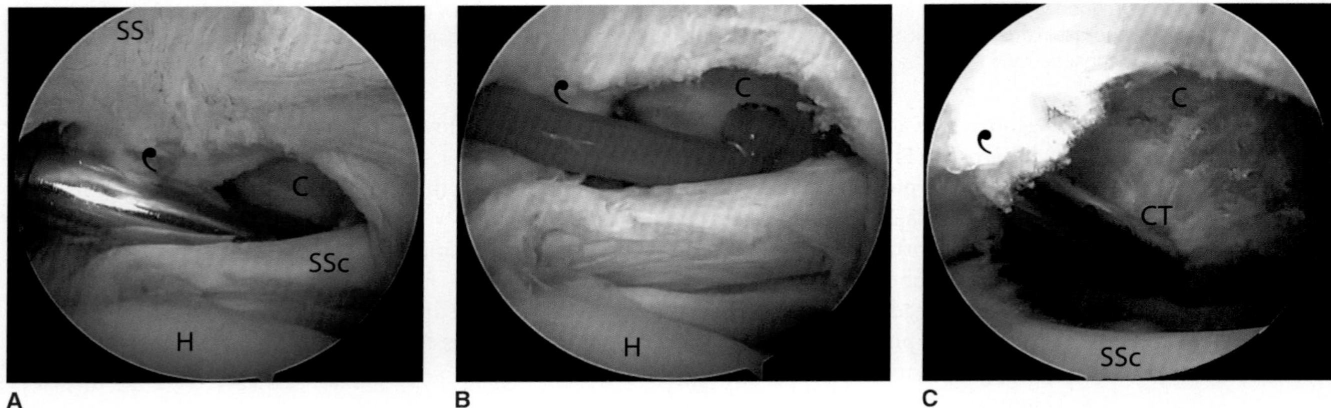

Figure 16-6 | Working in the subcoracoid space (left shoulder) requires repositioning of instruments posterior **(A and B)** and anterior **(C)** to the comma tissue (*black comma symbol*). Work with a 30-degree scope **(A and B)** until the interval has been opened and landmarks defined. A 70-degree scope improves the view **(C)** for working anterior to the tendon. C, coracoid; CT, conjoint tendon; H, humeral head; SS, supraspinatus tendon; SSc, subscapularis tendon.

- Once the anatomic landmarks have been identified, switching to a 70-degree scope allows an excellent view of the entire subcoracoid space (Figs. 16-6C and 16-7B) and lesser tuberosity footprint (Fig. 16-7F).
- The comma tissue is preserved (Figs. 16-6 and 16-7) because this tissue:
  - Acts as a "rip stop" for sutures of the upper tendon
  - Aids in reduction of the supraspinatus when a retracted anterosuperior tear exists
- As needed, instruments are used either anterior (Fig. 16-6A and B) or posterior (Fig. 16-6C) to the comma to expose the coracoid, conjoint tendon, subscapularis tendon, and lesser tuberosity by removing pathologic fibrofatty and bursal tissue.

Repair Techniques

- All subscapularis tendon tears where there has been fiber failure from the footprint (Fig. 16-7F) are repaired. Abrasive wear of the tendon (Fig. 16-7E) or linear, longitudinal tearing without failure at the tendon insertion can occasionally be treated by subcoracoid decompression (Fig. 16-7) alone.
  - Subcoracoid stenosis (coracohumeral distance <6 mm) (Fig. 16-7B) is treated by removing any coracoid tip osteophyte with a burr (Fig. 16-7C).
  - The end point of this step occurs when the posterior coracoid is coplanar with the conjoint tendon and there exists 7-10 mm of space between the coracoid and the subscapularis tendon (Fig. 16-7D).
- Lesser tuberosity bone bed preparation is critical when repairing the subscapularis.
  - All soft tissue remnants are removed with electrocautery (Fig. 16-8A).
  - The "charcoal" bone is removed with a burr on reverse or a ring curette (Fig. 16-8B) to expose healthy bone to maximize the chances of healing of the repair.

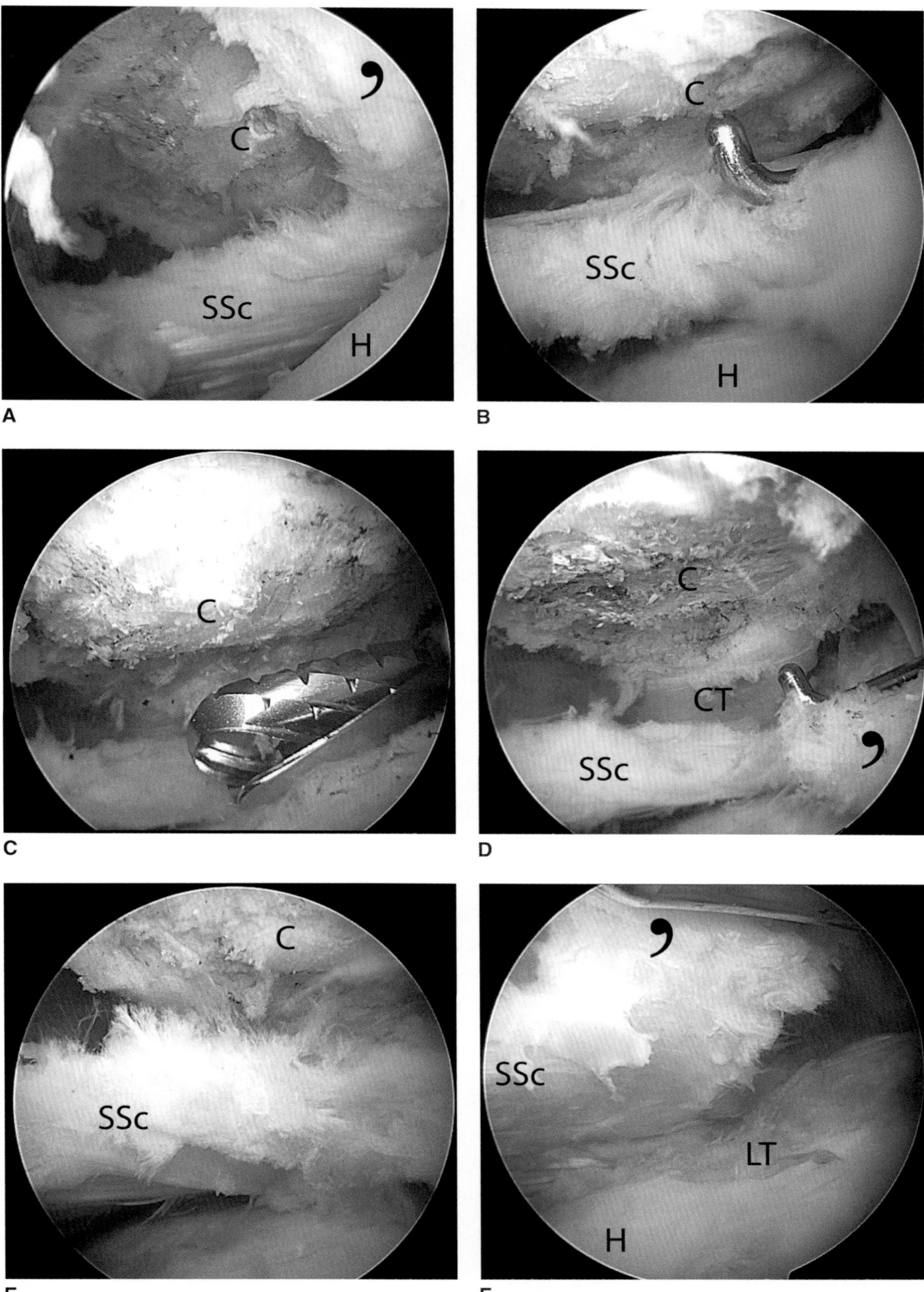

Figure 16-7 | Coracoplasty technique (right shoulder, 30 degree **(A)** and 70 degree **(B-F)** views). **A.** The rotator interval has been opened while preserving the comma tissue (*black comma symbol*) to show a coracoid **(C)** tip osteophyte. **B.** Before coracoplasty, less than a 3-mm coracohumeral interval is present with upper subscapularis (SSc) fraying **(E)** from impingement on the osteophyte. **C.** A high-speed burr is used to perform the coracoplasty from an ASL working portal with the instrument anterior to the comma. **D.** The end point of coracoplasty is a 7- to 10-mm coracohumeral interval and the conjoint tendon (CT) coplanar with the coracoid. **F.** Internal rotation and the posterior lever push bring the lesser tuberosity (LT) bone into the working space. H, humeral head.

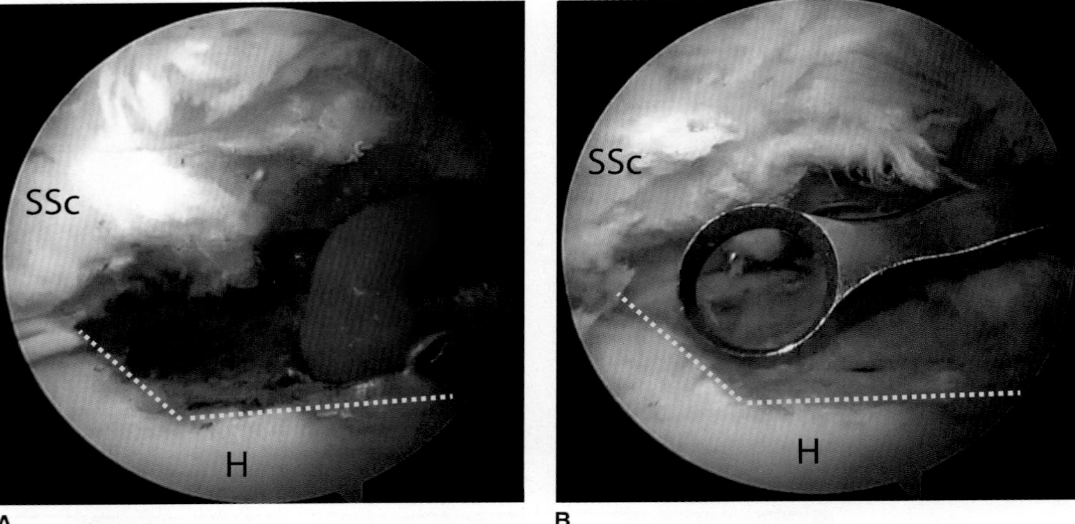

Figure 16-8 | Lesser tuberosity bone bed preparation (right shoulder) viewing with a 70-degree arthroscope and working from an ASL portal. The typical, "sharp angled" appearance of the superomedial border of the lesser tuberosity articular margin is outlined in *dotted yellow*. **A.** Electrocautery is used to remove soft tissue remnants. **B.** Ring curette (shown) or burr on reverse is used to remove the "charcoal" bone leaving a healthy bone bed with a sharp articular margin. H, humeral head; SSc, subscapularis.

Retracted Subscapularis Tears

- Most retracted subscapularis tendon tears can be repaired primarily or to a slightly (~5 mm) medialized bone bed[5]; however, a three-sided release may be necessary (Fig. 16-9).
  - The comma tissue is identified and protected.
  - A traction suture is placed at the junction of the comma and upper tendon border (Fig. 16-13A and B) through the ASL portal but maintained outside of the cannula.
  - Anterior (Fig. 16-9A) and superior (Fig. 16-9B) releases involve skeletonizing the coracoid from lateral (tip) along the neck to the base to release adhesions between the subscapularis tendon and the bone.
    - A combination of electrocautery and shaver is used (Fig. 16-9A).
    - The subscapularis is freed from the deep fascia and conjoint tendon, if necessary, respecting the proximity of the musculocutaneous nerve.
    - A 30-degree elevator is used bluntly under the neck of the coracoid (Fig. 16-9B) to lyse adhesions in this area (it is unnecessary and risky to dissect medial to the neck).
  - Posterior release (Fig. 16-9C) involves freeing adhesions between the subscapularis and the scapula.
    - Blunt dissection with a 15-degree elevator is used typically, as this is a relatively avascular plane.

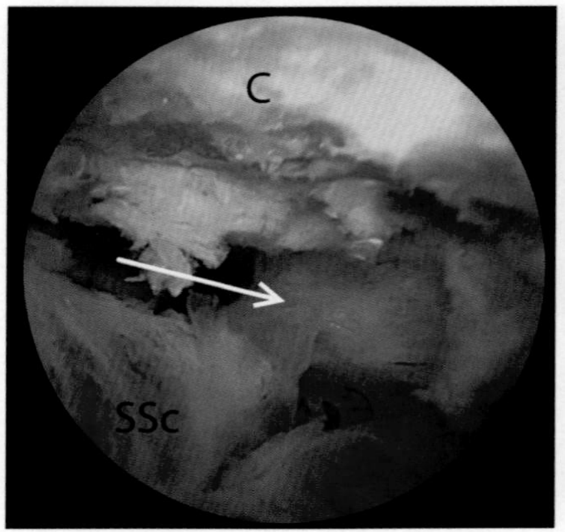

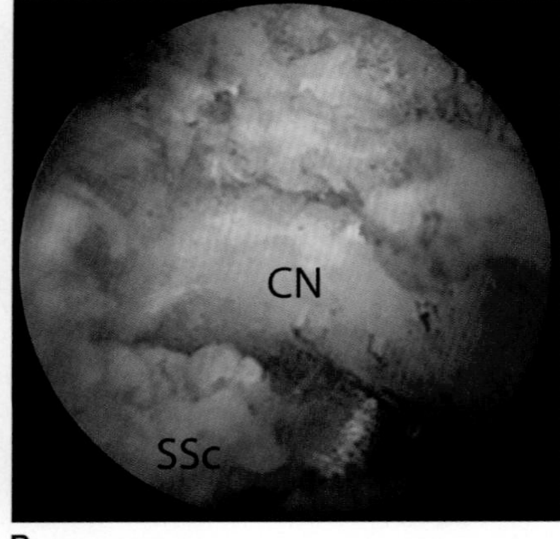

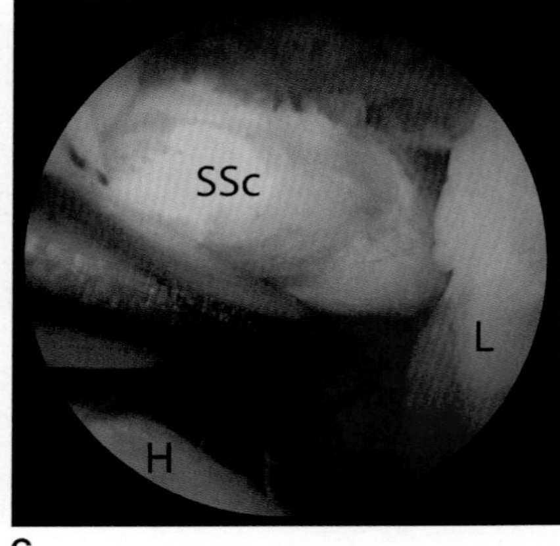

Figure 16-9 | Left shoulder 70-degree arthroscopic views showing three-sided subscapularis releases. **A.** The anterior release involves lysis of adhesions between the coracoid (**C**) and the subscapularis tendon (SSc). A shaver from anterosuperior is used to resect adhesions in this area (*white arrow*). **B.** A 30-degree arthroscopic elevator bluntly releases adhesions between the tendon and the coracoid neck (CN). **C.** A 15-degree elevator is used to free the posterior subscapularis from the anterior scapula. H, humeral head; L, anterior labrum.

Partial-Thickness and Full-Thickness Upper Subscapularis Tears

- Tears of the upper 50% of the subscapularis tendon (Fig. 16-10A) fixed with a single anchor (Fig. 16-10B) represent the majority of repairs in our practice.
  - A tape suture secured with a knotless, threaded suture anchor (eg, FiberTape and SwiveLock, Arthrex, Inc., Naples, FL) is a very efficient construct (SpeedFix, Arthrex, Inc., Naples, FL).[6]
    - Usually the tape suture is passed antegrade (Fig. 16-10C and D) (eg, Scorpion suture passer, Arthrex, Inc., Naples, FL) through the ASL portal.
    - The anchor (Fig. 16-11) is placed through the ASL portal or through an accessory anterior portal, depending on the best angle of approach (Fig. 16-11).
  - Sutures (no. 2 FiberWire, Arthrex, Inc., Naples, FL) from a high biceps tenodesis construct can be used to suture the upper subscapularis tendon (Fig. 16-12).
    - The tenodesis socket is placed slightly medial at the top of the groove (Fig. 16-12D) so that the tendon is compressed against the lesser tuberosity (Fig. 16-12F).
    - One FiberWire limb from each suture pair is passed antegrade using a Scorpion through the ASL portal.
    - The sutures are tied with a six-throw surgeon's knot[7] with a double-diameter knot pusher (6th Finger, Arthrex, Inc., Naples, FL).
    - This is most commonly done as a single-portal technique.

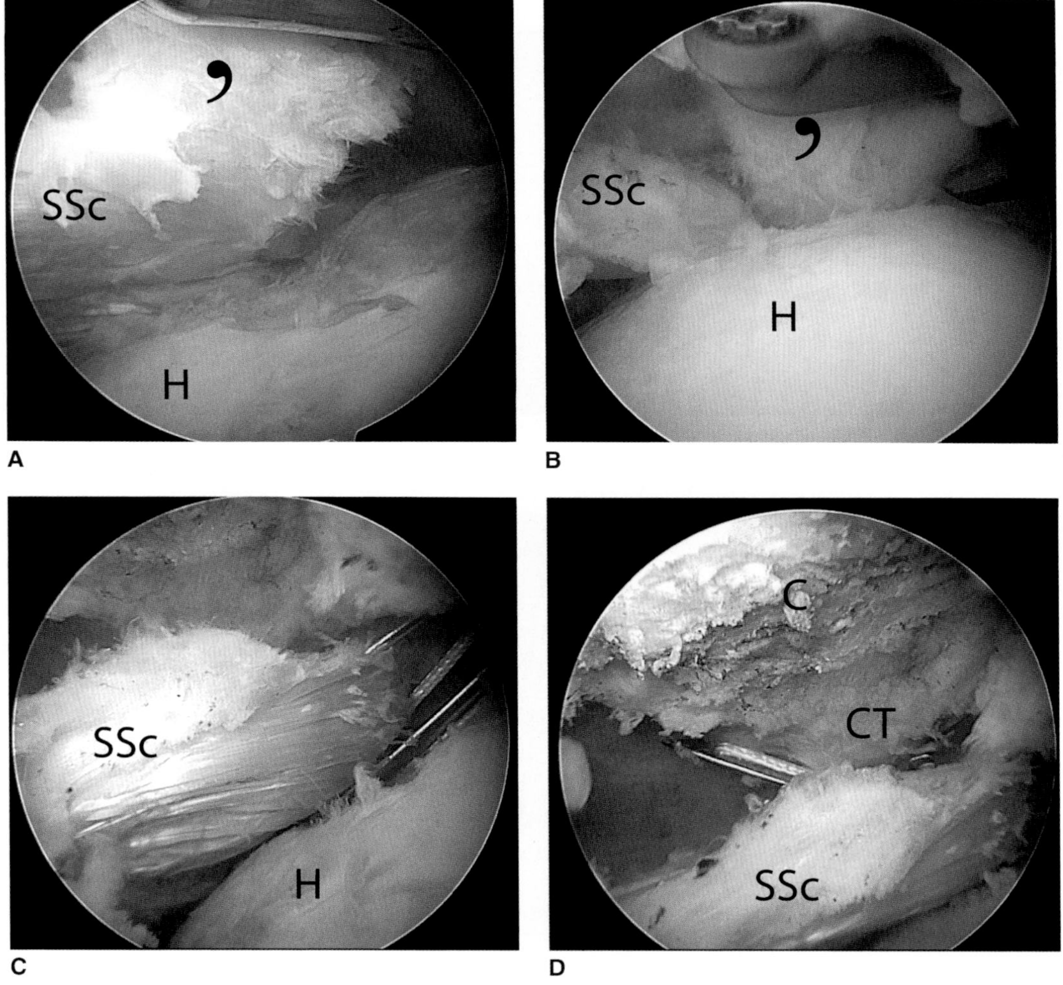

Figure 16-10 | SpeedFix upper subscapularis repair (right shoulder). **A.** 70-degree view demonstrates the subscapularis (SSc) tear and **(B)** final anatomic repair (30-degree view) with preserved comma tissue (*black comma symbol*). **(C)** A FiberTape suture is passed through the ASL working portal with a Scorpion suture passer **(D)**. Care must be taken to not fire the Scorpion needle against the coracoid **(C)** or into the conjoint tendon (CT). The suture tails are retrieved out of the anterior portal, threaded through the eyelet of the anchor, and secured using a SwiveLock anchor **(E)**. After the FiberTape has been cut **(F)**, the final construct is very low profile (70 degrees view). C, coracoid; CT, conjoint tendon; H, humeral head; LT, lesser tuberosity.

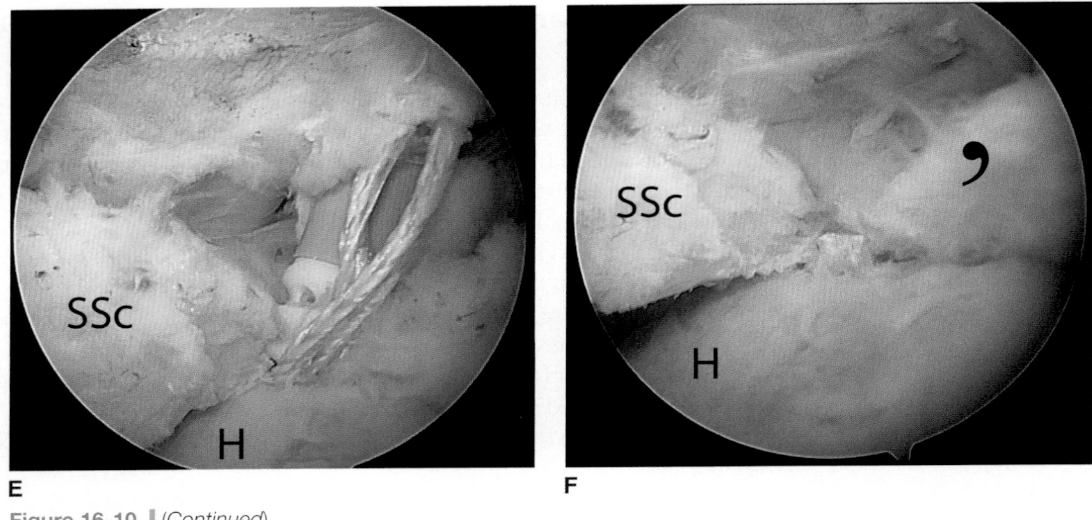

Figure 16-10 | (*Continued*)

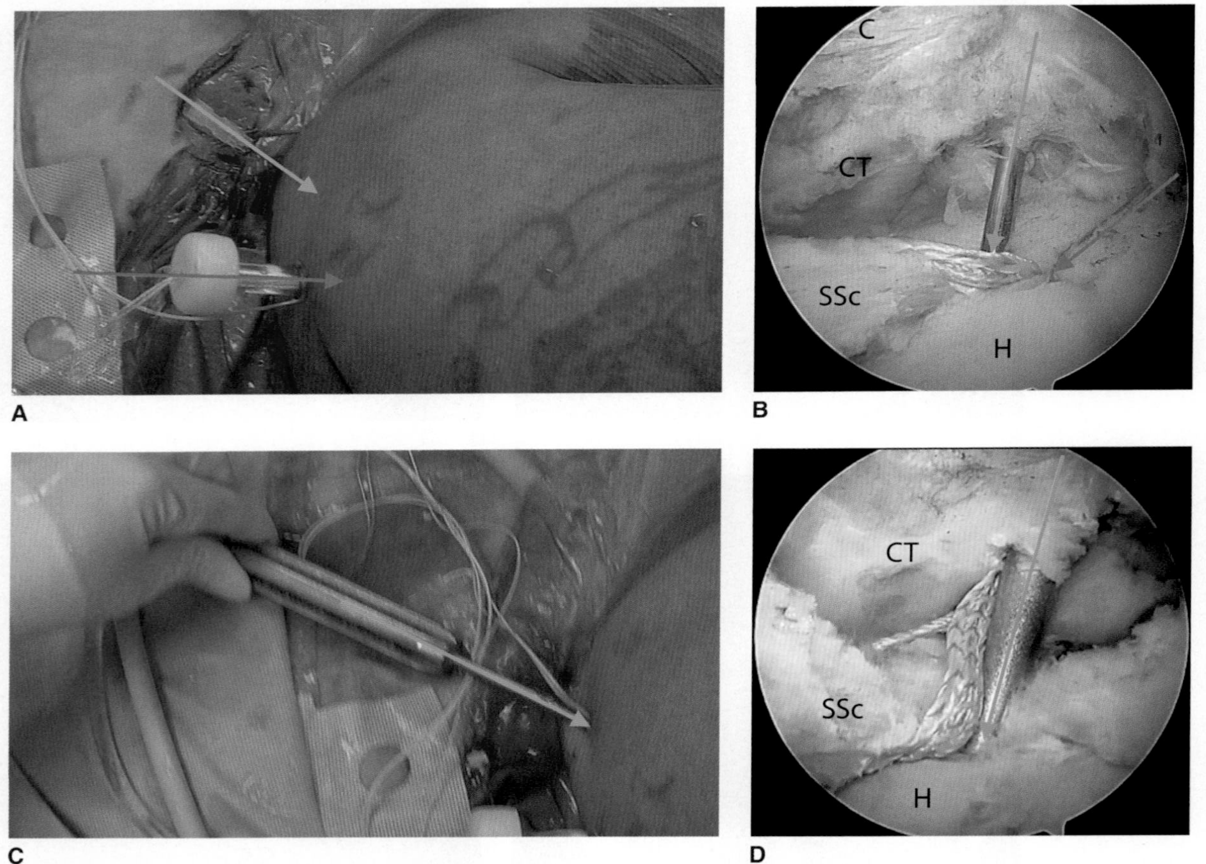

Figure 16-11 | Right shoulder external **(A and C)** and 70-degree arthroscopic **(B and D)** views demonstrate how an accessory anterior portal often is required to gain the appropriate angle to the lesser tuberosity (*green arrows*). This angle often results in instruments being used very close to the patient's face **(C)** because of the retroversion of the proximal humerus. Depending on the patient's anatomy, an ASL portal (*red arrow*) also can provide a good angle of approach for upper subscapularis anchor placement with rotation of the humerus. C, coracoid; CT, conjoint tendon; H, humeral head; SSc, subscapularis.

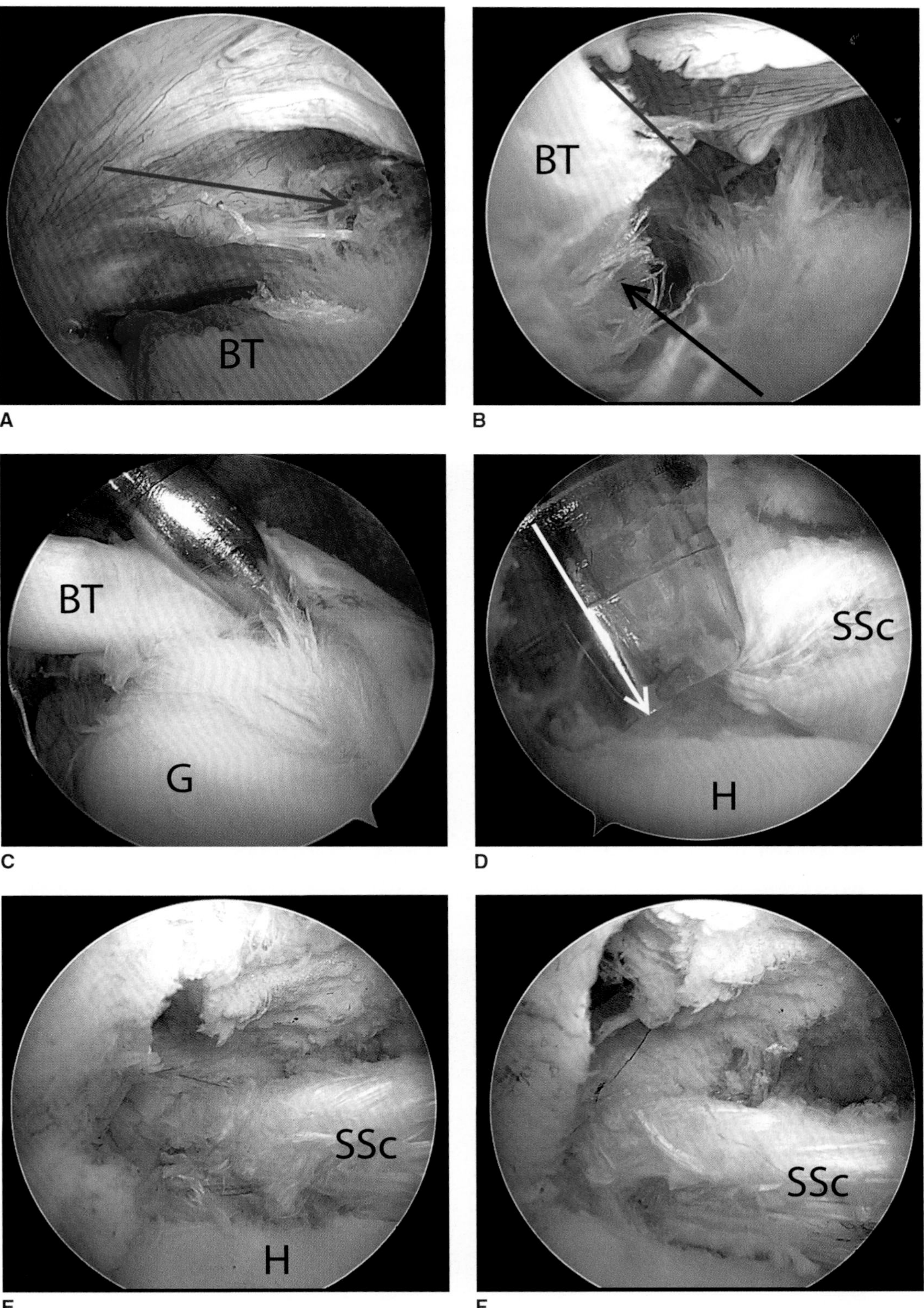

Figure 16-12 | Left shoulder upper subscapularis tear repaired using biceps tenodesis construct sutures. **A.** 70-degree view down the bicipital groove shows medial side wall high-grade tearing (*blue arrows*) and **(B)** abrasive wear (*black arrow*) of the medial biceps tendon (BT). Additionally, this patient had a type 2 SLAP tear with a displaceable biceps root **(C)**. An arthroscopic biceps tenodesis **(D)** was performed, with the tenodesis socket placed slightly medially at the top of the groove (*white arrow* shows guide pin for a cannulated reamer). After the tenodesis screw has been placed, no. 2 FiberWire sutures (typically 2 pairs of sutures) are then available to be passed **(E)** and tied for subscapularis (SSc) repair **(F)**. G, glenoid; H, humeral head.

Multiple Anchor and Double-Row Repairs

Larger subscapularis tears may require additional anchors and/or linked, double-row fixation.

- Two medial suture anchors are used for tears larger than 50% of the superoinferior length of the lesser tuberosity (rule of thumb: one double-loaded suture anchor [5.5 or 4.5 mm BioComposite FT CorkScrew (Arthrex, Inc., Naples, FL)] is used for each linear centimeter of tear).
  - The inferior medial anchor can be placed transtendon for nonretracted tears (Fig. 16-13A and B), from lateral to the retracted edge (ensure a good angle of approach using spinal needle), or by coming "over the top" of the superior border of the subscapularis (Fig. 16-14C).
  - In the case of two medial anchors, sutures can be passed and tied using a double-pulley construct (Fig. 16-14F and J), in a horizontal mattress fashion (Fig. 16-13C and D) or as simple sutures.
- Linked, double-row repairs of the subscapularis may require novel constructs, as the "real estate" for lateral row anchors can be limited.
  - Double-row repair should be attempted for large (50%-100% bare lesser tuberosity) tears (Fig. 16-14B), particularly those that are full thickness from medial to lateral and retracted.

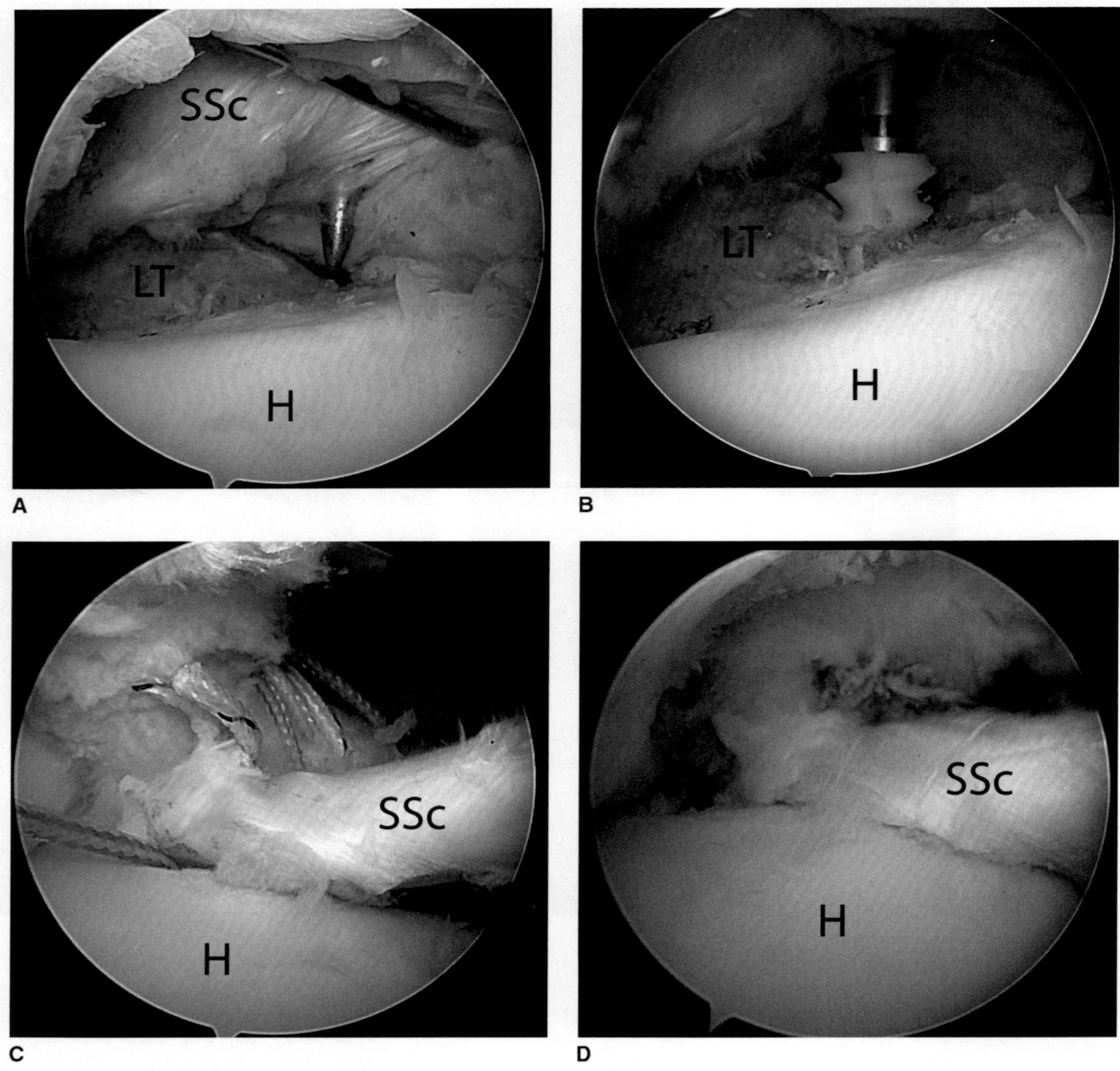

Figure 16-13 | Left shoulder single-row subscapularis (SSc) repair with two medial anchors. **A.** 70-degree view showing a bone socket being punched transtendon with the lower medial anchor **(B)** also being inserted in this fashion. The sutures from both medial anchors have been passed **(C)** in mattress fashion and then tied using a double-diameter knot pusher. The final construct **(D)** shows an anatomic repair. H, humeral head; LT, lesser tuberosity.

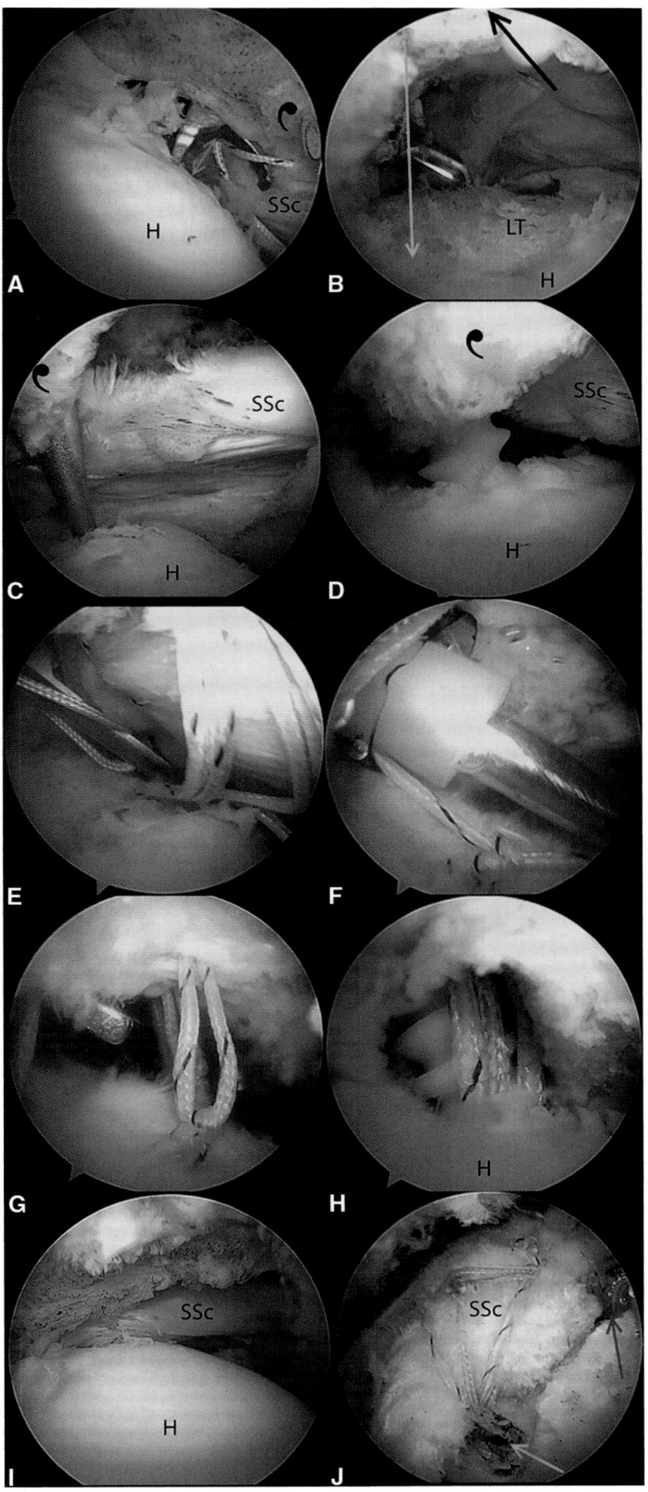

Figure 16-14 | Left shoulder showing a linked, double-row subscapularis repair (SpeedBridge). **A.** In this case, even with a posterior lever push, there was limited working space (*red double arrow*) anteriorly. A traction suture placed at the junction of the comma tissue (*black comma symbol*) and the upper subscapularis (SSc) is being retrieved out of an accessory anterior portal. **B.** The working space (*green double arrow*) has been dramatically improved with anteriorly directed traction (*black arrow*) from the traction suture. Nearly the entire lesser tuberosity (LT) has bare bone. **C.** The punch for the lower medial anchor is being brought in superior to the subscapularis tendon. This anchor also can be placed transtendon. **D.** The superomedial anchor is inserted at the superomedial aspect of the LT. **E.** Antegrade lower medial anchor suture passage using a Scorpion from the ASL portal. **F.** The final six-throw surgeon's knot is tied in the subcoracoid space completing a medial double-pulley construct (*white sutures* from each anchor tied together as a double mattress). **G.** The *blue sutures* from each anchor passed and tied as standard horizontal mattresses. Half of the suture limbs were retrieved and fixed laterally to SwiveLock anchors **(H)**. The final 70-degree intra-articular **(I)** and subacromial **(J)** views of the repair show anatomic restoration of the footprint. In this case, because the biceps tendon had been chronically torn, the bicipital groove was unobstructed for placement of inferior (*orange arrow*) and superior (*blue arrow*) lateral row anchors. H, humeral head.

- If a SpeedFix upper tendon repair has not fully restored the footprint, the FiberTape suture can be left long and secured laterally into a biceps tenodesis construct or another SwiveLock anchor as a linked, double-row construct.[8]
- If the LHB tendon has been chronically torn and retracted (or with tenotomy), there may be adequate room for a true SutureBridge or SpeedBridge (Arthrex, Inc., Naples, FL) repair with two lateral row knotless anchors (Fig. 16-14).

- In the case of planned LHB tenodesis, most of the subscapularis repair can be completed up to placement of an inferolateral row anchor. Then the biceps tenodesis can be completed with the tenodesis anchor (BioComposite SwiveLock Tenodesis or Bio-Tenodesis, Arthrex, Inc., Naples, FL) serving as the superolateral row anchor.

Postoperative Care

Arthroscopic rotator cuff repair allows postoperative rehabilitation that prioritizes tendon-to-bone healing over early, aggressive shoulder range of motion, as the risk of stiffness is low.[9,10]

- 0-6 weeks: Sling immobilization
  - Three times daily passive external rotation of shoulder with the arm at the side (PVC cane) to 0 degrees (larger, full-thickness subscapularis tears) or 30 degrees (small, partial-thickness subscapularis tears).
  - Isolated subscapularis tears or other at-risk patients (calcific tendonitis, adhesive capsulitis, concomitant labral repair) perform early, closed chain, passive overhead motion (table slide)
- 6-12 weeks: Sling is discontinued and full passive range of motion (ROM) is added.
  - Full passive external rotation (ER) stretching is begun.
  - Rope and pulley overhead and behind back internal rotation stretches are begun.
  - Arm can be used for light activities of daily living below shoulder level.
- 3-6 months: Full active overhead ROM and strengthening
  - Rubber band strengthening is initiated.
  - No heavy overhead lifting and no acceleration of arm in sport is allowed.

References

1. Brady PC, Narbona P, Adams CR, et al. Arthroscopic proximal biceps tenodesis at the articular margin: evaluation of outcomes, complications, and revision rate. *Arthroscopy.* 2015;31(3):470-476.
2. Sheean AJ, Hartzler RU, Denard PJ, Lädermann A, Hanypsiak BT, Burkhart SS. A 70° arthroscope significantly improves visualization of the bicipital groove in the lateral decubitus position. *Arthroscopy.* 2016;32(9):1745-1749.
3. Hartzler RU, Burkhart SS. Medial biceps sling takedown may be necessary to expose an occult subscapularis tendon tear. *Arthrosc Tech.* 2014;3(6):e719-e722.
4. Lo IK, Burkhart SS. The comma sign: an arthroscopic guide to the torn subscapularis tendon. *Arthroscopy.* 2003;19(3):334-337.
5. Denard PJ, Burkhart SS. Medialization of the subscapularis footprint does not affect functional outcome of arthroscopic repair. *Arthroscopy.* 2012;28(11):1608-1614.
6. Denard PJ, Burkhart SS. A new method for knotless fixation of an upper subscapularis tear. *Arthroscopy.* 2011;27(6):861-866.
7. Burkhart SS, Lo IK, Brady PC. *Burkhart's View of the Shoulder: A Cowboy's Guide to Advanced Shoulder Arthroscopy.* Philadelphia, PA: Lippincott Williams & Wilkins; 2006:48-52.
8. Denard PJ, Lädermann A, Burkhart SS. Double-row fixation of upper subscapularis tears with a single suture anchor. *Arthroscopy.* 2011;27(8):1142-1149.
9. Koo SS, Parsley BK, Burkhart SS, Schoolfield JD. Reduction of postoperative stiffness after arthroscopic rotator cuff repair: results of a customized physical therapy regimen based on risk factors for stiffness. *Arthroscopy.* 2011;27(2):155-160.
10. Huberty DP, Schoolfield JD, Brady PC, Vadala AP, Arrigoni P, Burkhart SS. Incidence and treatment of postoperative stiffness following arthroscopic rotator cuff repair. *Arthroscopy.* 2009;25(8):880-890.

Chapter 17

Arthroscopic Biceps Tenodesis

JASON P. ROGERS
W. STEPHEN CHOATE
JOHN M. TOKISH

Sterile Instruments/Equipment

- Standard arthroscopic shoulder set, including a SutureLasso (Arthrex, Naples, FL) or equivalent and an arthroscopic grasper with ability to lock
- 30-degree arthroscope
- Bipolar radiofrequency (RF) thermal ablation device. Our preference is the 90-degree wand.
- Two clear, plastic cannulas: one 7-mm Twist-In and one 8-mm Twist-In (Arthrex, Naples, FL)
- Power drill for anchor placement
- Free no. 2 nonabsorbable sutures
- SwiveLock (Arthrex, Naples, FL), 4.75- × 19.1-mm biocomposite knotless anchor. We use a larger-diameter anchor in poor-quality bone.

Positioning

- The patient is positioned in the lateral decubitus position (Fig. 17-1).
  - All bony prominences are carefully padded, including the contralateral elbow (radial and ulnar nerves), greater trochanter, fibular head (peroneal nerve), and ankle malleoli.
- See Chapter 1 for full description.

Surgical Approach

- Accurate identification and marking of bony anatomy prior to starting the case is paramount for success in establishing portals.
  - Important landmarks include the posterolateral acromion edge, acromioclavicular joint, coracoid tip, scapular spine, clavicle (posterior border specifically), and lateral midacromion.
- Standard posterior, anterior interval (midglenoid), and lateral portals are used. An accessory "falciform" portal can be used for direct access to the bicipital groove.
  - The posterior viewing portal is positioned 2-3 cm inferior from and just medial to the posterolateral corner of the acromion.
  - The anterior interval portal is established lateral to the coracoid tip (never medial to avoid neurovascular structures) and halfway between acromioclavicular joint and anterolateral border of the acromion.
    - An "outside-in" technique with a spinal needle under direct visualization from posterior portal is used.
    - The anterior capsule is dilated with a hemostat to facilitate access in and out of the joint.

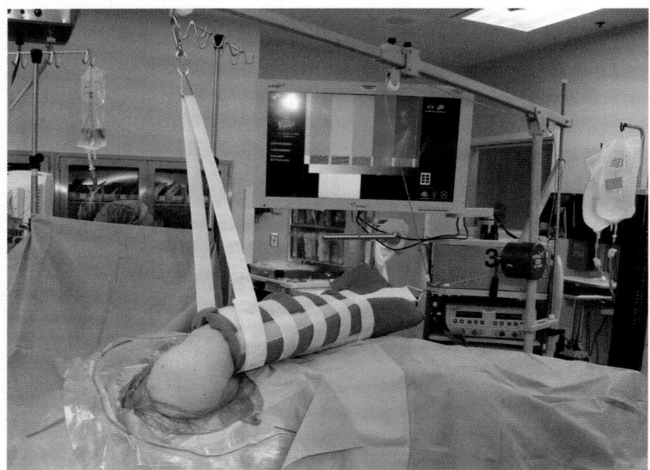

Figure 17-1 | Patient positioned in left lateral decubitus with lateral arm holder in place. White axillary straps provide lateral force, distracting the glenohumeral joint. Longitudinal traction is applied with weights off the end. Moving the weights to the middle pulley will provide abduction of the glenohumeral joint.

- The lateral portal is placed 3 cm off the lateral border of the acromion and exactly halfway between the anterior and posterior corners of the lateral acromion for a true "50-yard line" position.
  - The portal typically is established after the intra-articular portion of case is complete, and the arthroscope is in the subacromial space (Fig. 17-2).

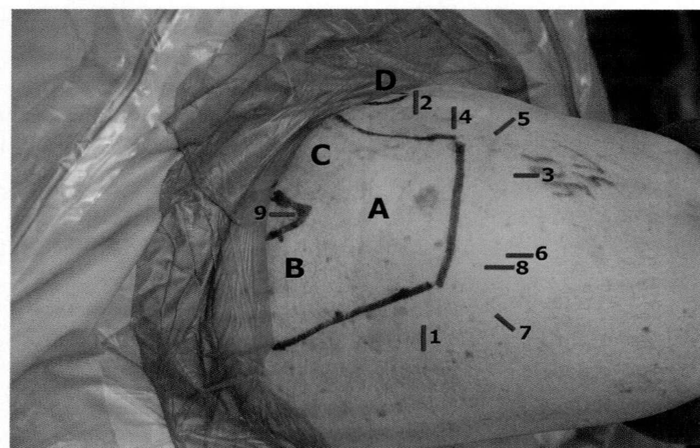

Figure 17-2 | The patient is in lateral decubitus position with sterile drapes in place and bony anatomy with all working portals marked. The typical portals used for shoulder arthroscopy include posterior (*1*), anterior central (may move distal for true midglenoid portal) (*2*), anterolateral (*3*), anterosuperior (*4*), anterosuperior-lateral (*5*), posterolateral (*6*), posterior 7 o'clock (*7*), Wilmington (*8*), and Neviaser (*9*).

- Glenohumeral joint
  - Following portal placement, intra-articular evaluation is performed in a systematic manner.
  - In the absence of instability or planned labral repair, the standard anterior interval portal is established and a probe is introduced into the joint (Fig. 17-3).

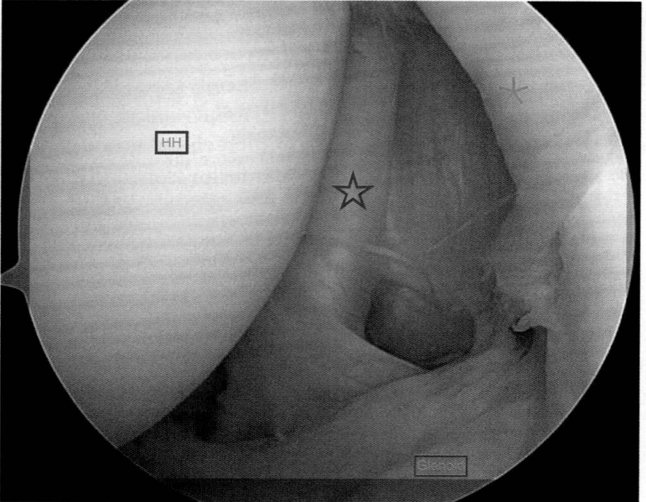

Figure 17-3 | Rotator interval. HH, humeral head; star, subscapularis; asterisk, LHBT.

- Diagnostic evaluation of the long head of the biceps tendon (LHBT) should assess for tearing, subluxation, tenosynovitis, and/or superior labral pathology. All such findings are indications to perform a biceps tenodesis (Figs. 17-4 to 17-6).

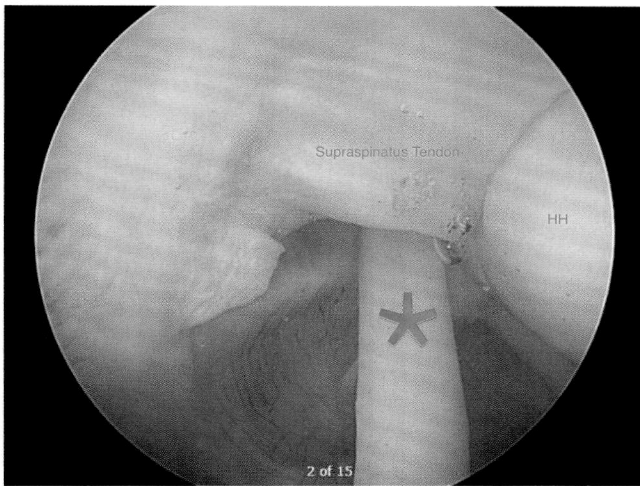

Figure 17-4 | Biceps sling. HH, humeral head; asterisk, LHBT.

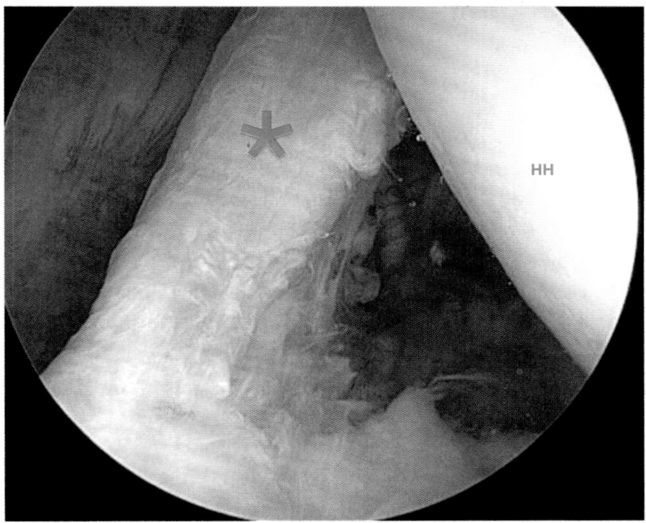

Figure 17-5 | Long head biceps tendon tearing intra-articularly without associated rotator cuff tear. HH, humeral head; asterisk, LHBT.

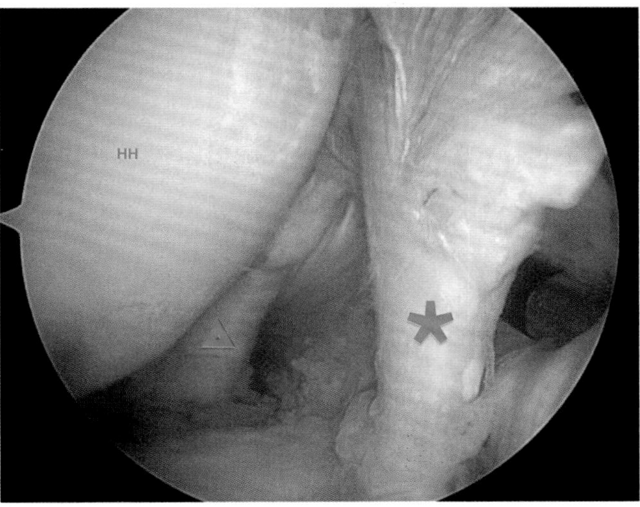

Figure 17-6 | Intra-articular long head biceps tendon tear with flattening in setting of concomitant massive, retracted rotator cuff tear. Triangle, subscapularis tendon; HH, humeral head; asterisk, LHBT.

- The intertubercular portion of the tendon is pulled into the joint for inspection. The anchor attachment at the superior labrum is probed for signs of instability and trauma (>5 mm of separation from the articular glenoid margin, detachment with positive peel back, local synovitis, or chondral damage) (Figs. 17-7 and 17-8).

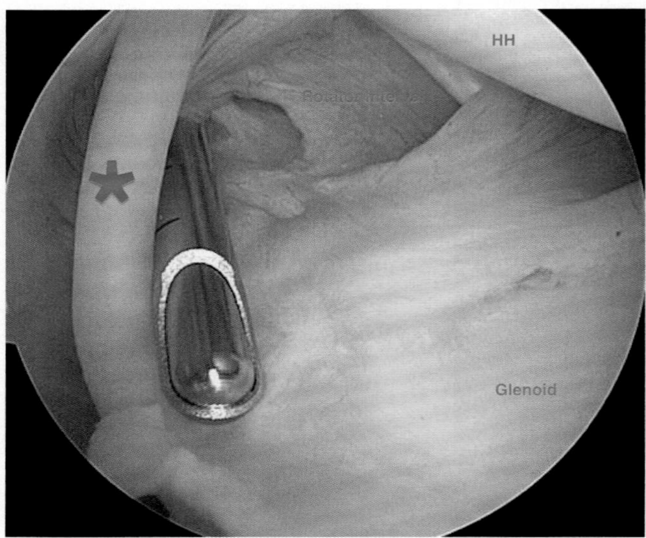

Figure 17-7 | Long head biceps tendon is delivered into the joint, using a probe or shaver, for further evaluation during the diagnostic portion of the case. HH, humeral head; asterisk, LHBT.

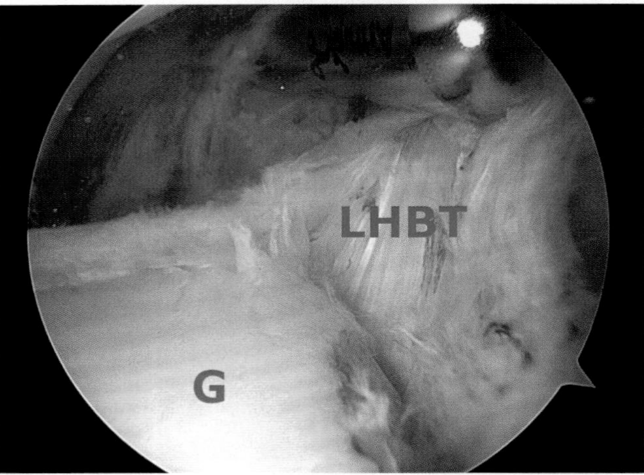

Figure 17-8 | Superior labral anterior to posterior (SLAP) tear type II. Shaver retracting LHBT. G, glenoid; LHBT, long head of the biceps tendon.

- Only 56% of the LHBT can be viewed from within the joint. This can be optimized with an arm position of 40 degrees abduction, 30 degrees forward flexion, and 90 degrees of elbow flexion.[1]

- Once LHBT pathology is confirmed and correlated with preoperative examination findings, the tendon is tenotomized. Care is taken to cut flush at the biceps-glenoid labrum interface to avoid leaving a stump of tissue. Otherwise, the residual stump is debrided or ablated.
  - Hypertrophic superior labral or residual biceps stump tissue can make passing sutures difficult during a concomitant rotator cuff repair.
- We prefer using curved Mayo scissors through the anterior interval portal, as shown in Figure 17-9, for the tenotomy. An RF ablation wand is an alternative option.

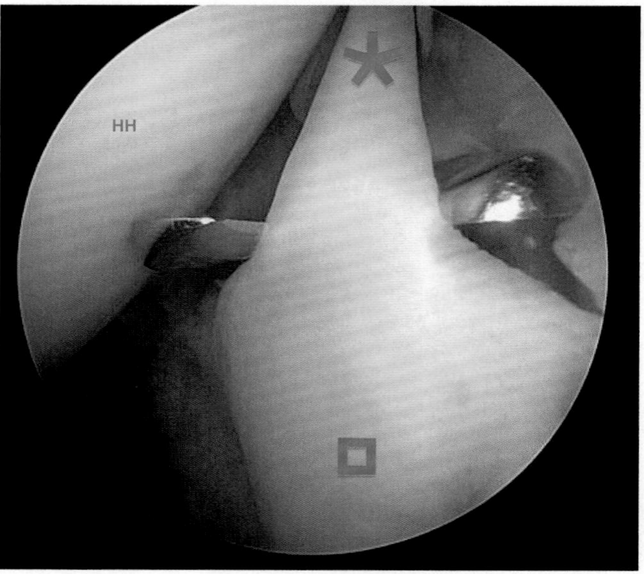

Figure 17-9 | Biceps tenotomy with Mayo scissors through the anterior interval portal. HH, humeral head; asterisk, LHBT; square, superior labrum.

- If anatomic tensioning of the biceps is desired for the tenodesis ("tension assured"), the tendon is identified, stitched, and fixed at its resting length in the subdeltoid space prior to intra-articular tenotomy.
- In the setting of a normal intra-articular examination but clinical suspicion for biceps pathology, the tendon can be left intact and the examination for pathology is completed in subdeltoid space. This often includes opening the bicipital groove for inspection.
  - LHBT pathology may be isolated to the distal aspect of the intertubercular groove in a watershed zone.[2]
- Subacromial/subdeltoid space
  - Once the intra-articular portion of the procedure is complete, the arthroscope is redirected through the posterior portal into the subacromial space.
  - The trocar tip is used to localize the coracoacromial ligament (CAL) and then swept laterally and posteriorly into the subdeltoid recess, avoiding the hypervascular medial bursal tissue.
  - The lateral working portal is established.
    - We strive to use the same portals to treat every patient; however, with isolated biceps pathology and no rotator cuff tearing, the lateral portal can be moved more anterior along the lateral edge of the acromion.
    - Our preference is to be 3 to 4 cm off the lateral edge of the acromion at the "50-yard" mark.
  - With the camera viewing up toward the CAL and acromial undersurface, the shaver is introduced through lateral portal and localized.
  - The camera is then turned down toward the rotator cuff, and bursectomy is performed.
    - We believe the keys to successful work in the subacromial/subdeltoid space are maintaining visual clarity and maximizing the working space.
    - Care is taken to protect the underlying cuff tissue, particularly in the setting of extensive scar and hypertrophied bursal tissue.
    - Shaving medial to the cuff myotendonous junction can provoke bleeding and is avoided.
    - Bursal tissue is cleared to the posterolateral corner to expose the infraspinatus/teres minor tendons and then moved laterally into the subdeltoid recess.
    - Using a shaver or thermal ablator, the subdeltoid recess is opened from the posterolateral corner to the subscapularis anteriorly. Adhesions and bursal connections to the humerus are important to resect without violating the deltoid fascia (Fig. 17-10).

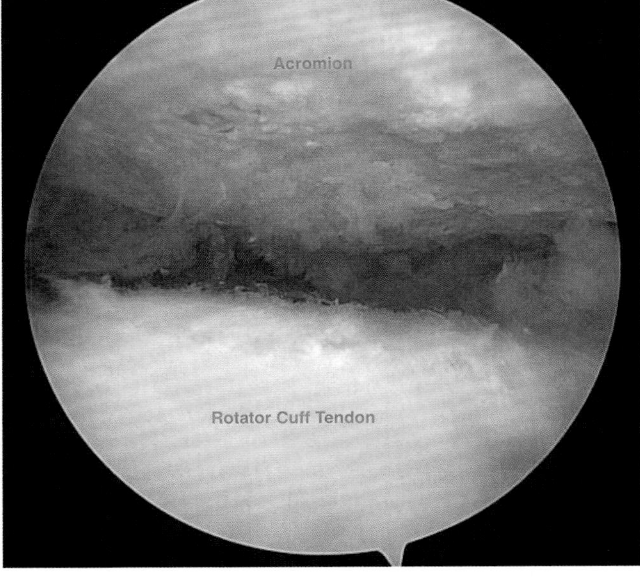

Figure 17-10 | Wide view of the subacromial space from the posterior portal after bursectomy.

- Following creation of a "room with a view," the bicipital groove and LHBT are localized.
  - External rotation of the shoulder is helpful in bringing these structures into view when the arthroscope is in the posterior portal.
  - The scope is driven anteriorly, looking down the humerus toward the pectoralis major tendon. The falciform ligament can be an important landmark to help locate the bicipital groove as it crosses over the groove in the inferior aspect of the space.
  - Other landmarks that can be helpful are the ascending branches of the anterior humeral circumflex vessels, which are visible lateral to the biceps. The conjoined tendon runs roughly parallel to the biceps and can be distinguished from it by the fact that it is "off the bone" as opposed to the biceps, which is "on the bone."
  - A straightforward method to finding the biceps is to begin at the CA ligament and follow this to the coracoid. The coracoid is then used to locate the conjoined tendon, which is followed inferiorly. The biceps is lateral to this in the distal aspect of the space.
  - Additional bursectomy should be carried out with a shaver or RF wand as necessary until the transverse fibers of the falciform ligament (upper border of pectoralis major tendon) are in view.
- An RF wand is used to dissect out the biceps, open up the transverse humeral ligament, and free the tendon from groove.
  - Bleeders can occur in the groove, usually lateral to the tendon.
- When using "tension-assured" method, the tendon remains at its native resting length and the working side of the 90-degree RF wand should be pointed away from the tendon while clearing out the groove. Working from posterior to anterior, the wand can be used to retract and push the tendon anteriorly as the groove borders are gradually exposed.
- If the LHB tendon has already been cut, a soft tissue locking grasper is inserted through the anterior portal, the free tendon end is grasped and then directed anterior and medial to the groove, out of harm's way (Figs. 17-11 and 17-12).

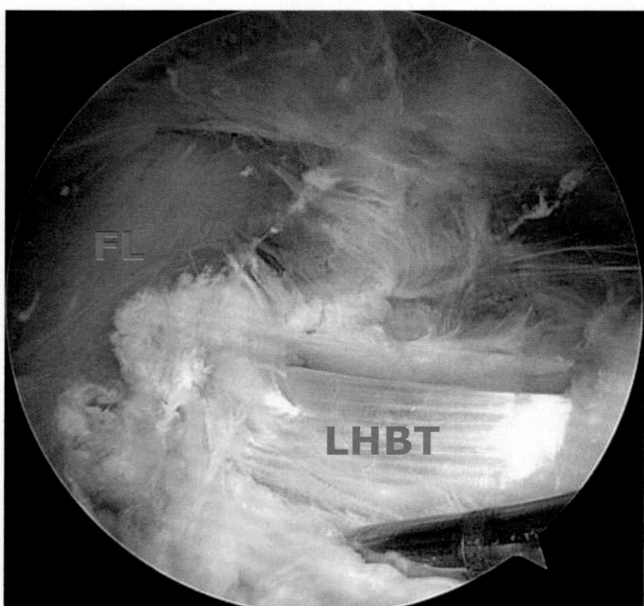

Figure 17-11 | Subdeltoid LHBT being dissected. Long head biceps tendon is adjacent to the probe. The falciform ligament is distal to the tip of the probe, and transverse humeral ligament is to the right of this view. FL, falciform ligament; LHBT, long head of the biceps tendon.

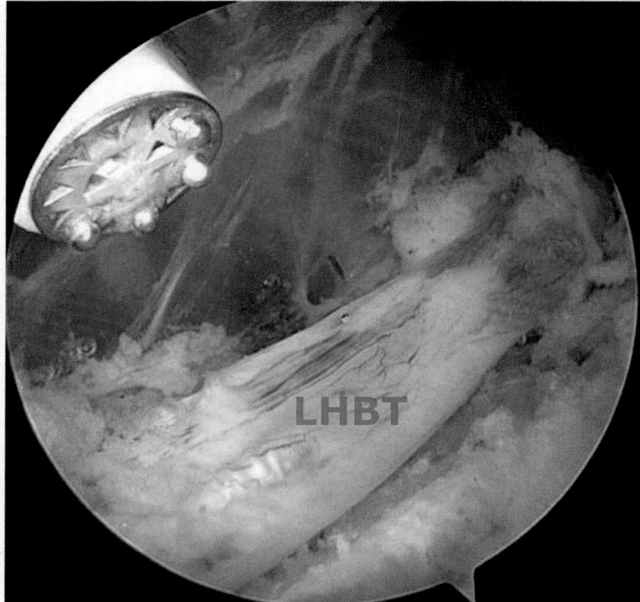

Figure 17-12 | LHBT is freed from tenosynovium, in subdeltoid space. LHBT, long head of the biceps tendon.

- For direct access to the bicipital groove, we recommend establishing an accessory, "falciform" portal at this juncture.
  - For localization, a line is dropped from anterolateral corner of the acromion down the anterolateral humerus, and a spinal needle is brought in directly over the LHBT, just above the falciform ligament, using "outside-in" technique.
  - An 8-mm translucent cannula is inserted to facilitate access (Figs. 17-13 and 17-14).

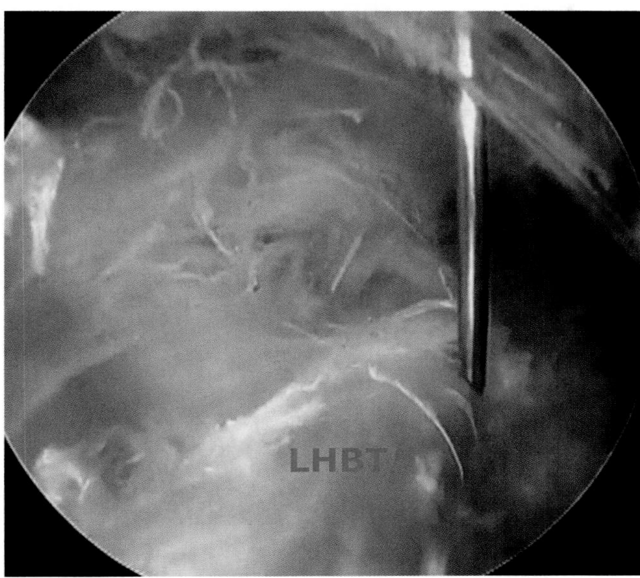

Figure 17-13 | Spinal needle used to establish the falciform portal. LHBT is at the tip of the needle, which is perpendicular to the groove. LHBT, long head of the biceps tendon.

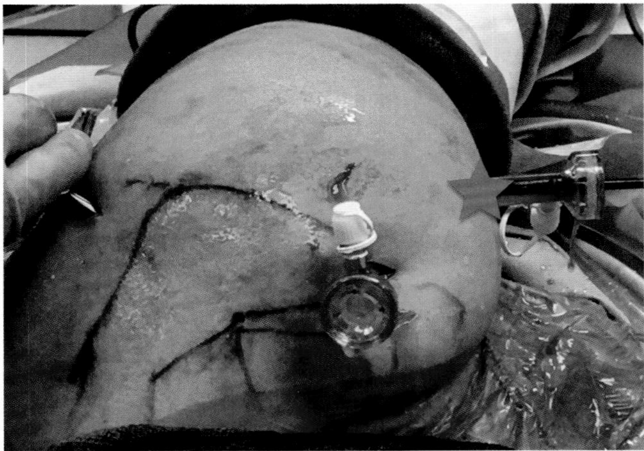

Figure 17-14 | RF wand in falciform portal (marked with *star*). The other cannula pictured is in the anterosuperior-lateral (ASL) portal and will be used to grasp the cut LHBT.

Biceps Tenodesis Techniques

- "Tension assured" fixation
  - After exposure of the groove, anchor position is located in the lower third of the groove above the pectoralis major tendon.
  - Using no. 2 nonabsorbable suture, two "lasso-loop" stitches are passed to secure the tendon at the level of the future anchor position (Figs. 17-15 and 17-16).[3]
  - A pilot hole for knotless anchor tenodesis is created in the groove center using an appropriately sized awl or power drill with bone tap for hard bone.
  - The groove is gently decorticated with a rasp or motor shaver just distal to the anchor site in preparation for tendon-to-bone healing (Fig. 17-17).
  - The free suture ends from the "lasso-loop" stitches are loaded through the anchor eyelet and pulled to bring the tendon flush to the anchor.

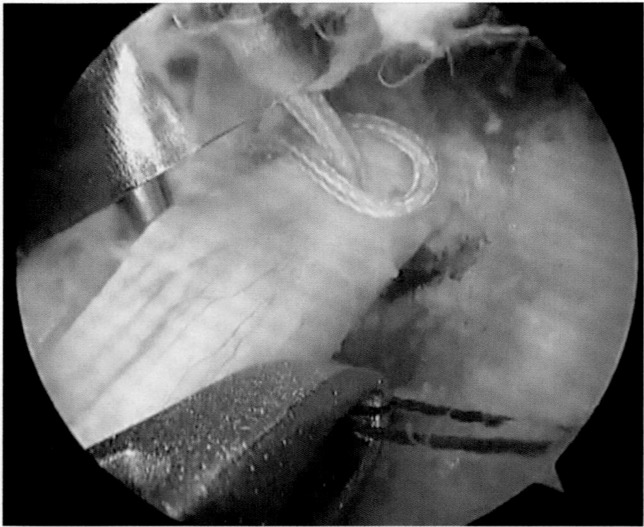

Figure 17-15 | "Lasso-loop" stitches are used to secure the LHBT. A BirdBeak is used to pierce the tendon midsubstance and retrieve the free no. 2 suture, to execute the "lasso loop."

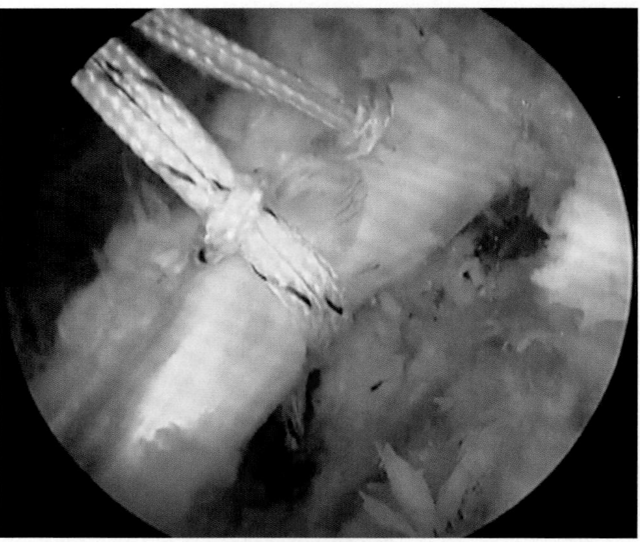

Figure 17-16 | Two lasso loops in place.

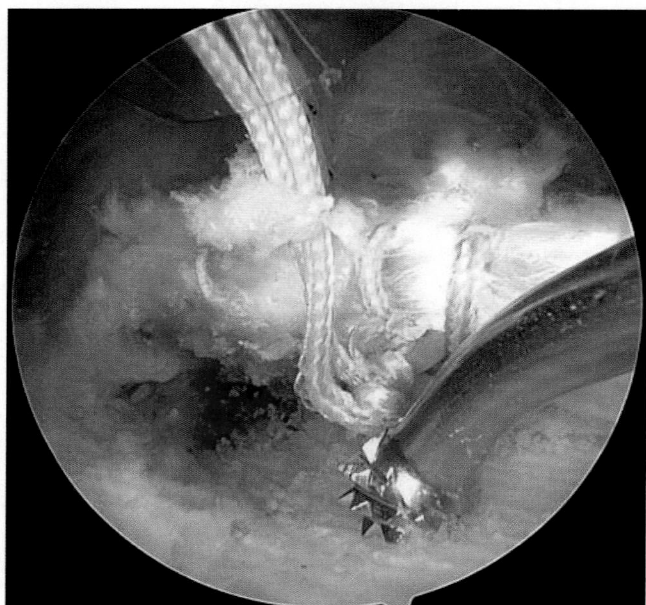

Figure 17-17 | Rasp is used to prepare the bony bed for biceps healing, just distal to anchor position. Sutures are delivered from falciform cannula to aid in LHBT retraction.

- The anchor-tendon unit is then deployed down the "falciform" cannula, tensioned, and fixed into the pilot hole.
- The biceps is cut just above (proximal to) the sutures, with care not to cut the suture or cut so closely that the stitch can loosen (Figs. 17-18 and 17-19).
- The arthroscope is replaced in the joint, and the LHBT is cut from the labrum and the free tendon is retrieved and discarded.

- Fixation for the preemptively tenotomized LHBT
  - The bicipital groove is located and opened as previously described.
  - The cut tendon is controlled with a locking grasper and subluxated anteromedially from the groove.
  - After groove preparation and adequate hemostasis, the location for anchor placement is selected as with the "tension-assured" technique, and the tendon is brought back to the groove center.

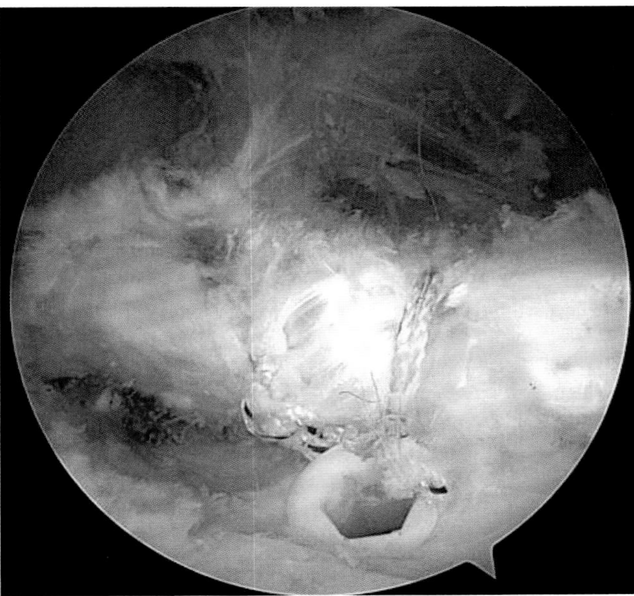

Figure 17-18 | The vented anchor is in place utilizing the lasso loops, at anatomic tension.

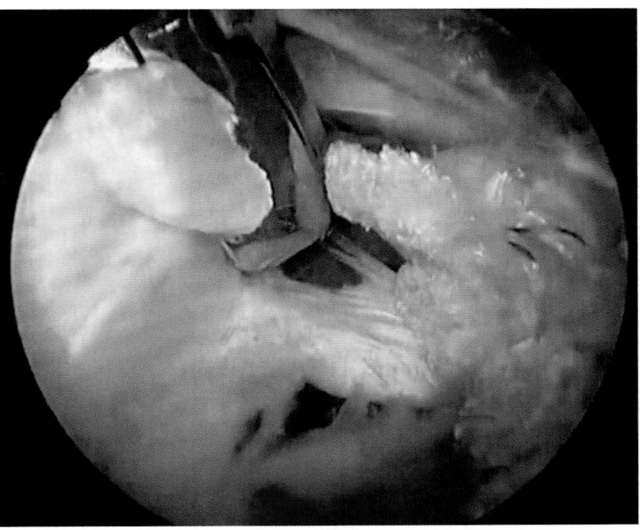

Figure 17-19 | Arthroscopic biters are used to amputate the fixed tendon just above the proximal suture and the anchor.

- To establish the appropriate length-tension relationship, the tendon is marked 25 mm from the cut end, and the "lasso-loop" stitches are passed at that level for tenodesis at the proximal groove.
  - Anatomic study has shown that, on average, 25 mm of tendon length can be measured from the superior labral attachment to the top of the groove (intra-articular). An additional 31 mm of tendon lies between the top of the groove to the lower border of the subscapularis.[4]
- Following localization of the tenodesis site and suturing of the tendon, the final tenodesis steps are completed, as previously outlined.
- The grasper from the anterior cannula is used to provide countertension and facilitate suture passage.

- In some cases, we use a forked biotenodesis screw for alternative fixation.
  - This method saves the time necessary to mobilize and suture the tendon.
  - It is ideal for smaller tendons, which can be completely "straddled" by the anchor fork (Fig. 17-20).

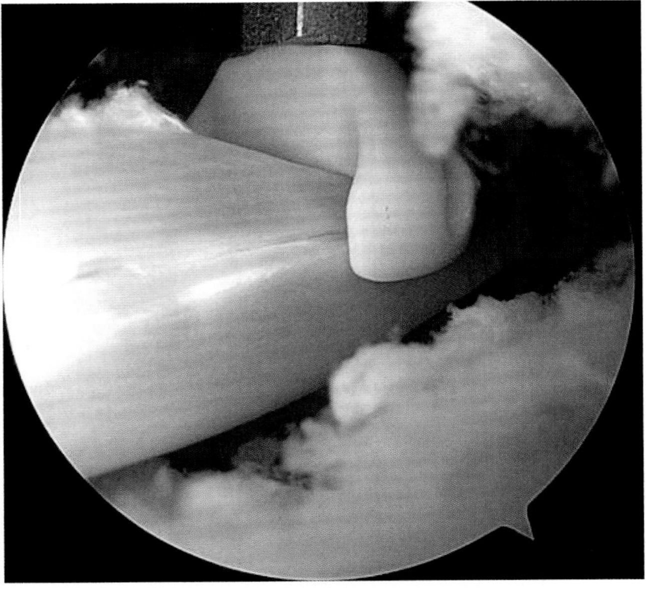

Figure 17-20 | Forked biotenodesis screw straddling LHBT in preparation for interference fit into the bone tunnel.

- The length of the anchor should be taken into account when setting tension and advancing the anchor; travel of the tendon into bone with the screw must be accounted for to avoid overtensioning.
- The screw can cut into tendon during advancement, and, without suture fixation, premature amputation can occur.

References

1. Hart ND, Golish SR, Dragoo JL. Effects of arm position on maximizing intra-articular visualization of the biceps tendon: a cadaveric study. *Arthroscopy*. 2012;28(4):481-485.
2. Saithna A, Longo A, Leiter J, Old J, MacDonald P. Shoulder arthroscopy does not adequately visualize pathology of the long head of biceps tendon. *Orthop J Sports Med*. 2016;4(1):1-6.
3. Lafosse L, Van Raebroeckx A, Brzoska R. A new technique to improve tissue grip: "the lasso-loop stitch". *Arthroscopy*. 2006;22(11):1246.
4. Denard P, Dai X, Hanypsiak B, Burkhart S. Anatomy of the biceps tendon: implications for restoring physiological length-tension relation during biceps tenodesis with interference screw fixation. *Arthroscopy*. 2012;28(10):1352-1358.

Suggested Readings

Arce G. Arthroscopic suprapectoral biceps tenodesis. In: Ryu R, Angelo R, Abrams J, eds. *The shoulder: AANA Advanced Arthroscopic Surgical Techniques*. 1st ed. Thorofare, NJ: SLACK Incorporated and AANA; 2016.

Snyder S. Biceps tendon. In: Snyder S, ed. *Shoulder Arthroscopy*. 3rd ed. Philadelphia, PA: Lippincott Williams & Wilkins; 2014.

Chapter 18
Open Subpectoral Biceps Tenodesis

MOLLY A. DAY
BRIAN R. WOLF

Introduction/Indications

- Tendinopathy of the long head of the biceps brachii tendon (LHBT) can be associated with a number of shoulder conditions, including rotator cuff pathology, superior labral tears, subacromial impingement, or glenohumeral arthritis.
- Biceps tenodesis involves detachment of the LHBT from the superior labrum and reattachment to the proximal humerus.
- Biceps tenodesis is indicated for partial-thickness tear, tendon subluxation, superior labrum anterior to posterior (SLAP) tears, and failed nonoperative management of bicipital tenosynovitis.
- Advantages of tenodesis are protection of the length-tension relationship of the biceps, thereby maintaining elbow flexion and supination strength; avoidance of muscle atrophy and cramping; and prevention of the cosmetic deformity associated with biceps tenotomy.

Relevant Anatomy

- The LHBT originates at the superior aspect of the glenoid fossa and labrum at the supraglenoid tubercle.
- Although there is some anatomic variation, it usually attaches in the posterior aspect of the superior labrum and attaches directly to the supraglenoid tubercle.
- The tendon is encased within a synovial sheath in the glenohumeral joint and courses through the bicipital groove in the proximal humerus to join the lateral head of the biceps muscle. Therefore, the LHBT is an intra-articular (but extrasynovial) structure, passing an average of 35 mm over the head of the humerus and into the bicipital groove, becoming extra-articular.
- The tendon makes a 30- to 40-degree turn into the bicipital groove, where it is stabilized by the biceps pulley (composed of fibers from the coracohumeral and superior glenohumeral ligaments) and contributions from the subscapularis and supraspinatus tendons.
- The average length of the LHBT from the supraglenoid tubercle to the musculotendinous junction is 11.2-13.8 cm, and the average diameter is 6 mm.
- The tendon's blood supply arises from the brachial and deep brachial arteries distally and the branches of the anterior humeral circumflex artery proximally; much of the intra-articular portion of the LHBT is poorly vascularized.

Pathogenesis

- The LHBT is at risk of injury, irritation, and degenerative changes because of its constrained course within the bicipital groove and its proximity to the acromion and rotator cuff, which subjects it to intra- and extra-articular restraints, possible subacromial impingement, and constant sliding of the tendon during shoulder motion.

- The biomechanical importance of the LHBT as a stabilizer of the glenohumeral joint continues to be controversial. Its primary function is at the elbow, where it acts as a flexor and supinator.
- Disorders of the LHBT can be classified as degenerative, inflammatory, traumatic, and instability.

Patient Evaluation/Examination

- The most common complaint is anterior shoulder pain over the bicipital groove radiating to the biceps muscle.
  - Pain at night and with rotation of the abducted arm also is common.
  - Pain may be exacerbated by lifting with the elbow extended and the shoulder externally rotated.
  - Pain may radiate down the arm and even to the hand, but this referred pain should not be confused with cervical radiculopathy, which may require further investigation.
- Physical examination should include evaluation for any clinical deformity of the biceps, palpation of the LHBT in the bicipital groove through the subpectoral triangle, and range of motion and strength of the shoulder and elbow.
- The most common physical finding is point tenderness over the LHBT in the bicipital groove.
- To localize the bicipital groove, the arm is internally rotated 10 degrees (the position in which the groove generally faces anteriorly) and palpated 7 cm below the acromion.
- Several provocative tests have been described for the diagnosis of LHBT; individually they have poor specificity, but can be diagnostic when used together.
  - Speed test
  - Yergason test
  - Biceps instability test

Imaging Evaluation

- Imaging for biceps tendinopathy often is difficulty and nonspecific; it may be helpful to rule out associated pathology.
- Plain radiographs may show acromial spurring or calcification in the bicipital groove.
- Ultrasound is cost-effective and noninvasive and can be used to test for LHBT tearing, dynamic subluxation and instability, and fluid in the tendon sheath but is highly operator dependent.
- MRI may show increased signal within the LHBT and concomitant labral and/or rotator cuff pathology.

Sterile Equipment and Instruments

- 30-degree arthroscope
- Handheld arthroscopic biter
- Radiofrequency probe
- Army-Navy retractors
- Right-angle clamp
- Tenodesis button (Arthrex, Naples, FL)
- 2.7-mm drill
- Nonabsorbable no. 2 suture

Biceps Tenodesis Technique

- After preparation and draping, the patient is positioned in the beach-chair position, and general anesthesia is administered (Video 18-1).
- A diagnostic arthroscopic examination is done first.
  - The arm is positioned in 30 degrees of forward flexion, 40 degrees of abduction, and 90 degrees of elbow flexion (Hart).
- If the biceps tendon is torn, severely frayed, or subluxing into the subscapularis, arthroscopic tenotomy is done.
  - LHBT is released from attachment at the superior labrum with a handheld biter or a radiofrequency wand. The LHBT is retracted from the glenohumeral joint by extending the elbow.

- For the open tenodesis, a 3- to 4-cm vertical incision is made on the proximal-anterior medial arm at the level of the inferior border of the palpable pectoralis major tendon.
  - One-third of the incision should lie over the level of the tendon, and two-thirds should extend inferior to the tendon
- The skin and subcutaneous tissue are incised sharply, and dissection is carried down to the level of the fascia.
- The brachial fascia is identified as it blends into the fascia overlying the pectoralis tendon.
  - This interface is opened sharply at an oblique angle consistent with the inferior aspect of the pectoralis.
- An Army-Navy retractor is used to retract the inferior border of the pectoralis major tendon superiorly, and the arm is internally rotated to allow palpation of the bicipital groove and the biceps tendon.
- A second retractor is used to hold the short head of the biceps tendon medially, with care taken to protect the musculocutaneous nerve.
- Blunt dissection proceeds until the LHBT is exposed within the bicipital groove.
  - The LHBT often is covered with tenosynovium, which should be dissected off the tendon.
- The biceps tendon is drawn into the wound and retrieved with a right-angle clamp.
- The LHBT is prepared at the level of the musculotendinous junction with locking no. 2 permanent sutures such that two equally long suture tails are attached to the LHBT.
  - The sutures are passed through the LHBT from ~2 cm distal to the musculotendinous junction to ~1 cm proximal.
  - One limb of suture is then woven through a 2-hole biceps tenodesis button by passing the suture down through the first hole and back up through the second hole. The other limb is passed through the cortical button holes in the opposite direction, and the excess proximal LHBT above the sutures is excised.
- The bicipital groove is prepared with electrocautery to expose the underlying bone.
  - A small curet or rasp can be used to stimulate punctate bleeding in the groove where the tenodesis will occur underneath the distal pectoralis tendon, which is retracted superiorly.
- A 2.7-mm drill is centered in the anterior humeral cortex within the bicipital groove and drilled through the anterior cortex at the level of the inferior border of the pectoralis major tendon insertion.
  - The drill is angled slightly distal to proximal and aimed toward the center of the humeral canal. Care is taken not to penetrate through the posterior cortex.
- A deployment device inserted through the tunnel in the anterior cortex is used to deploy the tenodesis button with the sutures attached into the intramedullary canal of the humerus. The button will flip 90 degrees in the canal to catch on the anterior cortex, similar to fixation buttons commonly used for anterior cruciate ligament surgery or distal biceps tendon repairs.
- Both limbs of the sutures exiting the humeral cortex are passed through the biceps tendon again, this time from posterior to anterior.
- The sutures are tensioned, drawing the biceps tendon down to firmly appose the biceps tendon to the anterior cortex of the proximal humerus.
- The two limbs of the sutures are tied together to complete the tenodesis.
  - The musculotendinous junction of the LHBT should sit approximately at the inferior border of the pectoralis tendon after tenodesis is complete; the soft tissues are then allowed to fall back into position.
- The wound is irrigated and closed in layers.

Postoperative Care/Rehabilitation

- The arm is immobilized for 4-6 weeks.
- Physical therapy is started at 2 weeks, focusing on range of motion, including pendulum exercises, passive forward flexion, and external rotation.
- Typically, resisted biceps flexion or supination is avoided for 6-12 weeks to allow healing of the tenodesis.
- At 12 weeks, gradual progression to full activity is begun as tolerated.

Chapter 19

Anatomic Reconstruction of Acromioclavicular Joint Injuries

BRADLEY P. JAQUITH
ANTHONY A. MASCIOLI
THOMAS (QUIN) THROCKMORTON

Indications

- Rockwood classification (Fig. 19-1)
  - Types I and II—conservative treatment
  - Types IV, V, and VI—operative treatment
  - Type III—controversial[1-3]
- Surgical options[4]
  - Intra-articular fixation
  - Extra-articular coracoclavicular (CC) repair
  - Ligamentous reconstruction
  - Arthroscopic reconstruction

Preoperative Evaluation

- Routine physical examination of the shoulder
- Standard radiographic shoulder series
  - Anteroposterior.
  - True anteroposterior (Grashey).
  - Axillary lateral—necessary for diagnosis of type IV acromioclavicular (AC) separation (Fig. 19-2).
  - Bilateral Zanca view (beam directed 10-15 degrees cephalad) may be useful.
  - MRI is not typically obtained unless other shoulder pathology is suspected.

Sterile Instruments/Equipment

- Sterile drapes, including impervious stockinette and 4-in elastic bandage wrap for forearm and hand
- Three strands of large braided suture, for example, FiberTape or SutureTape (Arthrex Inc., Naples, FL)
- Nitinol wire
- Guide wires and reamers
- PEEK screws

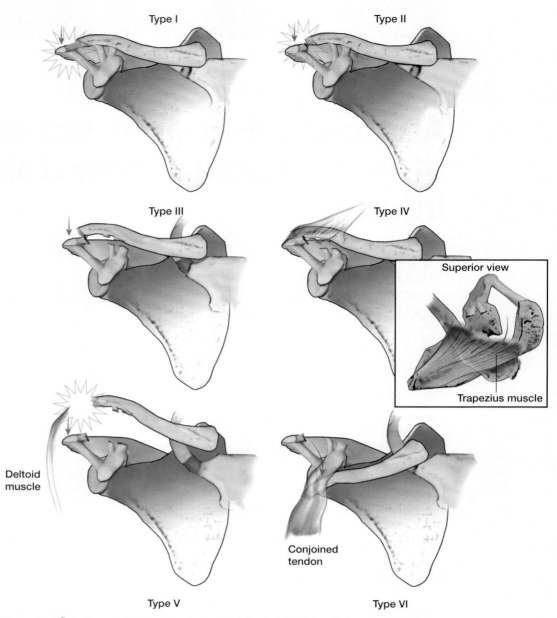

Figure 19-1 | Rockwood classification of acromioclavicular joint dislocations.

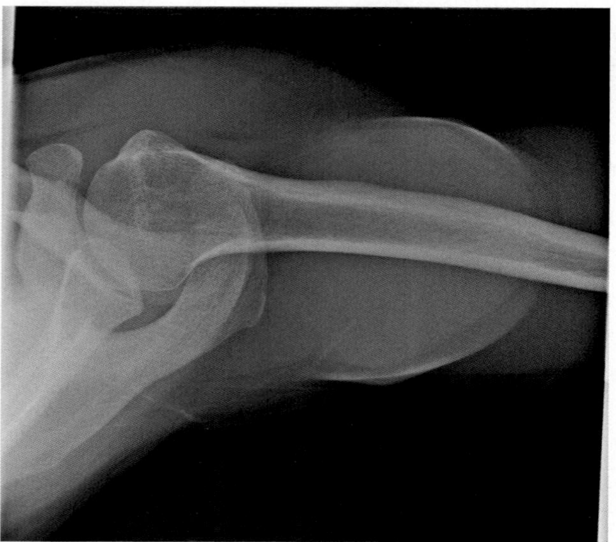

Figure 19-2 | Type IV acromioclavicular separation demonstrating posterior displacement of the clavicle referable to the acromion.

Patient Positioning

- Beach-chair position (Fig. 19-3)

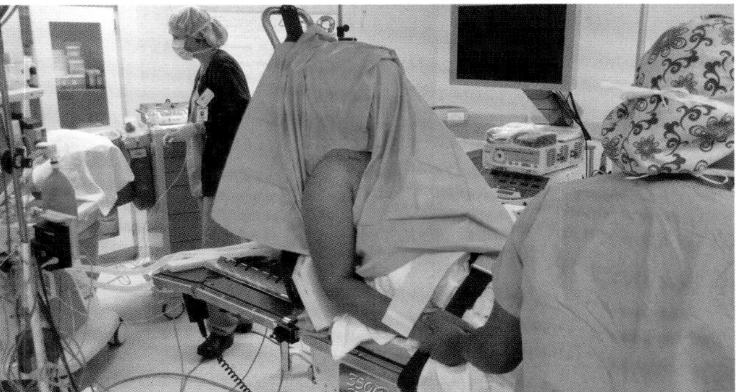

Figure 19-3 | Beach-chair position.

- Entire ipsilateral extremity prepared and draped circumferentially to allow freedom of movement and facilitate reduction
- Padded Mayo stand available to rest arm on

Surgical Approach

- Incision is made from lateral end of the clavicle to the coracoid (Fig. 19-4).
- Sharp dissection is carried down to the deltotrapezial fascia, and medial and lateral flaps are raised (Fig. 19-5).
- The deltotrapezial fascia is incised to allow access to the distal 5 cm of the clavicle (Fig. 19-6).
    - The deltotrapezial fascia is repaired at closure with no. 2 braided suture.

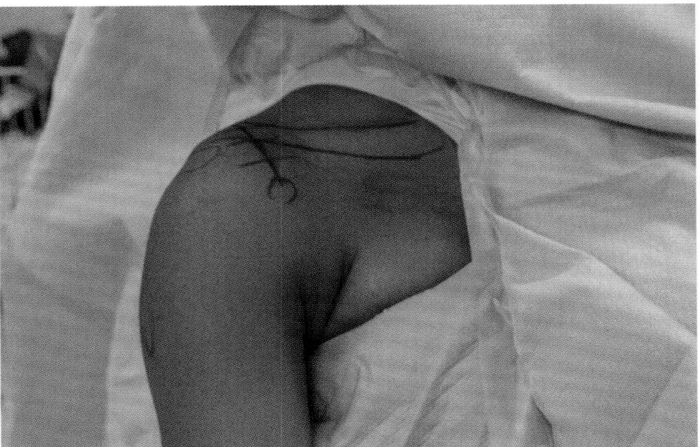

Figure 19-4 | Incision from the lateral end of the clavicle to the coracoid.

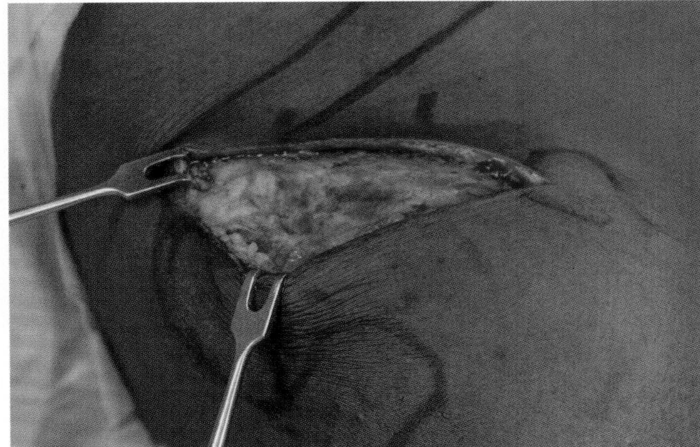

Figure 19-5 | Sharp dissection down to the deltotrapezial fascia; medial and lateral flaps raised.

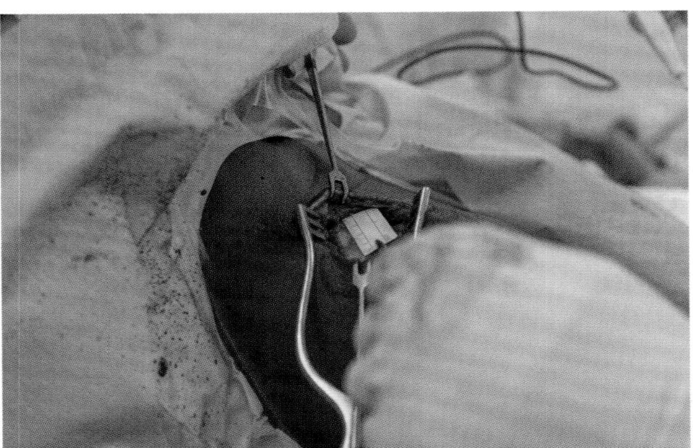

Figure 19-6 | Deltotrapezial fascia incised to allow access to distal clavicle.

- Subperiosteal flaps are raised to expose the superior and inferior surfaces of the clavicle (Fig. 19-7).

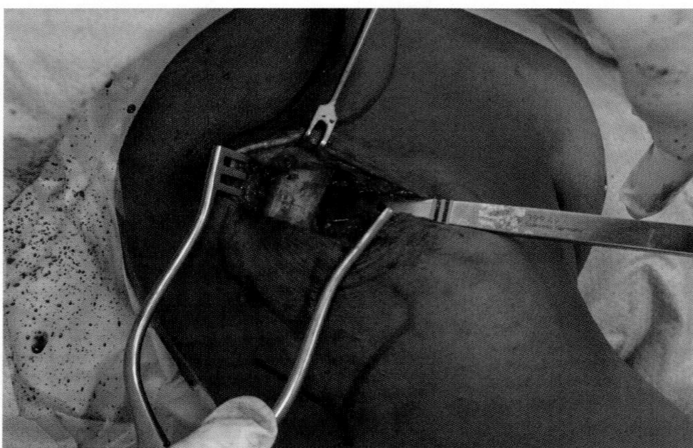

Figure 19-7 | Subperiosteal flaps raised to expose superior and inferior clavicular surfaces.

- Resection of the distal clavicle allows better viewing and debridement of any scar tissue, which allows easier reduction, especially in chronic cases. Resection of the distal clavicle has been shown to reduce failure rates and is recommended by some because of the high likelihood of AC arthritis associated with these injuries.
- Dissection is carried deep to the deltoid to identify the coracoid. Medial and lateral subperiosteal flaps are raised from the coracoid (Fig. 19-8).

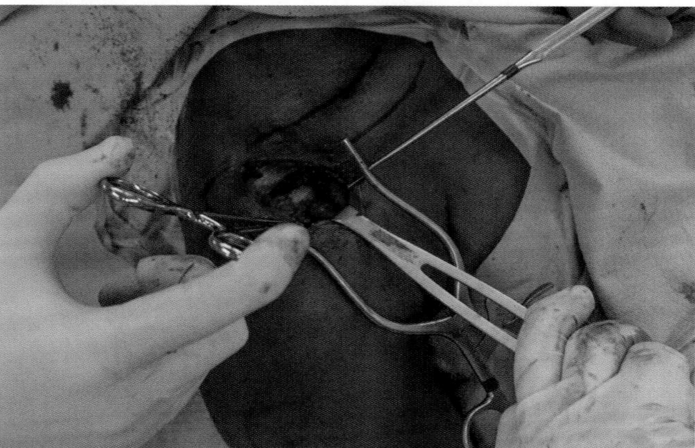

Figure 19-8 | Medial and lateral flaps raised from the coracoid.

Graft Passage and Reduction

- A suture passer with a nitinol wire is passed around the inferior aspect of the coracoid and left in place for graft passage.
- The conoid and trapezoid tubercles are identified. A guidewire is placed in each tubercle and reamed to the appropriate size of the graft (Fig. 19-9A-C).
- The graft is prepared and sized on the back table, and each end is whipstitched (Fig. 19-10).
  - Multiple graft choices are available, including semitendinosus, gracilis, peroneus longus, and toe extensor tendons, which can be allograft or autograft.[4]
  - Pretensioning similar to the process used in anterior cruciate ligament (ACL) reconstruction may be considered to optimize the graft.
- Three strands of heavy braided suture (Fibertape, Arthrex Inc., Naples, FL) are also prepared with the graft.

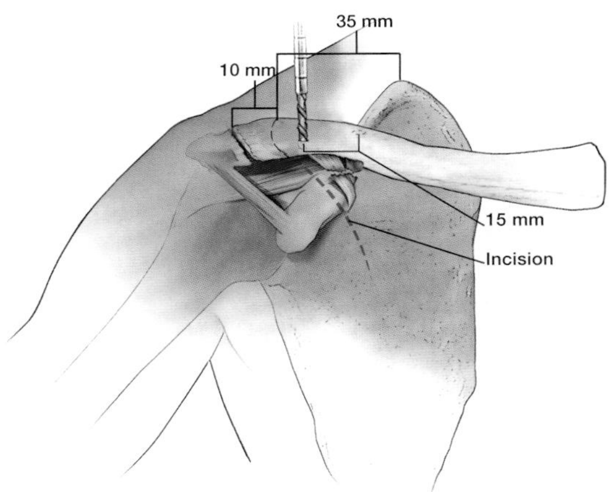

A

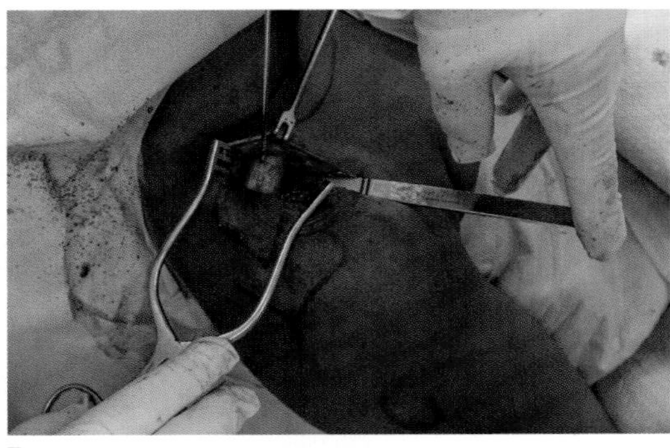

B

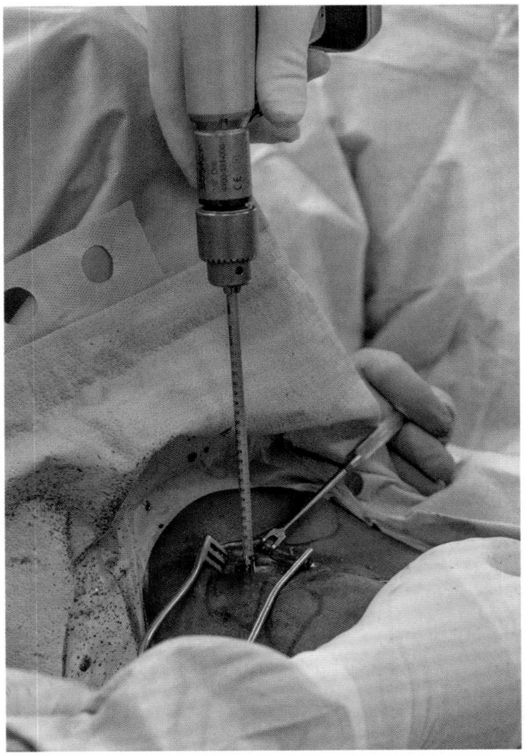

C

Figure 19-9 | A. Conoid and trapezoid tubercles identified. **B.** Guidewire placed in each tubercle, which is reamed to size of graft **(C)**.

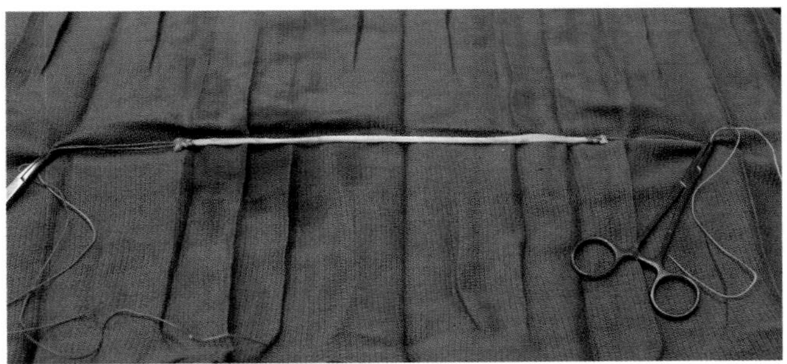

Figure 19-10 | Prepared graft with each end whipstitched.

- The suture passer with the nitinol wire is used to pass the graft around the coracoid (Fig. 19-11).
- The limbs of the graft are crossed and brought through the two drill holes in the clavicle (Fig. 19-12A-C).

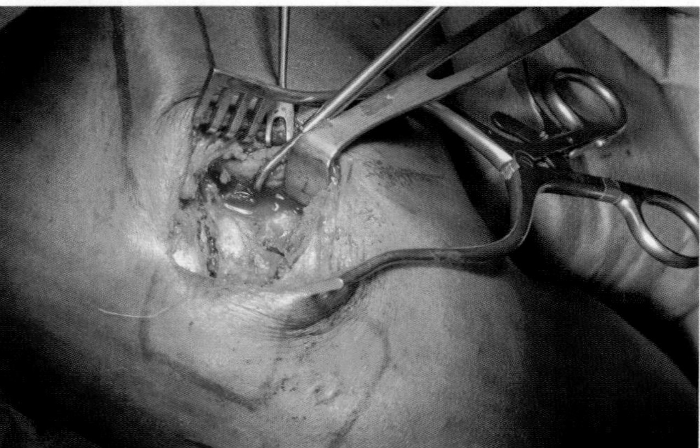

Figure 19-11 | Suture passer used to pass graft around the coracoid.

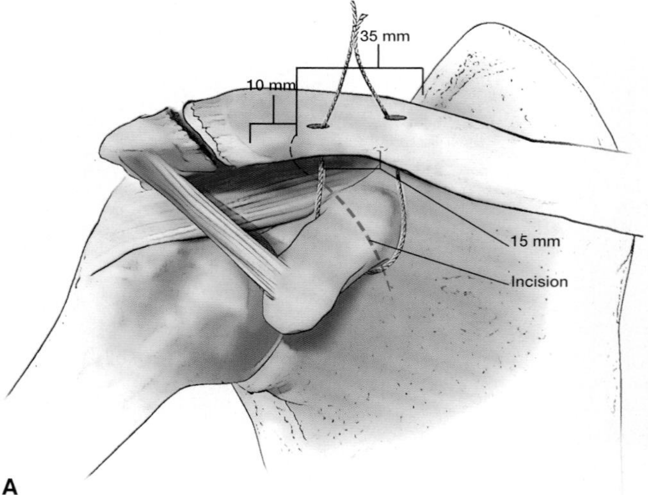

A

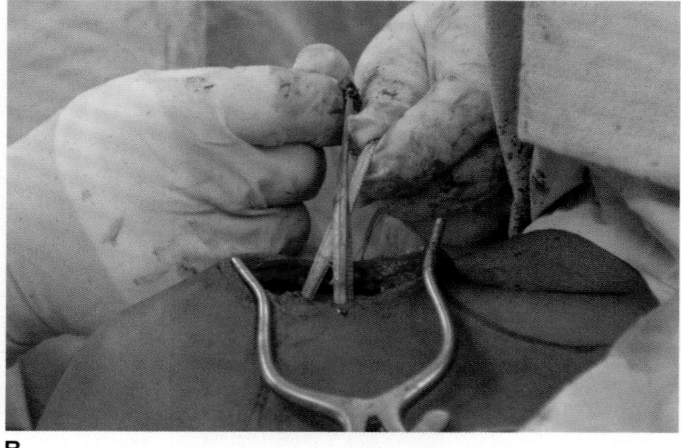

B

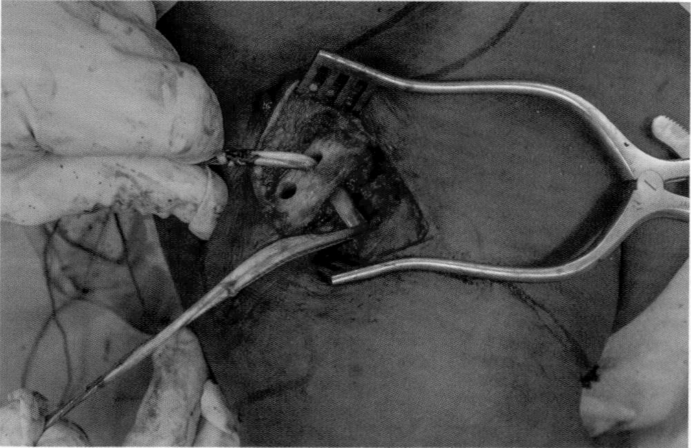

C

Figure 19-12 | **A-C.** Limbs of graft crossed and passed through drill holes in the clavicle.

- One of the sutures is also brought through each drill hole, while the other two are passed posteriorly to the clavicle.
- The arm is supported on a padded Mayo stand, and the AC joint is reduced with manual pressure.
- The sutures are tied to provide provisional fixation.
  - The use of nonbiologic fixation in addition to the graft may allow the graft to mature under tension and provides strong backup fixation.[5]

- The graft is tensioned and held, while appropriately sized PEEK screws are placed in each of the drill holes (Fig. 19-13A and B).

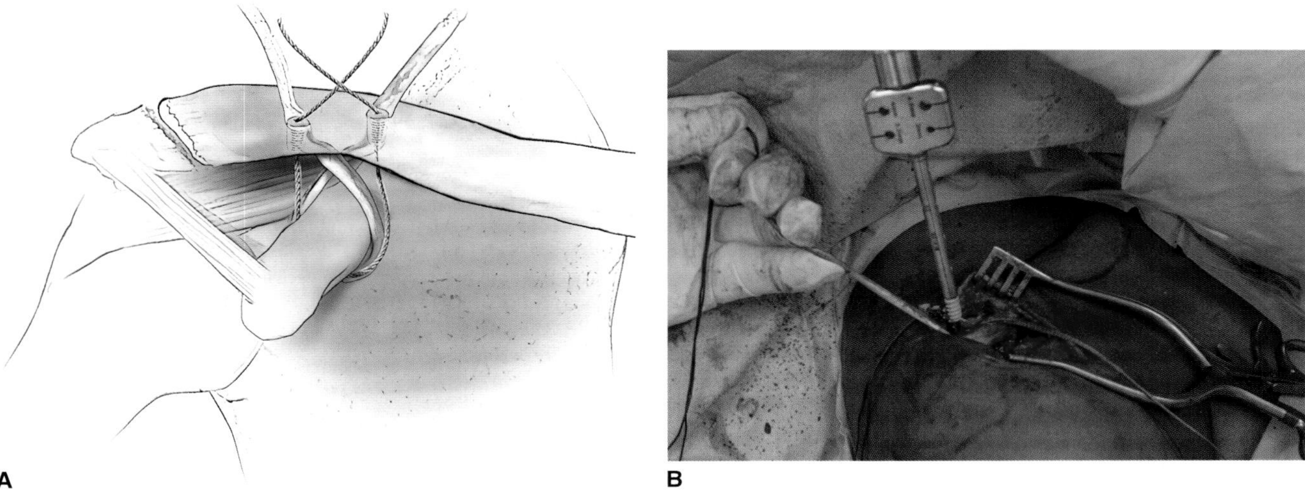

Figure 19-13 | A and B. Graft tensioned and PEEK screws placed in drill holes.

- The medial limb of excess graft is excised, and the lateral limb can either be excised or used for superior AC capsule reconstruction.
  - To reconstruct the superior capsule, the lateral limb is brought over the superior AC joint and sutured in place (Fig. 19-14A and B).

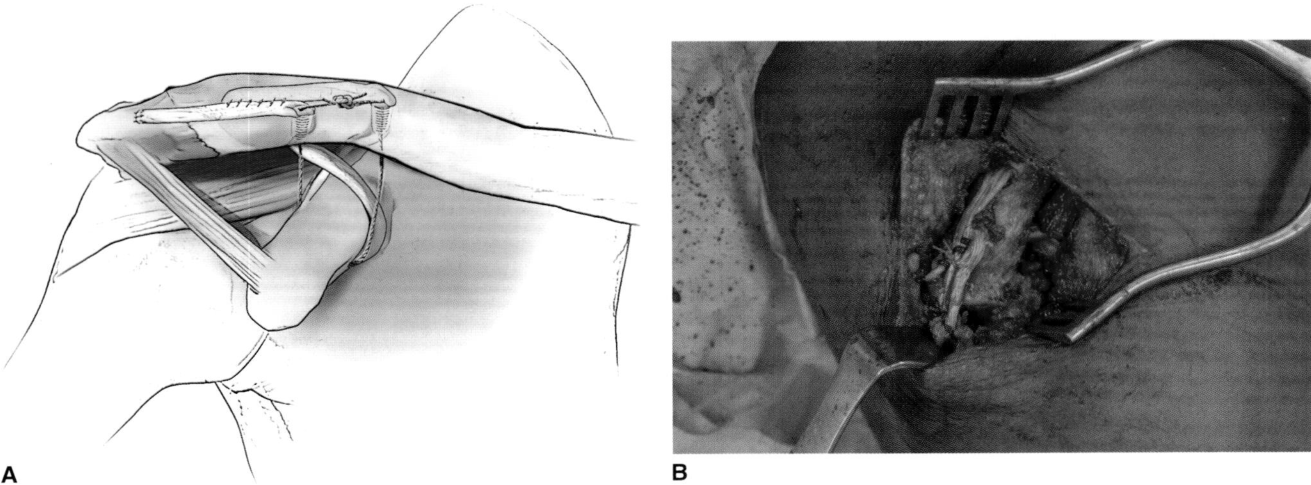

Figure 19-14 | A and B. Lateral limb of graft brought over superior AC joint and sutured in place.

- Video 19-1 demonstrates intraoperative stability of an AC joint reconstruction.

Postoperative Protocol

- Strict sling immobilization for 6 weeks following surgery.
  - An important concept in rehabilitation of AC joint reconstructions is that gravity will provide a constant force acting to disrupt the repair.
  - The sling should firmly support the elbow and even slightly elevate the shoulder to minimize gravitational stress on the reconstruction.

- Patients are trained in Codman exercises to be done twice daily to minimize shoulder stiffness but are otherwise encouraged to wear the sling as instructed full time.
- Active-assisted and passive range of motion are instituted at 6 weeks, with active range of motion, strengthening, and return to sport-specific activities beginning at 12 weeks.

References

1. Li X, Ma R, Bedi A, Dines DM, Altchek DW, Dines JS. Management of acromioclavicular joint injuries. *J Bone Joint Surg Am.* 2014;96(1):73-84.
2. Schlegel TF, Burks RT, Marcus RL, Dunn HK. A prospective evaluation of untreated acute grade III acromioclavicular separations. *Am J Sports Med.* 2001;29(6):699-703.
3. Simovitch R, Sanders B, Ozbaydar M, Lavery K, Warner JJP. Acromioclavicular joint injuries: diagnosis and management. *J Am Acad Orthop Surg.* 2009;17(4):207-219.
4. Grutter PW, Petersen SA. Anatomical acromioclavicular ligament reconstruction: a biomechanical comparison of reconstructive techniques of the acromioclavicular joint. *Am J Sports Med.* 2005;33(11):1723-1728.
5. Biggers MD, Mascioli AA, Mauck BM, Azar FM, Smith RA, Throckmorton TW. Analysis of mechanical failures after anatomic acromioclavicular joint reconstruction. *Curr Orthop Pract.* 2015;26(5):526-529.

Chapter 20
Principles of Elbow Arthroscopy

MICHAEL D. CHIU
JASON L. KOH

Indications for Elbow Arthroscopy

- Evaluation of painful elbow
- Capsular release for contractures and stiffness[1]
- Removal of loose bodies[2]
- Treatment of early degenerative changes[2]
  - Osteophyte debridement of olecranon and coronoid fossae
    - Valgus extension overload
- Treatment of osteochondral lesions of the radial head
- Treatment of osteochondritis dissecans of the capitellum
- Lateral epicondylitis debridement and release or repair
- Fractures of the radial head
- Partial synovectomy

Contraindications

- Altered anatomy—congenital or prior surgical procedures[3]
  - Ulnar nerve transposition
- Bony ankylosis or extensive fibrous ankylosis[1]
  - Precludes safe introduction of arthroscope by impeding joint distension
- Local active soft tissue infection[3]

Advantages of Elbow Arthroscopy

- Minimally invasive[4]—decreased postoperative pain and faster return to activity
- Superior articular cartilage visualization

Disadvantages

- Risk of neurovascular (NV) injury[3,5] and technically more challenging

Anesthesia, Positioning, and Setup

- Anesthesia
  - General: minimal risks; complete muscle relaxation; allows postoperative neurologic examination[6]
  - Regional: more risk involved; limited patient tolerance to positioning; decreased postoperative nausea[6]

- Patient positioning: supine, prone, or lateral decubitus
  - Supine position
    - Adequate access to anterior and posterior compartments
    - Easier anesthesia airway management and open surgery conversion
  - Prone or lateral decubitus position (Fig. 20-1)

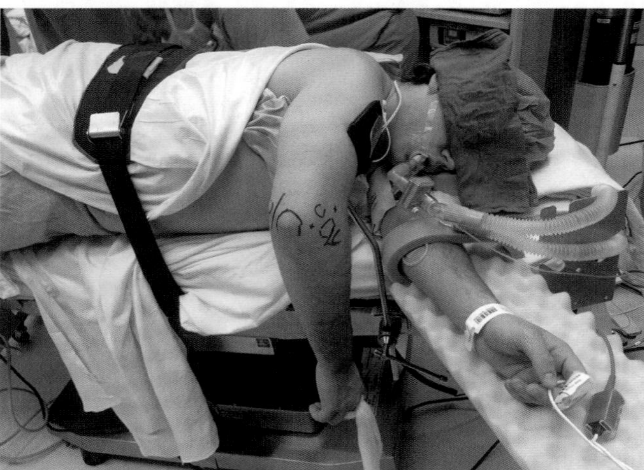

Figure 20-1 | Lateral decubitus patient positioning with noted airway accessibility. Operative shoulder is abducted, with elbow flexed and upper arm supported by a padded bolster placed proximally. Surgical landmarks, ulnar nerve, and portals are drawn out for illustration purposes.

    - Prone position: superior access to the posterior compartment; facilitates elbow manipulation, relaxes anterior NV structures
    - Lateral decubitus position: similar advantages with improved airway access by anesthesia team
- Setup
  - Shoulder abducted, elbow flexed (Fig. 20-1)
  - Padded bolster placed high on arm along with tourniquet
    - Allows anterior soft tissue relaxation
    - Accommodates more elbow flexion for visualization
  - Bony landmarks marked on skin
    - Done *before* joint distension
    - Ulnar nerve is *evaluated for subluxation*
  - Sterile limb positioner may be beneficial (Fig. 20-2)

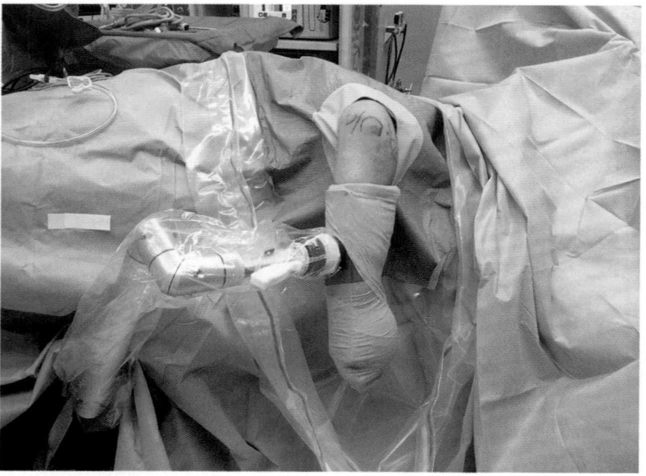

Figure 20-2 | A limb positioner device can be useful to maintain the elbow in various positions, especially when no surgical assistant is available.

- Arthroscopic tower, monitor, and pump are positioned directly opposite the surgeon across the table (Fig. 20-3)

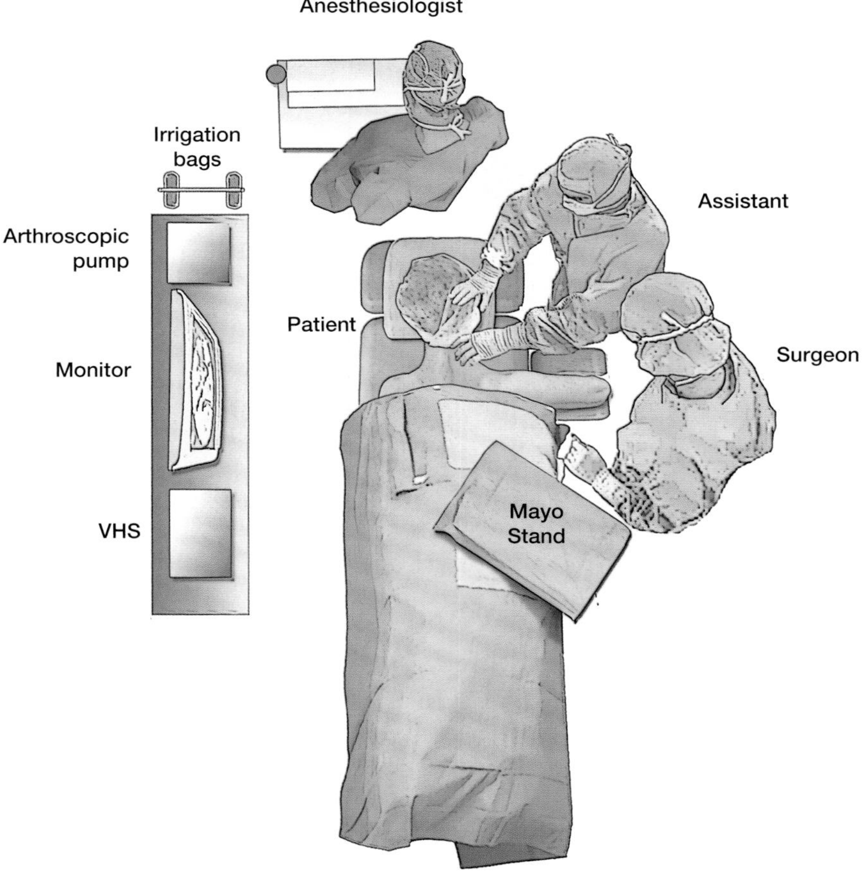

Figure 20-3 | Setup in the operating room (prone position depicted).

Surgical Landmarks and Common Portal Sites

- Anteromedial (AM) Portal (Fig. 20-4)
  - 2 cm distal and 2 cm anterior to medial humeral epicondyle[3,7]
  - Excellent visualization of anterior compartment and capsule
  - Anterior branch of medial antebrachial cutaneous nerve (MACN) and median nerve at risk
    - MACN is superficially within 6 mm.[3]
    - Median nerve is within 14 mm (mean 6.5 mm).[3,5]
      - Brachialis muscle protects median nerve in *elbow flexion*
    - Ulnar nerve subluxation or transposition is checked before portal placement.
- Proximal-Medial (PM) or Superomedial Portal (Fig. 20-4)
  - 2 cm proximal to medial humeral epicondyle[3,7]
    - A trocar is introduced anterior to the intermuscular septum and directed toward the radial head.
    - Contact is maintained along the anterior cortex of the humerus.
  - Excellent visualization of anterior compartment
  - Median nerve potentially at risk
    - Aiming cannula distally and *parallel* to the median nerve in sagittal plane makes *PM portal safer than AM portal*[3]
- Distal Anterolateral (DAL) Portal (Fig. 20-5)
  - 3 cm distal and 2 cm anterior to lateral humeral epicondyle[3,7]
  - Located anteriorly in sulcus between radial head and capitellum

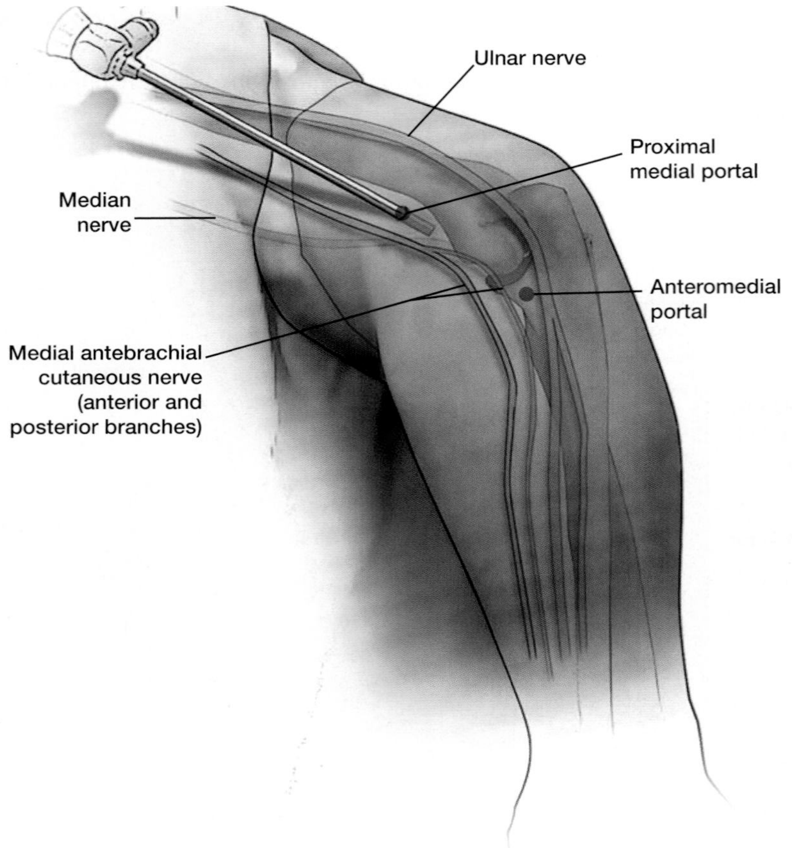

Figure 20-4 | The proximal-medial or superomedial portal (arthroscope depicted) and anteromedial portal, with proximity to important nerves.

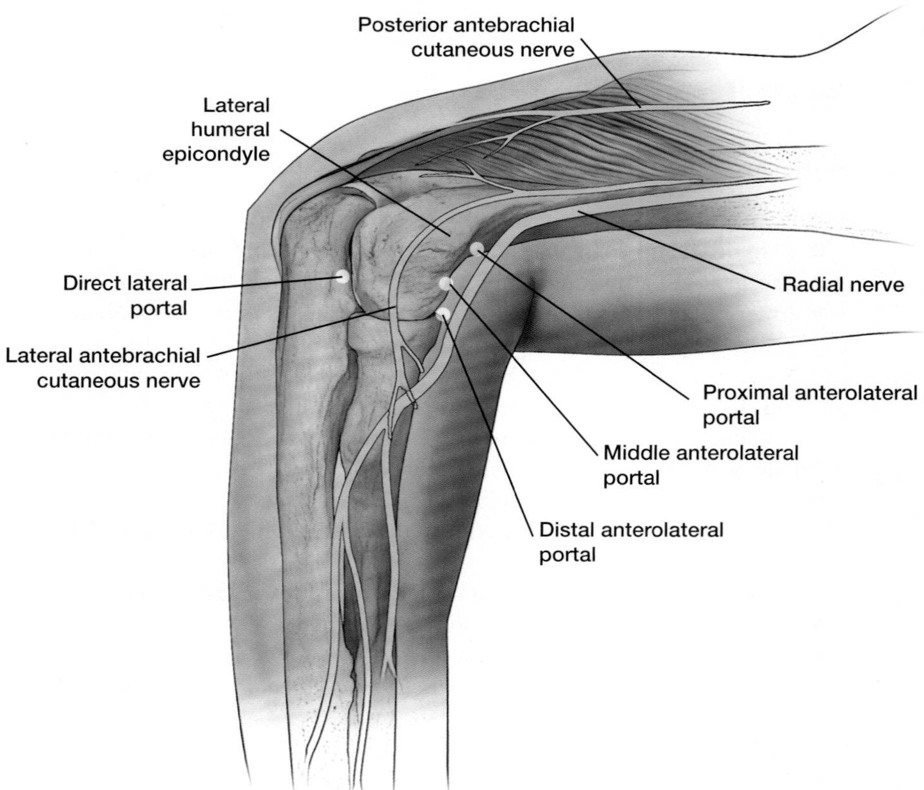

Figure 20-5 | The three proximal, middle, and distal anterolateral portals; the direct-lateral portal in the "soft spot"; and relevant structures.

- Adequate visualization of coronoid process, trochlea, coronoid fossa, medial capsule, and any medial plica
- Posterior antebrachial cutaneous nerve (PACN), posterior interosseous nerve (PIN), and radial nerves at risk[3,7]
  - PACN—2 mm from cannula.
  - PIN—1-13 mm away from cannula.
    - Increased distance with forearm pronation
  - Radial nerve can pass within 3 mm of cannula.
- Middle Anterolateral (MAL) Portal (Fig. 20-5)
  - Located 1 cm proximal and anterior to the lateral humeral epicondyle[3,7]
  - Safer than DAL portal[8]
- Proximal Anterolateral (PAL) Portal (Fig. 20-5)
  - 2 cm proximal and 1 cm anterior to lateral humeral epicondyle[3,7]
  - *Safest* of anterolateral portals[8]
  - Excellent visualization due to proximal location, especially of the radiohumeral joint[3,9]
- Posterolateral (PL) Portal (Figs. 20-6 and 20-7)

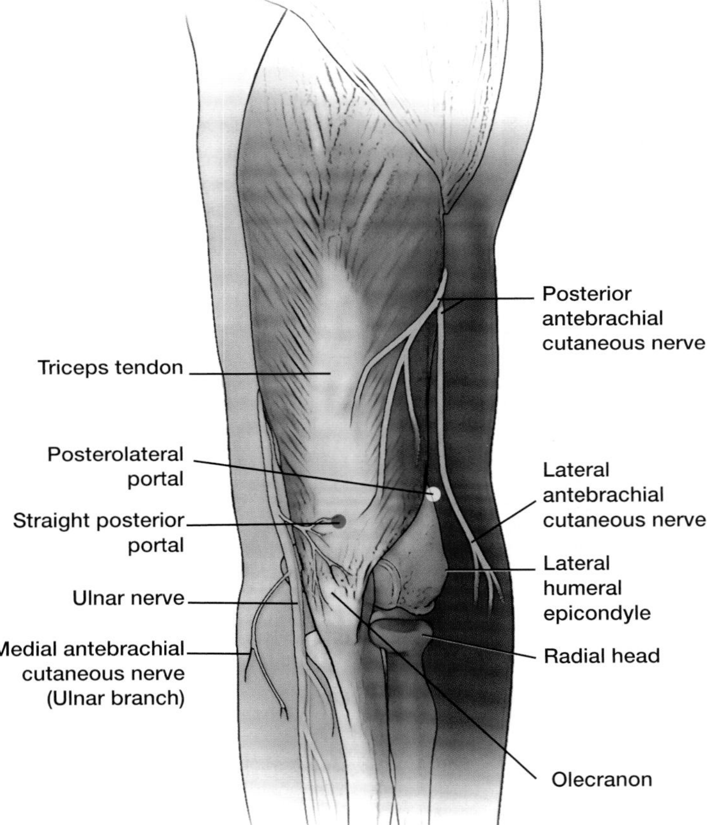

Figure 20-6 | The straight-posterior and posterolateral portal locations with surrounding pertinent anatomy.

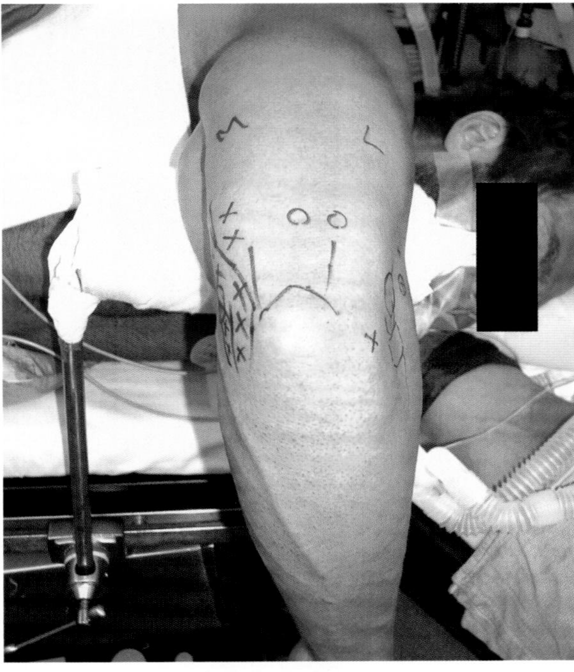

Figure 20-7 | Posterior surface of the right elbow with patient in lateral decubitus position and arm over a padded bolster. Note ulnar nerve subluxation, medial and lateral markings, straight-posterior and posterolateral portals (*circled*), and direct-lateral portal (X in "soft spot").

  - 2-3 cm proximal to the olecranon tip, along the lateral border of the triceps tendon.
    - Directed toward the olecranon fossa.[3,7]
  - Allows visualization of the posterior trochlea and olecranon tip and fossa.
    - Posterior capitellum is poorly visualized.
  - PACN and ulnar nerves at risk.[3,7]
    - PACN passes within 25 mm of portal.
    - Ulnar nerve passes ~25 mm from portal.
      - No risk if trocar *remains lateral* to the posterior midline.
  - Minimizes risk of NV injuries relative to other lateral portals.[9]

- Straight-Posterior (P) Portal (Figs. 20-6 and 20-7)
  - 2-3 cm proximal to the olecranon tip, transtriceps tendon, with trocar directed toward the olecranon fossa.[3,7]
  - Working portal in olecranon osteophyte for resection or loose body removal.
  - Ulnar nerve is at risk with *medial violation* of the posterior midline.
- Direct-Lateral (DL) or Midlateral Portal (Figs. 20-5 to 20-7)
  - Located centrally in the "soft spot" of the triangle: lateral epicondyle, radial head, and olecranon[3,7]
  - Useful for distension and as a working portal to access the posterior capitellum and the radiocapitellar (RC) and radioulnar (RU) joints.
  - PACN passes within 7 mm of the portal.[3]

Diagnostic Arthroscopy

- The joint is distended through the DL portal.
  - 15-20 mL are used.
  - This increases the distance between NV structures and the joint.
- Anterior Compartment
  - It is *safer to start more proximally* (PM vs AM portal risks).
  - *Caution should be exercised during debridement of anterolateral tissue* because of the proximity of the radial nerve and PIN (Fig. 20-8).

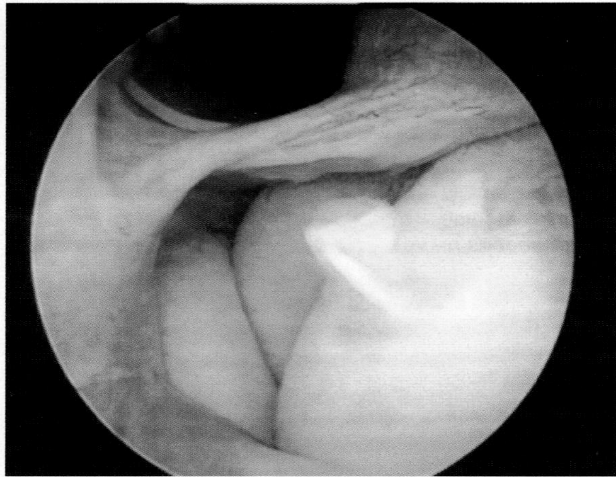

Figure 20-8 | Arthroscopic assessment from proximal-medial portal, with visualization of radiocapitellar adhesions.

  - The anterior capsule is stripped off the humerus *proximally* to increase the working space in elbow contractures.
  - Loose bodies in the proximal anterior humerus and radiocapitellar joint are removed (Fig. 20-9).

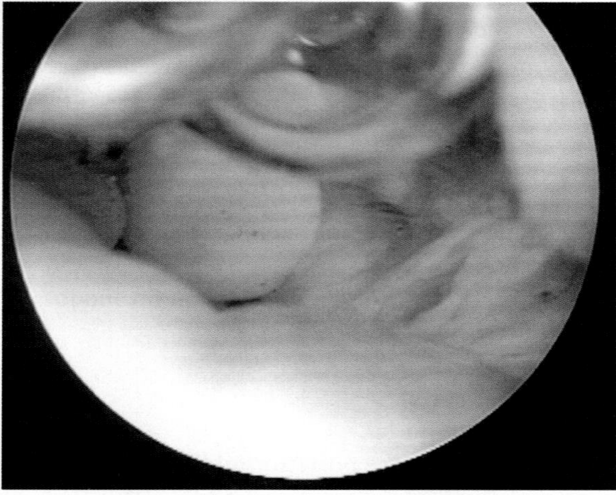

Figure 20-9 | Arthroscopic view of anterior compartment demonstrating a loose body.

- Posterior Compartment
  - Gentle blunt dissection with blunt trocar in olecranon fossa improves visualization.
  - A 2.7-mm arthroscope in the DL portal is directed into the olecranon fossa.
    - This provides good visualization of the olecranon and posterior radiocapitellar joint (Fig. 20-10).

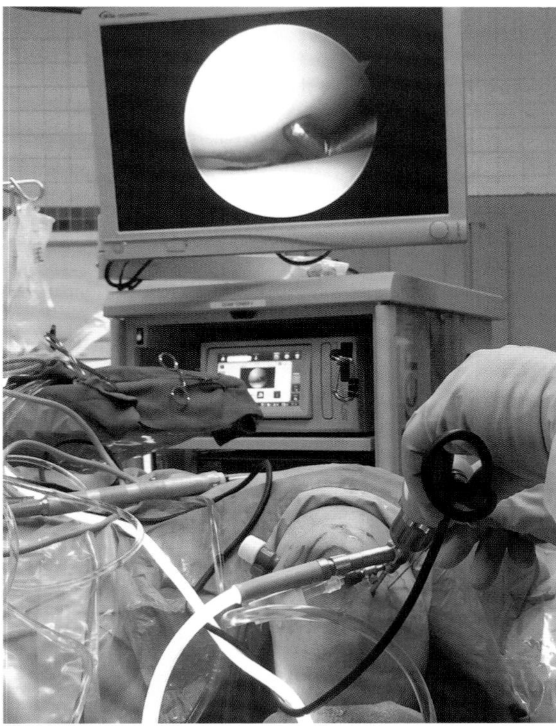

Figure 20-10 | Radiocapitellar joint visualization and evaluation with a probe, using a 2.7-mm arthroscope in the direct-lateral portal.

    - Extreme *caution is required in the posteromedial elbow* because of the proximity of the ulnar nerve (Fig. 20-11)
    - Loose bodies in the posterolateral gutter are removed.

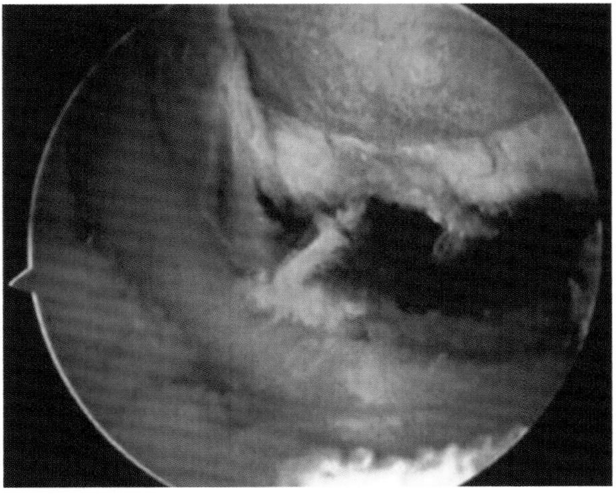

Figure 20-11 | Ulnar nerve seen in posteromedial elbow following careful debridement of surrounding soft tissue.

Pearls and Pitfalls

- Thoughtful preparation in positioning and setup; arm secured for stability.
- Exsanguination and distension of the joint after landmarks are drawn.
- Only skin is incised; subcutaneous tissues are spread with blunt trocars.
- Proximal portals reduce NV injury.
- Suction is minimized near the capsule and nerves.
- Portals are closed to avoid fistulas and postoperative infection.

Acknowledgment

Arianna P. Selagea for medical illustrations.

References

1. Koh J, Cook A. *Chapter 33: Surgical Techniques of the Shoulder, Elbow, and Knee in Sports Medicine*. 1st ed. Philadelphia, PA: Elsevier; 2008:327-334.
2. Phillips BB, Strasburger S. Arthroscopic treatment of arthrofibrosis of the elbow joint. *Arthroscopy*. 1998;14:38-44.
3. Baker CL, Jones GL. Arthroscopy of the elbow. *Am J Sports Med*. 1999;27(2):251-264.
4. Timmerman L, Andrews JR. Arthroscopic treatment of posttraumatic elbow pain and stiffness. *Am J Sports Med*. 1994;22:230-235.
5. Marshal PD, Faiclough JA, Johnson SR, et al. Avoiding nerve damage during elbow arthroscopy. *J Bone Joint Surg Br*. 1993;75-B:129-131.
6. Canale ST, Phillips BB. *Chapter 49: Campbell's Operative Orthopaedics*. 10th ed. Philadelphia, PA: Elsevier; 2002:2613-2665.
7. O'Driscoll SW. Arthroscopic treatment for osteoarthritis of the elbow. *Orthop Clin North Am*. 1995;26:691-706.
8. Field LD, Altchek DW, Warren RF, et al. Arthroscopic anatomy of the lateral elbow: a comparison of three portals. *Arthroscopy*. 1994;10:602-607.
9. Stothers K, Day B, Regan WR. Arthroscopy of the elbow: anatomy, portal sites, and a description of the proximal lateral portal. *Arthroscopy*. 1995;11:449-457.

Chapter 21
Arthroscopic Treatment of OCD of the Capitellum

SHERWIN S. W. HO
JOHN R. MILLER

Sterile Instruments/Equipment

- 30-degree arthroscope
  - 2.7-mm arthroscope for working in direct lateral compartment
  - 4.0-mm arthroscope for routine anterior and posterior compartments; inflow is from cannula of the arthroscope, and, because it is larger, it allows better inflow, joint distension, and hemostasis
- Self-locking limb positioner (eg, Arthrex Trimano, Smith & Nephew SPIDER)
- 2.9-mm full-radius shaver blade without teeth
- Microcurettes
  - Allows better movement in tight lateral compartment
- Small joint obturator and cannulas
- Small slotted cannula
- 5.5-mm disposable cannula with stop cock
- Microfracture awls
- Smooth .062-in Kirschner wire
- Sterile tourniquet
- 1.6- and 2.0-mm smooth drills
- 1.6- or 2.0-mm absorbable nails for osteochondritis dissecans (OCD) fixation (1.6 mm most commonly used)

Positioning

- Prone for patients under 150 lb (Fig. 21-1)
  - Keeps body and table away from smaller arms
- Lateral decubitus for patients over 150 lb (Fig. 21-2)
- Self-locking limb positioner allows control of arm within tight space between elbow and table.

Surgical Approach

- Diagnostic arthroscopy is done with anteromedial, anterolateral, posterior, and posterolateral portals.
  - Direct lateral and accessory lateral portals are created specifically for management of OCD lesions of capitellum.
  - An inflow pump system allows better visualization while working with 2.7-mm arthroscope in the lateral compartment.
  - To obtain adequate fluid pressure, pump pressure can be increased to 90-100 mm Hg to offset the small diameter of the 2.7-mm arthroscope.

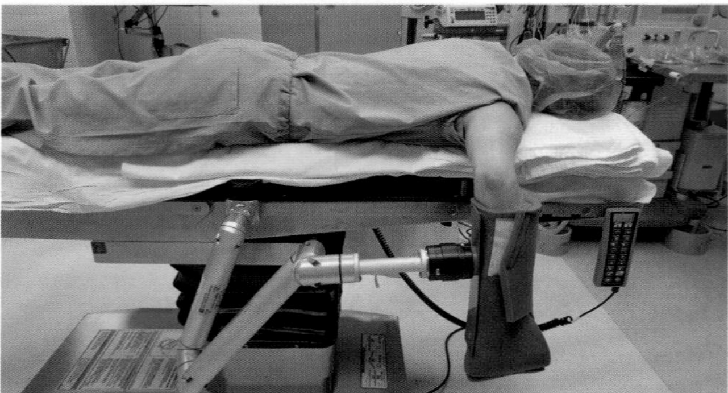

Figure 21-1 | Prone positioning with self-locking limb positioner improves working space in smaller patients.

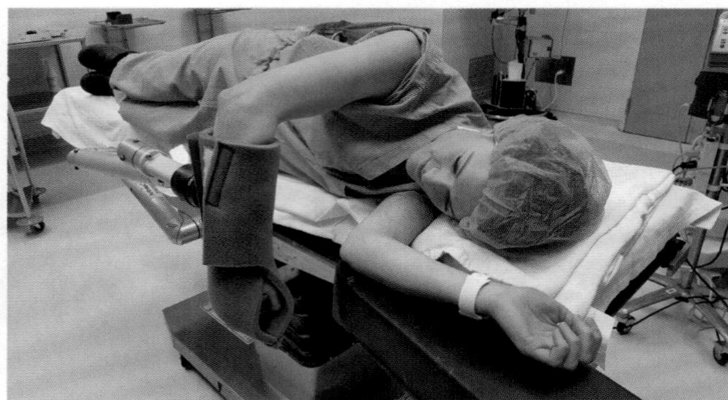

Figure 21-2 | Lateral decubitus positioning preferred for larger patients or those with difficult airways.

- OCD fragment are identified, and the competency of the overlying cartilage is evaluated.
  - Although uncommon, fragments over 1 cm in diameter and with sufficient underlying bone may be suitable for fixation.
  - Small, multifragmented, and/or inadequate underlying bone should be removed.
  - Typically there is loose, unstable cartilage overlying the lesion, which is easily recognized arthroscopically.
  - However, lesions with intact overlying articular cartilage but unstable underlying bone require careful probing to identify soft, ballotable articular cartilage indicating location of the lesion.
- For grade I or II chondral lesions, in situ drilling with a .062-in smooth Kirschner wire should be considered.

Debridement/Microfracture

- This is recommended for OCD fragments that are not suitable for fixation (most grade III and IV elbow OCD lesions).
- Unstable cartilage flaps are removed with a shaver and curettes (Fig. 21-3).
- The base of the OCD lesion is debrided of overlying fibrous tissue (Fig. 21-4).

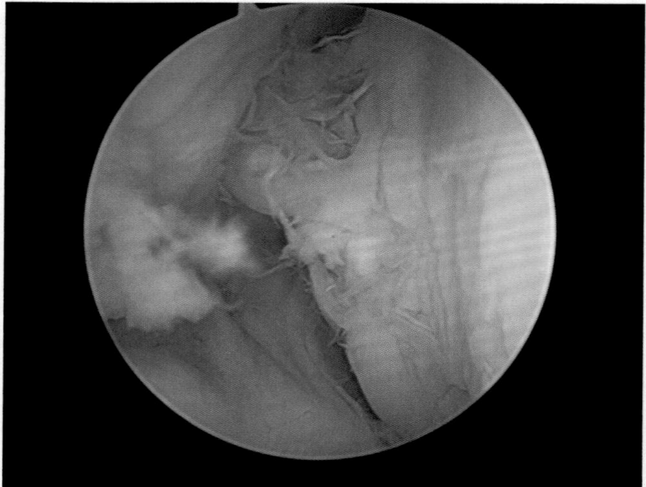

Figure 21-3 | Loose, unstable cartilage overlying capitellar OCD. Most lesions are easily identifiable arthroscopically, but some require careful use of a probe to localize the defect.

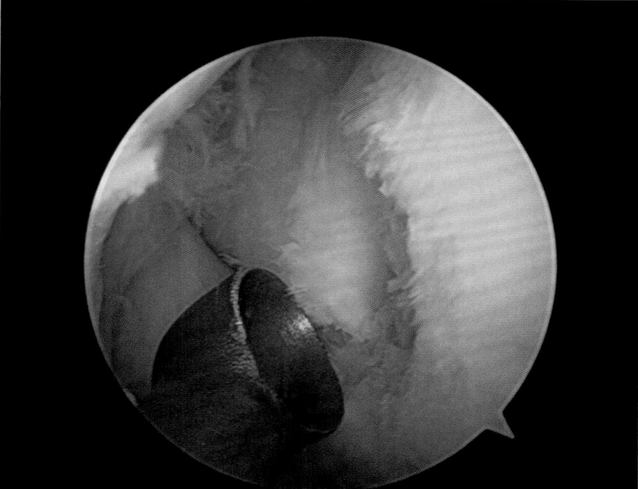

Figure 21-4 | Fibrous tissue under OCD fragment should be debrided with a curette and/or shaver.

- Care is taken to avoid removing excess subchondral bone.
- Loose or unstable cartilage edges that can propagate into loose bodies or chondral flaps should be removed.

- After a healthy bone base is obtained, microfracture of the capitellum is done to promote fibrocartilage healing (Fig. 21-5).

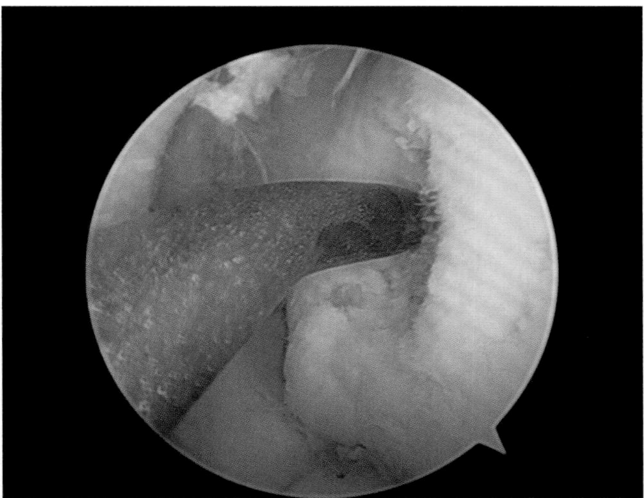

Figure 21-5 | Microfracture of the base of the lesion to stimulate fibrocartilage healing.

- Microfracture awls usually are adequate for bone marrow stimulation.
- Chronic, avascular lesions may require the use of a .062-in Kirschner wire for deeper drilling.
  - Drilling is performed perpendicular to the cartilage surface to avoid chondral penetration. This may require additional incisions or skin punctures to obtain correct trajectory.

OCD Fixation

- If the OCD fragment appears suitable for fixation, templating is recommended before surgery (Fig. 21-6).

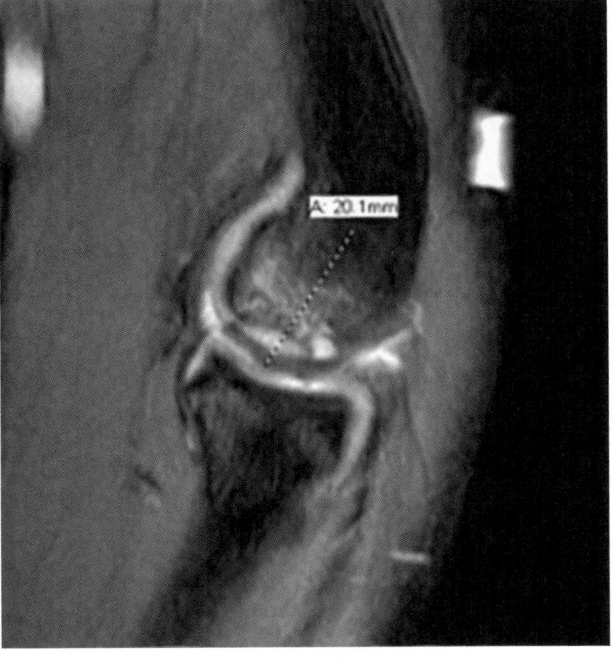

Figure 21-6 | Template of proposed OCD fixation.

- The length of the proposed nail/fixation device is templated on MRI images.
- The maximal length of the nail is used for fixation while avoiding the opposite cortex or physis.
- The number of nails that will fit within the OCD fragment is estimated (ideally 2).

- The recipient capitellar lesion is prepared with microcurettes and a 2.9-mm full-radius shaver without teeth (Fig. 21-7).
  - The surrounding border of articular cartilage should be smooth and stable.
  - It is helpful to microfracture the base of the lesion to assist with healing after fixation (Fig. 21-8).

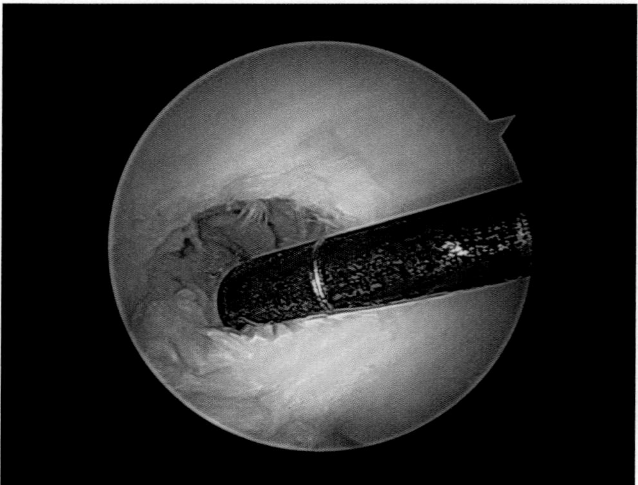

Figure 21-7 | OCD lesion is opened to reveal fibrous tissue overlying base.

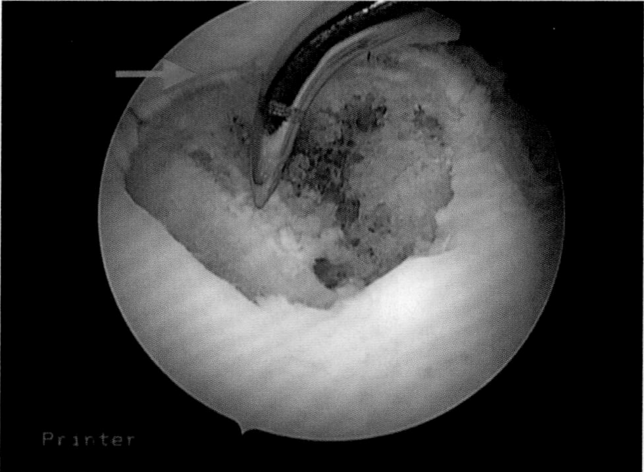

Figure 21-8 | Base of recipient lesion is debrided and prepared with microfracture to improve healing potential. Note that the OCD lesion remains hinged to the base (*arrow*) to allow easier reduction.

- The recipient lesion often needs to be deepened and enlarged to allow the OCD fragment to be fully seated and avoid difficulty with reduction.
- If possible, the defect should be left hinged to the surrounding cartilage because complete detachment will increase the difficulty of reduction and fixation (Fig. 21-9).

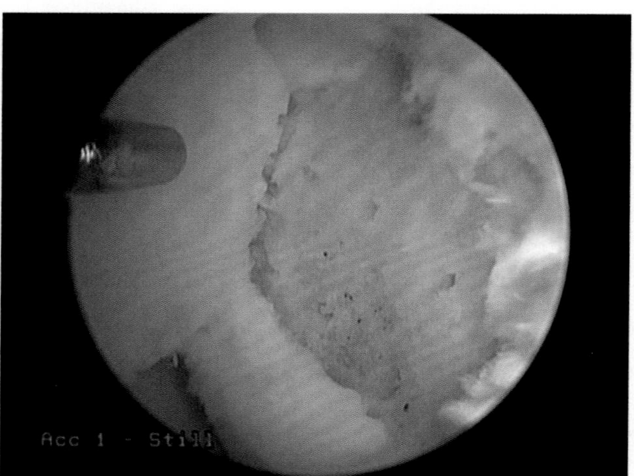

Figure 21-9 | Hinged OCD lesion beneath probe remains attached to remaining articular cartilage to prevent difficult reduction of a detached fragment.

- A 1.5-in 25-gauge needle is used to identify percutaneous placement of fixation nails perpendicular to the joint surfaces
- A small stab wound is made with a no. 11 blade scalpel, and a drill or insertion cannula with impactor is placed percutaneously against the OCD lesion.
- A nail length is selected that will place fixation barbs well within the capitellum and past the base of the lesion while avoiding open physes.
  - Often the physis will be penetrated to afford adequate strength of fixation.
  - Smooth, nonthreaded, bioabsorbable nails generally do not result in growth arrest.

- When using nails, we recommend overdrilling with a 2.0-mm drill for a 1.6-mm nail, unless the underlying bone is atypically osteoporotic.
  - This avoids difficulty when inserting the nail.
- A skilled assistant is necessary when inserting nails to manage the arthroscope and inflow.
- The guide for a 1.6-mm nail is placed over the fragment (Fig. 21-10).

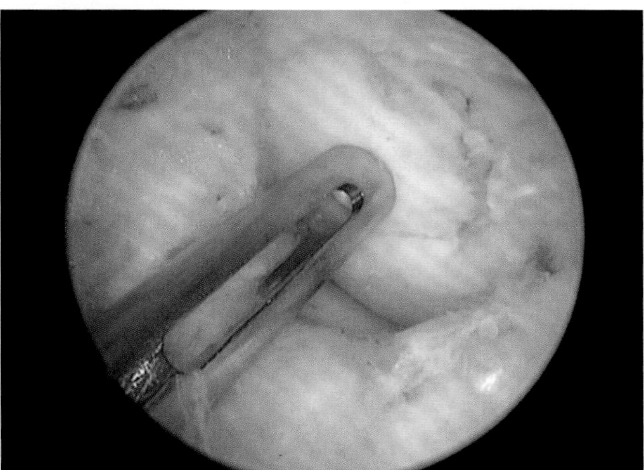

Figure 21-10 | Guide is placed perpendicular to reduced articular cartilage surface. Percutaneous placement of the guide may be required to obtain correct trajectory.

  - If the fragment remains proud, it is tapped gently with the guide and inserter to further reduce the fragment.
  - Repetitive or aggressive impaction of the fragment should be avoided to prevent chondrocyte damage.
  - If the fragment cannot be fully reduced, the guide is removed and the recipient lesion is prepared further.
- Once the lesion is appropriately reduced with the guide in place, inflow is turned off.
  - The backflow of fluid can displace the nail out of the guide during insertion.
- The nail is placed carefully in the guide to avoid the nail being washed out of the inserter (Fig. 21-11).

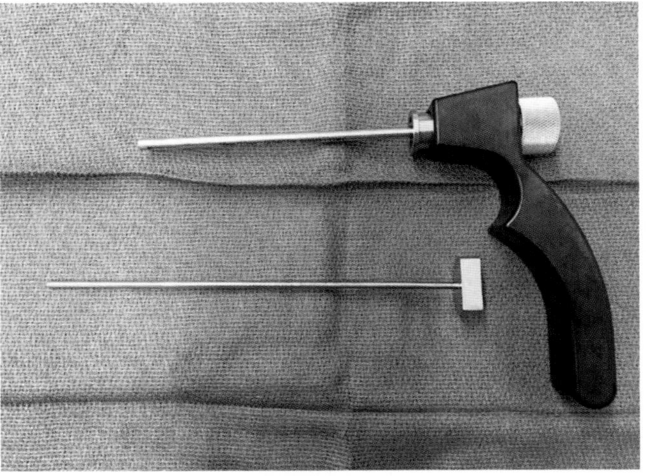

Figure 21-11 | Example of an arthroscopic OCD fixation system.

  - A small needle driver is used to place the nail in the end of the inserter and is covered with a finger (Fig. 21-12).
  - The finger is replaced with the impactor, and the nail is pushed until its tip is positioned in the slot of the guide (Fig. 21-13).
- The inflow is turned on to observe nail insertion through the open slot in insertion guide (Fig. 21-14).

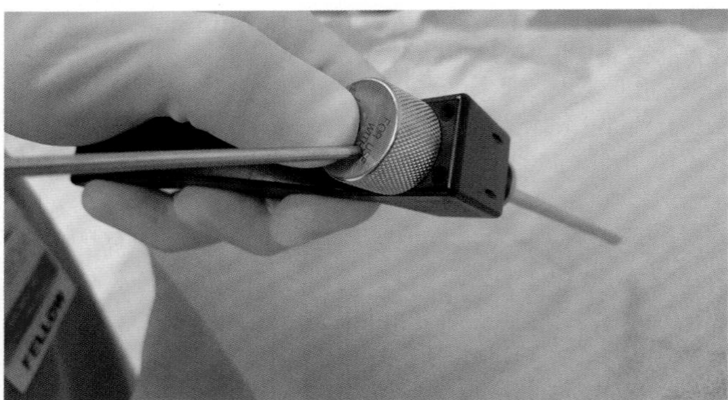

Figure 21-12 | After placement of fixation nail into the device, the surgeon's finger should be held over the opening to prevent backing out of the nail due to backflow through slots in the guide.

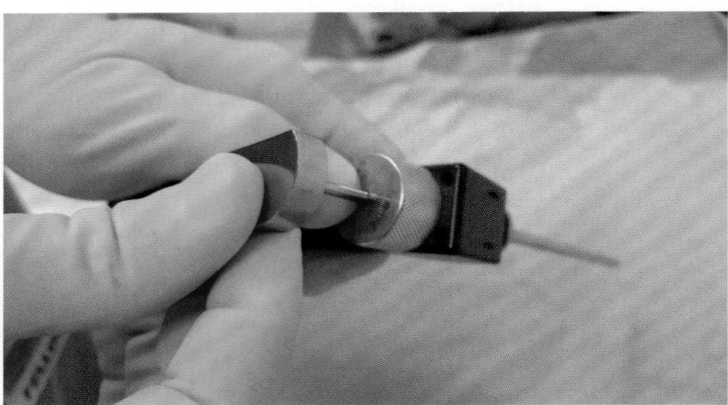

Figure 21-13 | The surgeon's finger is carefully replaced with impactor to prevent the nail from backing out of the guide.

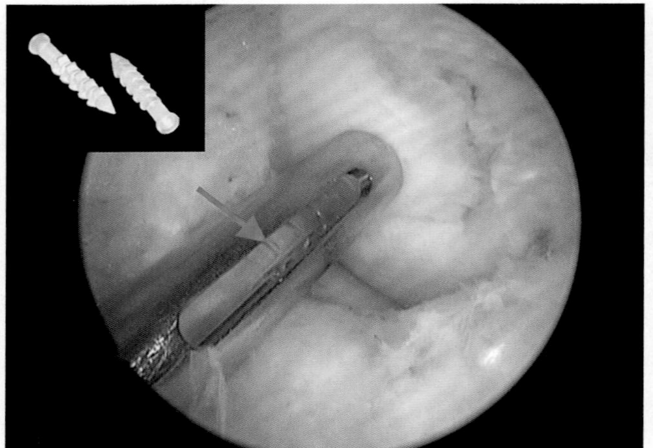

Figure 21-14 | Fixation nail (shown in **inset**) is visualized through slot in guide to ensure proper insertion (barbs of transparent nail noted with *arrow*).

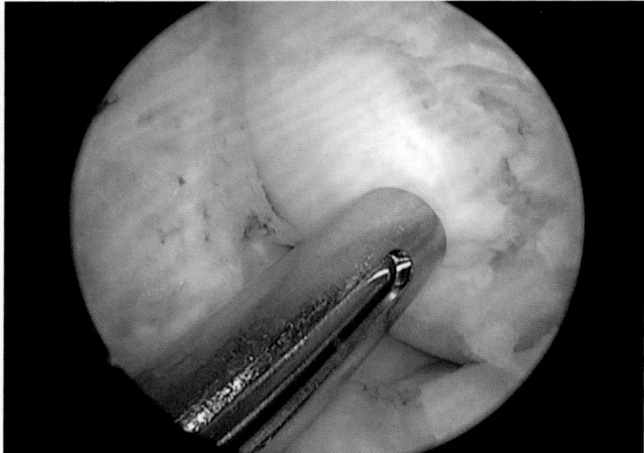

Figure 21-15 | The nail is impacted into the lesion with care to avoid fragmentation or loss of reduction.

- The nail is tapped into the fragment until the head of the nail is flush with the articular cartilage (Fig. 21-15).
- After the nail is seated with the 1.6-mm impactor, a 2.0-mm impactor can be used to further seat the head of the nail at or slightly below the level of surrounding articular cartilage (Fig. 21-16).

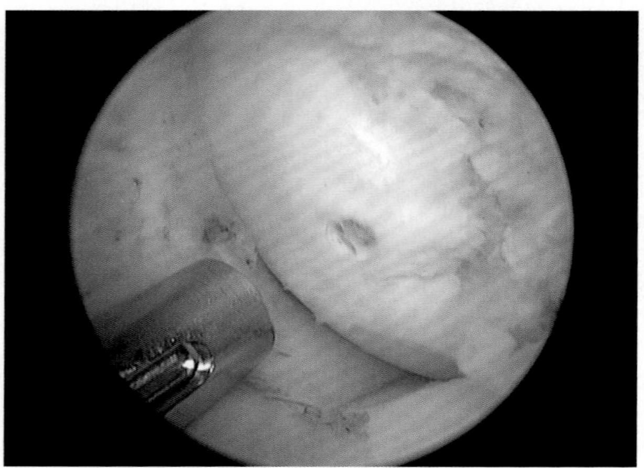

Figure 21-16 | The nail should be slightly countersunk to the articular surface after insertion.

- These steps are repeated for each additional nail.
  - Most lesions will have space for only one or two nails.
  - The OCD lesion should be level with, if not countersunk to, intact articular cartilage.

Chapter 22

Arthroscopic Treatment of Valgus Extension Overload

DJURO PETKOVIC
FRANK ALEXANDER
CHRISTOPHER S. AHMAD

Equipment (Figs. 22-1 and 22-2)

- Nonsterile tourniquet
- Articulating arm holder (if supine)
- Lateral elbow positioner (if lateral position)
- Beanbag (for lateral position)
- 4.0-mm 30-degree arthroscope
- 2.7-mm arthroscope as needed
- 3.5- and 4.5-mm mechanical shavers
- Electrocautery device
- Switching stick(s)
- Fully threaded and partially threaded graspers
- Blunt-tipped elevator
- Osteotomes (one-fourth in both straight and curved)
- Articulating retractor
- 60-cc syringe with normal saline and 18-G needle
- 10-cc syringe containing lidocaine with epinephrine

Positioning

- For an isolated arthroscopy case (no ligament reconstruction), the following positioning is preferred (Fig. 22-4).
- Lateral decubitus position with a beanbag.
  - All bony prominences, such as the femoral condyles and fibular head, are padded.
  - An axillary roll is placed underneath the contralateral axilla.
- The shoulder is at 90 degrees of forward elevation and in slight abduction.
- The ipsilateral humerus is supported with a lateral elbow positioner as high as possible.
- The elbow positioner is secured on the table in such a way to avoid interference with elbow range of motion. This can be achieved by securing the positioner to the table at the level of the nipple and angling it slightly proximally. Maximal flexion and extension of the elbow is ensured with positioning (Figs. 22-3 and 22-4).
- The contralateral elbow is in 90 degrees of flexion on an arm rest positioned as high as possible.
- A nonsterile tourniquet is placed on the ipsilateral arm.
- Positioning of the beanbag and any instruments anterior to the chest of the patient is minimized to avoid obstructing the arthroscopic instrumentation to the elbow.
- After the patient is positioned, instruments entering the elbow from the various portals and at various elbow flexion angles should be simulated to verify optimal setup and unobstructed path of instruments.

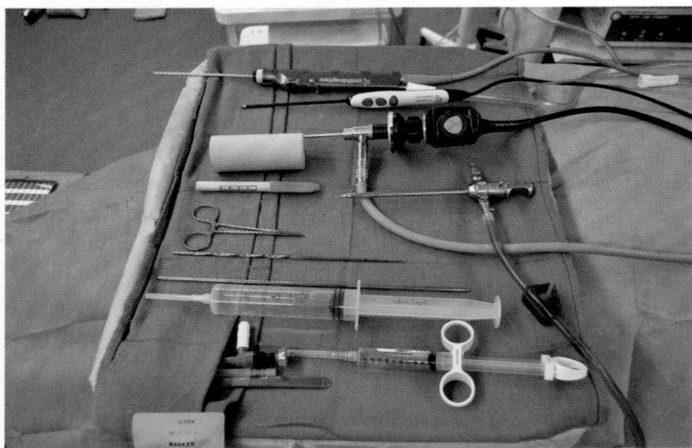

Figure 22-1 | Instruments to have available on the Mayo stand. From **top** to **bottom**: mechanical shaver, electrocautery, 30-degree arthroscope, Esmarch bandage, marking pen, trocar and metal cannula for arthroscope, straight clamp, probe, switching stick, saline injection, lidocaine injection, cannula, spinal needle, no. 11-blade scalpel.

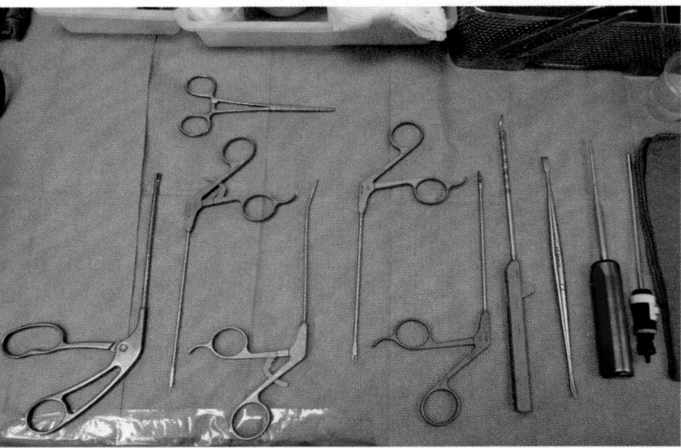

Figure 22-2 | Other instruments to have available include graspers, retractors, elevators, osteotomes, and an alternative sized shaver.

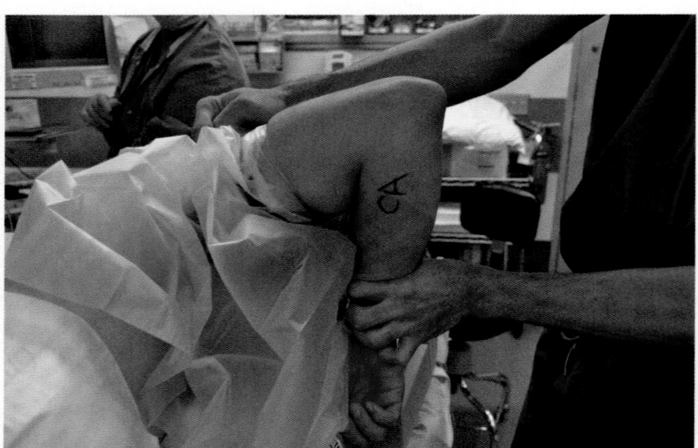

Figure 22-3 | Patient in lateral position and tourniquet placed. Note the ample exposure for further draping and the unobstructed full elbow flexion.

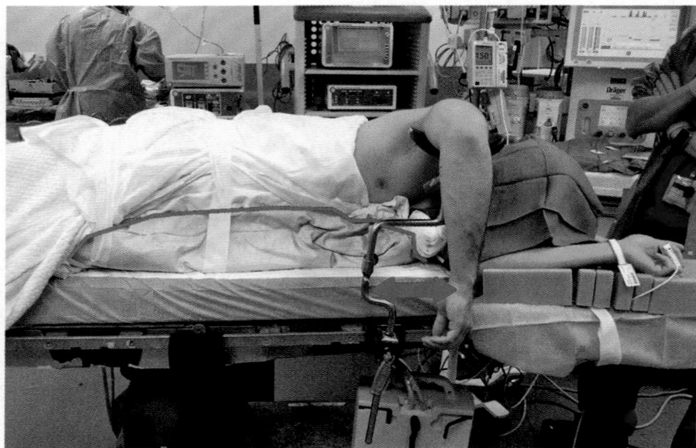

Figure 22-4 | Patient in the lateral position with lateral elbow positioner and beanbag. Note the low level of the beanbag (see *red line*), thus avoiding any interference with the trajectory of surgical instruments. Also, note that the elbow positioner is secured to the table in such a way that plenty of space exists between the shaft of the positioner and the patient's hand (*red double arrow*), thus allowing unobstructed full elbow flexion.

Alternative Positioning

- For arthroscopy in conjunction with a procedure requiring a supine position (such as an ulnar collateral ligament [UCL] reconstruction, ulnar nerve transposition, or other open procedure), the following positioning is recommended (Fig. 22-5).
  - The patient is placed supine with an articulating arm holder on the contralateral side, secured to the table at the level of the patient's contralateral knees.
  - If associated open procedures are warranted, arthroscopy is done first followed by the open procedure.
  - Once arthroscopy is complete, the arm is disengaged from the articulating arm holder and is placed on a hand table on the ipsilateral side of the operating table.
- The remainder of this technique is presented from the perspective of lateral positioning, but similar principles apply to supine positioning regarding planning, instrumentation, and strategy.

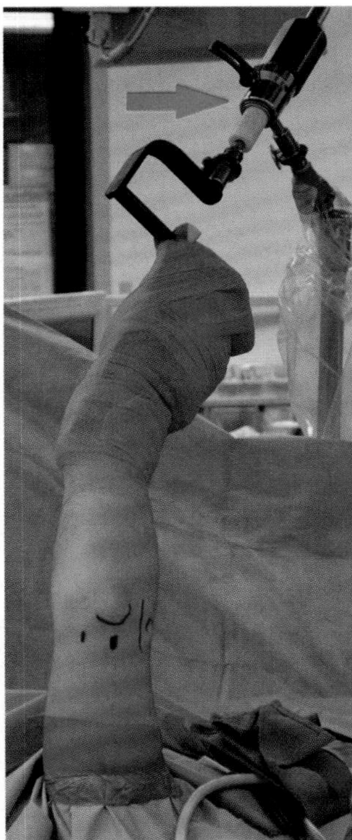

Figure 22-5 | Patient prepared and draped with arm suspension positioning device for arthroscopy before UCL reconstruction. An articulating arm holder fixed to the contralateral side of the OR table (*red arrow*) suspends the arm across the patient's body.

Planning

- Before surgery, history, physical examination, and imaging confirm the diagnosis.
  - The history should be consistent with a story of posterior elbow pain.
  - Physical examination findings consistent with valgus extension overload (VEO) include pain with provocative maneuvers, tenderness at the posteromedial olecranon, and pain with forced elbow extension.
  - Imaging should confirm an osteophyte at the posteromedial olecranon.
- It is important to determine the location of the ulnar nerve and whether it subluxes on dynamic examination. This can influence whether it is safe to use a standard anteromedial portal and also may affect any potential vulnerability of the nerve when working in the posteromedial aspect of the elbow. Knowledge of the location of the ulnar nerve is especially important after previous elbow surgery, such as UCL reconstruction, in which the nerve may have been transposed anteriorly. This information should be obtained from previous operative reports.
- Preoperative CT scanning with 2-D and 3-D reconstructions helps identify the precise location of the osteophytes (Fig. 22-6A-C). During arthroscopy, some osteophytes may be encased in soft tissue and not easily identified.
- An essential component of good surgical planning is appropriate patient counseling. Many patients with VEO have concomitant insufficiency or will later develop insufficiency of the UCL. Patients should be made aware that they can experience UCL dysfunction and may eventually require UCL reconstruction.

Portal Placement

- Before marking the portals, the following structures are outlined (Figs. 22-7 and 22-8).
  - Olecranon
  - Lateral epicondyle
  - Radial head
  - Medial epicondyle
  - Path of the ulnar nerve
- Next, the various portals are outlined.
  - Anteromedial (AM) portal: 2 cm proximal to the medial epicondyle and 1 cm anterior to intermuscular septum. This portal can be 1-13 mm from the medial antebrachial cutaneous nerve (MABCN).[1]

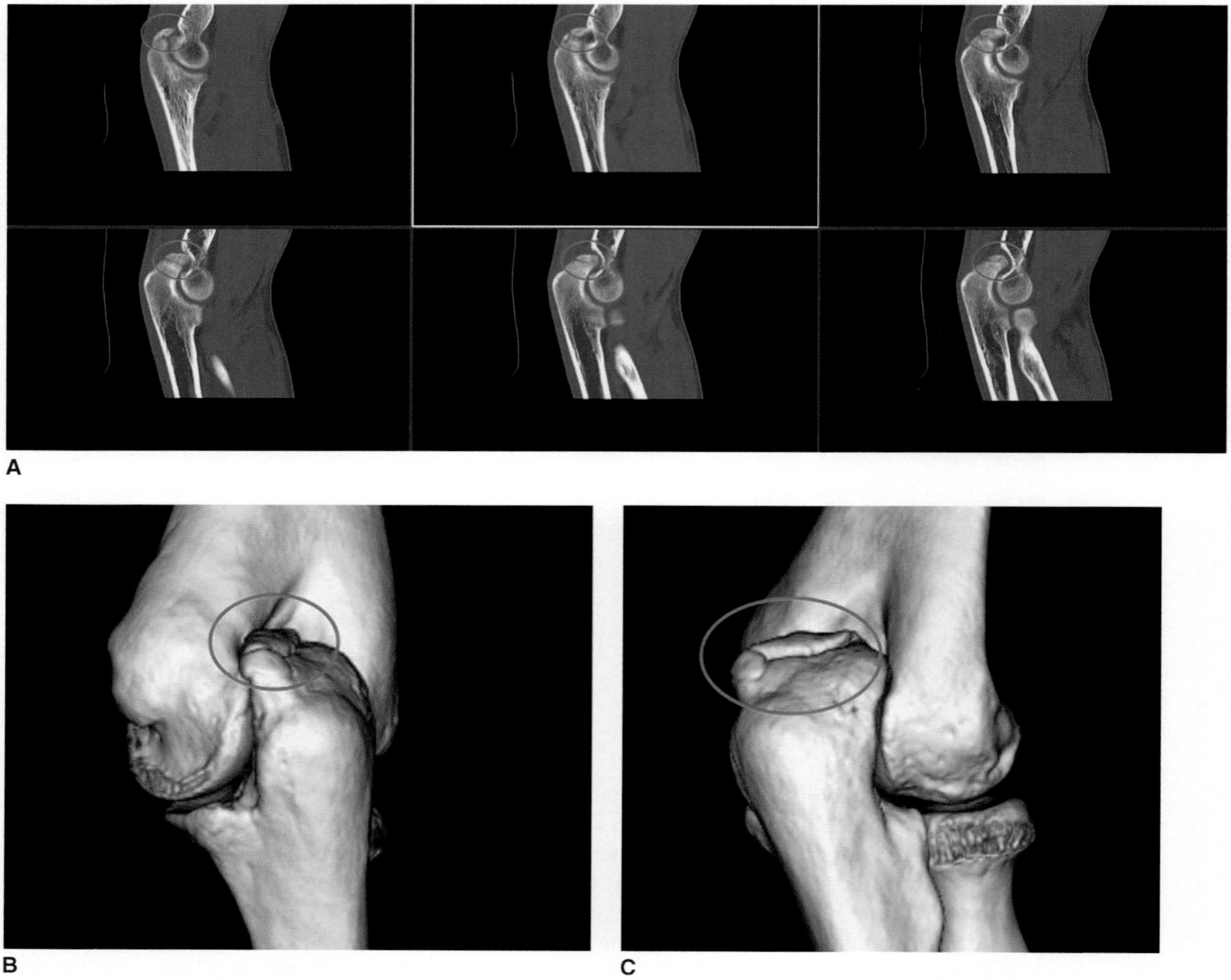

Figure 22-6 | **A.** Multiple cuts of the sagittal CT scan demonstrating olecranon osteophytes within the *red circles*. **B and C.** 3-D reconstructions of the CT of the right elbow showing the prominent olecranon osteophytes within the *red circles*.

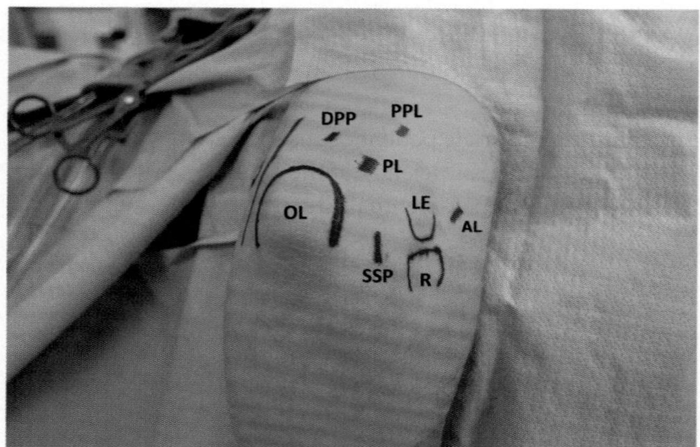

Figure 22-7 | Posterolateral view of the elbow. OL, olecranon; R, radial head; LE, lateral epicondyle; SSP, soft spot portal; DPP, direct posterior portal; PL, posterolateral portal; PPL, proximal posterolateral portal; AL, anterolateral portal.

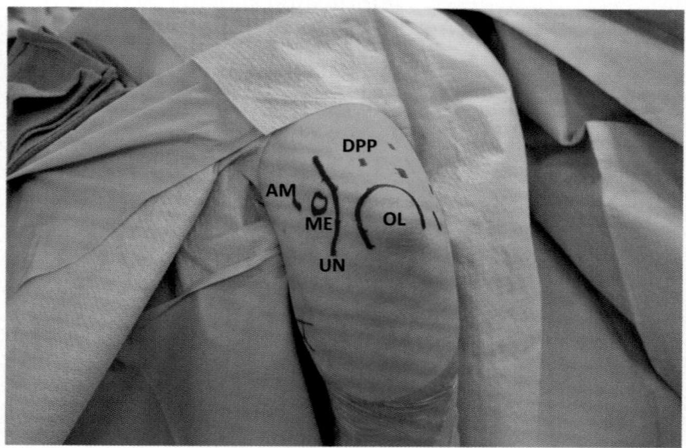

Figure 22-8 | Posteromedial view of the elbow. DPP, direct posterior portal, AM, anteromedial portal; O, olecranon; UN, ulnar nerve; ME, medial epicondyle.

- Anterolateral (AL) portal : 1 cm anterior and proximal to the lateral epicondyle. This portal is established with needle localization.
- Posterolateral (PL) portal: 1 cm proximal to the olecranon tip and adjacent to the lateral border of the triceps.
- Accessory proximal posterolateral portals (PPL): proximal to the PL portal for retractor insertion, typically 3 cm proximal to the olecranon tip and along the lateral border of the triceps tendon.
- Direct posterior portal (DPP): located 2-3 cm proximal to the tip of the olecranon in the midline of the triceps. This portal can be established under direct vision with a spinal needle to ensure a good angle and access to the olecranon tip.
- Soft spot (SS) portal: also known as the direct lateral portal, placed in the recess formed between the olecranon tip, radial head, and lateral epicondyle.

Procedure

- The arm is exsanguinated with an Esmarch bandage, and the tourniquet is inflated.
- The joint is insufflated with normal saline.
- Through the AM portal, anterior diagnostic arthroscopy, including valgus stress test of the UCL, is done.
- The AL portal is established under direct vision with an outside-in technique.
- Posterior diagnostic arthroscopy is carried out through the PL portal; an accessory PL portal can be established for a retractor as needed.
- A direct posterior (DPP) working portal is established, and loose bodies are debrided and removed. The olecranon osteophyte tip is removed (the viewing portal and working portal can be switched to the DPP and PL portals, respectively, as needed).
- Contouring of the bony surfaces, including the posteromedial olecranon and fossa (viewing portal PL and working portal DPP), is completed.
- A soft spot working portal (SSP) is established, and loose bodies are debrided and removed from the radiocapitellar joint as needed.

Anterior Elbow Joint Arthroscopy

- Arthroscopy begins in the anterior portal if there is any anterior elbow pathology.
- Often in VEO, the pathology is isolated to the posterior compartment, and it is reasonable to start arthroscopy from the posterior aspect of the joint, so that the anterior compartment arthroscopy can be skipped.
  - This often is done when patients have had prior ulnar nerve transposition and an AM portal is contraindicated.
- If starting arthroscopy from the anterior aspect of elbow joint, an 18-gauge needle is introduced through the SS portal and the joint is distended with ~30 mL of sterile saline until resistance is encountered (Fig. 22-9).

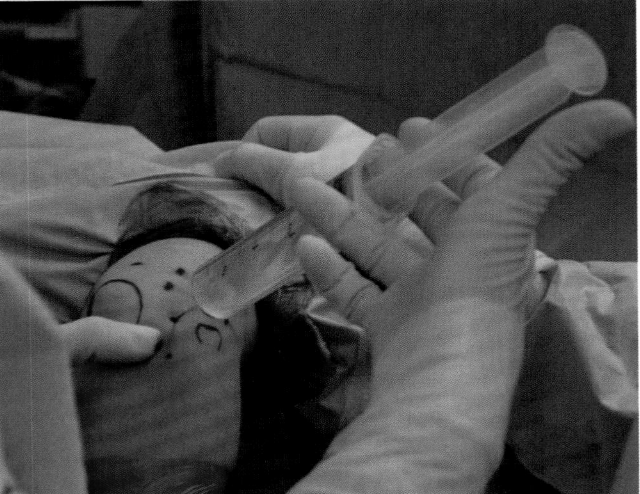

Figure 22-9 | The elbow joint is insufflated with a 60-cc syringe through an 18-gauge needle in the soft spot portal.

- Insufflation increases the distance between the neurovascular structures and the joint surfaces during introduction of the arthroscopic trocar. The nerve-to-bone distance increases about 12 mm for the median nerve and 6 mm for the radial nerve.[2]
- Insufflation also confirms that the joint is entered when fluid returns from the trocar.
- An assistant maintains pressure on the syringe during joint entry.

- The first portal for standard arthroscopy is the AM portal, located 2 cm proximal to the medial epicondyle and ~1 cm anterior to the intermuscular septum.
  - Palpating the septum usually is possible and helps with accurate placement of the portal. The MABCN along with the ulnar nerve is at risk with this portal.
  - A no. 11-blade scalpel is used to incise skin only, avoiding deep penetration to prevent iatrogenic nerve injury.
  - A small hemostat clamp is used to spread bluntly down to the capsule to avoid injury to the MABCN.
  - It is important to ensure that the dissection is anterior to the intermuscular septum to avoid ulnar nerve injury.
  - A blunt-tipped trocar is used to feel along the anterior humerus toward the radiocapitellar joint.
  - The anterior capsule is penetrated with the blunt trocar (Fig. 22-10). Fluid will exit the cannula.
  - The needle is removed from the SSP once joint entry is confirmed.

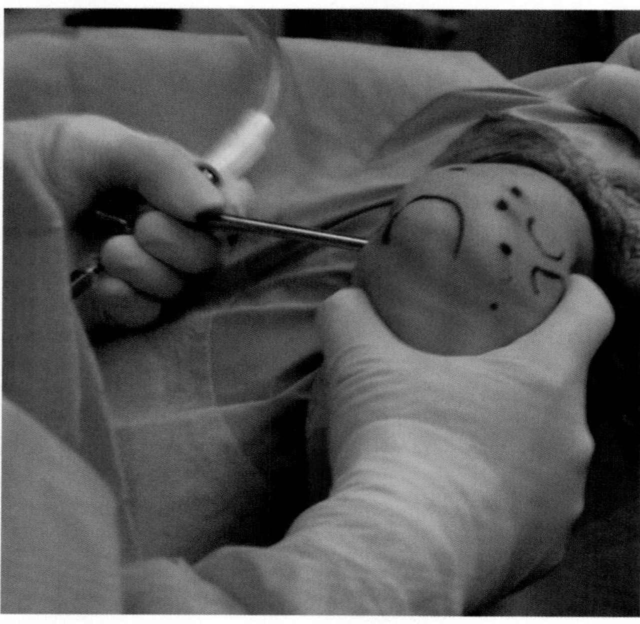

Figure 22-10 | The anterior elbow joint is entered through the anteromedial portal with a blunt trocar and arthroscopic cannula. Counter pressure is applied to stabilize the elbow.

- Anterior arthroscopy.
  - The arm is maintained in 90 degrees of flexion.
  - Evaluation for:
    - Loose bodies.
    - Articular cartilage damage.
    - Synovitis.
    - Anterior radiocapitellar joint.
    - The radial head is evaluated for osteochondral lesions with pronation and supination.
    - An 18-gauge spinal needle from the AL portal can be used as outflow and help with visualization.
- If a working portal is required, an AL portal is established.
  - The correct site and trajectory are localized with a spinal needle.
  - A no. 11-blade scalpel is used to incise the skin only to avoid injury to any superficial nerves.
  - A small hemostat clamp is used to bluntly spread through the capsule into the elbow joint from the AL portal.
  - A 3.5-mm shaver is used in the anterior aspect of elbow joint for any debridement.

- A switching stick guides passage of the camera into the AL portal for an alternative view of elbow joint, especially the medial side.
- Consideration should be given to using an articulating retractor through a proximal AL portal to retract soft tissues as needed in the anterior compartment.
- The coronoid tip and fossa are evaluated for osteophytes.
- The articular cartilage of the trochlea is evaluated for any chondral lesions.
- The UCL insufficiency test, aka arthroscopic valgus stress test, can be checked at this point.
  - The ulnohumeral articulation is viewed from the AL portal.
  - The interval between the coronoid process and the medial trochlea is assessed.
  - On valgus stress, ≥3-mm increase in the interval is positive for valgus instability.

Posterior Elbow Joint Arthroscopy

- If starting arthroscopy from the posterior elbow in patients without anterior elbow pathology, the portal sites are injected with lidocaine with epinephrine. There is no need to insufflate the joint; examination can safely proceed without endangering neurovascular structures.
- A posterolateral (PL) portal is established as the viewing portal (Fig. 22-11) with outside-in technique.

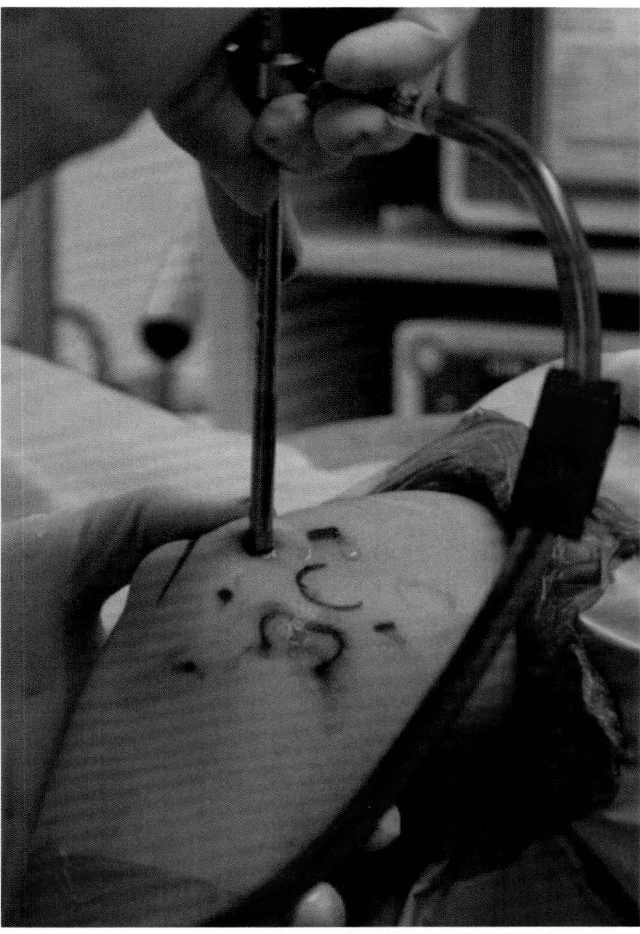

Figure 22-11 | The PL portal is established by incising the PL portal site; a blunt trocar through a metal cannula allows penetration of the posterior capsule and joint entry. This is the main posterior viewing portal.

  - An incision is made through the skin with a no. 11-blade scalpel.
  - A cannula with a blunt trocar is introduced through the PL portal; then the trocar is removed and the arthroscope is inserted through the cannula.
- The elbow is maintained in 30-45 degrees of flexion to relax the triceps.
- This should allow access to the posteromedial osteophytes of the olecranon, loose bodies, and any chondromalacia.

- While viewing from the PL portal, instruments (shaver and osteotome) are inserted through the DPP.
  - The DPP portal is established with a spinal needle, and then a no. 11-blade scalpel is used to make an incision through the skin and triceps (Fig. 22-12).
  - The DPP portal will serve as the working portal and potentially as the viewing portal if needed to place the grasper through the PL portal.
- The first goal is to create an adequate working space for viewing.
  - A mechanical shaver can be used to debride synovium and soft tissues in the olecranon fossa.
  - In the posterior compartment, a 4.5-mm shaver is preferred; the size of the shaver is adjusted as needed (Fig. 22-13).

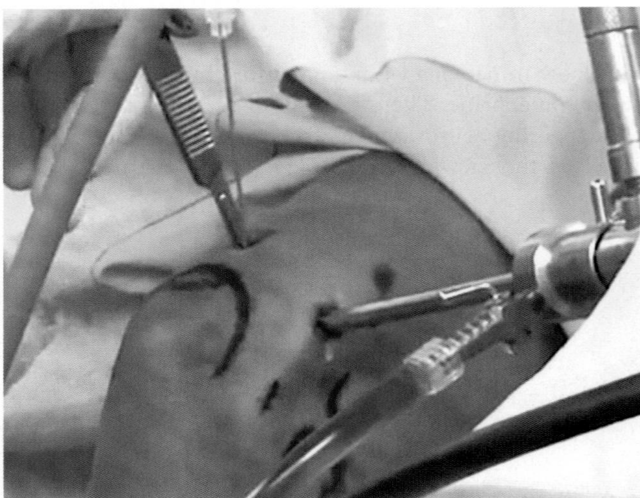

Figure 22-12 | While viewing from the PL portal, a spinal needle is used to localize the optimal position of the DPP portal. Once this is found, the DPP site is incised down through the capsule with a no. 11-blade scalpel.

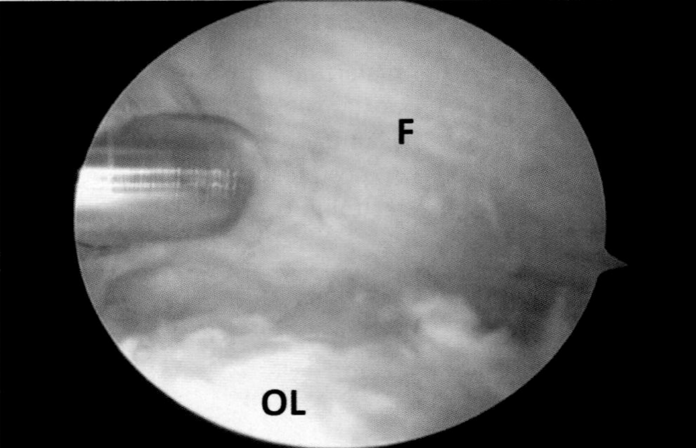

Figure 22-13 | A mechanical shaver is inserted from the DPP portal while viewing from the PL portal. This is used to debride synovium and debris and gain enough room for adequate visualization. OL, olecranon; F, olecranon fossa.

  - It is important to flex and extend the elbow to confirm the olecranon and trochlea and their orientation.
  - Once the olecranon tip is seen, cautery can be used to remove all the soft tissue on the olecranon for enhanced viewing (Fig. 22-14).
- Osteophytes encased in soft tissue are debrided with a shaver and cautery, exposing the pathologic olecranon tip (Fig. 22-15).
  - When using cautery, the instrument is activated in short bursts if working medially to avoid irritation and damage to the ulnar nerve.

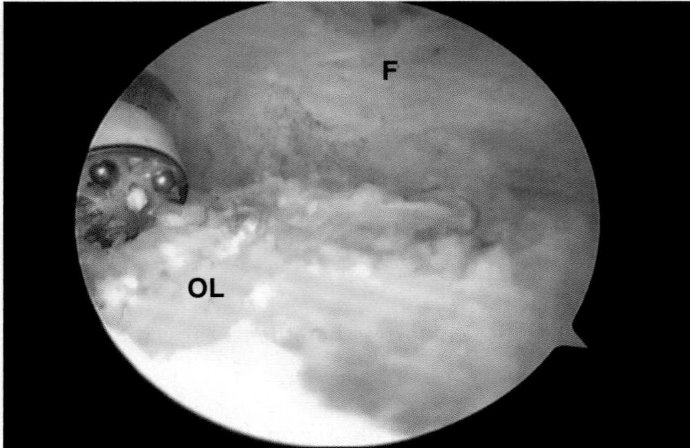

Figure 22-14 | Cautery is used to remove soft tissues from the olecranon tip. OL, olecranon; F, olecranon fossa.

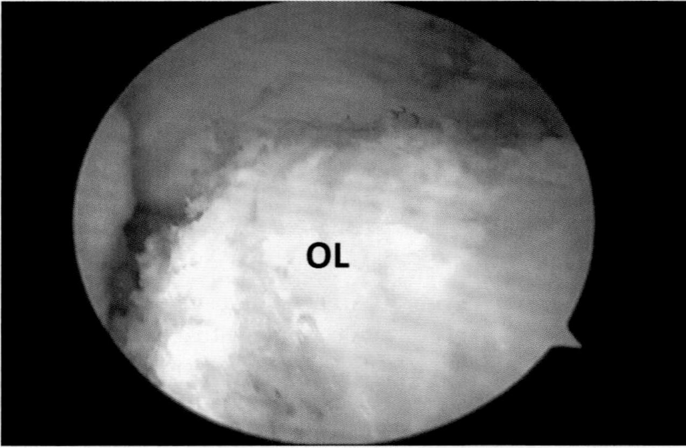

Figure 22-15 | The olecranon (OL) is cleared of soft tissues to allow appreciation of its exact shape.

- Once the bony surfaces are shelled out, an elevator or oscillating shaver can be used to define the border between normal bone and osteophyte (Fig. 22-16A and B).
  - KEY TIP: If difficulty is encountered in distinguishing the boundary of normal and abnormal bone, the quality of bone can be used as a guide. Abnormal bone tends to be softer while normal bone is more dense, and this differentiation can be made by palpation with probes and shavers.

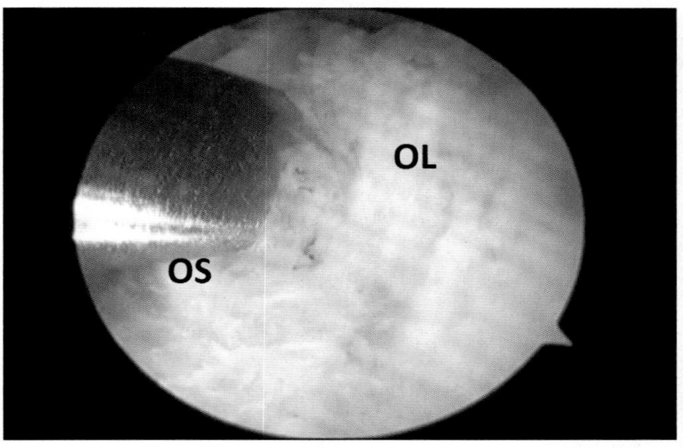

A

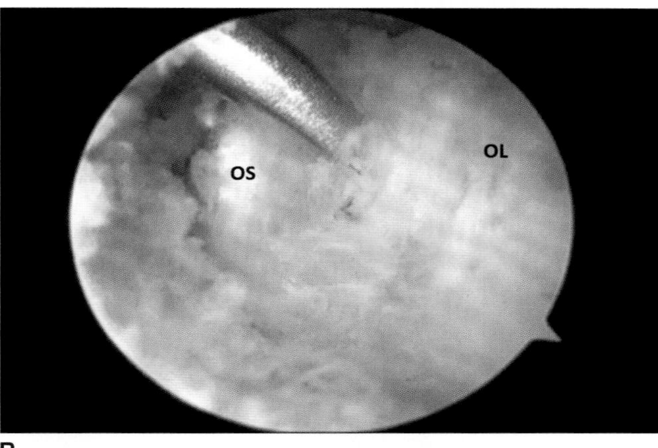

B

Figure 22-16 | **A and B.** A blunt elevator is used to define the junction between pathologic osteophyte (OS) and normal olecranon bone (OL).

- If a clear plane cannot be developed, a small straight osteotome can be used to gently tap and loosen the osteophyte (Fig. 22-17).

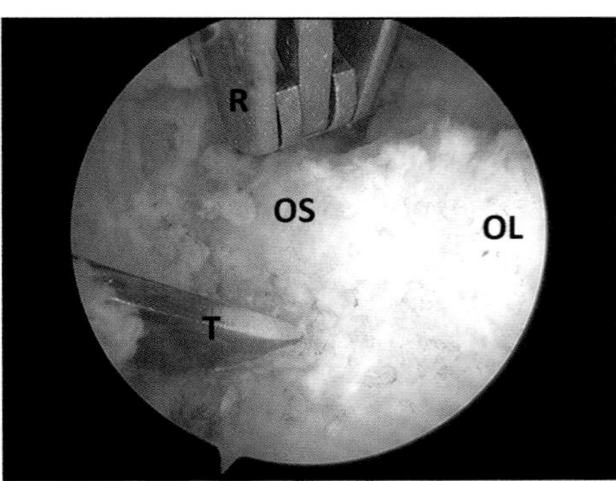

Figure 22-17 | Looking from the posterolateral portal, this image shows what can be done if an osteophyte will not separate with blunt probing alone. While protecting the soft tissues with an articulating retractor (R) from the PPL portal, a 1/4-in or .25-in straight osteotome (T) is introduced from the DPP portal at the junction of the soft pathologic osteophyte (OS) and the larger normal olecranon bone (OL).

- A motorized shaver can be used to decrease its size and facilitate removal of the osteophyte through an arthroscopic portal (Fig. 22-18A and B).
- The osteophyte is released from surrounding soft tissues (Fig. 22-19A-C).
- KEY TIP: Rather than remove the osteophyte from the DPP portal, which has dense fibrous triceps tendon, the camera is moved to the DPP portal, and the PL portal is expanded as needed and used as the working portal (Fig. 22-20).
- The osteophyte is removed with a ratcheted grasping device from the PL portal (Fig. 22-21).
- The olecranon is further contoured with a shaver or burr (Fig. 22-22A and B).
  - KEY TIP: The exact amount of resection is controversial; in general, resection should be very conservative, removing only pathologic bone and leaving all native olecranon.
  - Excessive bone removal from the posterior olecranon can lead to excessive stress in the UCL as well as pain and instability.
  - Studies have shown that resection of as little as 3 mm of the posteromedial olecranon can lead to increased strain on the UCL with valgus stress.[3]
  - An assistant can flex and extend the elbow to expose different aspects of the olecranon and distal humerus, thus optimizing the trajectory of the instruments.
- A curved retractor placed through the PPL portal can be used to retract medial soft tissues or to protect the ulnar nerve (Fig. 22-23).

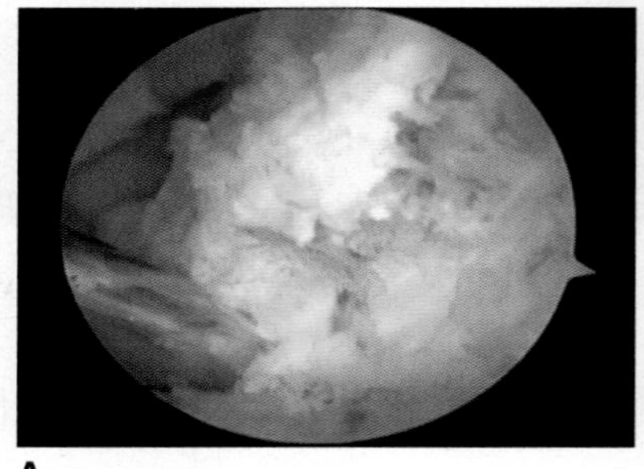

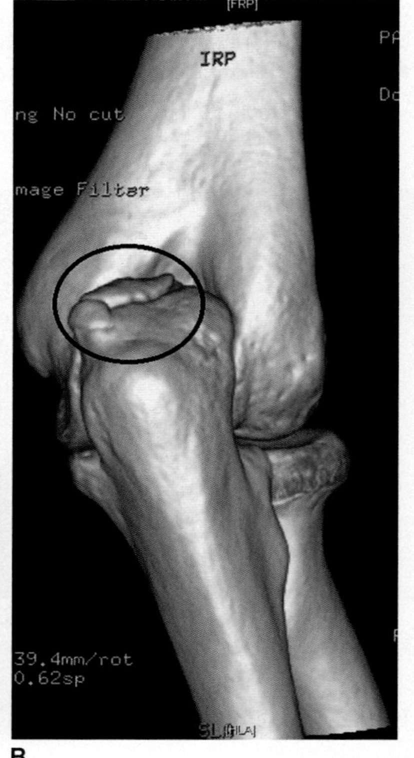

A B

Figure 22-18 | A motorized shaver can be used to release the osteophyte (OS) from the surrounding tissues **(A)**. As the boundaries of the osteophyte become more evident, the contour of the osteophyte (*black circle*) resembling that of the preoperative CT scan **(B)** becomes visible.

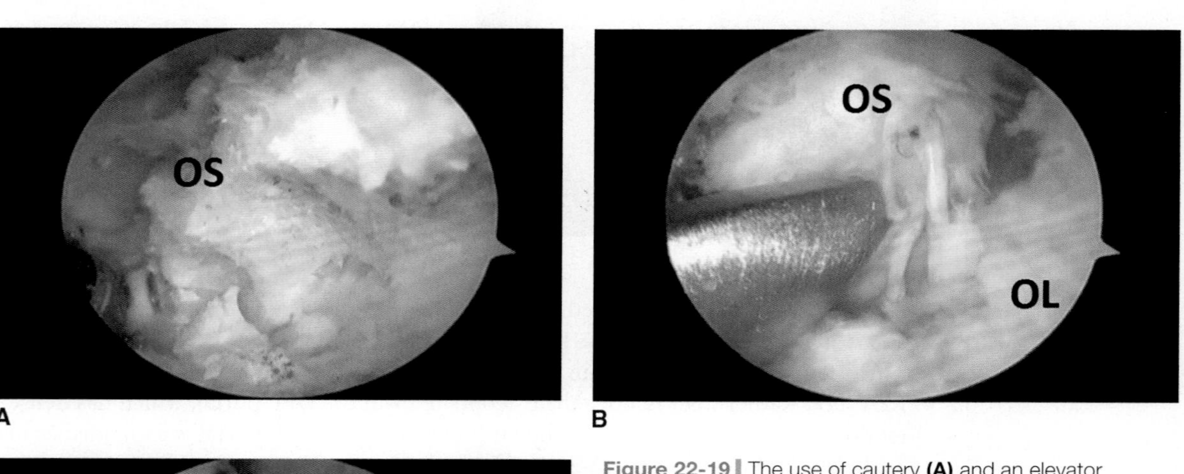

A B

OS

C

Figure 22-19 | The use of cautery **(A)** and an elevator **(B and C)** to free the main fragment of the osteophyte (OS) from the surrounding soft tissue and normal olecranon (OL) bone.

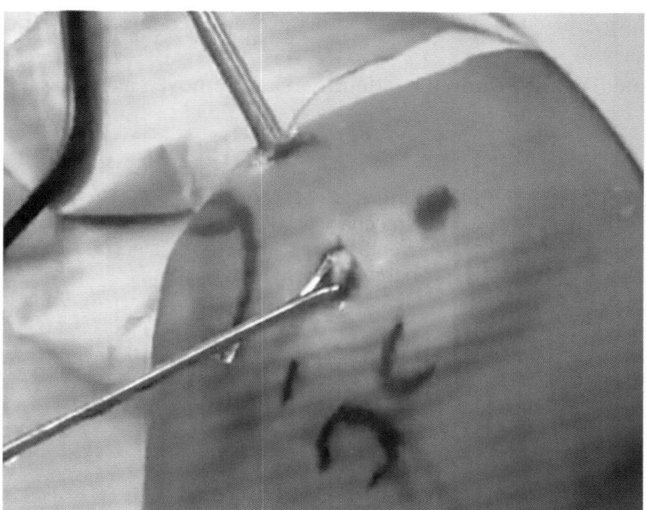

Figure 22-20 | Switching of the portal sites. The camera is introduced through the DPP portal, and the grasping instrument is introduced through the PL portal to avoid difficulty in removing the osteophyte past the triceps fascia.

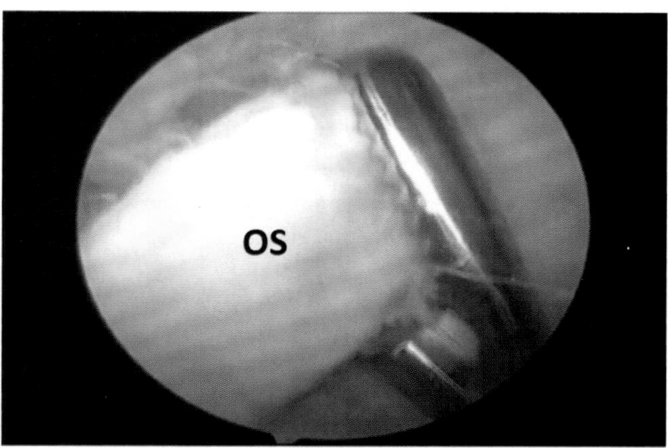

Figure 22-21 | Switching the viewing portal to the DPP portal, an articulating grasper is introduced through the PL portal to grasp and remove the osteophyte (OS).

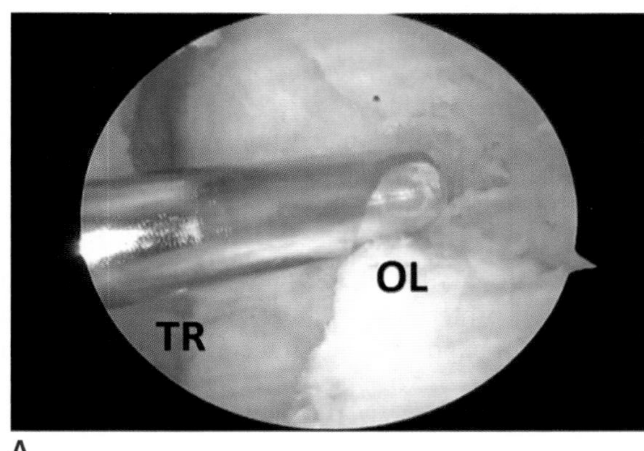

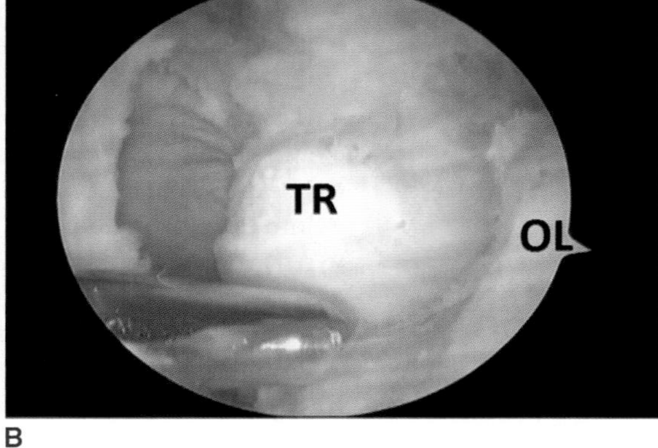

Figure 22-22 | A mechanical shaver is used to help debride any residual osteophyte located on the proximal and medial olecranon. Elbow extension **(A)** and flexion **(B)** can be used to expose different areas of the olecranon and humerus. OL, olecranon; TR, Trochlea.

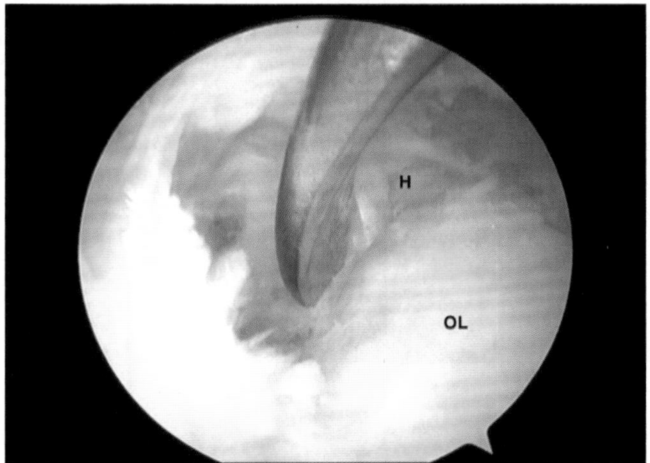

Figure 22-23 | An articulating retractor is introduced from the PPL portal to retract the soft tissues in the posteromedial gutter. This allows protection of the ulnar nerve and safe work in this area of the elbow while using instruments from the PL portal. OL, olecranon; H, distal medial humerus.

- Once the osteophyte is removed, the humeral chondral surface can be examined for a "kissing lesion," which can be debrided as necessary.
- Any residual osteophytes in the posteromedial gutter should be identified and removed as necessary (Fig. 22-24).

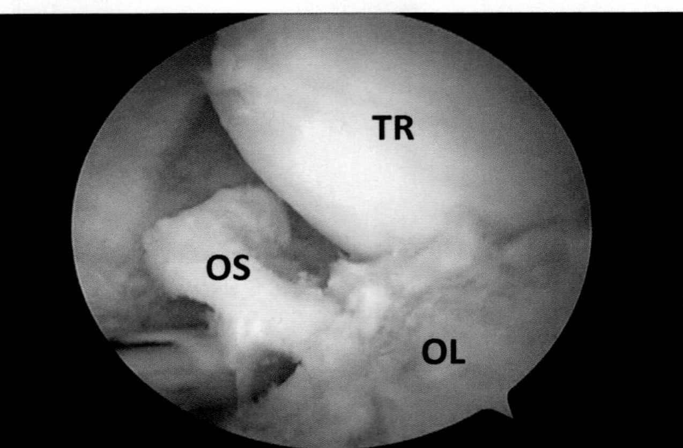

Figure 22-24 | Viewing from the PL portal, a mechanical shaver is used to debride and eventually remove residual osteophytes (OS) in the posteromedial aspect of the elbow. OL, olecranon; TR, trochlea.

- KEY TIP: Protection of the ulnar nerve when working in the posteromedial aspect of the elbow joint is essential to avoid complications.
    - The ulnar nerve is just superficial to the capsule in the posteromedial gutter.
    - Use of suction in this area of capsule should be avoided to prevent pulling of the soft tissues into the mouth of the shaver or other instrumentation.
    - If cautery is necessary, only short bursts are used. An assistant should be monitoring the forearm and hand for any twitching, which can be a sign of ulnar nerve irritation.
    - Use of the burr is avoided because of the turbulence created and the possibility of pulling the nerve into the rotating burr tip.
    - An articulating retractor introduced through the PPL portal is effective for retraction of the nerve.
    - If the ulnar nerve cannot be adequately protected with an articulating retractor, an open posteromedial incision should be considered for exposure and protection of the ulnar nerve under direct vision.
- In the olecranon fossa, the area should be further debrided to restore the natural contour of anatomic fossa (Fig. 22-25).
    - Fibrous tissue and any remaining osteophytes in the olecranon fossa can be removed with a mechanical shaver.

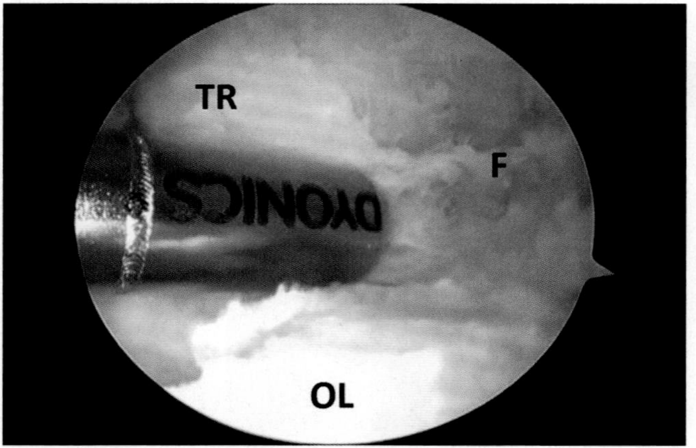

Figure 22-25 | Debridement of the olecranon fossa to restore the anatomic fossa. The viewing portal is the PL portal, while the shaver is in the DPP portal. OL, olecranon; TR, trochlea; F olecranon fossa.

- A "soft spot" portal (SSP) is created to treat any pathology in the radiocapitellar joint (Fig. 22-26)
  - A more distal position allows visualization of the posterior radiocapitellar joint.
  - The SSP portal is located in the center of the triangle formed by the lateral epicondyle, the tip of the olecranon, and the radial head.
  - This is the same spot commonly used to aspirate or insufflate the joint.
  - This portal can be as close as 6 mm from the lateral antebrachial cutaneous nerve,[1] so it is important to be cautious with this incision.
  - Pathologic radiocapitellar plica can be removed in this position.

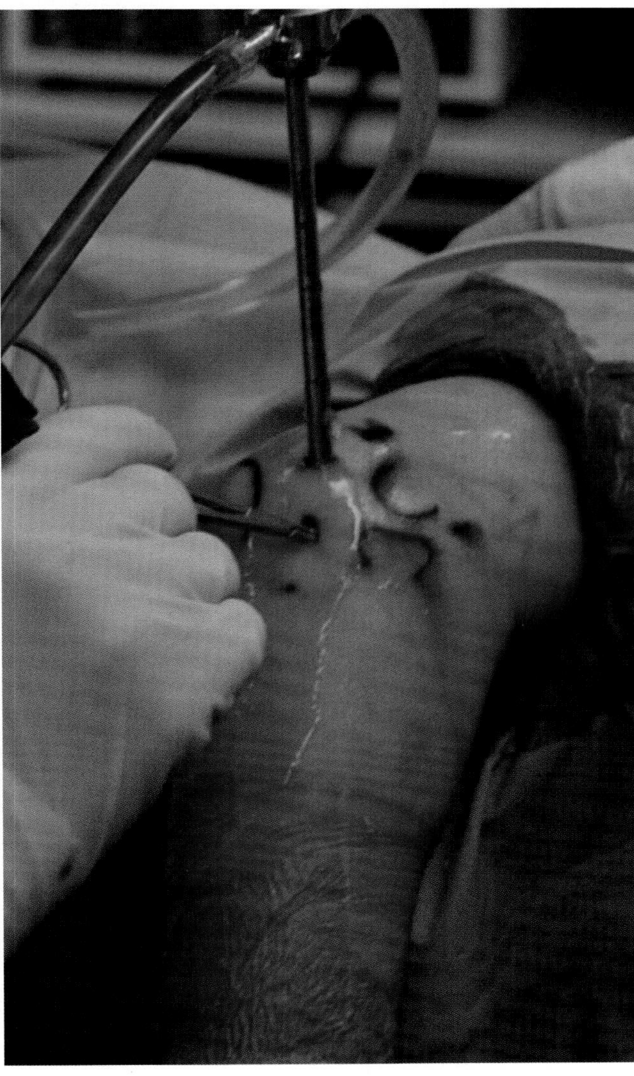

Figure 22-26 | An effective method to access the radiocapitellar joint. The camera is in the PL portal looking distally at the radiocapitellar joint, and the working portal is the SSP portal.

- KEY TIP: For access to the loose bodies in the PL elbow, the following suggestions should be kept in mind:
  - Large loose bodies should be removed through the PL or SSP portals because removal through the DPP portal requires going through the triceps, which will provide resistance.
  - Progressive flexion allows visualization of cartilage lesions on the anterior capitellum.
  - Osteochondral lesions, if present, are located in the posterior radiocapitellar joint and are best accessed through the SSP portal.
  - The most commonly missed lesions are loose bodies in the posterior radiocapitellar joint.
  - Competition between instruments can be problematic because the working distance between the PL and SSP portals is small; alternative viewing portals should be established as needed.

- An intraoperative radiograph can be used to determine the adequacy of resection and confirm that no excessive resection has been performed.
- The osteophyte locations should match the preoperative plan (Fig. 22-27A and B).
- Manipulation under anesthesia can be used as needed to gain range of motion.

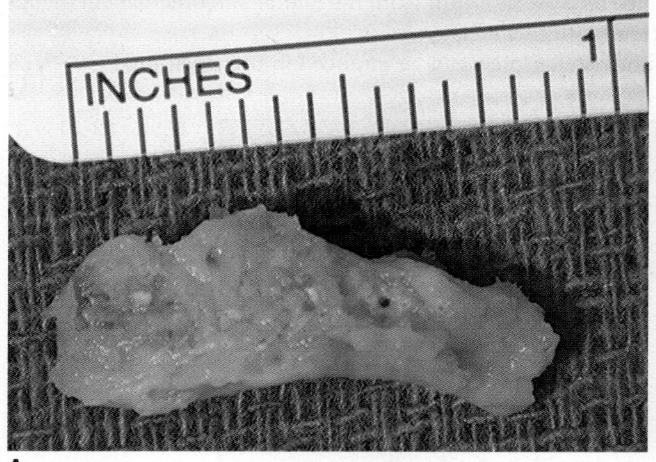

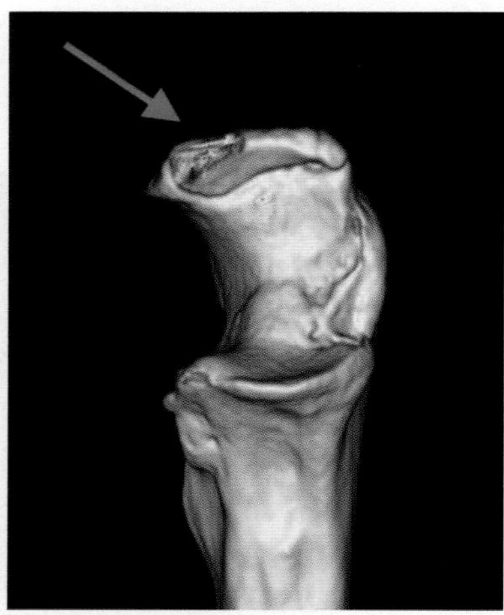

Figure 22-27 | The excised osteophyte **(A)** and the associated 3-D CT scan **(B)** showing the position of the osteophyte (*red arrow*) on the ulna.

Postoperative Protocol

- A soft compressive dressing and sling are worn for comfort for 1 week.
- Active elbow flexion is begun immediately.
- Focused exercises
  - Elbow range-of-motion restoration.
  - Flexor-pronator strength.
  - General strengthening and conditioning for throwing, including the entire kinetic chain.
    - Rotator cuff, periscapular muscles, core strengthening, and lower extremity.
  - At 6 weeks, a progressive throwing program is begun.
  - Return to sports is allowed at 3-4 months.

References

1. Unlu MC, Kesmezacar H, Akgun I, Ogut T, Uzun I. Anatomic relationship between elbow arthroscopy portals and neurovascular structures in different elbow and forearm positions. *J Shoulder Elbow Surg*. 2006;15(4):457-462.
2. Miller CD, Jobe CM, Wright MH. Neuroanatomy in elbow arthroscopy. *J Shoulder Elbow Surg*. 1995;4(3):168-174.
3. Kamineni S, Hirahara H, Pomianowski S, et al. Partial posteromedial olecranon resection: a kinematic study. *J Bone Joint Surg Am*. 2003;85(6):1005-1011.

Chapter 23

Ulnar Collateral Ligament Reconstruction: Modified Jobe Technique

CHRIS S. WARRELL
JAMES R. ANDREWS

Sterile Instruments/Equipment

- Tourniquet
- Blunt and sharp tendon strippers (if a gracilis autograft is needed)
- Metzenbaum scissors
- Sharp dissection scissors
- Bovie electrocautery
- Bipolar electrocautery
- Right-angle retractors
- Baby Hohmann retractors
- Vessel loops
- Key elevator
- One-fourth-in osteotome and/or small burr (if posteromedial olecranon osteophytes are present)
- Drills—3.5 mm (for palmaris autograft) and 4.0 mm (for gracilis autograft)
- Curettes—no. 1 and no. 2 curved and straight
- Mineral oil
- Hewson suture passer (Smith & Nephew)

Positioning

- The patient is positioned supine on a standard operating table.
- The operative arm is placed on a hand table.
- A nonsterile tourniquet is placed as proximal on the operative extremity as possible.
- If a palmaris longus tendon autograft is to be harvested, we recommend marking out the course of the tendon preoperatively while the patient is able to perform active wrist flexion and opposition of the thumb and small finger.
- The elbow is flexed to 30-45 degrees while operating on the medial elbow.
- Surgical towels placed under the elbow and wrist permit an optimal degree of elevation for hand placement during dissection and drilling.
- If need for a gracilis autograft is anticipated, the contralateral lower extremity is prepared and draped.
    - A large bump or triangle placed under the foot allows necessary flexion, external rotation, and abduction of the leg to perform dissection at popliteal fossa.

Surgical Approach

- ***Autograft Harvest***
  - The ipsilateral palmaris longus tendon is harvested using a three-incision technique (Fig. 23-1).[1,2]

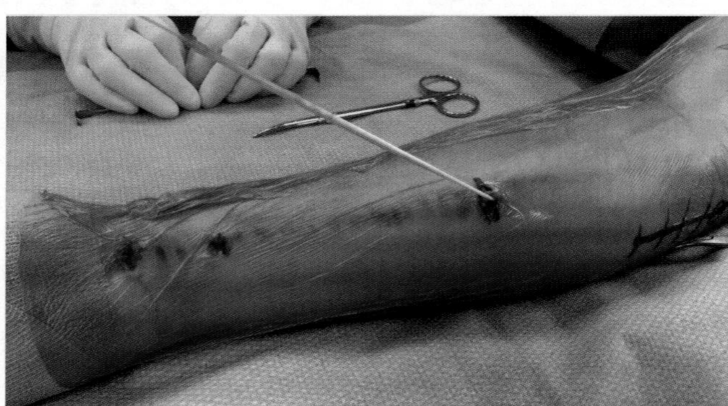

Figure 23-1 | The palmaris longus tendon is harvested using a three-incision technique. (Copyright James R. Andrews.)

    - Three separate 1-cm transverse incisions are made over the volar forearm: one just proximal to the wrist crease, a second 3-5 cm proximal to the first, and a third ~15 cm proximal to the first.
    - A hemostat is used to bluntly free up the tendon at each incision.
    - A hemostat is placed deep to the tendon at each incision to ensure that the correct structure is being harvested, while the nearby flexor tendons and median nerve are protected.
    - The wrist is flexed by an assistant while the tendon is transected at the distal incision.
    - The hemostat is used to deliver the transected tendon out of the second incision.
    - The end of the tendon is whipstitched using a size 0 absorbable braided suture.
    - In-line traction is placed on the tendon, and its course proximally is confirmed with palpation.
      - If there is any doubt regarding the location of the tendon proximally, the most proximal incision can be delayed until this time.
    - The tendon is drawn out of the most proximal incision. Traction can be placed on the tendon, and muscle can be bluntly or sharply removed if additional tendon length is required.
      - A minimal length of 15 cm is recommended.
    - The tendon is transected at the proximal incision and taken to the back table, where the proximal end is whipstitched with size 0 absorbable braided suture.
  - When necessary, the contralateral gracilis tendon is harvested through a minimally invasive posteromedial knee incision.[3-5]
    - A 2- to 3-cm transverse incision is made at the medial aspect of the popliteal fossa, directly over the gracilis tendon.
    - Dissection with Metzenbaum scissors is performed to identify and isolate the gracilis tendon.
    - A loop of suture is placed around the gracilis tendon to enable traction and further local dissection of the tendon.
    - An atraumatic tendon stripper is used proximally to bluntly separate the tendon from the muscle.
    - A sharp tendon stripper is then passed over the tendon distally to free the tendon from its insertion at the pes anserinus.
    - The tendon is taken to the back table for further preparation.

- ***Superficial Dissection***
  - A slight V-shaped, two-armed incision is made at the medial elbow, centered directly over the medial epicondyle and extending 3 cm proximal and 6 cm distal to the medial epicondyle (Fig. 23-2).

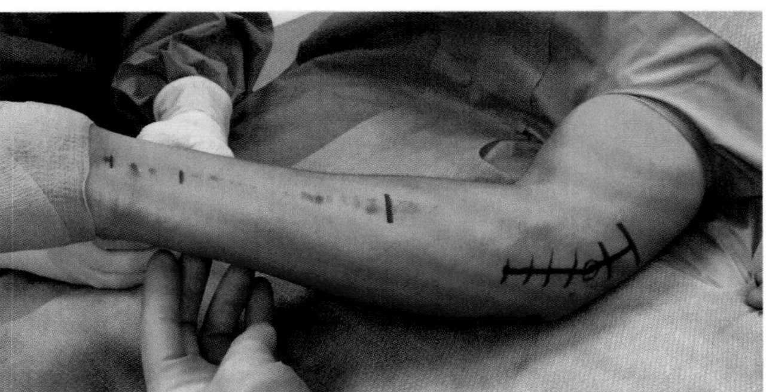

Figure 23-2 | The incision at the medial elbow is centered over the medial epicondyle and extends ~9 cm in length. (Copyright James R. Andrews.)

  - The branches of the medial antebrachial cutaneous nerve (MABCN), which are variable in their course about the medial elbow[6] (Fig. 23-3) are identified, mobilized, and protected.
    - The most constant branch of the MABCN is often found in the distal aspect of the incision ~3 cm distal to the medial epicondyle.

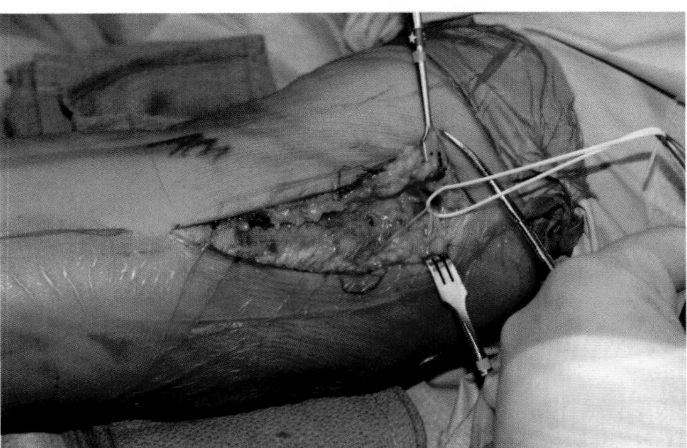

Figure 23-3 | Branches of the medial antebrachial cutaneous nerve are identified and protected. (Copyright James R. Andrews.)

  - Dissection of the branches of the MABCN must be carried as far proximal as the incision allows to ensure necessary mobility throughout the procedure.
  - A vessel loop is placed around each branch of the MABCN to allow gentle mobilization throughout the procedure.
- ***Ulnar Nerve Release***
  - The ulnar nerve is released along its course from the arcade of Struthers proximally to its path between the two heads of the flexor carpi ulnaris (FCU) distally.
  - It is safest to begin the dissection proximal to the Osborne ligament, where the nerve is more easily identified and mobilized.
  - A vessel loop is placed around the nerve to allow gentle mobilization during further dissection.
  - Care must be taken to identify and protect the first two branches of the ulnar nerve.[7,8]
    - The first (posterior) branch typically arises just distal to the medial epicondyle.
    - The second (anterior) branch typically arises where the nerve courses between the two heads of the FCU.
    - Dissection along the medial, more superficial side of the ulnar nerve usually is safest and will help avoid iatrogenic injury to these branches.
    - Thorough dissection of these branches is required to ensure safe mobilization of the ulnar nerve throughout the procedure.
  - Distally, the ulnar nerve is released by splitting the superficial fascia of the FCU in line with its muscular fibers.
  - A key elevator is used to split the flexor carpal ulnaris (FCU) muscle in line with its fibers, preferably along the raphe between the humeral and ulnar heads of the muscle.

- The deep FCU aponeurosis is a common site of unrecognized or residual nerve compression and should be completely released, distally, well under the muscle.
- The small vessels that travel with the nerve and course along the floor of the cubital tunnel are carefully cauterized to maintain hemostasis.

- ***Ulnar Nerve Transposition Sling***
  - With the ulnar nerve mobilized and retracted posteriorly, the medial intermuscular septum is easily identified.
  - The medial intermuscular septum is bluntly separated from the triceps muscle and sharply divided at the most proximal aspect of the incision for a length of 4-5 cm.
  - A no. 15 scalpel is used to separate a 3-5 mm wide strip of the distal intermuscular septum from the humerus (Fig. 23-4).
  - The distal insertion into the superior aspect of the medial epicondyle is left intact.
    - If the distal insertion is disrupted, it may be sutured back to the periosteum or fascia overlying the flexor-pronator mass.
  - Several small vessels run along the septum and often require use of electrocautery for hemostasis.

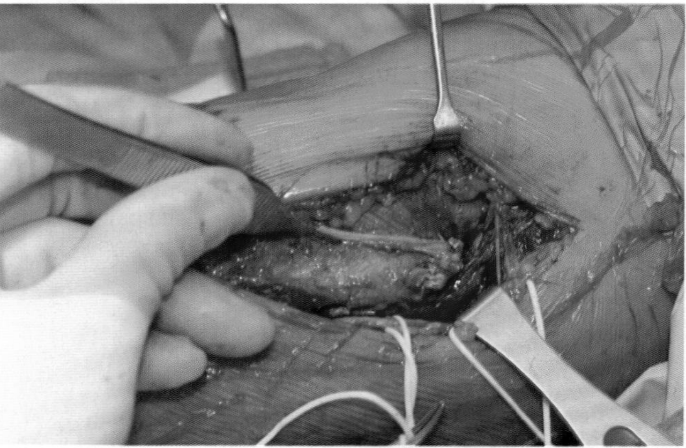

Figure 23-4 | A strip of the medial intermuscular septum is dissected to create a sling for the ulnar nerve transposition performed at the end of the procedure. (Copyright James R. Andrews.)

- ***Posterior Arthrotomy***
  - If preoperative imaging reveals posteromedial olecranon osteophytes or posterior loose bodies, an arthrotomy may be necessary.
  - A 1- to 2-cm posterior arthrotomy is made perpendicular to the long axis of the arm (Fig. 23-5).

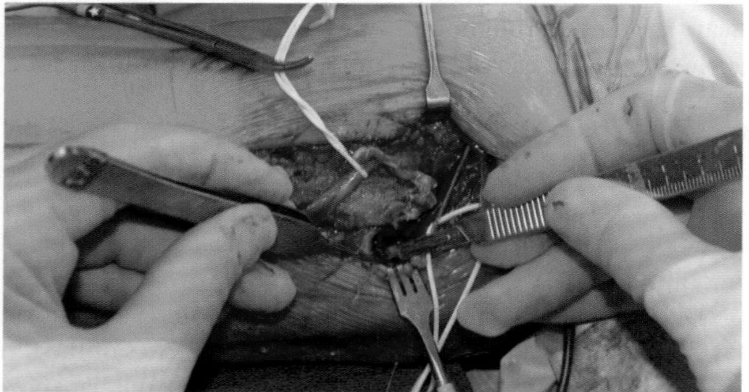

Figure 23-5 | A posterior arthrotomy is performed if preoperative imaging suggests the presence of posteromedial olecranon osteophytes and/or posterior loose bodies. (Copyright James R. Andrews.)

  - Osteophyte removal is performed with use of a 1/4 in osteotome, rongeur, and/or burr.
    - Great care is taken to avoid overresection of native olecranon and alteration of elbow kinematics.[9-11]
  - The arthrotomy is closed with size 0 absorbable braided suture.
    - This closure also allows tightening of the posterior band of the ulnar collateral ligament (UCL).
- ***Exposure of Injured UCL***
  - The raphe between the anterior bundle of the UCL and overlying flexor digitorum superficialis (FDS) muscle is identified at the level of the sublime tubercle.
  - A no. 15 blade scalpel is used to sharply elevate the FDS muscle off of the UCL.
    - Retraction placed on the FDS with a right-angled retractor can aid in identification of the raphe and ease elevation.

- Elevation proceeds in a retrograde fashion from the sublime tubercle of the ulna to the medial epicondyle.
- The UCL sweeps upward to the medial epicondyle, and care must be taken not to cut into the ligament.
- There are small branches from the ulnar recurrent vessels near the origin of the UCL, which often require hemostasis by electrocautery.

- The native UCL is inspected to determine the extent of injury, including tears, avulsions, calcification and/or abnormal laxity.
  - Calcification should be excised as it may alter ligament kinematics and/or cause injury to the reconstructed ligament.
  - If preoperative imaging reveals significant calcification and suggests the need for extensive native ligament debridement, a larger autograft (gracilis) may be required.[12]
- The anterior band of the native UCL is split longitudinally in line with its fibers (Fig. 23-6).

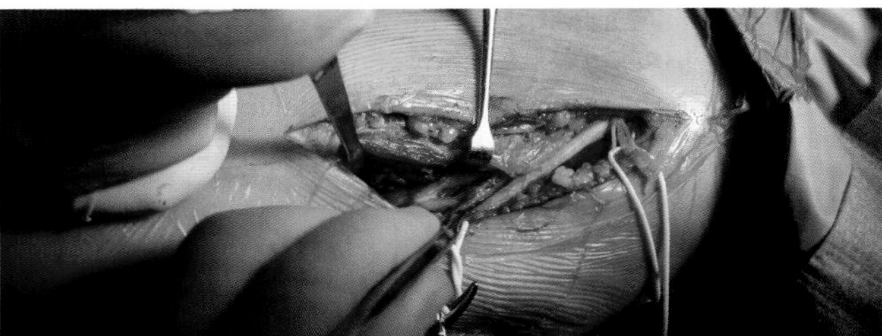

Figure 23-6 | The native UCL is split to allow visualization of the ulnohumeral joint during drilling. (Copyright James R. Andrews.)

- The undersurface of the UCL is examined to document partial thickness injury to the deeper, more substantial layer of the ligament.
- The ulnohumeral joint can be inspected through the UCL split and examined for pathology.

- ***Ulnar Tunnel Preparation***
  - With the joint line now visible through the UCL split, the ulnar tunnel is created first.
  - A small, blunt Hohmann retractor is carefully placed over the anterior border of the ulna to gain exposure.
    - Care must be taken to avoid overretraction and injury to the ulnar nerve anterior motor branch to the FCU.
  - The first drill hole is started at the posterior edge of the sublime tubercle, ~1 cm distal to the ulnohumeral joint line, aiming anterior and parallel to the joint line (Fig. 23-7A).
  - A hemostat is placed in the first drill hole to aid in triangulation when drilling the second hole.
  - The second ulnar drill hole is started at the anterior edge of the sublime tubercle and is aimed posterior to converge on the hemostat in the first drill hole at a right angle (Fig. 23-7B).
    - A bone bridge of 6-9 mm is left between the two ulnar drill holes.

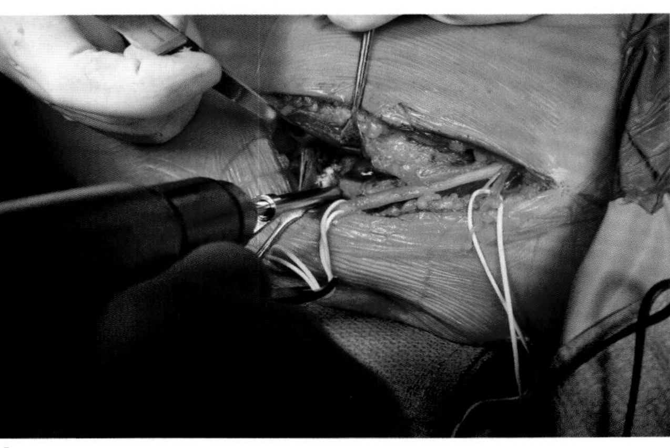

A

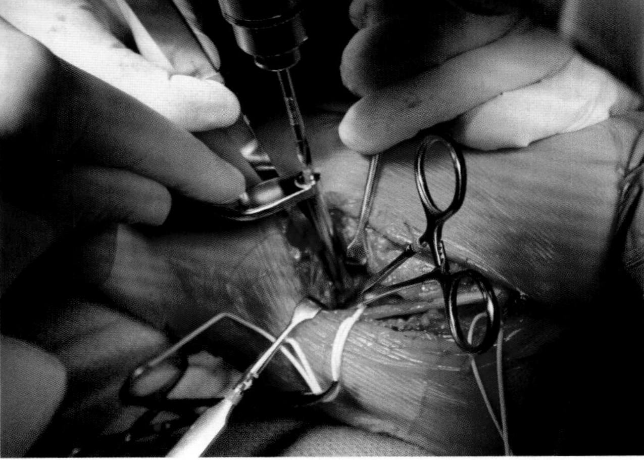

B

Figure 23-7 | A. The first ulnar drill hole is started at the posterior edge of the sublime tubercle, ~1 cm distal to the ulnohumeral joint line, aiming anterior and parallel to the joint line. (Copyright James R. Andrews.) **B.** The second ulnar drill hole is started at the anterior edge of the sublime tubercle and is aimed posterior to converge on the hemostat in the first drill hole at a right angle. (Copyright James R. Andrews.)

- A no. 1 curved curette is used to further connect the drill holes and remove debris.
  - No. 2 curved curette is used when necessary.
- The ulnar tunnel is irrigated with sterile saline to clear debris.
- If intraoperative fracture of the ulnar tunnel occurs, an interference screw or suture anchor technique can be considered.[13-15]
  - Alternatively, drill holes can be made more distal on the sublime tubercle.

- ***Humeral Tunnel Preparation***
  - Three separate unicortical drill holes are made to create a Y-shaped tunnel configuration in the medial epicondyle.
  - Care must be taken to create a tunnel that is deep (lateral) enough to minimize risk of intraoperative and/or postoperative fracture.
  - A 3.5-mm drill is sufficient to create a tunnel that will allow passage of a palmaris longus autograft.
    - A 4.0-mm drill may be required if a gracilis autograft is used, but great care must be exercised in tunnel placement as risk of fracture increases with larger grafts/tunnels.
  - The first humeral drill hole is made in a retrograde fashion, starting at the origin of the UCL for aiming posterior and superior (Fig. 23-8A) for an intraosseous distance of 7-10 mm.
    - Take care to avoid starting the entry tunnel too posterior.
  - A straight curette is placed in the first drill hole to aid in triangulation when drilling the second and third holes.
  - The second and third holes are drilled in an antegrade fashion.
    - While the transposition sling is protected, the posteromedial epicondyle is cleared of soft tissue with electrocautery.
    - Having an assistant push down on the wrist to place valgus stress across the elbow and deliver the medial epicondyle will permit better access for drilling.
    - Starting at the posterior aspect of the medial epicondyle, the second and third holes are drilled to converge on the curette placed in the first hole (Fig. 23-8B and C).
      - One is posterosuperior and one is posteroinferior, and at least a 1 cm bone bridge should separate the tunnels.
  - No. 1 and/or no. 2 straight and curved curettes are used to further connect the drill holes.
  - The humeral tunnel is irrigated with sterile saline to clear debris.

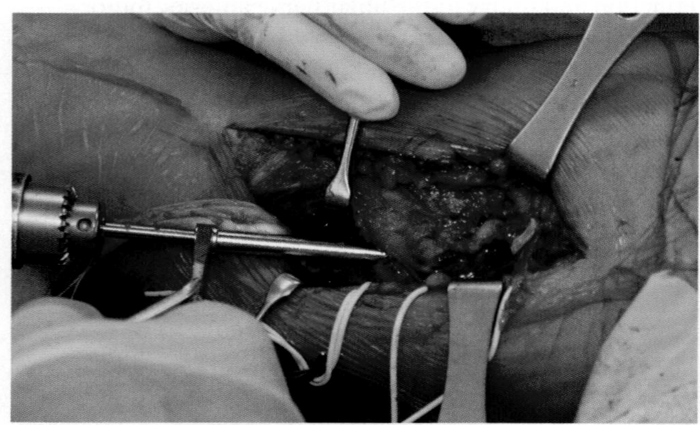

A

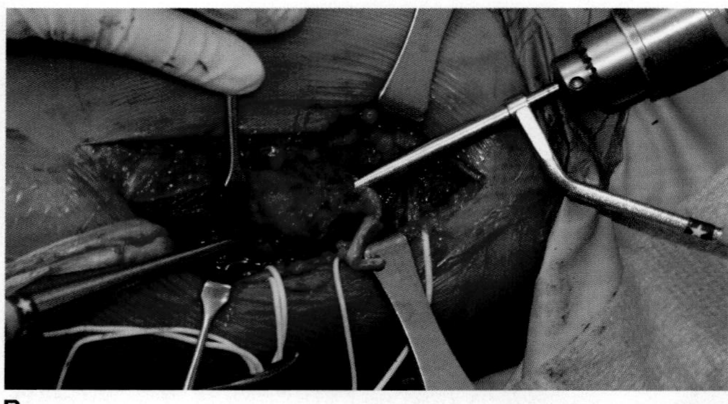

B

C

Figure 23-8 | A. The first humeral drill hole is made in a retrograde fashion, starting at the origin of the UCL and aiming posterior and superior. (Copyright James R. Andrews.) **B.** The second humeral drill hole is started at the posterosuperior aspect of the medial epicondyle, aiming to converge on the curette placed in the first drill hole. (Copyright James R. Andrews.) **C.** The third humeral drill hole is started at the posteroinferior aspect of the medial epicondyle, aiming to converge on the curette placed in the first drill hole. (Copyright James R. Andrews.)

- ***UCL Repair and Reconstruction***
  - Prior to passage of the graft, the split in the native ligament is repaired.
    - Work proceeds distal to proximal, leaving an unrepaired portion near the medial epicondyle for an entry point for the graft.
    - Ligament tissue is imbricated with size 0 nonabsorbable braided suture, thereby tightening the native ligament.
  - A Hewson suture passer is curved and used to pass the graft through the ulnar tunnel until limbs of equal length are present on both sides.
  - The limbs of the graft are crossed and passed in a retrograde direction through the humeral tunnel using the Hewson suture passer.
    - A figure-of-eight configuration is created with the inferior limb exiting the superior tunnel and the superior limb exiting the inferior tunnel (Fig. 23-9).
    - Mineral oil can be used to ease passage of the graft.
    - If the graft is long enough to span the joint a third time, a suture loop can be passed with the graft through the superior humeral tunnel to enable passage of one limb back through the tunnel in an antegrade fashion.

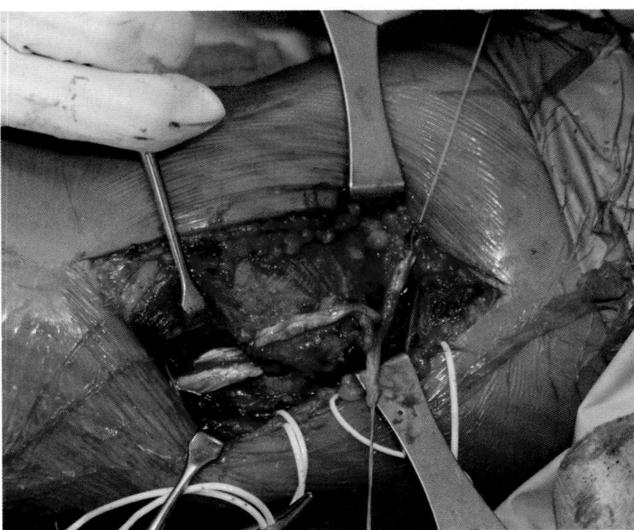

Figure 23-9 | A figure-of-eight configuration is created with the inferior limb exiting the superior humeral tunnel and the superior limb exiting the inferior humeral tunnel. (Copyright James R. Andrews.)

  - The elbow is placed in 20-30 degrees flexion, and a slight varus stress is placed across the elbow.
  - The graft is tensioned by an assistant and the limbs are sutured together, side to side, at the posterior aspect of the medial epicondyle, as well as to the periosteum of the medial epicondyle (Fig. 23-10).
  - The portion of the graft spanning the joint is sutured together, as well as to the underlying native ligament using size 0 nonabsorbable braided suture (Fig. 23-11).

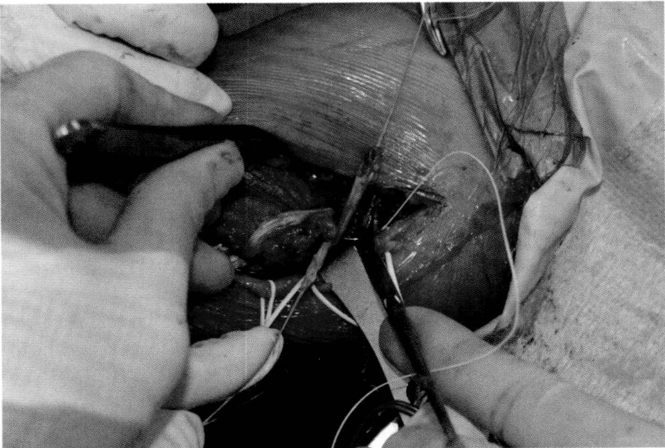

Figure 23-10 | The graft is tensioned and sutured together at the posterior aspect of the medial epicondyle. (Copyright James R. Andrews.)

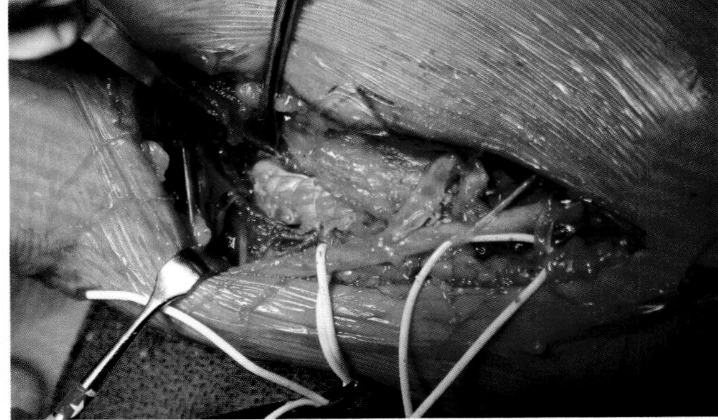

Figure 23-11 | The portion of the graft spanning the joint is sutured together, as well as to the underlying native UCL. (Copyright James R. Andrews.)

    - This provides further tension to the graft and creates a more anatomic reconstruction.
  - Excess graft is resected with a no. 15 scalpel.
- ***Ulnar Nerve Transposition***
  - An anterior subcutaneous ulnar nerve transposition is performed in all cases as dictated by our exposure of the ligament.
  - The ulnar nerve is placed anterior to overlie the flexor-pronator mass.
  - The sling from the medial intermuscular septum is laid loosely over the nerve and sutured to the fascia of the flexor-pronator mass with size 3-0 nonabsorbable braided suture (Fig. 23-12).
    - Make sure the sling is loose, as contracture can be expected during the first few months of the healing process.

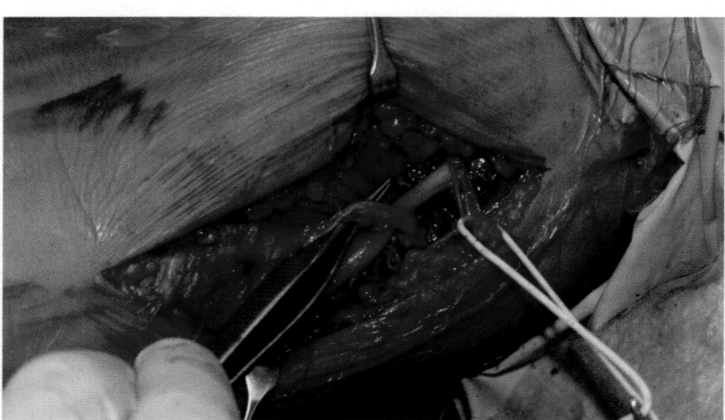

Figure 23-12 | The sling from the medial intermuscular septum is laid loosely over the nerve and sutured to the fascia of the flexor-pronator mass. (Copyright James R. Andrews.)

  - The cubital tunnel is closed and the medial triceps and remaining intermuscular septum are approximated with size 0 nonabsorbable braided suture to prevent any subluxation of the nerve.
    - A 2- to 3-cm opening is left for passage of the nerve between the two heads of the FCU.
  - The elbow is taken through gentle range of motion to ensure there is no compression or tethering of the nerve.
- ***Wound Closure and Postoperative Care***
  - The wound is thoroughly irrigated with sterile normal saline.
  - The tourniquet is let down, and meticulous hemostasis is achieved with electrocautery.
  - A single Hemovac drain is placed, exiting proximal to the wound and with caution to avoid the ulnar nerve.
  - The wound is closed in a layered fashion.
  - Soft dressings are placed.
  - A posterior long-arm splint is placed with the elbow in 90 degrees of flexion.
  - A sling is provided for comfort.
  - The Hemovac drain is removed before leaving the recovery unit or on postoperative day 1.
  - The splint is removed 5-7 days after surgery and aggressive range of motion of the elbow is started.
  - Throwing athletes follow a standardized 4-phase rehabilitation protocol as described by Wilk et al.[16-18]

References

1. Azar FM, Andrews JR, Wilk KE, et al. Operative treatment of ulnar collateral ligament injuries of the elbow in athletes. *Am J Sports Med.* 2000;28(1):16-23.
2. Bruce JR, Andrews JR. Ulnar collateral ligament injuries in the throwing athlete. *J Am Acad Orthop Surg.* 2014;22(5):315-325.
3. Kodkani PS, Govekar DP, Patankar HS. A new technique of graft harvest for anterior cruciate ligament reconstruction with quadruple semitendinosus tendon autograft. *Arthroscopy.* 2004;20:e101-e104.
4. Prodromos CC, Han YS, Keller BL, et al. Posterior mini-incision technique for hamstring anterior cruciate ligament reconstruction graft harvest. *Arthroscopy.* 2005;21:130-137.
5. Wilson TJ, Lubowitz JH. Minimally invasive posterior hamstring harvest. *Arthrosc Tech.* 2013;2(3):e299-e300.
6. Lowe JB III, Maggi SP, Mackinnon SE. The position of crossing branches of the medial antebrachial cutaneous nerve during cubital tunnel surgery in humans. *Plast Reconstr Surg.* 2004;114(3):692-696.
7. Ng ZY, Mitchell JH, Fogg QA, et al. The anatomy of ulnar nerve branches in anterior transposition. *Hand Surg.* 2013;18(3):301-306.
8. Tubbs RS, Custis JW, Salter EG, et al. Quantitation of and landmarks for the muscular branches of the ulnar nerve to the forearm for application in peripheral nerve neurotization procedures. *J Neurosurg.* 2006;104(5):800-803.

9. Andrews JR, Heggland EJH, Fleisig GS, et al. Relationship of ulnar collateral ligament strain to amount of medial olecranon osteotomy. *Am J Sports Med.* 2001;29(6):716-721.
10. Kamineni S, Hirahara H, Pomianowski S, et al. Partial posteromedial olecranon resection: a kinematic study. *J Bone Joint Surg Am.* 2003;85-A(6):1005-1011.
11. Kamineni S, ElAttrache NS, O'Driscoll SW, et al. Medial collateral ligament strain with partial posteromedial olecranon resection. A biomechanical study. *J Bone Joint Surg Am.* 2004;86-A(11):2424-2430.
12. Dugas JR, Bilotta J, Watts CD, et al. Ulnar collateral ligament reconstruction with gracilis tendon in athletes with intraligamentous bony excision: technique and results. *Am J Sports Med.* 2012;40(7):1578-1582.
13. Ahmad CS, Lee TQ, ElAttrache NS. Biomechanical evaluation of a new ulnar collateral ligament reconstruction technique with interference screw fixation. *Am J Sports Med.* 2003;31(3):332-337.
14. Hechtman KS, Zvijac JE, Wells ME, et al. Long-term results of ulnar collateral ligament reconstruction in throwing athletes based on a hybrid technique. *Am J Sports Med.* 2011;39(2):342-347.
15. Dines JS, ElAttrache NS, Conway JE, et al. Clinical outcomes of the DANE TJ technique to treat ulnar collateral ligament insufficiency of the elbow. *Am J Sports Med.* 2007;35(12):2039-2044.
16. Wilk KE, Arrigo C, Andrews JR. Rehabilitation of the elbow in the throwing athlete. *J Orthop Sports Phys Ther.* 1993;17(6):305-317.
17. Wilk KE, Azar FM, Andrews JR. Conservative and operative rehabilitation of the elbow in sports. *Sports Med Arthrosc Rev.* 1995;3(3):237-258.
18. Wilk KE, Arrigo C, Andrews JR, et al. Rehabilitation following elbow surgery in the throwing athlete. *Operat Tech Sports Med.* 1996;4:114-132.

Chapter 24
Posterolateral Rotatory Reconstruction

BRIAN J. KELLY
LARRY D. FIELD

Sterile Instruments/Equipment

- Sterile tourniquet
- Tendon stripper (if using autograft)
- 4-mm round burr
  - Used to create bone tunnels for graft passage
- 1.5-mm round burr or drill bit
  - Used to create bone tunnels for suture passage
- Curved awl
  - Used to connect ulnar bone tunnels to facilitate graft passage
- Hewson suture passer
- No. 2 braided, nonabsorbable suture (surgeon preference)
- Implants
  - Tendon allograft (if not using autograft)
  - Suture anchors (if performing an open or arthroscopic ligament repair)
- Arthroscopic instruments
  - 4-mm 30-degree arthroscope
  - Interchangeable cannulas
  - Retrograde suture retriever
  - Suture grasper
  - Arthroscopic knot pusher
- Suture for skin closure (surgeon preference)
- Dressing and splint material

Positioning

- The patient is positioned supine on a regular operating room table.
- The arm is placed on an arm board.
  - Alternatively, the arm can be positioned across the patient's chest.
- The extremity is prepared and draped according to surgeon preference such that the entire upper extremity is exposed.
- A sterile tourniquet is placed on the upper arm.

Surgical Approach

- The surgical approach is the same for all of the open reconstruction and repair techniques. There may be slight variation in the amount of dissection necessary depending on the location of bone tunnels.
- The incision begins 2-3 cm proximal to the lateral epicondyle and extends 8-10 cm distally toward the subcutaneous border of the ulna (Fig. 24-1).

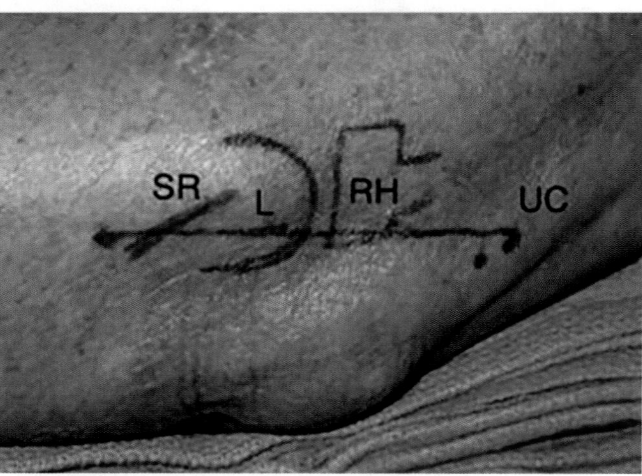

Figure 24-1 | An 8-cm skin incision is marked over the Kocher interval using the supracondylar ridge (SR), lateral epicondyle (L), radial head (RH), and ulnar crest (UC) as palpable landmarks.

- The Kocher approach is used.
  - The interval between the anconeus and extensor carpi ulnaris (ECU) muscles is identified, and the fascia is opened with a scalpel. The interval often can be defined by a thin fat stripe that is seen through the deep fascia (Fig. 24-2).
  - The anconeus is elevated from distal to proximal to facilitate the clearest distinction from the underlying lateral ulnar collateral ligament (LUCL).
  - The anconeus muscle is retracted posteriorly to expose the supinator crest, which is the ulnar attachment site of the LUCL (Fig. 24-3).
  - The ECU muscle fibers are sharply dissected from the LUCL, and the muscle is elevated anteriorly along with some of the common extensor origin (Fig. 24-3).
  - The lateral epicondyle and supracondylar ridge are cleared of soft tissue to obtain the exposure necessary for drilling the humeral bone tunnels. This often requires elevation of some of the common extensor origin and triceps muscle.

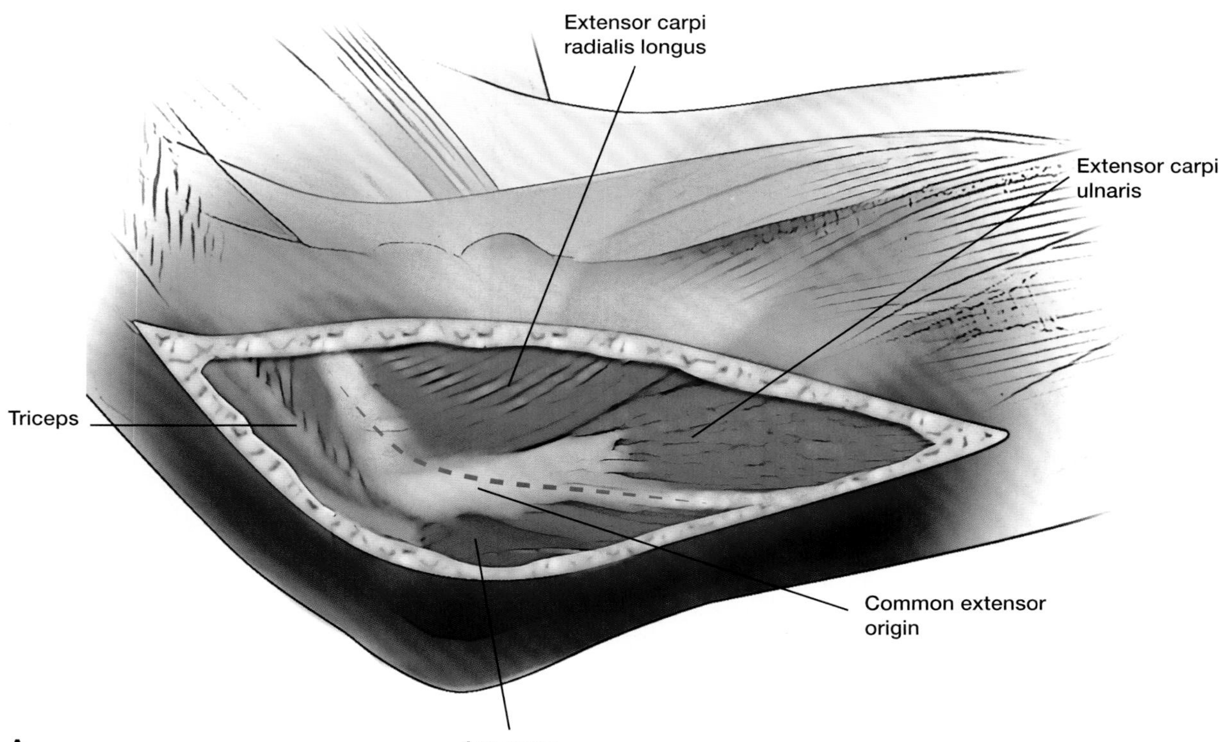

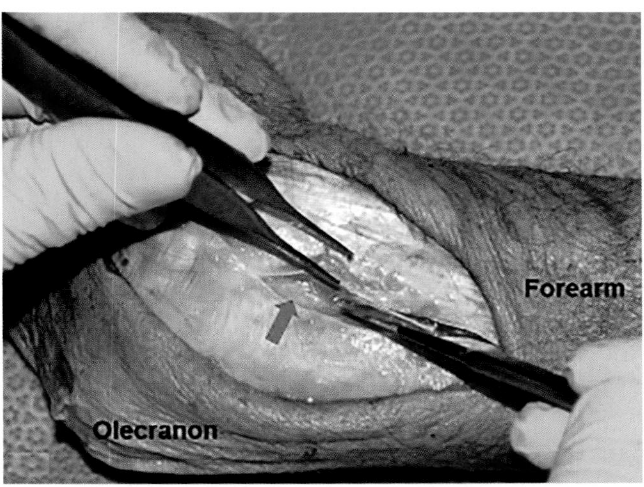

Figure 24-2 | Illustration **(A)** and intraoperative photo **(B)** show the incision made in the deep fascia between the ECU and the anconeus muscles. This interval often can be identified by a fat stripe deep to the fascia (*red arrow*). The dissection is continued proximally between the ECRL and the triceps to expose the supracondylar ridge.

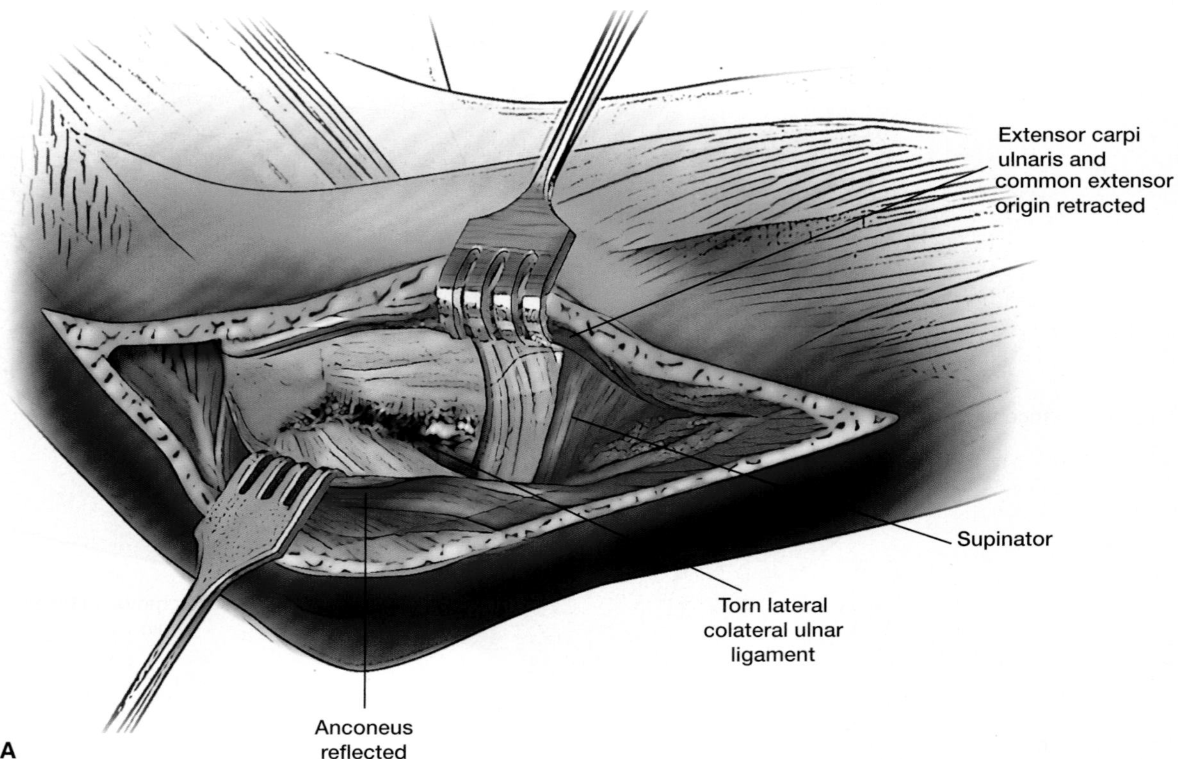

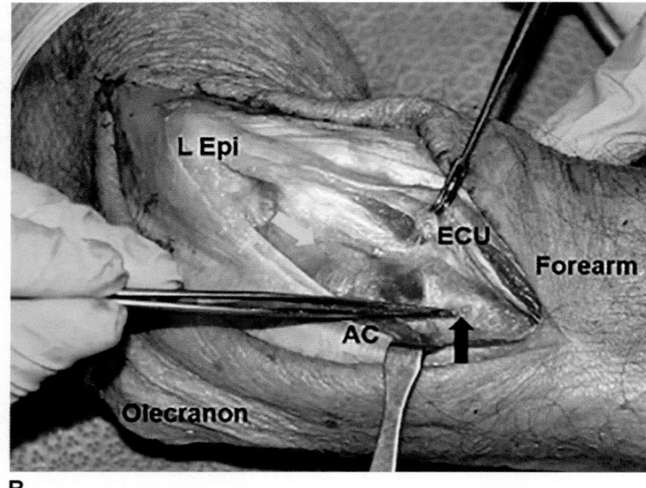

Figure 24-3 | Illustration **(A)** and intraoperative photo **(B)** show the anconeus (AC) reflected posteriorly and the ECU reflected anteriorly to reveal the LUCL (*yellow arrow*) and supinator crest (*black arrow*). L Epi, lateral epicondyle.

Graft Options

- Palmaris longus autograft
- Gracilis autograft
- Semitendinosus autograft
- Plantaris autograft
- Multiple allograft options

Docking Technique[1-5]

- Ulnar tunnel preparation
  - The first hole is created with a 4-mm burr near the tubercle on the supinator crest; this should be distal to the radial head–neck junction to ensure the most stable construct (Fig. 24-4).
  - The second hole is created with a 4-mm burr at the proximal aspect of the supinator crest near the insertion of the annular ligament. A sufficient bone bridge of 15-20 mm is maintained between the two tunnels (Fig. 24-4).

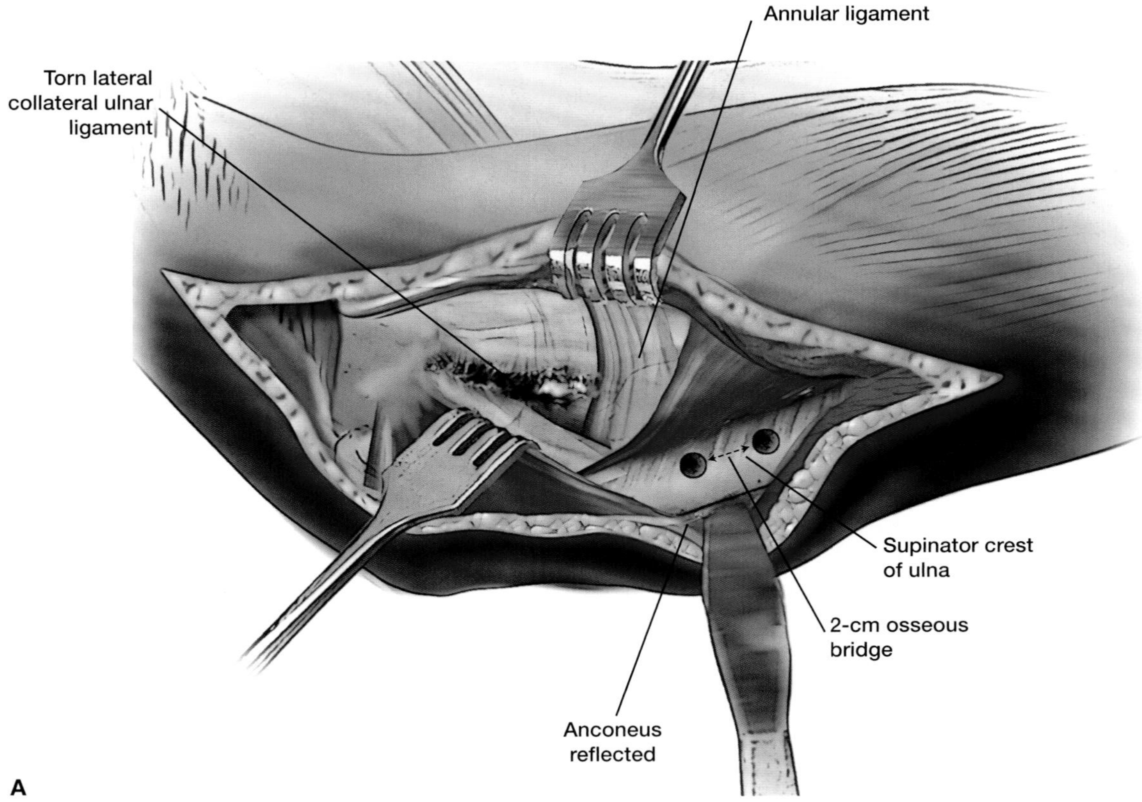

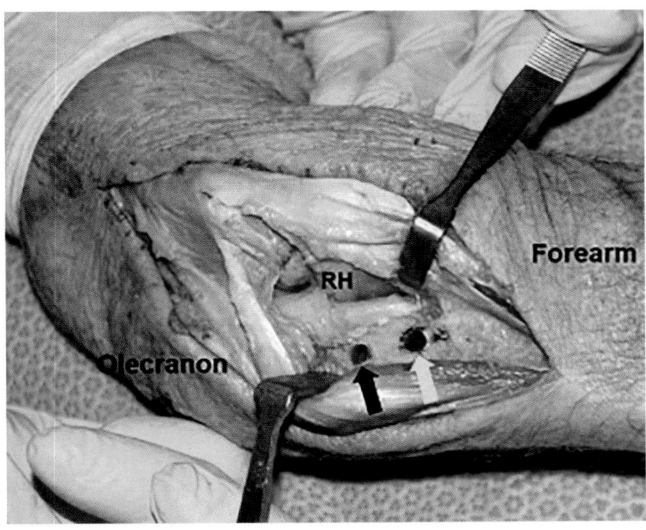

Figure 24-4 | Illustration **(A)** and intraoperative photo **(B)** show the proximal and distal ulnar holes, which are created along the supinator crest with a 4-mm burr, leaving at least a 15- to 20-mm bone bridge. It is important that the distal hole (*yellow arrow*) is distal to the radial head–neck junction to ensure the most stable construct. The proximal hole (*black arrow*) is located near the insertion of the annular ligament. RH, radial head.

- While the supinator tubercle may be palpable only ~50% of the time, the distal tunnel should be placed ~15 mm distal to the proximal margin of the radial head.[6,7]
- These holes do not need to be drilled deeper than the cortex. A curved awl is used to create an osseous tunnel connecting the two holes while taking care not to violate the bone bridge.

- Humeral tunnel preparation
  - Identification of the isometric point is facilitated by passing a suture through the two ulnar tunnels and tying it to itself. The proximal end of the suture is held over the lateral epicondyle while the elbow is flexed and extended. The location where the suture does not move during the range of motion is the isometric point (Fig. 24-5). It is typically located anterior and inferior to the center of the lateral epicondyle.[1]
  - A 4-mm burr drilled to a depth of 15 mm is used to create the humeral docking site at the isometric point (Fig. 24-6).

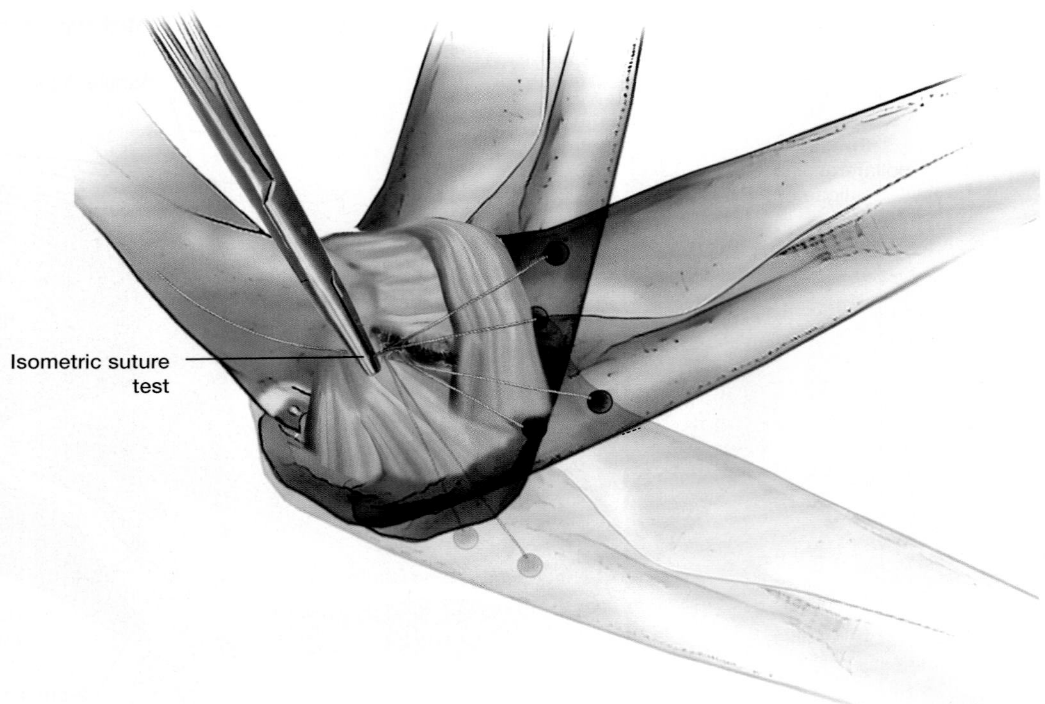

Figure 24-5 | Identification of the isometric point. A suture is passed through the two ulnar tunnels and tied to itself. The proximal end of the suture is held over the lateral epicondyle with a hemostat while the elbow is flexed and extended. The location where the suture does not move during the range of motion is the isometric point.

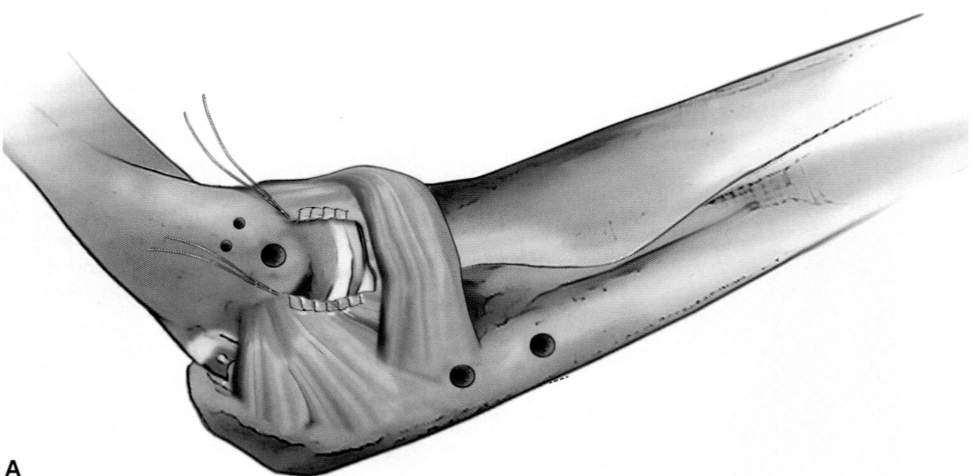

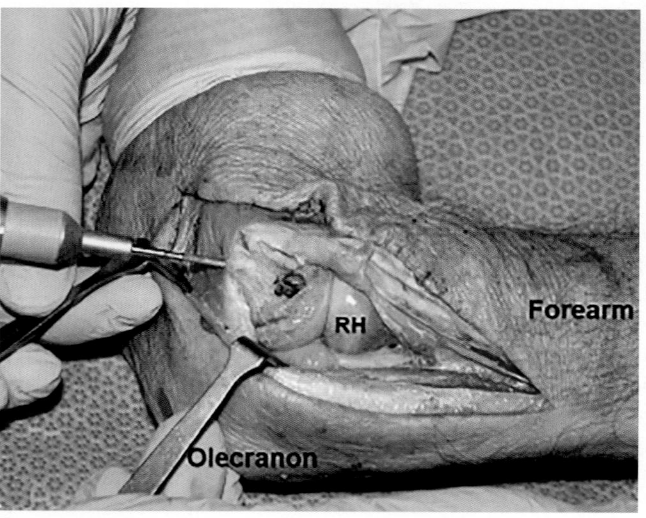

Figure 24-6 | Illustration **(A)** and intraoperative photo **(B)** show the humeral bone tunnels. A 4-mm burr is used to make the larger tunnel at the previously identified isometric point (marked on lateral epicondyle with skin marker). A 1.5-mm burr is used to make the proximal holes for suture passage; these are angled toward the isometric point to facilitate suture passage. A bone bridge of at least 10 mm is left between all three holes. In the illustration, the Krackow sutures through the anterior and posterior capsule can also be seen. RH, radial head.

- A 1.5-mm burr or drill bit is used to drill two additional holes to a depth of 15 mm angled toward the isometric point tunnel and with bone bridges of at least 10 mm between each of the three holes (Fig. 24-6).
  - A Hewson suture passer is used to pass a looped suture from each of these holes, exiting from the humeral docking tunnel; these will be used to facilitate graft passage and the optional capsular repair/plication.
- Capsular repair/plication
  - The capsule is often patulous, and it can be repaired and tightened in conjunction with graft passage.
  - The capsule, with any residual LUCL, is incised linearly along its fibers.
  - A nonabsorbable suture is passed through the anterior capsular tissue in a Krackow configuration, leaving two free suture limbs at the proximal extent. This technique is repeated through the posterior capsular tissue (Fig. 24-6A).
- Graft passage and tensioning
  - One limb of the graft is prepared with a no. 2 nonabsorbable suture in a Krackow or whipstitch configuration. This limb is passed through the ulnar tunnel from distal to proximal with a Hewson suture passer.
  - The sutures through the posterior limb of the graft and the two suture limbs that were passed through the posterior capsule are shuttled through the more posterior humeral tunnel using the looped suture passed during humeral tunnel preparation. The posterior limb of the graft is then docked in the humerus.
  - The elbow is placed in full pronation while tension is placed on both limbs of the graft. The arm can be cycled through multiple flexion-extension arcs to eliminate creep from the graft. The elbow is brought to rest in 40 degrees of flexion and full pronation.
  - The free, anterior limb of the graft is placed next to the humeral tunnel and the length of graft necessary to maintain adequate tension is visualized and marked with a skin marker (Fig. 24-7).

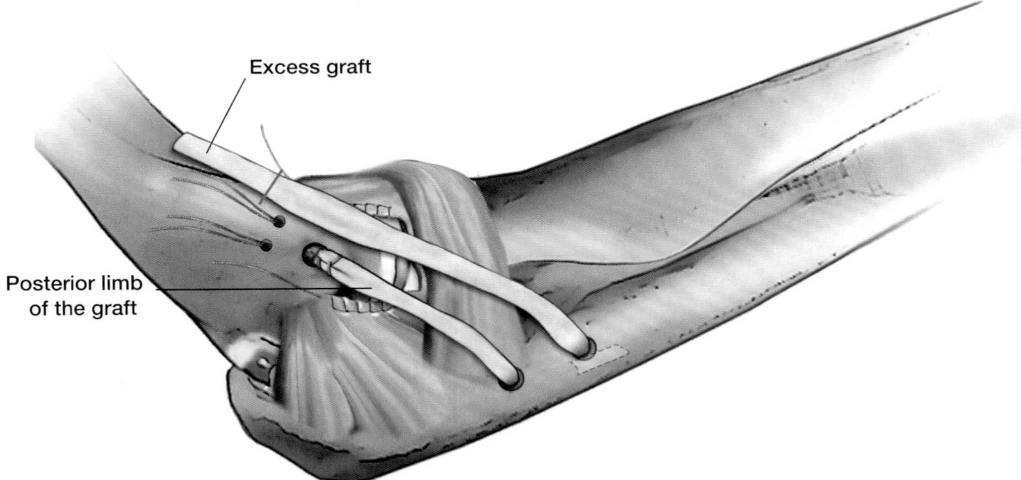

Figure 24-7 | The posterior limb of the graft is docked in the humeral tunnel. The free, anterior limb of the graft is tensioned and placed next to the isometric point tunnel to estimate the length of graft necessary. The excess graft is excised.

  - A no. 2 nonabsorbable suture is used to prepare this limb of the graft in a Krackow or whipstitch configuration ending at the level marked in the previous step. The residual graft is excised.
  - The sutures through the anterior limb of the graft and the two suture limbs that were passed through the anterior capsule are shuttled through the more anterior humeral tunnel using the looped suture passed during humeral tunnel preparation. The anterior limb of the graft is then docked in the humerus (Fig. 24-8).
  - The elbow is placed in 40 degrees of flexion and full pronation while an axial load and valgus stress are applied. The sutures are tied over the humeral bone bridge while in this position; the capsular sutures are tied first, followed by the graft sutures. Excess nonabsorbable suture can be used to suture the two limbs of the graft together as they exit the humeral tunnel (Fig. 24-9).

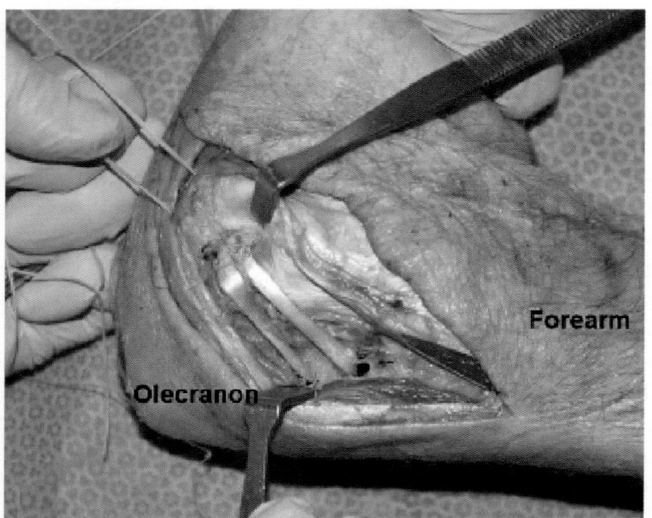

Figure 24-8 | The anterior limb of the graft is docked into the humeral tunnel by shuttling the sutures through the anterior suture-passing tunnel with a Hewson suture passer.

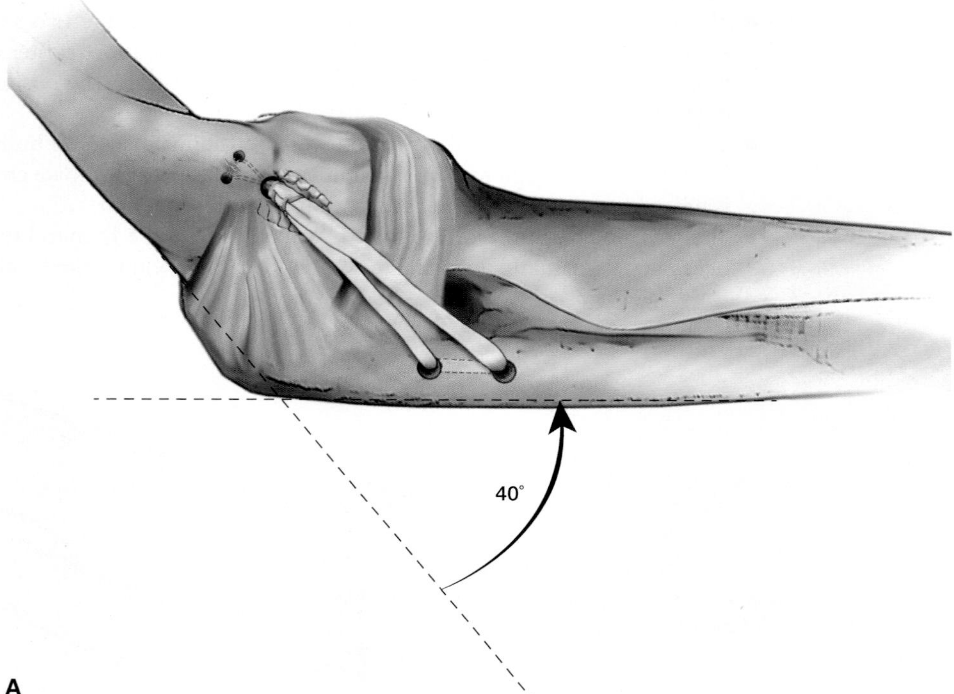

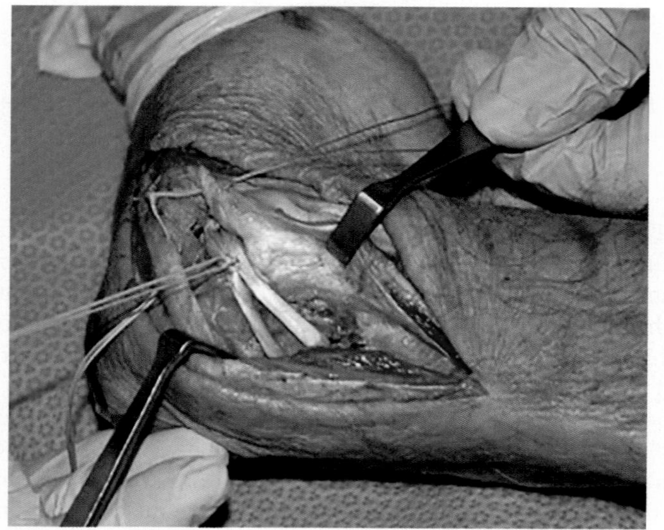

Figure 24-9 | Illustration **(A)** and intraoperative photo **(B)** show the final graft construct with the suture limbs tied over the supracondylar ridge between the two proximal bone tunnels. The graft is tensioned and tied with the elbow in 40 degrees of flexion and full pronation while an axial load and valgus stress is applied. The intraoperative photo shows an additional nonabsorbable suture used to suture the two limbs of the graft together as they exit the humeral tunnel.

- Wound closure
  - The tourniquet is deflated, hemostasis is achieved, and the wound is irrigated.
  - The anconeus and ECU fascia is closed with absorbable suture.
  - The subcutaneous tissue and skin are closed according to surgeon preference.

Figure-8 Yoke Technique[5,8]

- Ulnar tunnel preparation
  - The first hole is created with a 4-mm burr near the tubercle on the supinator crest; this should be distal to the radial head–neck junction to ensure the most stable construct (Fig. 24-4).
  - The second hole is created with a 4-mm burr at the proximal aspect of the supinator crest near the insertion of the annular ligament. A sufficient bone bridge of 15-20 mm is maintained between the two tunnels (Fig. 24-4).
  - While the supinator tubercle may be palpable only ~50% of the time, the distal tunnel should be placed ~15 mm distal to the proximal margin of the radial head.[6,7]
  - These holes do not need to be drilled deeper than the cortex. A curved awl is used to create an osseous tunnel connecting the two holes while taking care not to violate the bone bridge.
- Humeral tunnel preparation
  - Identification of the isometric point is facilitated by passing a suture through the two ulnar tunnels and tying it to itself. The proximal end of the suture is held over the lateral epicondyle while the elbow is flexed and extended. The location where the suture does not move during the range of motion is the isometric point (Fig. 24-5). It typically is located anterior and inferior to the center of the lateral epicondyle.[1]
  - A 4-mm burr drilled to a depth of 15 mm is used to create the humeral docking site at the isometric point.
    - This hole needs to be widened somewhat with the burr to accept three passes of the graft.
  - A 4-mm burr is used to drill two additional holes to a depth of 15 mm and separated from each other and from the humeral docking site by at least 10 mm (Fig. 24-10).

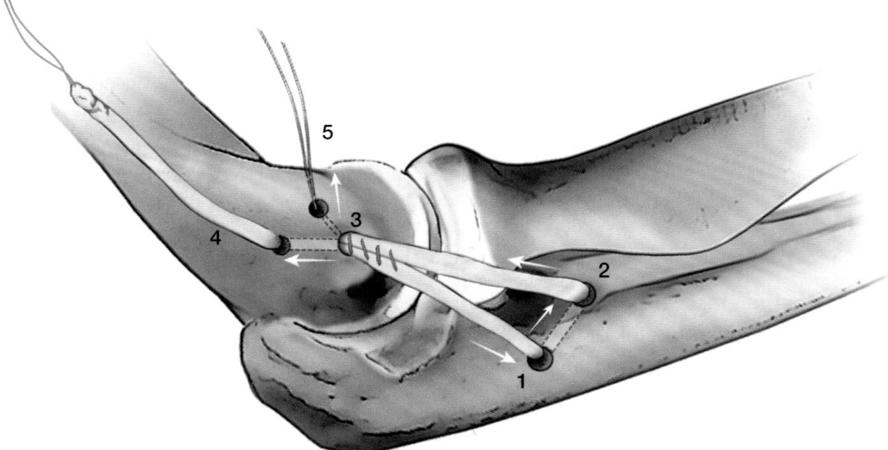

Figure 24-10 | The first humeral bone tunnel is made with a 4-mm burr at the identified isometric point; this tunnel is slightly widened to accept three passes of the graft. Two proximal tunnels are also drilled with a 4-mm burr to create three holes separated by bone bridges of at least 10 mm. The graft is initially passed through the ulnar tunnel (*1-2*). The sutures through the graft are then passed through the anterior humeral tunnel (*3-5*) and the anterior limb advanced to the isometric point. The residual long limb of the graft is passed through the posterior humeral tunnel (*3-4*). A "yoke stitch" is then placed to suture the two limbs of the graft together at the isometric point.

- Graft passage and tensioning
  - Both limbs of the graft are prepared with a no. 2 nonabsorbable suture in a Krackow or whipstitch configuration.
  - One limb of the graft is passed through the ulnar tunnel from proximal to distal with a Hewson suture passer. This limb is then pulled through with just enough length to reach the isometric point of the humerus. The sutures through the end of this graft limb are pulled through the anterior humeral tunnel with a Hewson suture passer to be used later to reinforce the reconstruction.

- The remaining long limb of the graft is passed through the isometric point and out the posterior humeral tunnel with a Hewson suture passer.
- The two limbs are tied together at the isometric point in a side-to-side configuration using no. 2 nonabsorbable suture. This is called the "yoke stitch" (Fig. 24-10).
- The long limb of the graft is wrapped over the supracondylar ridge and then through the anterior humeral tunnel from proximal to distal with a Hewson suture passer; it will exit at the isometric point, leaving a tripled graft at this point.
- The long limb is passed through the ulnar tunnel from proximal to distal with a Hewson suture passer. If it is not long enough, it can be sutured to the posterior limb of the reconstruction in a side-to-side configuration (Fig. 24-11).
- The elbow is placed in 40 degrees of flexion and full pronation while an axial load and valgus stress are applied. While in this position, the sutures through each limb of the graft are tensioned and tied into the graft to complete the figure-8 construct (Fig. 24-11).

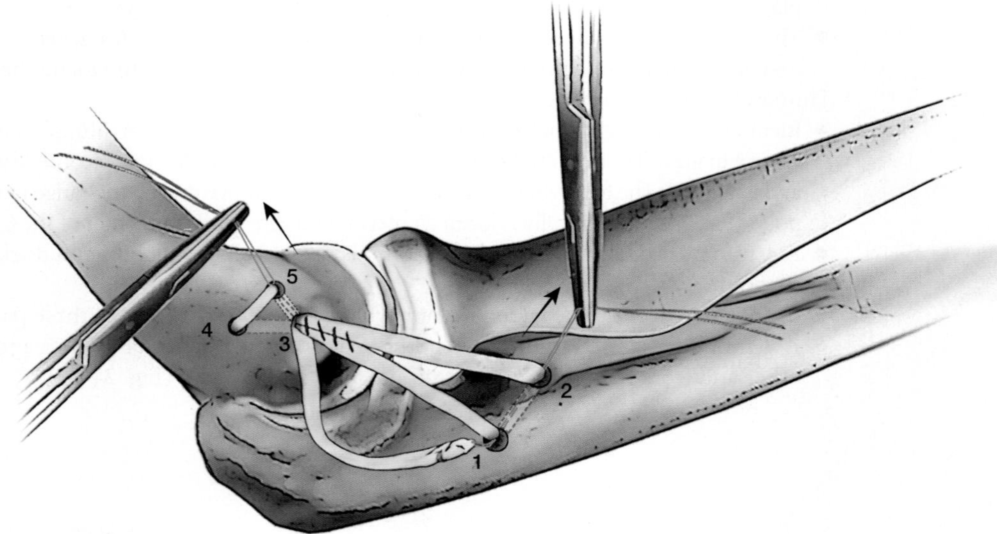

Figure 24-11 | The long limb of the graft is then passed over the supracondylar ridge and through the anterior humeral tunnel (*5-3*), exiting at the isometric point. It is then passed through the ulnar tunnel (*1-2*), and it is sutured back to the graft at whatever point it reaches. The sutures from the anterior limb of the graft are sutured into the long limb of the graft as it passes over the supracondylar ridge. The graft is tensioned and the sutures are tied with the elbow in 40 degrees of flexion and full pronation while an axial load and valgus stress are applied.

- Wound closure
  - The tourniquet is deflated, hemostasis is achieved, and the wound is irrigated.
  - The anconeus and ECU fascia is closed with absorbable suture.
  - The subcutaneous tissue and skin are closed according to surgeon preference.

Direct Repair[2,5,8,9]

- The LUCL is most commonly avulsed from the humeral origin, and if surgery is elected in the acute period, it often can be repaired.
- The surgical approach and dissection are the same as described for the reconstruction techniques.
- The proximal end of the avulsed ligament is identified, and a no. 2 nonabsorbable suture is placed through the ligament in a Krackow configuration.
  - These sutures can be passed through bone tunnels with a Hewson suture passer and tied over the supracondylar ridge (Fig. 24-12). The bone tunnels are made using a 1.5-mm burr or drill bit and are spaced 1 cm apart surrounding the isometric point.
  - Alternatively, one or two suture anchors loaded with nonabsorbable suture and placed at the isometric point can be used to repair the avulsed tendon origin. One limb from the suture anchor is passed through the ligament in a Krackow configuration; the second limb is passed through the ligament only once to allow reduction of the ligament to its origin.

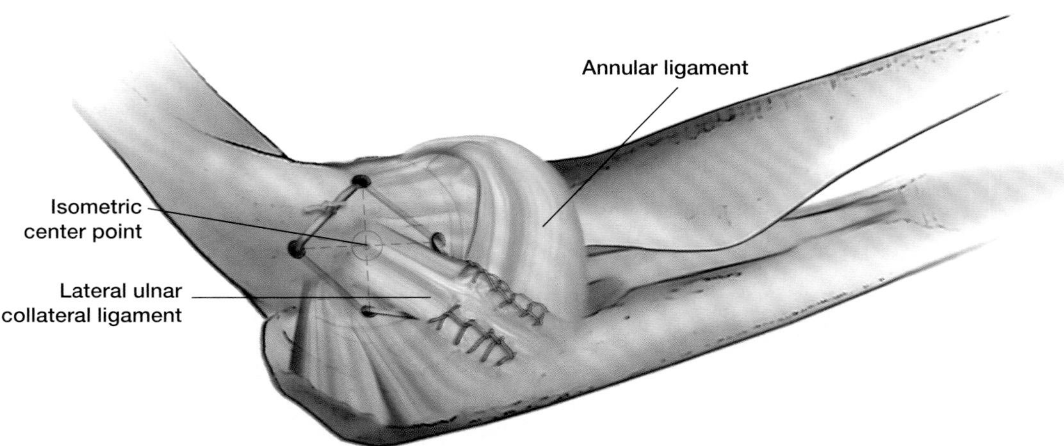

Figure 24-12 | A nonabsorbable suture has been passed through the ligament in a Krackow configuration. Bone tunnels are made using a 1.5-mm burr or drill bit and spaced 1 cm apart surrounding the isometric point. The sutures are passed through the bone tunnels and tied over the supracondylar ridge.

- The repair is always tensioned and tied with the elbow in 40 degrees of flexion and full pronation while an axial load and valgus stress are applied.

Arthroscopic-Assisted Repair[9-11]

- Positioning can be in the prone or lateral position, but we prefer the prone position. A tourniquet is placed high on the upper arm.
- A proximal anteromedial portal is made using standard techniques, taking care to make the skin incision anterior to the intermuscular septum to avoid the ulnar nerve.
- A diagnostic arthroscopy of the anterior compartment is conducted to inspect the radial head, annular ligament, radiocapitellar joint, coronoid, coronoid fossa, and trochlea. If any pathology in the anterior compartment needs to be treated, a proximal anterolateral portal can be created using an outside-in technique.
- A valgus load can be combined with supination to demonstrate posterolateral rotatory instability under direct arthroscopic observation. The radial head will subluxate posteriorly off the capitellum, consistent with injury to the LUCL. The annular ligament must also be assessed for damage, and a suture can be placed in it if necessary.
- A central posterior portal is established 3 cm proximal to the tip of the olecranon. A posterolateral portal is established at the same level but lateral to the triceps tendon. The posterior compartment is debrided to allow examination of the medial gutter, olecranon fossa, olecranon, and lateral gutter.
- The "drive-through sign" is present when an arthroscope in the central posterior portal can be moved from the lateral gutter to the medial gutter, across the ulnohumeral articulation. This finding should be eliminated after the LUCL repair is completed (Fig. 24-13).

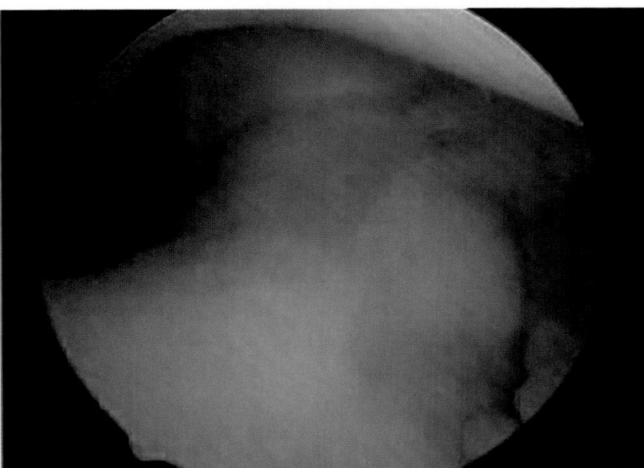

Figure 24-13 | The "drive-through sign" is present when the arthrocope in the central posterior portal can be easily moved from the lateral gutter to the medial gutter by passing across the ulnohumeral articulation (Courtesy of Dr. Felix H. Savoie, III.)

- The arthroscope is easily moved into the lateral gutter because of the incompetence of the LUCL complex. A bare area usually is present at the LUCL origin on the posterior aspect of the lateral epicondyle, usually directly lateral and slightly inferior to the center of the olecranon fossa. This area is debrided with an arthroscopic shaver to prepare the bone for insertion of a suture anchor. Care must be taken to stay close to the bone when debriding the lateral gutter to avoid inadvertently removing the remaining LUCL.
- A double-loaded suture anchor is inserted into the prepared LUCL origin through the posterolateral portal (Fig. 24-14).

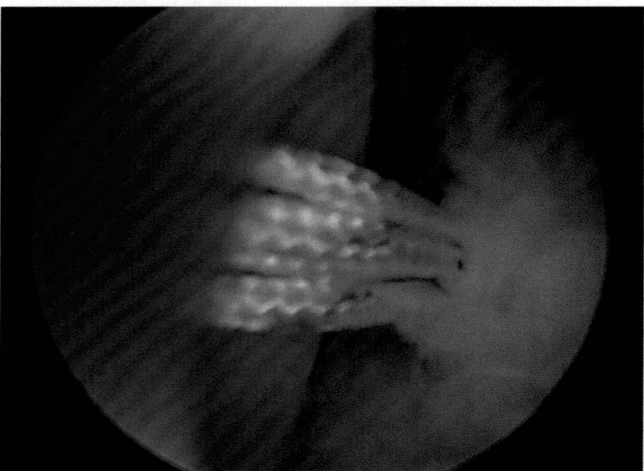

Figure 24-14 | With the arthroscope in the central posterior portal, the posterolateral portal is used to place a double-loaded suture anchor into the LUCL origin, just lateral to the olecranon fossa on the posterior aspect of the lateral epicondyle. (Courtesy of Dr. Felix H. Savoie, III.)

- A retrograde suture retriever (IDEAL suture passer, Depuy Mitek) is used to pass the sutures through the remaining LUCL tissue in a mattress configuration (Fig. 24-15). The LUCL tissue will be retracted distally and anteriorly from the origin.

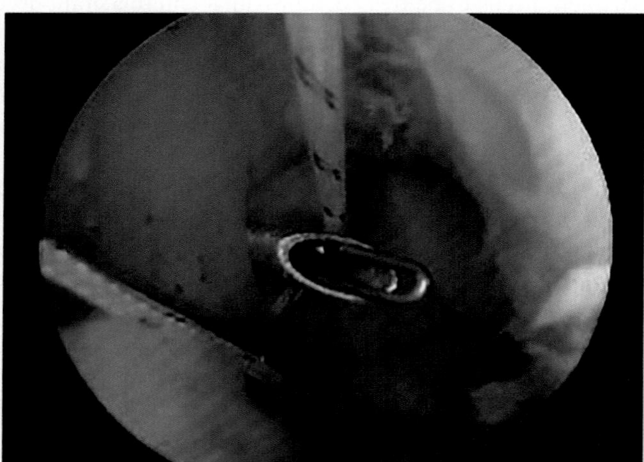

Figure 24-15 | A lateral "soft-spot" portal is used to pass a retrograde suture retriever through the remaining LUCL tissue, and sutures are retrieved in a mattress configuration. (Courtesy of Dr. Felix H. Savoie, III.)

- At this point, the ECRB origin is retracted anteriorly, and it is possible to identify the pathologic fibers on the undersurface of the ECRB and possibly common extensor tendon origin. The degenerative tendon has a gray fish-scale texture and appearance. The tendinous tissue is friable and is more easily scratched off bone than healthy fibers (Nirschl scratch test).
- Normal tendon fibers of the ECRL and EDC appear glistening white and smooth compared to the pathologic tissue and are infrequently involved.
- The pathologic tendon fibers of the ECRB (Fig. 26-9) are sharply excised. Flexing the elbow during this step removes unnecessary tension on the tissue and helps with visualization.
- Occasionally, fibers of the EDC are involved and should be excised back to normal-appearing tendon fibers.
- A sharp Freer elevator or curet can be used to debride any final remaining pathologic tendon from the ECRB footprint (Fig. 26-10).

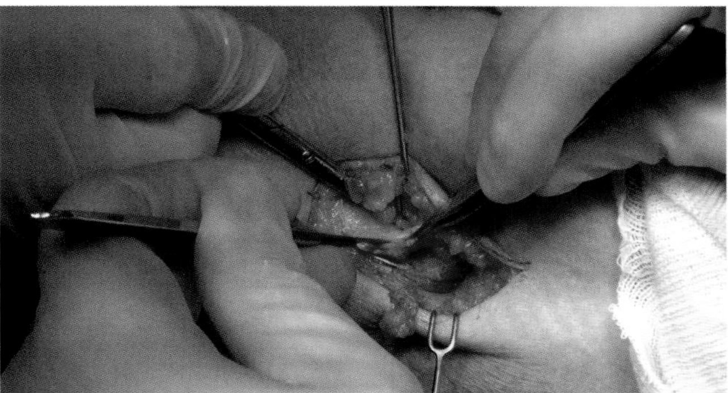

Figure 26-9 | The pathologic "fish-scale" tissue is excised sharply.

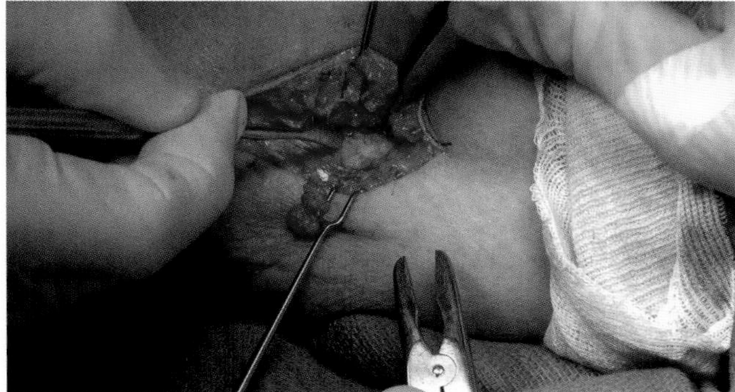

Figure 26-10 | A sharp Freer elevator is used to debride any remaining pathologic tissue.

- After the pathologic tissue is excised, the newly bare footprint of the ECRB is visible (Fig. 26-11). The lateral epicondyle is thoroughly inspected to avoid leaving pathologic tissue in place, which could lead to recurrence of symptoms.
  - The radiocarpal joint is inspected to make sure there is no synovitis or plica that needs to be excised (Fig. 26-12). The elbow is supinated and pronated to verify that the stability of the radiocapitellar joint has not been compromised. If posterolateral instability is present, the radial head will sublux posteriorly off the capitellum during forceful supination.

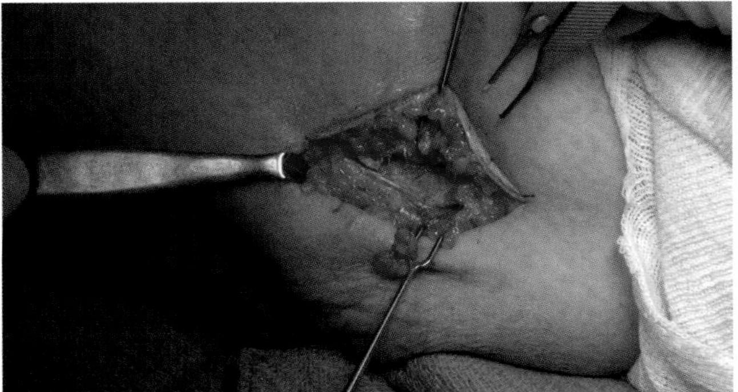

Figure 26-11 | When thorough excision is complete, the lateral epicondyle can be visualized.

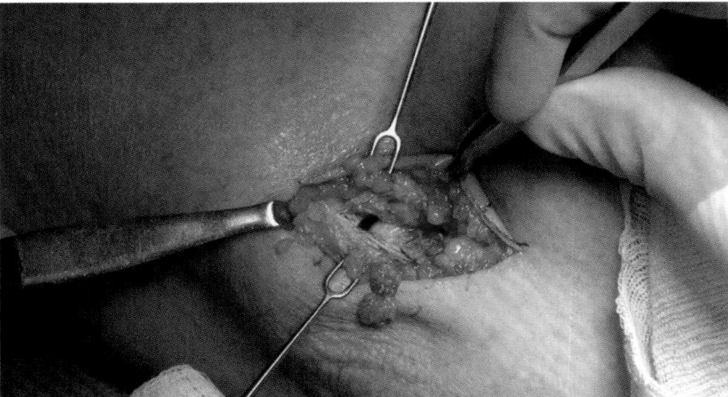

Figure 26-12 | The radiocapitellar joint is inspected and the elbow range of motion is tested for stability.

- If the patient has an especially prominent medial epicondyle, a small rongeur is used to perform a lateral epicondylectomy (Fig. 26-13), which will further debride the bony surface to provide a fresh bleeding surface for tendon healing (Fig. 26-14).

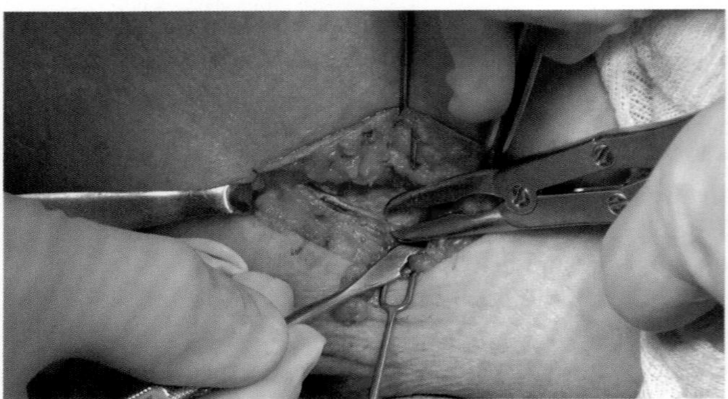

Figure 26-13 | If the lateral epicondyle is especially prominent, an epicondylectomy should be performed.

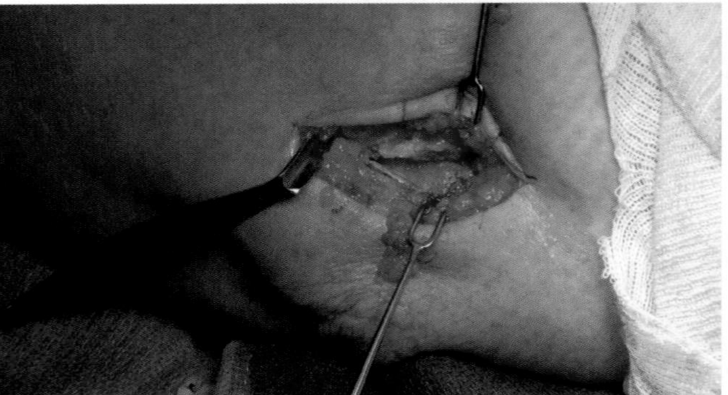

Figure 26-14 | The decorticated lateral epicondyle provides a bleeding surface for healing.

- The fascia is closed with a running, locking 2-0 Vicryl suture (Fig. 26-15). It is beneficial to perform the fascial closure with the elbow in extension to prevent overtightening of the supporting structures, which may lead to an elbow flexion contracture.

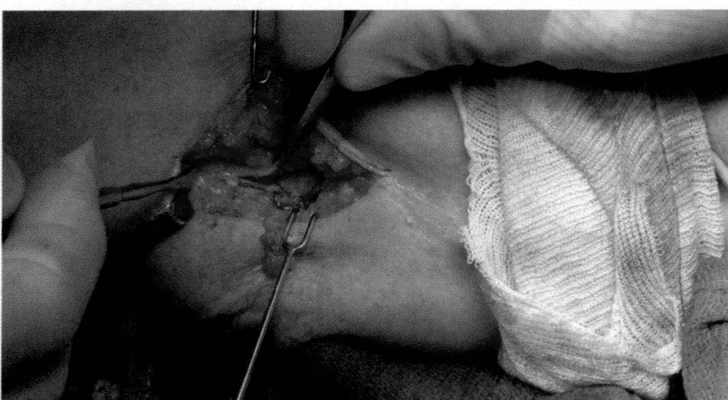

Figure 26-15 | Extensor tendon aponeurosis is closed side-to-side with an absorbable suture.

Postoperative Protocol

- Postoperatively, patients usually have a sense of soreness rather than the excruciating pain experienced preoperatively in most cases.
- Home range-of-motion exercises are performed for the first 6 weeks before a formalized therapy program is begun.
- Return to sports and unrestricted activities may take 3-6 months.

Outcomes

- At a 10- to 14-year follow-up, a 97% improvement rate and 8.9/10 patient satisfaction rating are reported after an open technique.[1]

Potential Complications

- To avoid iatrogenic elbow instability from excessive LUCL resection, the LUCL and capsule posterior to the equator of the radial head should not be excised.
- Symptoms may recur because of incomplete release of the ECRB or missed radial tunnel syndrome.
- Neurologic injury to the posterior interosseous radial nerve division or superficial sensory nerves can be caused by careless soft tissue retraction.

Reference

1. Dunn JH, Kim JJ, Davis L, et al. Ten- to 14-year follow-up of the Nirschl surgical technique for lateral epicondylitis. *Am J Sports Med.* 2008;36:261-266.

Chapter 27
One-Incision Distal Biceps Tendon Repair

MICHAEL D. MALONEY
RAYMOND J. KENNEY

Sterile Instruments/Equipment

- Tourniquet
- Seine, Army/Navy, and baby Bennett retractors
- Wire driver/drill
- 3.2-mm guidewire
- Acorn reaming drill bit
- Implants
  - Cortical button with insertion device
  - No. 2 nonabsorbable suture
  - Bioabsorbable tenodesis screw

Patient Positioning

- The patient is positioned supine and can remain on the stretcher or be transferred to an operating room table.
- A hand table should be used as the primary working surface for the operative extremity.
- A tourniquet can be applied high on the upper arm before preparation and draping, but a sterile tourniquet may be necessary for shorter arms.

Surgical Approach

- The incision is drawn over the midline volar forearm starting 2 cm distal to the elbow crease, extending distally about 3 cm (Fig. 27-1).

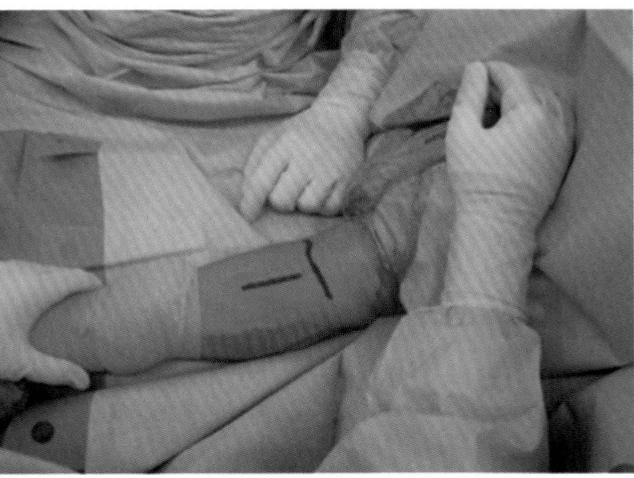

Figure 27-1 | Volar forearm/elbow showing markings for the distal elbow crease and the incision.

- The midline incision is made using a no. 15 blade scalpel, incising skin and dermis to the subcutaneous fat.
- The subcutaneous tissues are dissected, and the fascial plane between the flexor carpi radialis and the brachioradialis is identified.
- This plane is then carried down, carefully preserving the lateral antebrachial cutaneous nerve.
- A leash of vessels is identified within the fascial plane. Depending on the location of the vessels relative to the radial tuberosity, they may be preserved or ligated to adequately develop the plane.
- Blunt baby Bennett retractors are placed around the proximal radius, identifying the radial tuberosity. **Tip:** Pronosupinating the forearm while palpating the tuberosity will give the best idea of its orientation and position.
- At this point, it is important to maintain the forearm in supination to effectively expose and identify the radial tuberosity and to shift the posterior interosseous nerve away from danger.
- The radial tuberosity is identified and any remaining tissue is elevated with a key elevator and a rongeur.
- The distal biceps tendon is identified and mobilized with an Allis clamp (Fig. 27-2). It may be partially attached to the radial tuberosity, sitting relatively close to the native insertion or retracted proximal to the elbow. **Tip:** If retracted proximally, it may be necessary to make a second incision directly over the biceps muscle belly, tracing it distally to find the tendon.

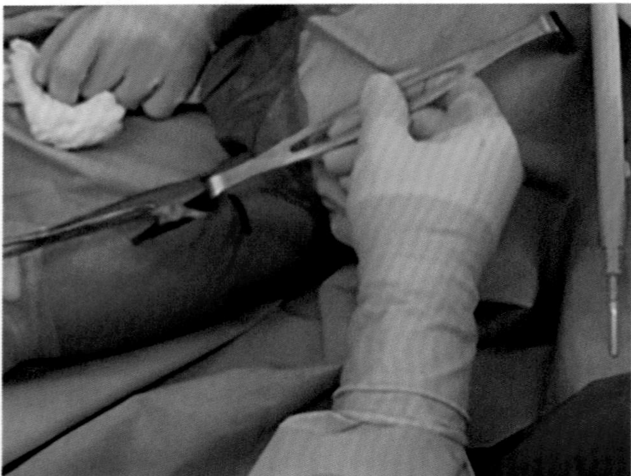

Figure 27-2 | Incision with distal biceps tendon mobilized with an Allis clamp attached to the end.

Tendon Preparation

- Once the tendon is mobilized, the distal end is prepared and trimmed such that it fits within an 8-mm sizing guide to ensure that it will be able to slide into the 8-mm tunnel. A smaller tendon will require a smaller tunnel, but the tunnel should be no larger than 8 mm in diameter.
- Using a no. 2 nonabsorbable suture, 5 or 6 whipstitches are passed up and back through the distal end of the tendon (Fig. 27-3).

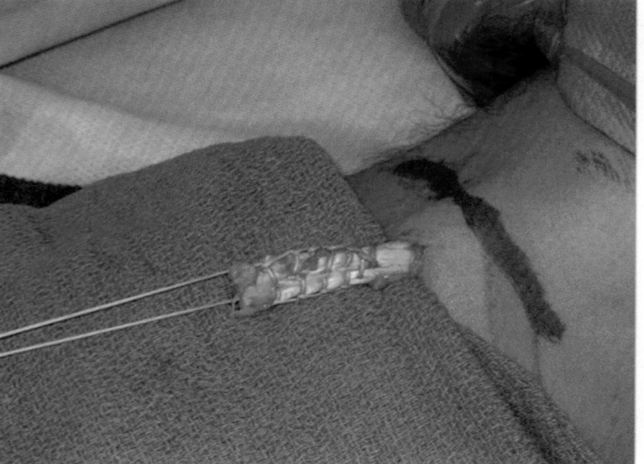

Figure 27-3 | Distal biceps tendon with suture fixation in place.

Radial Tuberosity and Tunnel Preparation

- Attention is taken to ensure any remaining soft tissue is debrided from the radial tuberosity.
- The 3.2-mm guidewire is placed centrally in the radial tuberosity, angled slightly radial to create the bone tunnel. **Tip:** Central placement on the tuberosity is critical because enough space is needed around all sides of the guidewire to avoid breaching one of the cortices with the acorn bit reamer and risk fixation failure of the bioabsorbable tenodesis screw (Fig. 27-4).
- Once adequate bony architecture has been verified on all sides of the pin, with enough room to allow for the acorn bit drill tip, the 3.2-mm guide pin is drilled bicortically and left in place.
- The acorn reaming drill bit is placed over the 3.2-mm guidewire, and only the near cortex of the radial tuberosity is drilled to create the bone tunnel for passage and seating of the distal end of the biceps tendon (Fig. 27-5).

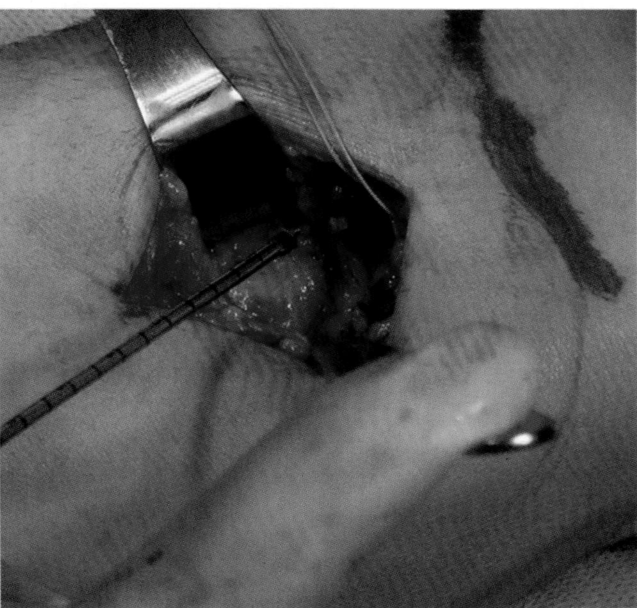

Figure 27-4 | Radial tuberosity as seen through the incision with 3.2-mm guide pin in the foreground.

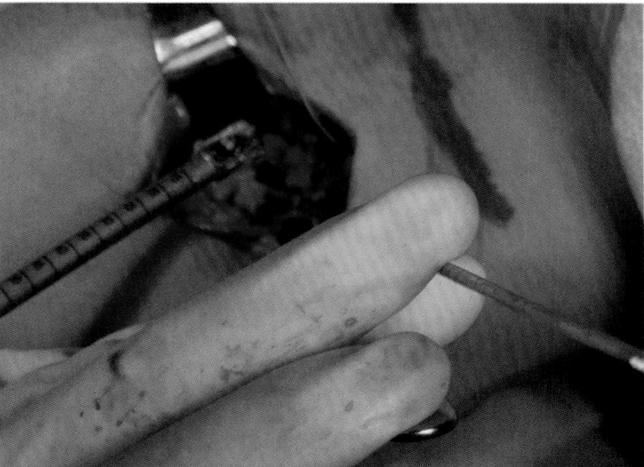

Figure 27-5 | The 3.2-mm guide pin remaining within the unicortical 8-mm tunnel after the reamer is removed.

Biceps Tendon Fixation

- The free ends of the no. 2 nonabsorbable suture exiting from the distal end of the biceps tendon are placed through the eyelets of the cortical button and then clamped (Fig. 27-6).

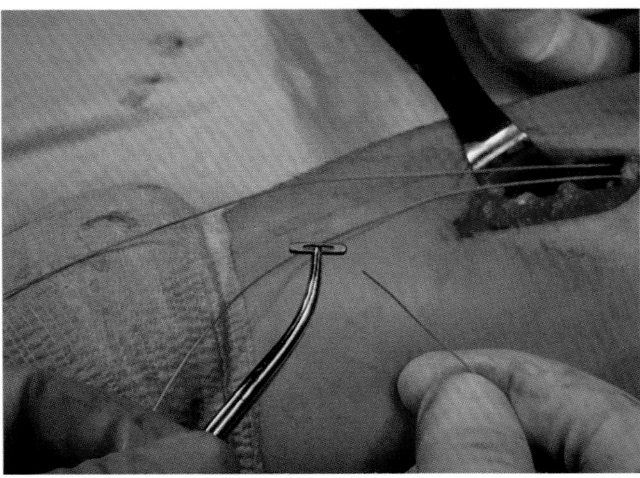

Figure 27-6 | Cortical button grasped with a snap showing the free end of the no. 2 nonabsorbable suture about to be passed through the eyelets.

- The threaded cortical button is placed on the insertion device, with tension kept on all sutures (Fig. 27-7).
- The cortical button is inserted into the tunnel and through the guidewire hole in the far cortex. The button is deployed with the insertion device remaining within the guidewire hole as the free ends of the no. 2 nonabsorbable sutures are tensioned, sliding each end sequentially through the button (Fig. 27-8).

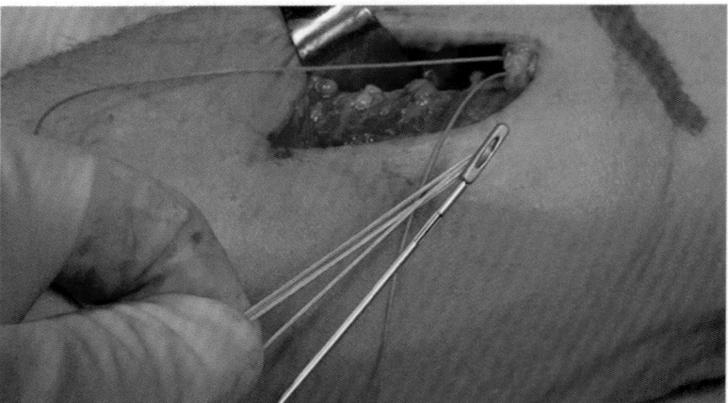

Figure 27-7 | Cortical button attached to the insertion device with free ends of no. 2 nonabsorbable suture passed through the eyelets.

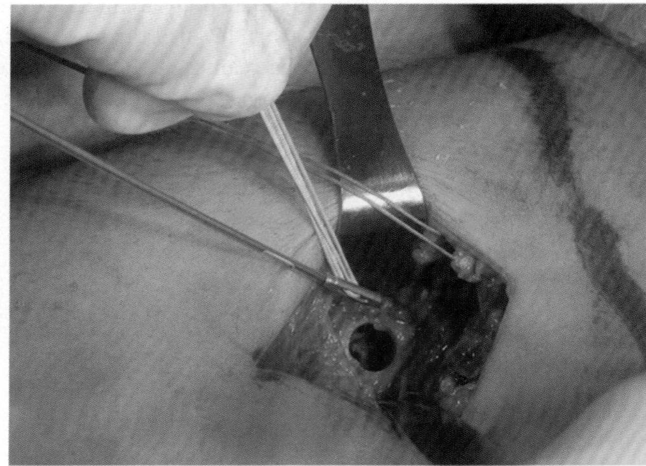

Figure 27-8 | Insertion of the cortical button.

- The distal end of the biceps tendon is then seated in the tunnel with the tension-slide technique (Videos 27-1 and 27-2).
- With the distal biceps tendon well seated in the tunnel, a bioabsorbable tenodesis screw is used for further fixation. One free limb of the no. 2 nonabsorbable suture is passed through the bioabsorbable tenodesis screw and through the top of the insertion driver (Fig. 27-9). The insertion driver is placed in the tunnel (Fig. 27-10), ideally placing the screw in the radial aspect of the bone tunnel and pushing the tendon posterior (Fig. 27-11).

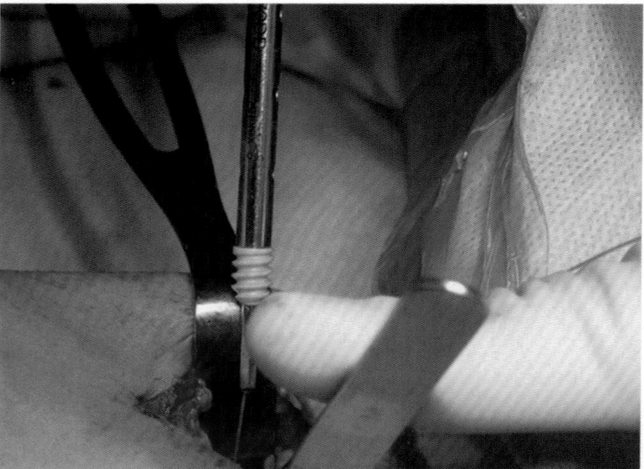

Figure 27-9 | Bioabsorbable tenodesis screw with one limb of the free no. 2 nonabsorbable suture through the center of the screw.

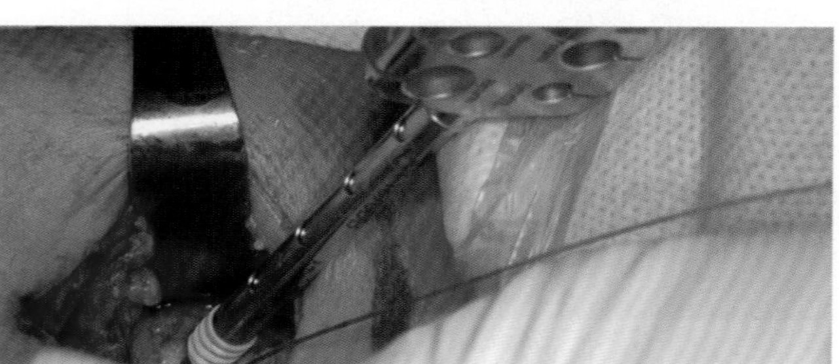

Figure 27-10 | Insertion of the bioabsorbable tenodesis screw within the 8-mm unicortical tunnel.

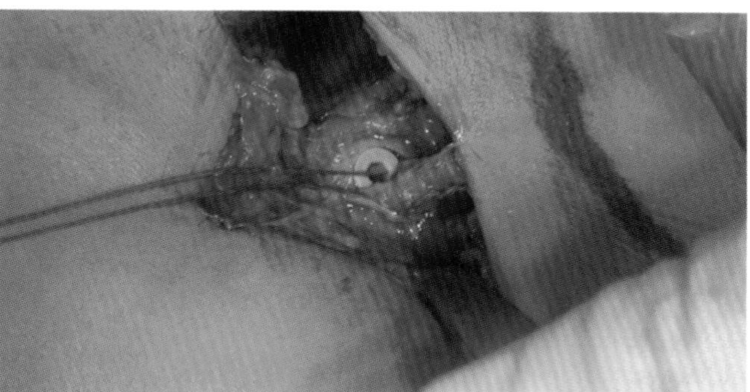

Figure 27-11 | Final fixation of the distal biceps tendon using a cortical button and bioabsorbable tenodesis screw.

- The two limbs of the no. 2 nonabsorbable suture are tied over the top of the bioabsorbable tenodesis screw and then cut.
- Thorough irrigation of the incision is performed to remove any bone debris from the tunnel preparation and drilling.
- The tourniquet is taken down, and any bleeding vessels are coagulated or tied off.
- The incision is closed with buried interrupted 2-0 Vicryl sutures for the subcutaneous tissues, and a running 3-0 Monocryl suture in a subcuticular fashion is used to close the skin. Steri-Strips are applied, and local anesthetic is injected around the surgical site.

Delayed Repair of Chronic Ruptures

- Repair of distal biceps tendon ruptures >4 weeks after injury may require an extensile anterior approach to the elbow to mobilize the tendon for delayed repair or tendon reconstruction.
- Interposition grafting may be required for tendon reconstruction if the distal biceps tendon cannot be adequately mobilized for primary repair.
  - Semitendinosus autograft can be woven through the proximal biceps muscle.
  - Achilles allograft can be sewn circumferentially around the proximal biceps muscle belly (Fig. 27-12).

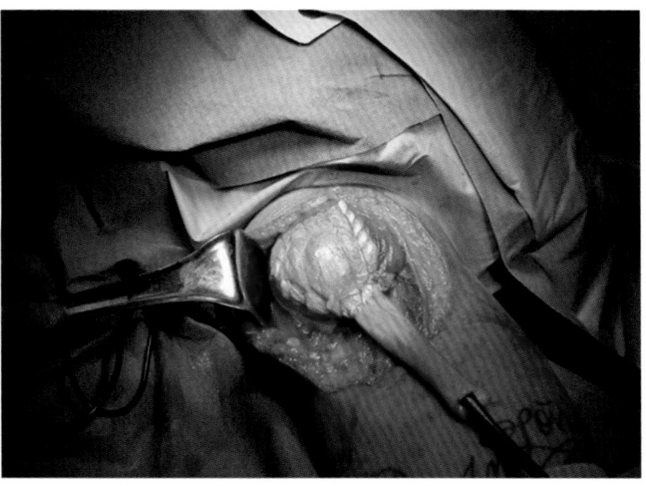

Figure 27-12 | Distal biceps tendon reconstruction using Achilles allograft sewn circumferentially around the biceps muscle belly.

Postoperative Care

- A sterile dressing is placed and a posterior slab splint with a lateral side strut is applied.
- Active flexion and extension as tolerated are permitted, but patients should lift nothing heavier than a coffee cup for the first 2 weeks.

Rehabilitation

- 5-7 days postoperatively:
  - The postsurgical dressing is removed, and a lighter dressing is applied.
  - A removable posterior long arm splint is fabricated with the elbow in 90 degrees of flexion with the forearm in neutral position. The splint is to be worn continuously.
  - Scar management and range of motion (ROM) are initiated.
  - Active assisted elbow extension and flexion (forearm must be supinated) and pronation and supination (elbow must be in as much flexion as possible, 100-120 degrees) are begun. **Tip:** The goal is full elbow ROM by 4 weeks postoperatively.
  - Full active shoulder, wrist, finger, and thumb ROM are maintained.
- 5-6 weeks postoperatively:
  - Grip and wrist progressive strengthening exercises are begun.
  - Posterior long arm splint wear is gradually decreased.
- 6-8 weeks postoperatively:
  - Progressive resistive exercises for the elbow are begun, and a gradual return to functional use of the arm as tolerated is allowed.

Suggested Readings

Bain GI, Prem H, Heptinstall RJ, Verhellen R, Paix D. Repair of distal biceps tendon rupture: a new technique using the Endobutton. *J Shoulder Elbow Surg.* 2000;9:120-126.

Balabaud L, Ruiz C, Nonnenmacher J, Seynaeve P, Kehr P, Rapp E. Repair of distal biceps tendon ruptures using a suture anchor and an anterior approach. *J Hand Surg Br.* 2004;29:178-182.

Darlis NA, Sotereanos DG. Distal biceps tendon reconstruction in chronic ruptures. *J Shoulder Elbow Surg.* 2006;15(5):614-619.

Mazzocca A, Bicos J, Arciero RA, Romeo AA, Cohen M, Nicholson G. Repair of distal biceps tendon ruptures using a combined anatomic interference screw and cortical button. *Tech Shoulder Elbow Surg.* 2005;6:108-115.

McKee MD, Hirji R, Schemitsch EH, Wild LM, Waddell JP. Patient oriented functional outcome after repair of distal biceps tendon ruptures using a single-incision technique. *J Shoulder Elbow Surg.* 2005;14:302-306.

Sethi P, Cunningham J, Miller S, Suuton K, Mazzocca A. Anatomical repair of the distal biceps tendon using the tension slide technique. *Tech Shoulder Elbow Surg.* 2008;9:182-187.

Sethi P, Obopilwe E, Rincon L, Miller S, Mazzocca A. Biomechanical evaluation of distal biceps reconstruction with cortical button and interference screw fixation. *J Shoulder Elbow Surg.* 2010;19(1):53-57.

Shields E, Olsen JR, Williams RB, Rouse L, Maloney M, Voloshin I. Distal biceps brachii tendon repairs: a single-incision technique using a cortical button with interference screw versus a double-incision technique using suture fixation through bone tunnels. *Am J Sports Med.* 2015;43(5):1072-1076.

Wiley WB, Noble JS, Dulaney TD, Bell RH, Noble DD. Late reconstruction of chronic distal biceps tendon ruptures with a semitendinosus autograft technique. *J Shoulder Elbow Surg.* 2006;15(4):440-444.

Chapter 28

Two-Incision Distal Biceps Repair

JULIAN J. SONNENFELD
BRIAN B. SHIU
WILLIAM N. LEVINE

Instruments/Equipment

- Sterile tourniquet
- Mini C-arm fluoroscopy
- Round or pineapple-shaped 4-mm burr
- Side-cutting 1-mm drill bit
- No. 2 looped nonabsorbable high-strength suture
- Kelly clamp
- Hewson suture passer
- Bipolar electrocautery

Positioning

- The patient is positioned supine with the arm placed across a hand table, and general or regional anesthesia is administered.
- A sterile tourniquet is placed on the upper arm and inflated before the incision is made.

Surgical Exposure

- The biceps tendon is palpated before the incision is made to confirm the location of the retracted tendon.
- An anterior approach is first used to locate the biceps tendon.
  - A single 2- to 3-cm transverse incision is made at the distal extent of the antecubital crease (Fig. 28-1).
    - The length of incision should allow enough space for finger palpation of the biceps tendon stump.
    - The incision should lie along the ulnar border of the brachioradialis muscle.
  - Dissection is performed down to the antebrachial fascia.
    - The traversing lateral antebrachial cutaneous nerve is identified.
  - Blunt finger dissection is used to facilitate biceps stump identification.
    - The biceps tendon will often be more superficial than expected.
    - Hematoma/seroma will likely be encountered before identifying the tendon.
  - An Allis clamp is used to grasp the tendon.
    - The distal tendon is carefully freed of adhesions and care is taken to ensure that the stump is not folded onto itself.

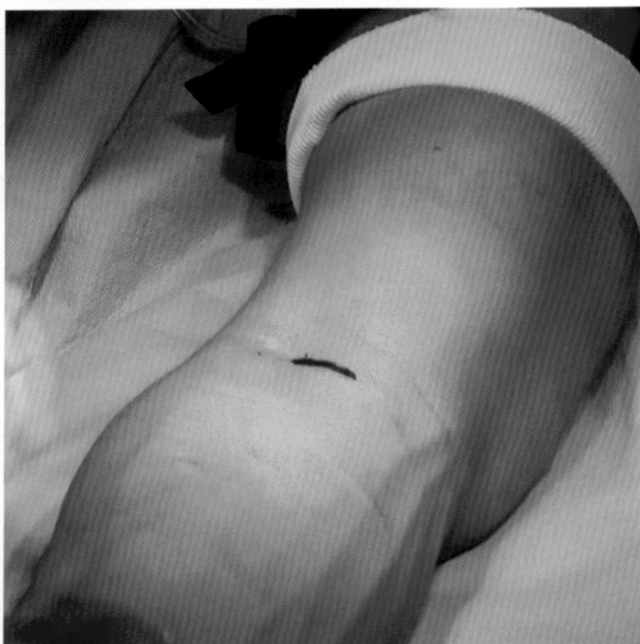

Figure 28-1 | A transverse 3-cm planned incision is drawn in the antecubital fossa in this patient who suffered an acute distal biceps rupture. (Courtesy of Columbia University Center for Shoulder, Elbow and Sports Medicine.)

- The distal end of the tendinotic biceps tendon is debrided (Fig. 28-2).
  - It may be difficult to insert the distal end of the tendon within the biceps footprint if the tendon edge is insufficiently trimmed.
- Two sutures (no. 2 looped nonabsorbable high-strength sutures) are passed 2.5 cm proximal to the distal edge of the tendon (Fig. 28-3).
  - A whipstitch technique is used to tubularize the distal portion of the tendon.
  - **Surgical Pearl:** Using blunt dissection along the entire length of the biceps will maximize tendon excursion. This should be done after the whipstitch is placed.
- The tendon can be sized at this point (typically 7 mm) to assist with estimating the size of the biceps docking site.

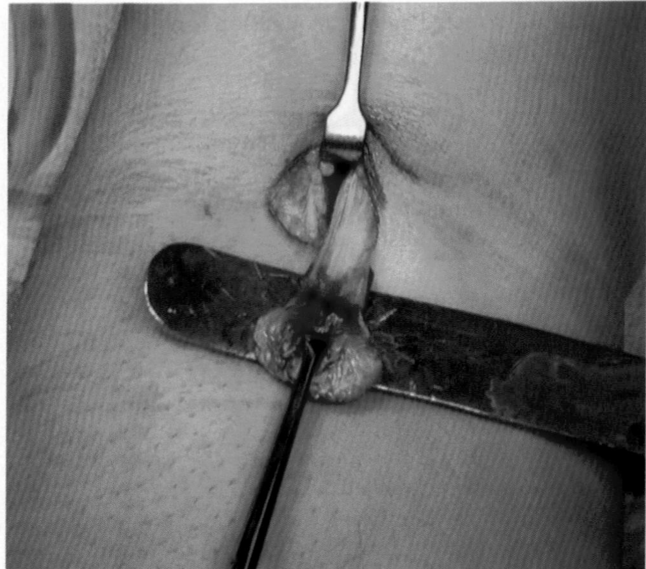

Figure 28-2 | The ruptured distal biceps is retrieved and brought outside the wound. Note the degenerative and widened distal extent of the tendon. (Courtesy of Columbia University Center for Shoulder, Elbow and Sports Medicine.)

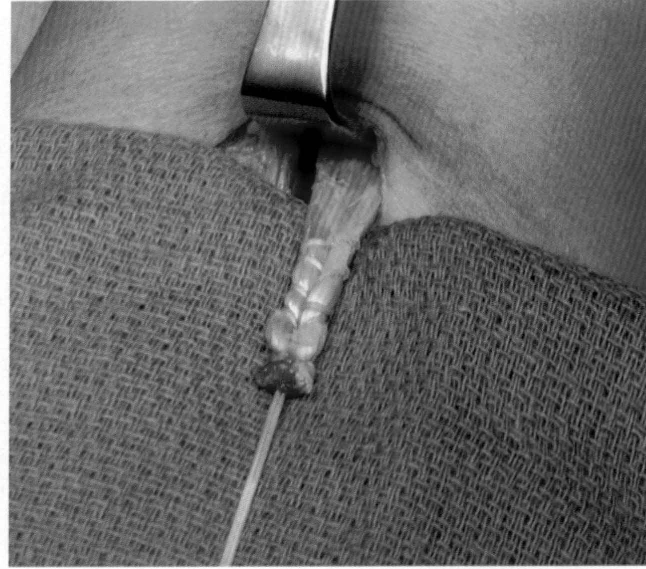

Figure 28-3 | The degenerative and widened distal 5 mm is excised and a running, locking nonabsorbable suture is placed to maximize control of the tendon and minimize suture pullout in line of the collagen fibers. (Courtesy of Columbia University Center for Shoulder, Elbow and Sports Medicine.)

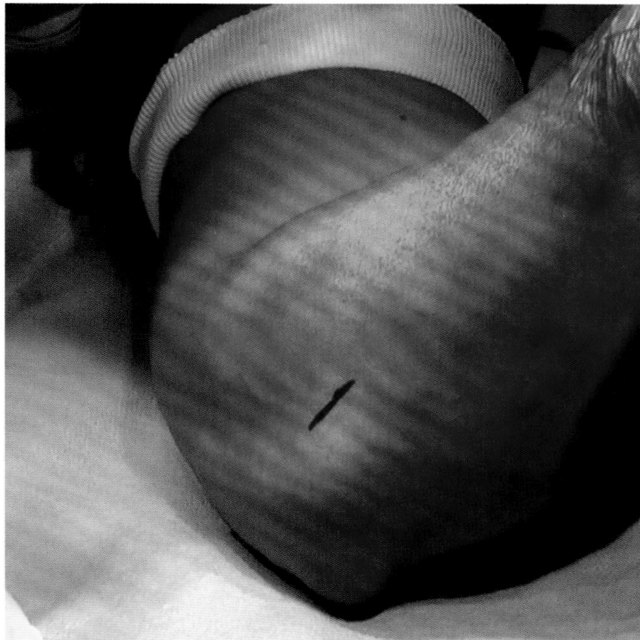

Figure 28-4 | A 3-cm marking is made on the dorsal forearm in anticipation of the second incision. (Courtesy of Columbia University Center for Shoulder, Elbow and Sports Medicine.)

- A second posterior forearm incision is used to expose the biceps tuberosity (Fig. 28-4).
  - **Surgical Pearl:** The expected incision should be drawn out and the location confirmed with a Kelly clamp from the anterior wound (Fig. 28-5).

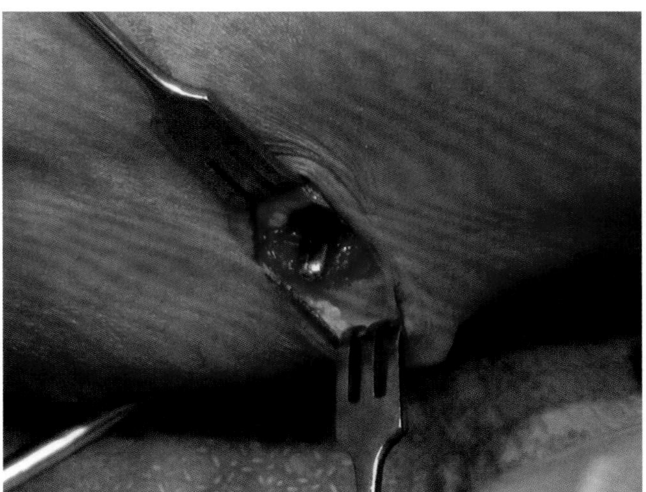

Figure 28-5 | The dorsal incision is made down to the muscle. A clamp is passed from the volar incision and brought out the dorsal incision. (Courtesy of Columbia University Center for Shoulder, Elbow and Sports Medicine.)

  - The incision lies between the radius and ulna and is centered 3-4 cm distal to the radiocapitellar joint.
  - In thin individuals, the radial tuberosity will be palpable along the ulnar border of the radius with the forearm in full supination.
- Blunt finger dissection is used to palpate down to the radial tuberosity through the anterior wound.
  - The radial tuberosity footprint is confirmed by pronating and supinating the forearm.
    - **Surgical Pearl:** A mini C-arm can be used to confirm the biceps footprint in patients with altered anatomy.
  - Any adhesions that may have developed since the time of injury are freed.
- A Kelly clamp is passed ulnar to the palpated biceps tuberosity with the curved portion of the clamp pointing laterally.

- The clamp is directed through the interosseous space while maintaining contact between the tip of the clamp and the radius to eliminate soft tissue bridges.
- **Pronation** of the forearm helps to protect the posterior interosseous nerve (PIN).

- The clamp should be advanced through the common extensor musculature and into the subcutaneous tissue to be seen tenting the skin over the dorsal aspect of the proximal portion of the forearm.
- The skin is incised over the site of prominence at the clamp; this should be ~3 cm long and carried through the common extensor musculature and supinator.
- With the forearm maximally pronated, the tuberosity is exposed with a muscle-splitting technique.
  - An elevator is used to lift any remnants of the biceps stump to prepare the radial tuberosity.
    - Pronating the forearm at this stage will also help to visualize the biceps footprint through the dorsal incision.
    - Fat will signify the biceps bursa, not proximity to the PIN—the nerve is relatively safe in this approach.

Preparation of the Radius

- A pineapple-shaped burr is used to create an oval trough in the radial tuberosity.
  - The trough should be wide enough for the tendon to be docked in the radius (this is on average 10 × 8 mm).
    - Depth should be ~5 mm.
    - The average size of the tendon is 7 mm.
    - The width of the burr can be used to guide resection amount.
  - A side-cutting burr is used to place two holes on the lateral side of the trough with at least a 7-mm bone bridge (Fig. 28-6).
    - These holes should be inset at least 5 mm from the docking edge to ensure an adequate bone bridge.

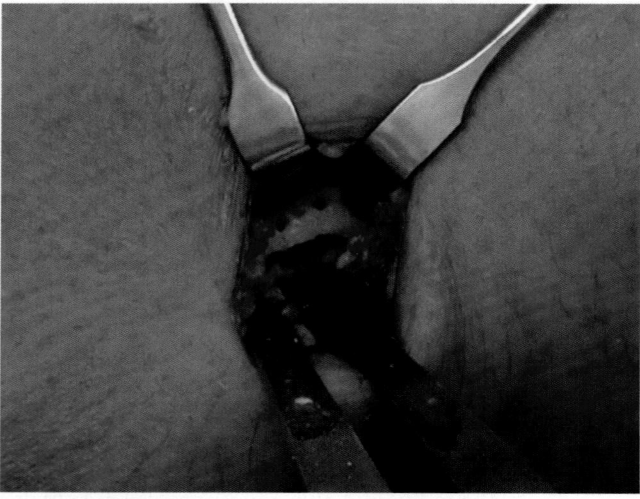

Figure 28-6 | A recipient socket is created with an acorn burr in the radial tuberosity. Three small drill holes are seen above the socket for later suture passage. (Courtesy of Columbia University Center for Shoulder, Elbow and Sports Medicine.)

Tendon Reattachment

- An index finger is placed down to the radial tuberosity through the anterior incision.
- A curved clamp is placed through the antecubital incision to find the plane adjacent to the ulnar border of the radius.
  - This curved clamp will be used to pull a shuttling suture proximally through the anterior incision.
- The nonabsorbable biceps sutures are loaded and shuttled through the distal aspect of the wound.
- A Hewson suture passer is used to pull each suture through each of the drill holes.
  - The forearm in full pronation for adequate visualization through the dorsal wound
    - The Hewson suture passer can be bent to 45 degrees at the tip to facilitate suture passage.

- Tension is placed on the sutures while pronating and supinating the forearm to help guide the tendon into the trough (Fig. 28-7).

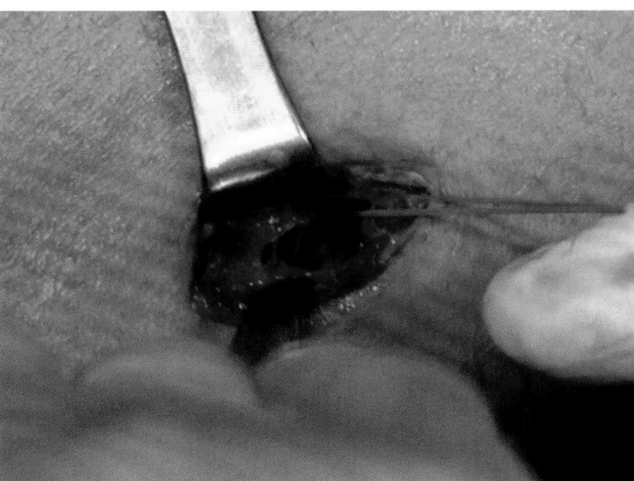

Figure 28-7 | The sutures from the biceps tendon are passed through the holes in the tuberosity. (Courtesy of Columbia University Center for Shoulder, Elbow and Sports Medicine.)

- The sutures should be tied and secured with at least six throws (see Fig. 28-8).
  - **Surgical Pearl:** Suture button fixation can be used as backup if there is failure of the bone bridge.

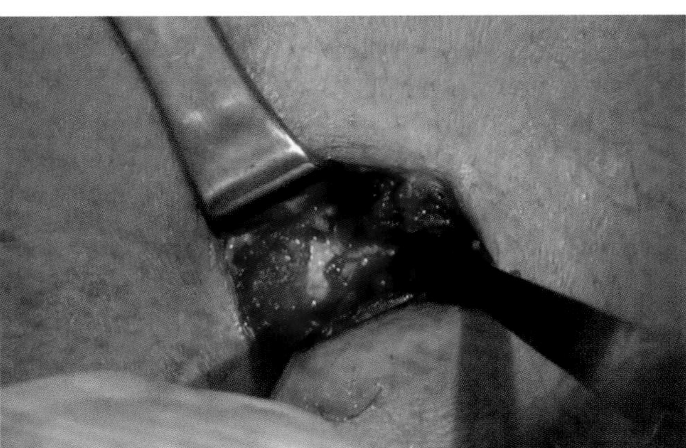

Figure 28-8 | Final repair of the repaired biceps tendon from the dorsal view. (Courtesy of Columbia University Center for Shoulder, Elbow and Sports Medicine.)

Closure

- Both incisions are copiously irrigated with normal saline to remove all bone debris and minimize the risk of heterotopic ossification.
- The tourniquet is deflated before closure to ensure adequate hemostasis.
- Fascia should be closed with 0 Vicryl (along the posterior incision only).
- 3-0 Biosyn (absorbable) sutures are used for subcutaneous skin (both incisions).
- 4-0 Biosyn (absorbable) sutures are used for skin (both incisions).

Postoperative Care

- It is important to assess the range of elbow extension in the operating room. Extension of the elbow should be limited beyond the angle at which the biceps tendon is felt to be excessively tight.
- A hinged elbow brace is placed to limit extension.
- Active elbow flexion is allowed starting 2 weeks postoperatively.
- Gradual elbow extension is progresses by 10 degrees weekly.
- Patient may begin elbow mobilization 2-3 days postoperatively.

Chapter 29
Triceps Tendon Repair

KATHRYN L. CRUM
MICHAEL C. CICCOTTI
MICHAEL G. CICCOTTI

Sterile Instruments/Equipment

- Tourniquet
- Self-retaining retractors
- Rasp
- 2-mm drill bit
- Ruler
- Rongeur
- Suture shuttling device (Hewson suture passer, Smith & Nephew, Andover, MA)
- Implants
  - Two no. 2 nonabsorbable sutures (preferably different colors)
  - Free needle
  - Two looped nonabsorbable sutures (FiberLink, Arthrex, Naples, FL)
  - Knotless suture anchor (4.75-mm BioComposite SwiveLock, Arthrex, Naples, FL)

Patient Positioning

- The patient is positioned either prone on chest rolls or in the lateral decubitus position on a beanbag, depending on surgeon preference.
  - We prefer prone on chest rolls.
- All bony prominences are carefully padded.
- The elbow should be positioned such that it can be held in a flexed position of 90 degrees, with freedom to extend as needed during the surgical repair.
  - With the patient prone, an arm holder is placed on the ipsilateral side of the bed at shoulder level such that the shoulder is in 90 degrees of abduction and neutral forward flexion.
  - A nonsterile tourniquet is placed proximally on the upper arm at the axilla to allow an adequate surgical field.
  - The upper arm is placed in the arm holder at the level of the tourniquet (Fig. 29-1).

Surgical Approach

- An 8- to 10-cm midline curvilinear incision is made over the posterior aspect of the elbow.
  - The incision starts 4-5 cm proximal to the tip of the olecranon and extends 4-5 cm distal to the tip of the olecranon.
  - The incision is gently curved to the radial side of the olecranon tip to prevent the healed incision from being in the area of direct contact when the elbow rests on a surface during daily activities.

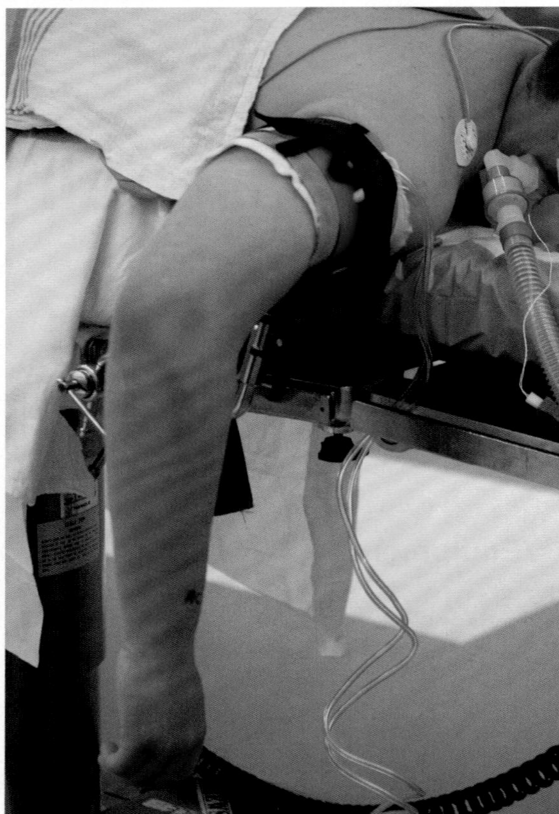

Figure 29-1 | Patient positioned prone on chest rolls with tourniquet and arm holder placed.

- Medial and lateral skin flaps are created.
  - The flaps should not be made too thin to avoid skin perforation and to provide adequate coverage with closure.
  - The ulnar nerve is palpated medially. The nerve is not routinely exposed, but great care is taken to protect it throughout the procedure.

Triceps Tendon and Olecranon Preparation

- The site of tendon injury is identified and prepared.
  - Often, the paratenon is violated. If it is intact, though, care is taken to incise it in its midline and gently elevate it off the remaining tendon for later closure.
  - The ruptured tendon often is surrounded by a serous or organizing hematoma. It may be tendinotic or bulbous, requiring some debridement.
  - Only the tendinotic tissue is debrided.
  - There may be some delamination between the deep medial head and more superficial lateral head that should be identified so as to include both with the repair.
  - The tendon is gently mobilized by freeing any surrounding adhesions.
  - The tendon footprint is identified and marked to aid in later suture passage.
- The tendon footprint on the olecranon is identified and prepared.
  - The proximal aspect of the tendon insertion begins ~12 mm distal to the tip of the olecranon.
  - This site is identified, and any remaining soft tissue is debrided from the bony footprint.
  - The exposed surface is gently rasped to create a vascular bed, with care taken not to decorticate the bone bed (Fig. 29-2).
  - The proximal olecranon periosteum is incised along the posterior ulnar border and elevated medially and laterally for later closure over the repair.

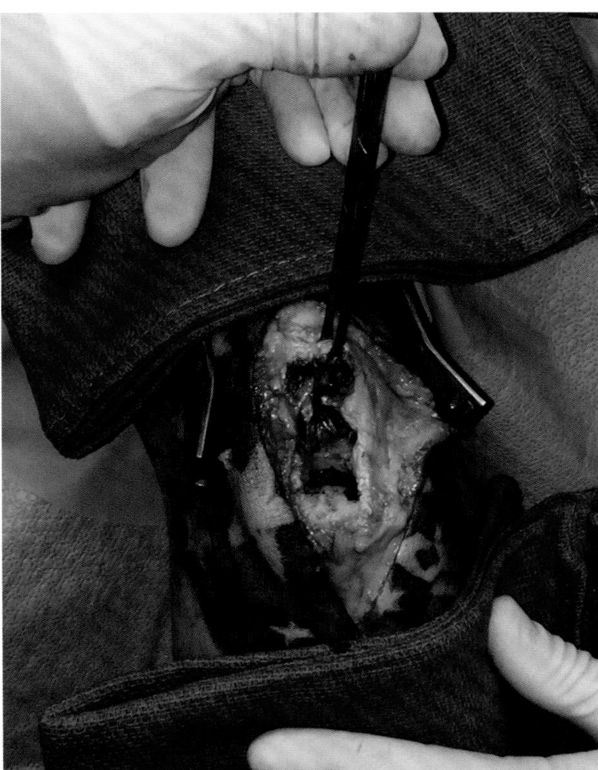

Figure 29-2 | The prepared triceps tendon and olecranon with corresponding footprint sites marked.

Repair Techniques

- Several techniques exist to repair the distal triceps tendon to the bone:
  - *Transosseous Cruciate Tunnels*[1]
    - This technique involves securing the tendon to the footprint by passing the sutures that have been placed in the tendon through crossing bone tunnels in the olecranon.
    - A no. 2 nonabsorbable suture is placed in a locking fashion (eg, Krackow/Bunnell) in the triceps tendon. The suture enters the previously demarcated footprint site on the medial tendon, passes along the medial edge proximally, and crosses to the lateral side and then distally along the lateral tendon edge to exit on the lateral half of the triceps footprint.
    - A 2-mm drill bit is used to create crossing bone tunnels in the olecranon.
    - The tunnels begin at the medial and lateral tendon footprint and extend distally to the contralateral cortical side on the dorsal ulna.
    - Care is taken when drilling from lateral to medial to protect the ulnar nerve.
    - A suture passer is used to retrieve each suture end through the tunnels from proximal to distal. The medial suture end is passed through the bone tunnels from medial to lateral, while the lateral suture end is passed from lateral to medial.
    - The sutures are then tied over the bone bridge with care to maintain the knot at the entrance of the distal lateral bone tunnel. This will ensure that the suture knot is less palpable and away from the ulnar nerve (Fig. 29-3).
  - *Standard Suture Anchor Repair*[2-4]
    - This technique involves placing two single-loaded suture anchors into the anatomic footprint on the olecranon.
    - One anchor is placed distally in the medial half of the olecranon footprint; the other anchor is placed distally in the lateral half of the olecranon footprint (Fig. 29-4A).
    - One suture limb of the medial anchor is placed in the medial half of the tendon in a Krackow fashion from distal to proximal 3-4 cm, then proximal to distal. One suture limb of the lateral anchor is passed in the same fashion through the lateral half of the tendon.

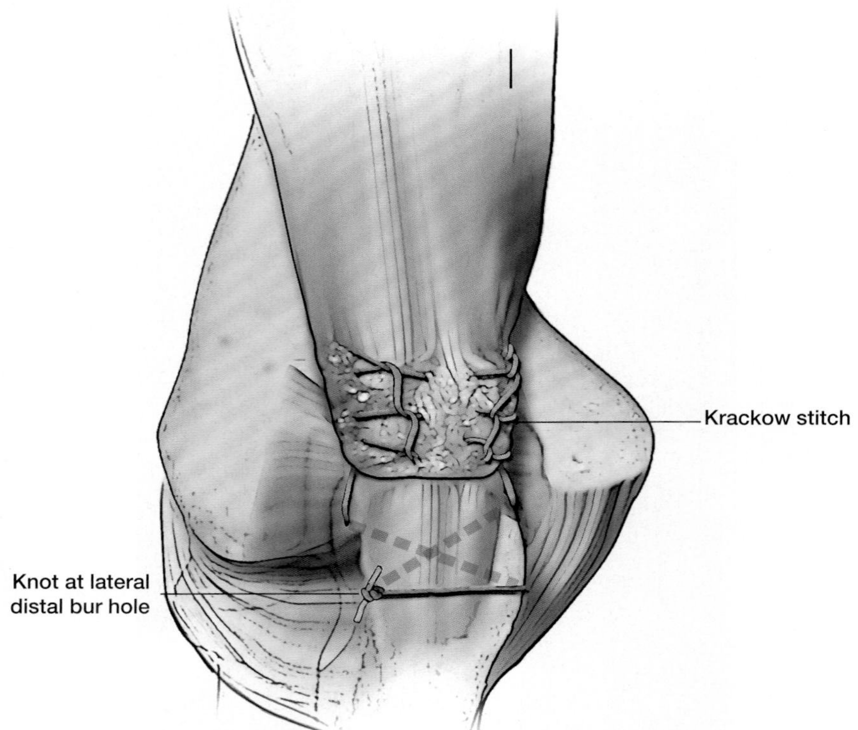

Figure 29-3 | Completed transosseous cruciate drill tunnel technique schematic. (SAGE Publishing From Petre BM, Grutter PW, Rose DM, Belkoff SM, McFarland EG, Petersen SA. Triceps tendons: a biomechanical comparison of intact and repaired strength. *J Shoulder Elbow Surg.* 2011;20:213-218, Figure 2, with permission.)

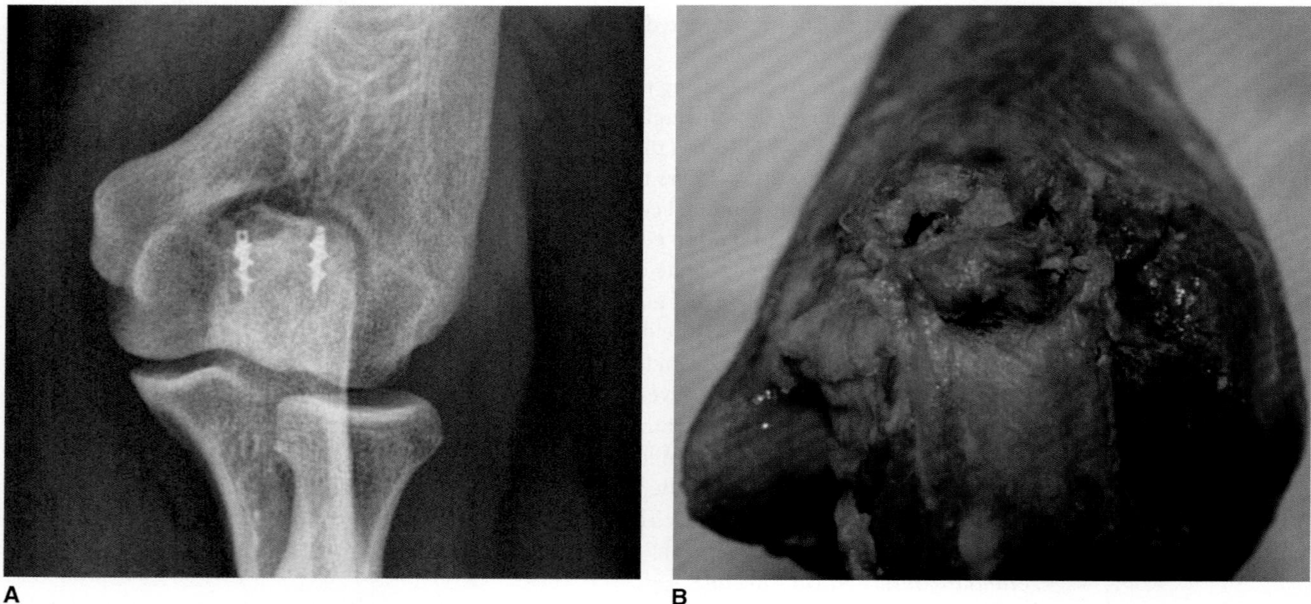

Figure 29-4 | A. Plain anteroposterior (AP) radiograph showing suture anchors placed in the olecranon. **B.** Completed standard suture anchor repair. (From Bava ED, Barber FA, Lund ER. Clinical outcome after suture anchor repair of complete traumatic rupture of the distal triceps tendon. *Arthroscopy*. 2012;28:1058-1063, Figure 1, with permission; Yeh PC, Stephens KT, Solovyova O, et al. The distal triceps tendon footprint and a biomechanical analysis of 3 repair techniques. *Am J Sports Med*. 2010;38:1025-1033, Figure 2, with permission.)

- The medial anchor Krackow-stitch limb is tied to the free suture end from that same medial anchor, while the lateral anchor Krackow-stitch limb is tied to the free suture end from that lateral anchor, thereby reducing the tendon to the olecranon (Fig. 29-4B).

- *Anatomic Transosseous Equivalent Repair*[5]
  - A single free no. 2 nonabsorbable suture is placed in a Krackow fashion along the medial edge of the triceps, distal to proximal, and then across the tendon and down the lateral side.
    - Both free ends should exit the posterior surface of the tendon ~1 cm proximal to the distal edge (Fig. 29-5A).

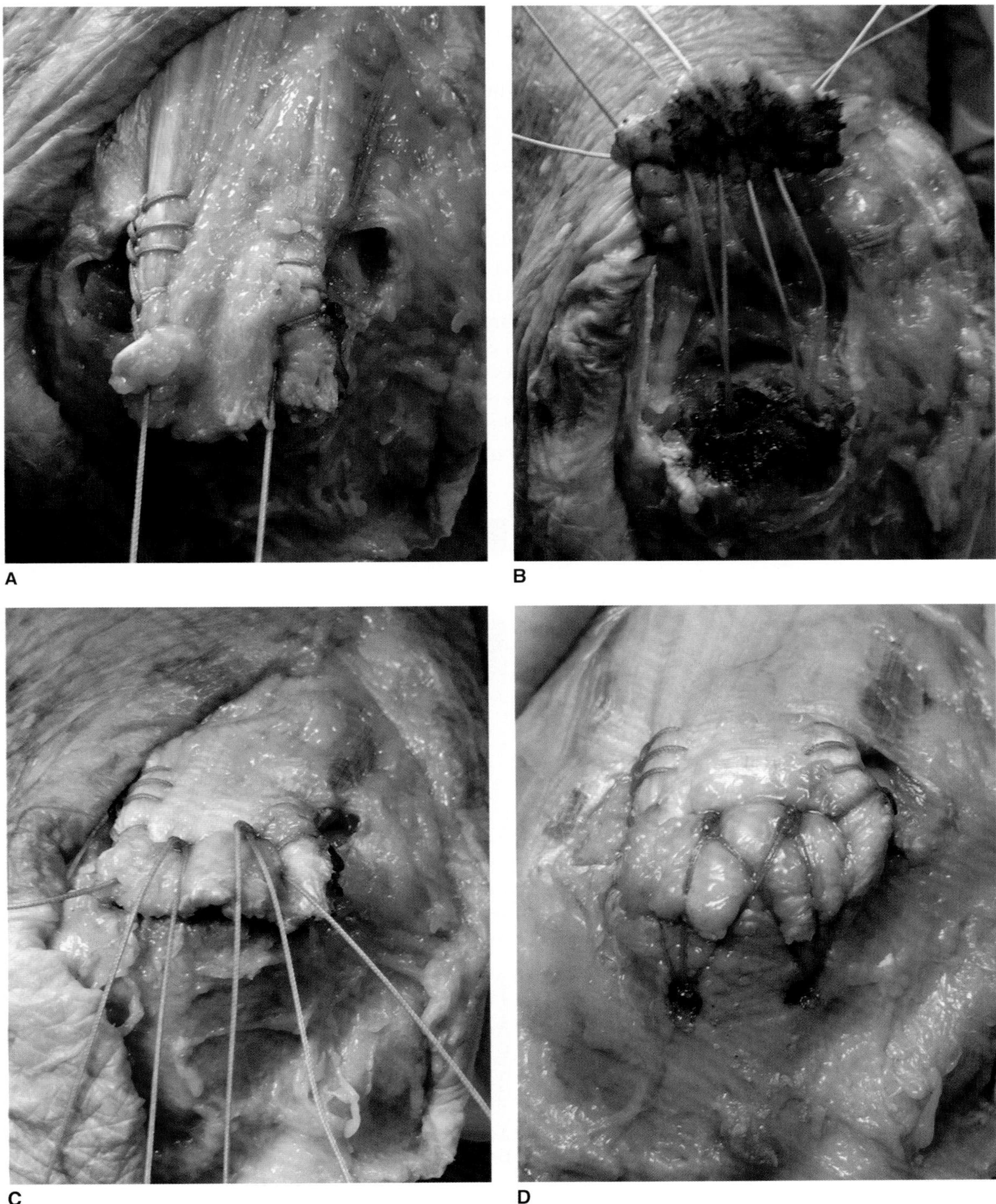

Figure 29-5 | A. The Krackow stitch placed from distal to proximal on the medial side, crossing over laterally, and then from proximal to distal on the lateral side. **B.** Suture anchors placed at the proximal olecranon footprint with all suture limbs passed through the proximal tendon footprint from anterior to posterior with 1 cm tissue bridge. **C.** Suture anchors are tied in mattress fashion reducing the proximal portion of the tendon and olecranon footprints. **D.** Completed anatomic transosseous equivalent repair with suture from each mattress stitch and the ipsilateral Krakow placed into a knotless anchor distal to the footprint. (From O'Donnell K, Rubenstein D, Ciccotti MG. Triceps tendon injury. In: Arciero R, Cordasco F, Provencher M, eds. *Shoulder and Elbow Injuries in Athletes: Prevention, Treatment and Return to Sport*. Philadelphia, PA: Elsevier; 2018, p. 489, Figure 7A-D, with permission.)

- Two single-loaded suture anchors are placed at the proximal margin of the anatomic tendon footprint on the olecranon.
  - These sutures are passed anterior to posterior, beginning 2 cm proximal to the tendon's distal edge at the proximal margin of the demarcated footprint on the tendon. The sutures should be passed in a horizontal mattress fashion with an ~1-cm tissue bridge between them (Fig. 29-5B).
- The suture limbs from each implant are then tied together reducing the proximal portion of the tendon footprint to the proximal portion of the olecranon footprint (Fig. 29-5C).
- The medial limb of the Krackow and a single limb from each suture anchor are then placed into a knotless suture anchor, which is implanted into the posteromedial olecranon 2 cm distal to the tendon.
- The lateral limb of the Krackow suture and the remaining suture limbs from each of the anchors are passed through a second knotless suture anchor that is then implanted on the posterolateral olecranon 2 cm from the tendon margin (Fig. 29-5D).

- *Knotless Anatomic Footprint Repair*[6-9]
  - This is our preferred technique for triceps tendon repair.
  - Functionally, it acts as a tension band construct and has demonstrated biomechanical superiority in comparison to alternative repair techniques.[6-8]
  - Patient positioning, surgical approach, triceps tendon preparation, and olecranon preparation are carried out as described earlier (pp. 223-224).
  - Two no. 2 nonabsorbable sutures, one lateral and one medial, are passed in a locking Krackow whipstitch fashion to secure the tendon.
    - Care is taken to ensure that the four limbs all begin and end at the proximal margin of the tendon footprint exiting through the deep anterior surface (Fig. 29-6).

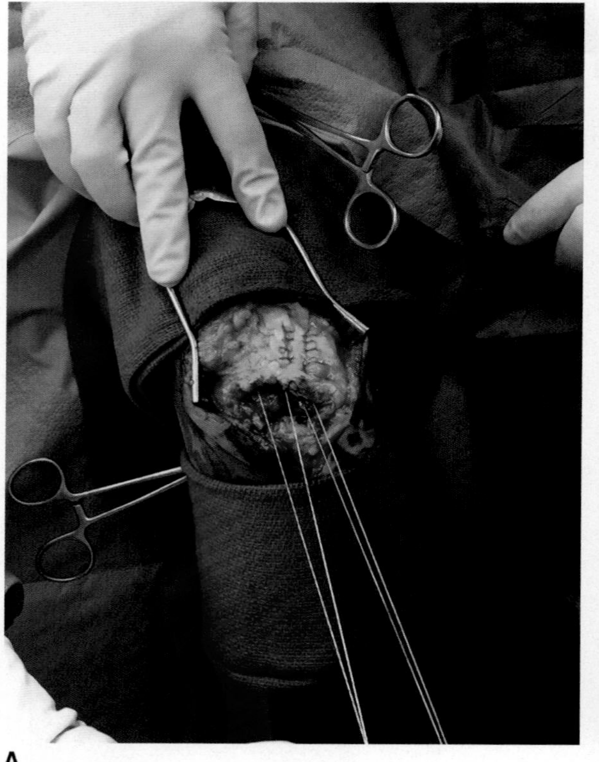
A

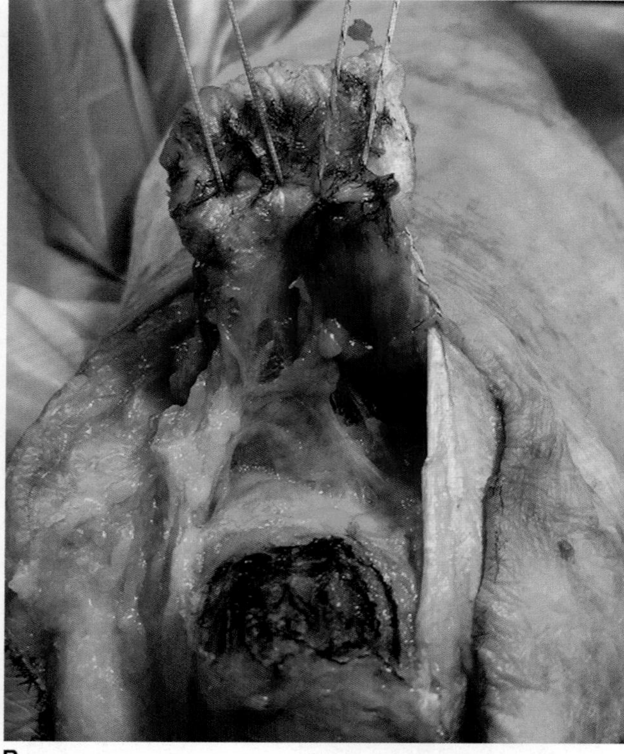
B

Figure 29-6 **A and B.** Medial and lateral Krackow stitches exiting on the deep surface of the triceps tendon at the level of the proximal footprint margin. Different-colored sutures facilitate management. (From O'Donnel K, Rubenstein D, Ciccotti MG. Triceps tendon injury. In: Arciero R, Cordasco F, Provencher M, eds. *Shoulder and Elbow Injuries in Athletes: Prevention, Treatment and Return to Sport*. Elsevier; 2018, p. 490, Figure 8, with permission.)

- The use of different color sutures medially and laterally aids greatly in suture management.

- A free needle is used to pass two looped nonabsorbable sutures (FiberLink, Arthrex, Naples, FL) one midway between the medial Krackow-stitch limbs and the other midway between the lateral Krackow-stitch limbs at the proximal margin of the footprint.
  - The loops should exit the superficial posterior tendon surface to aid in later suture shuttling.
  - Now three suture tails are on the deep anteromedial side and three on the deep anterolateral side (Fig. 29-7).

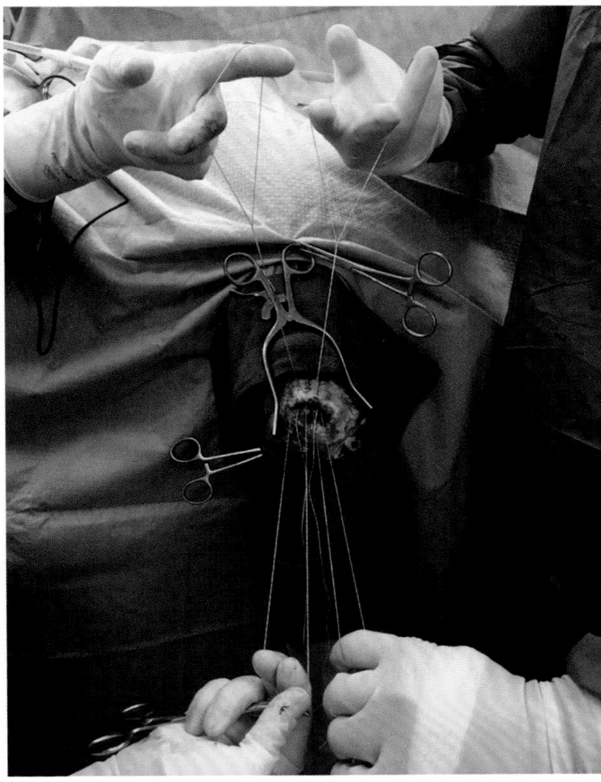

Figure 29-7 | The looped ends of suture exiting posteriorly midway between each Krakow stitch, which results in 3 medial and 3 lateral groups of sutures exiting on the deep anterior surface of the triceps tendon.

- The olecranon bone tunnels are created for preparation of the triceps bony footprint.
  - A 2-mm drill bit is used to create medial and lateral, longitudinal tunnels beginning at the proximal edge of tendon footprint on the olecranon and exiting distally and dorsally on the posteromedial and posterolateral surfaces of the ulna, respectively.
    - The drill bit should be angled appropriately at ~45 degrees in the sagittal plane from the longitudinal axis of the ulna to avoid penetration of the sigmoid notch (Fig. 29-8A and B).
    - Care is taken to slightly diverge these two longitudinal tunnels to provide room for the final knotless suture anchor.
  - A point on the central, dorsal surface of the ulna ~5-10 mm distal to the exit holes of the 2-mm drill tunnels is selected for placement of the knotless suture anchor.
    - This location is predrilled and tapped to facilitate placement of the implant in the hard ulnar bone.
      - Care is taken to angle away from the sigmoid notch.
- Suture shuttling is now carefully begun. This is facilitated by the different colored Krakow sutures.
  - The 3 medial suture limbs (2 from the medial Krackow stitch and 1 from the medial looped suture) are passed through the medial 2-mm ulnar tunnel from proximal to distal using a suture shuttling device or 22-gauge wire loop.

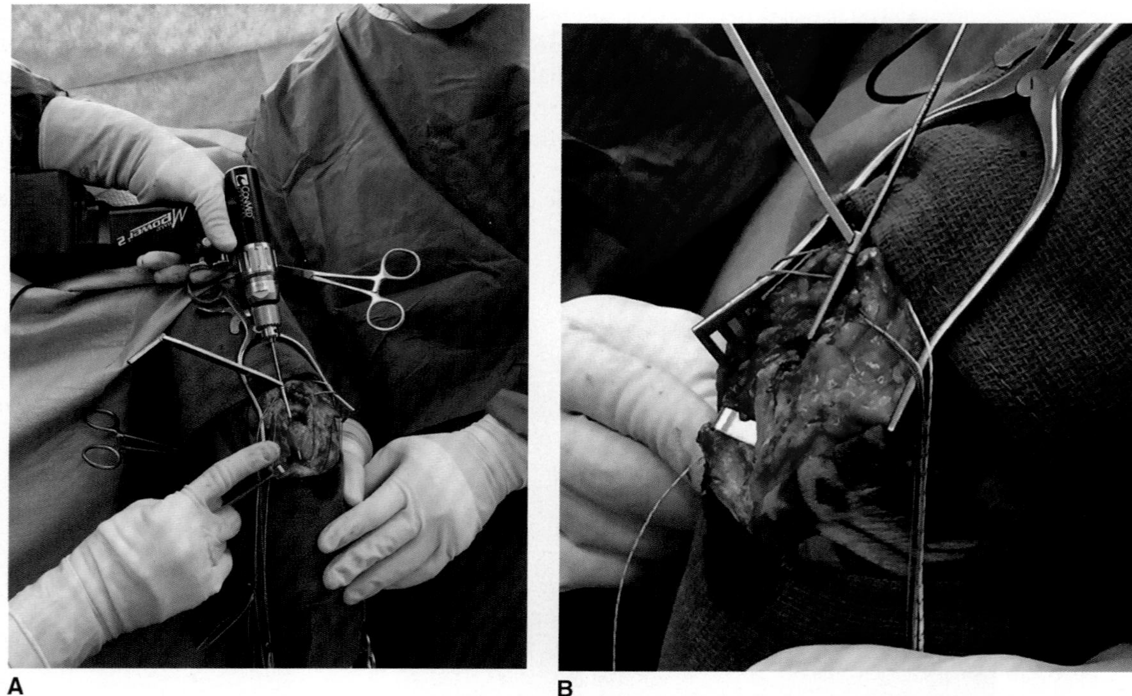

Figure 29-8 | A and B. Two views of the transosseous longitudinal tunnels that are started at the proximal margin of the footprint ~12 mm distal to the tip of the olecranon. The drill should be angled ~45 degrees in the sagittal plane from the longitudinal axis of the ulna, away from the sigmoid notch to avoid penetration of the articular surface.

- This step is repeated for the 3 lateral suture limbs through the lateral 2-mm ulnar drill tunnel.
- The sutures are all held firmly while the elbow is gently cycled to begin the process of compressing the tendon to the olecranon footprint.

- The footprint compression construct is now created.
  - One suture tail from the medial Krackow stitch and one tail from the lateral Krackow stitch are passed through the loop of the lateral looped suture (Fig. 29-9).

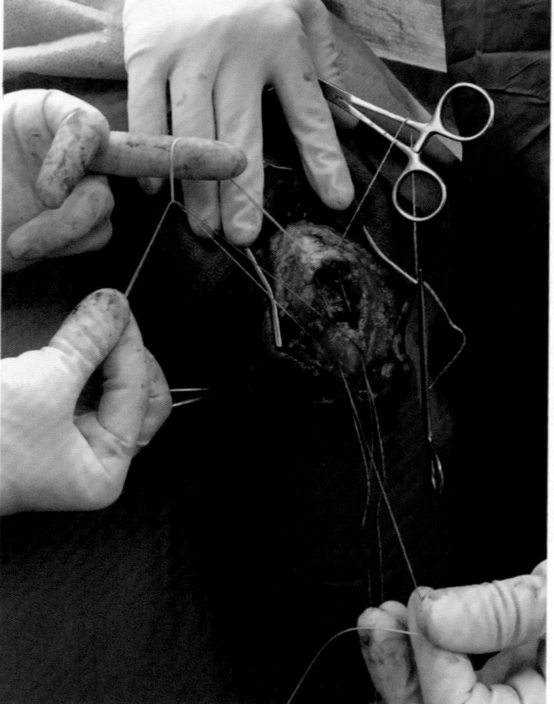

Figure 29-9 | One medial and one lateral Krakow stitch is passed through the medial looped suture proximal to the repair site. This is repeated on the lateral side.

- The looped suture is pulled distally, thereby shuttling the sutures back through the tendon and the lateral longitudinal drill tunnel.
- This step is repeated on the medial side with the remaining limb of each Krackow suture passed through the medial looped suture.
  - The medial looped suture is pulled distally, shuttling these sutures through the tendon and the medial longitudinal tunnel.
- The sutures are now in a "box-and-x" configuration to promote compression of the tendon and olecranon footprints[6] (Fig. 29-10).

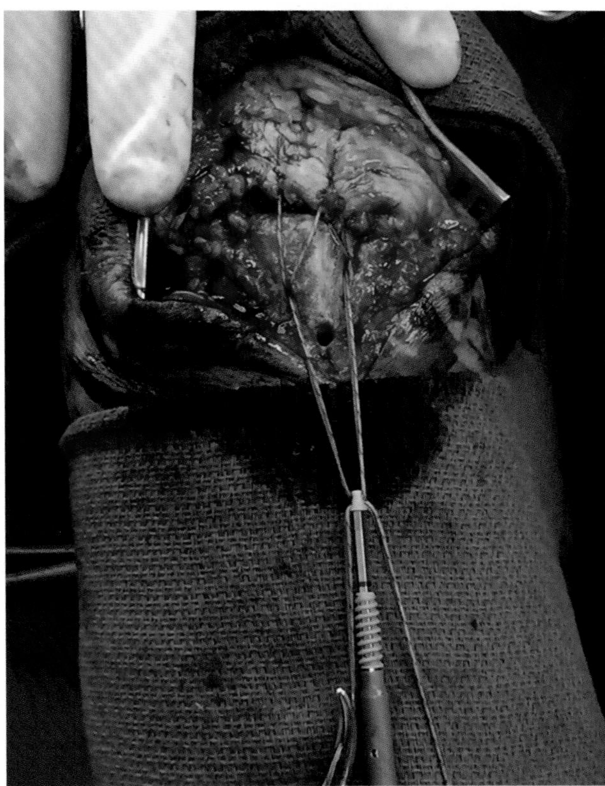

Figure 29-10 | Passage of the looped sutures distally results in the "box-and-x" configuration over the tendon footprint as the anchor is loaded and placed.

- The sutures are once again all held firmly while the elbow is gently moved through a range of motion to further facilitate tendon-to-olecranon compression.

- All four suture limbs are passed through the eyelet of the knotless suture anchor.
  - To decrease bunching, we recommend passing the two medial sutures from medial to lateral and the two lateral sutures from lateral to medial.
- The anchor is docked within the previously drilled and tapped hole, and the sutures are tensioned a final time to maximize compression.
- The elbow is gently moved through a range of motion, and the sutures are retensioned to ensure that no slack remains.
- The anchor is screwed into the olecranon with tension being held until the anchor is flush with the posterior ulnar cortex.
- The remaining excess suture limbs are cut flush with the cortex (Fig. 29-11).
- The periosteal flaps are approximated over the ulna.
- Any intact paratenon is closed over the triceps tendon and the repair site.
- Routine subcutaneous tissue and skin closures are then carried out.

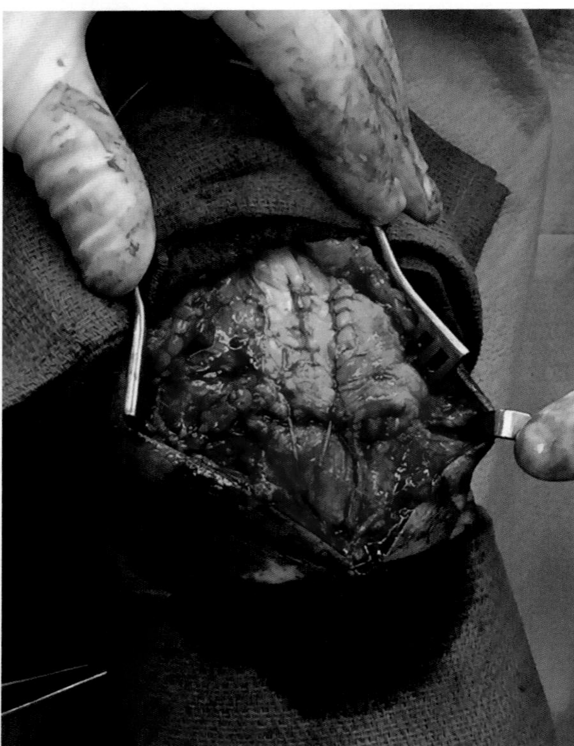

Figure 29-11 | The knotless anchor with all 4 Krackow suture limbs is inserted flush with the posterior ulnar cortex and the excess suture limbs are cut flush with the cortex, completing the repair.

Postoperative Protocol

- A posterior plaster, long arm splint with the elbow in 60 degrees of flexion and the forearm neutral, including the wrist, is applied and maintained for 10-14 days.
- Sutures are removed, and a hinged elbow brace is applied.
- Passive range of motion is initiated from full extension to 90 degrees of flexion. Motion is increased by 10 degrees/week until full elbow range of motion is obtained.
- During this time, leg, core, and cardio training may be initiated.
- Active range of motion begins at 8 weeks.
- Strengthening begins at 12 weeks.
- Return to sport- or work-related activities may require up to 4-6 months of rehabilitation.[10]

References

1. van Riet RP, Morrey BF, Ho E, et al. Surgical treatment of distal triceps ruptures. *J Bone Joint Surg Am.* 2003;85:1961-1967.
2. Bava ED, Barber FA, Lund ER. Clinical outcome after suture anchor repair of complete traumatic rupture of the distal triceps tendon. *Arthroscopy.* 2012;28:1058-1063.
3. Viegas SF. Avulsion of the triceps tendon. *Orthop Rev.* 1990;19:533-536.
4. Tsourvakas S, Gouvalas K, Gimtsas C, et al. Bilateral and simultaneous rupture of the triceps tendons in chronic renal failure and secondary hyperparathyroidism. *Arch Orthop Trauma Surg.* 2004;124:278-280.
5. Yeh PC, Stephens KT, Solovyova O, et al. The distal triceps tendon footprint and a biomechanical analysis of 3 repair techniques. *Am J Sports Med.* 2010;38:1025-1033.
6. Paci JM, Clark J, Rizzi A. Distal triceps knotless anatomic footprint repair: a new technique. *Arthrosc Tech.* 2014;3(5):e621-e626.
7. Clark J, Obopilwe E, Rizzi A, et al. Distal triceps knotless anatomic footprint repair is superior to transosseous cruciate repair: a biomechanical comparison. *Arthroscopy.* 2014;30:1254-1260.
8. O'Donnell KO, Ciccotti MG. In: Arciero RA, Cordasco FA, Provencher MT, eds. *Triceps Tendon Injury Shoulder and Elbow Injuries in Athletes: Prevention, Treatment, and Return to Play.* Philadelphia, PA: Elsevier; 2018:485-492.
9. Stucken C, Ciccotti MG. Distal biceps and triceps injuries in athletes. *Sports Med Arthrosc Rev.* 2014;22(3):153-163.
10. Finstein J, Cohen SC, DeLuca PF, et al. Triceps ruptures requiring surgical repair in national football players. *Orthop J Sports Med.* 2015;3(8):1-5.

Chapter 30
Principles of Hip Arthroscopy

JAMES B. COWAN
MARC R. SAFRAN

Preoperative Preparation

- Thromboembolic deterrent (TED) stockings are placed on both lower extremities 2 in below the level of the fibular head to avoid compression of the peroneal nerve.
- Hair on the operative extremity is trimmed medially to 1 in medial to the anterior superior iliac spine (ASIS), posterolaterally to the midbuttock, proximally to 2 in proximal to the inguinal crease and distally to 6-8 in distal to the inguinal crease.
- All preoperative imaging studies (XR, CT, and/or MRI) should be available for viewing in the OR.

Anesthesia

- Before surgery, the anesthesia plan is discussed with the appropriate anesthesia provider.
- Endotracheal intubation rather than a laryngeal mask airway is recommended.
- Muscular paralysis is induced.
- The goal is systolic blood pressure of ~100 mm Hg.

Patient Positioning, Fluoroscopy, Traction, and Draping

- Hip arthroscopy can be done with the patient in a supine or lateral position. We prefer supine positioning using a commercially available fracture table or table extension to provide traction.
- On the contralateral (non-operative) extremity, large pads are placed on the heel and dorsal and plantar aspects of the foot. On the operative extremity, a single pad is placed on the dorsal foot, and the foot and ankle are wrapped with self-adherent (Coban, 3M, St. Paul, MN) wrap to prevent slippage in the boot.
- Both feet are placed in the traction boots so that the heels are all the way down in the boot. The boot is closed as tightly as possible and secured with cloth tape.
- The patient is positioned so the operative extremity is against a well padded perineal post and then distally, so that the perineum abuts the post as well.
- The nonoperative extremity is abducted to 45 to 60 degrees and the operative extremity to 10 degrees. Both extremities should be placed in neutral rotation (patella facing ceiling) and alignment in the sagittal plane (no flexion or extension). Some surgeons prefer 15-20 degrees of internal rotation to place the femoral neck parallel to the ground and 10-20 degrees of hip flexion (Fig. 30-1).
- A clear nonsterile U-drape is placed from inferior to superior, on the far side of the umbilicus, medial to the ASIS, and as far posteriorly along the buttock as possible, and a clear nonsterile sheet is placed transversely at the level of the umbilicus.

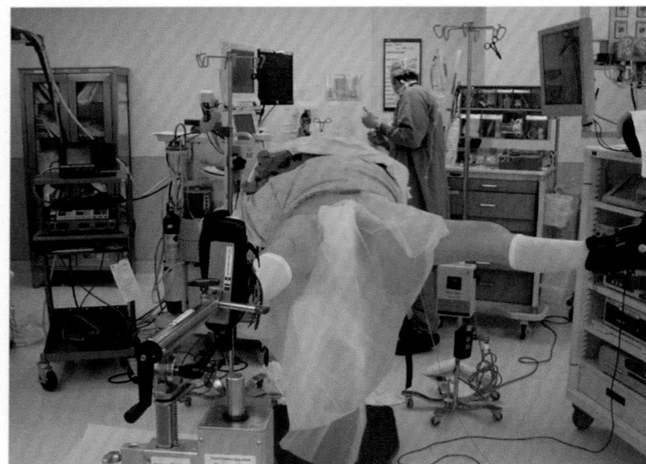

Figure 30-1 | Patient positioned supine for right hip arthroscopy. Note the perineal post is lateralized toward the operative hip. The operative hip is positioned in 10 degrees of abduction, as well as neutral rotation and neutral flexion/extension. The nonoperative hip is abducted 45-60 degrees to allow the fluoroscopic monitor to be positioned to assist with the surgery.

- The fluoroscopy machine should come between the patient's legs.
- Traction with just body weight is placed on the nonoperative extremity to help lateralize the operative extremity. Gross traction is placed on the operative extremity, followed by fine traction to subluxate the hip (usually10 to 50 lb of traction for 8-10 mm of hip joint distraction).

Approach and Arthroscopic Portals

- The anatomic structures are not outlined and no arthroscopic portals are made until traction is applied (Fig. 30-2).

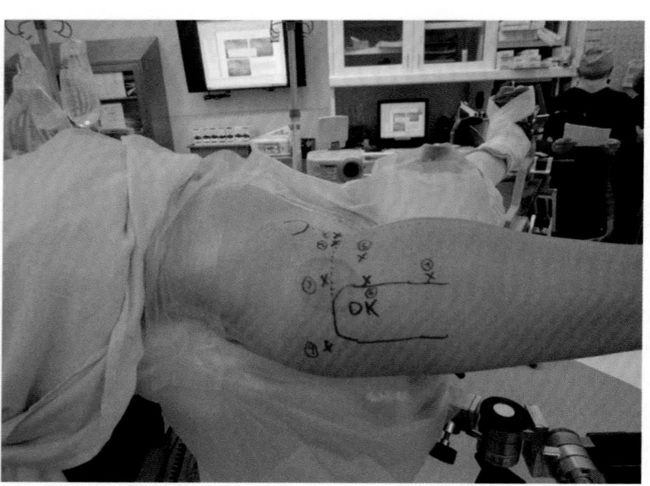

Figure 30-2 | Right hip with surgical marker outlining the greater trochanter, ASIS, and *#1* intersection of line going distal from ASIS and line going transverse at the tip of the greater trochanter, *#2* anterior portal, *#3* anterolateral portal, *#4* posterolateral portal, *#5* modified anterior or mid-anterior portal, *#6* distal anterolateral portal, and *#7* distal portal for endoscopic iliopsoas lengthening at the lesser trochanter.

- With standard sterile technique, an 18-gauge spinal needle is inserted at the site of the anterolateral portal (see below). The spinal needle should enter the hip joint between the femoral head and labrum (with the bevel facing away from the femoral head and the shaft adjacent to the femoral head) with a trajectory slightly convergent with the femoral neck and aiming toward the superior cotyloid fossa and medial sourcil (Fig. 30-3A).
- Once the spinal needle tip is intra-articular, the stylet is removed to eliminate the negative intra-articular pressure. Upon removal of the stylet, the quadriceps muscle will relax, indicating capsular and proprioceptive mechanoreceptor relaxation. Fluoroscopy should confirm intra-articular access with an air arthrogram (Fig. 30-3B).

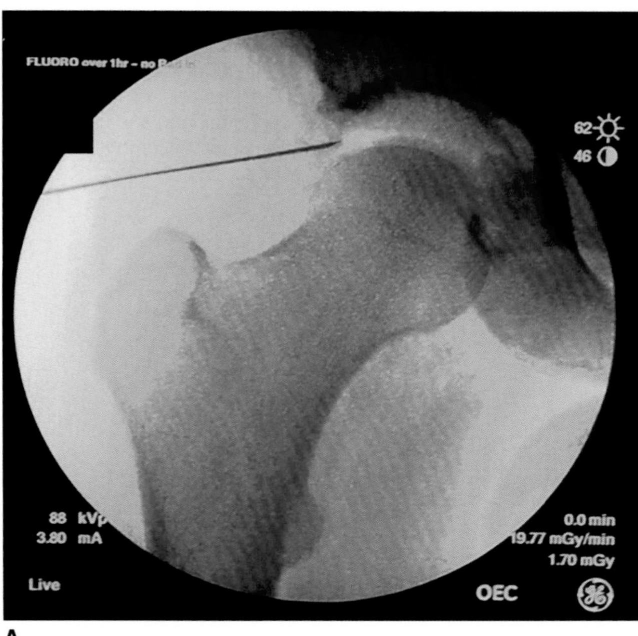

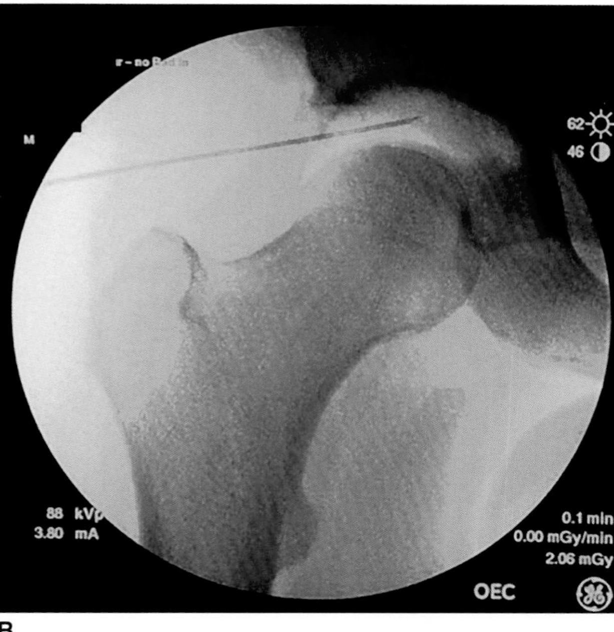

A **B**

Figure 30-3 | A. Fluoroscopic image of 18-gauge spinal needle entering at the site of the anterolateral portal with a trajectory slightly convergent with the femoral neck and aiming toward the superior cotyloid fossa and medial sourcil. **B.** Fluoroscopic image following spinal needle stylet removal showing air arthrogram that confirms intra-articular access has been achieved with the spinal needle.

- The amount of traction necessary is recorded, and then, traction is released for preparation and draping to reduce unnecessary traction time. After traction is released, an additional fluoroscopic image is taken to confirm that the hip is fully reduced or if there is residual subluxation.
- The operative field is prepared and draped according to the surgeon's preference, taking care to ensure that a wide surgical field is maintained from medial to the ASIS to the midbuttock laterally and from just distal to the umbilicus to the distal thigh (Fig. 30-4).

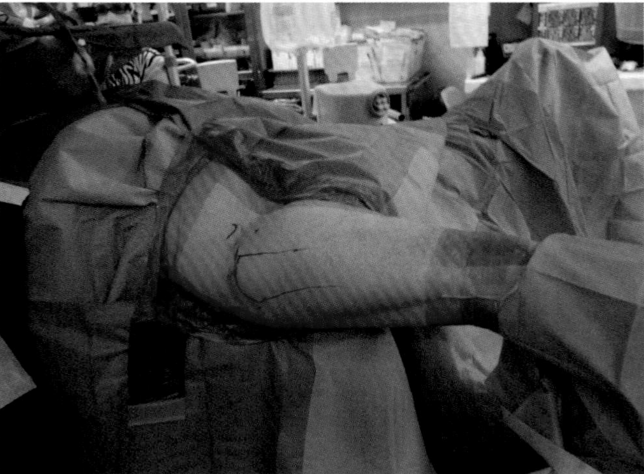

Figure 30-4 | Sterile draping of operative field for right hip arthroscopy.

Anterolateral Portal

- Location: 1-2 cm proximal and anterior to the tip of the greater trochanter. Trajectory for spinal needle localization is ~15 degrees cephalad and 20-30 degrees posteriorly.
- Uses: central compartment viewing (particularly anteriorly and superiorly) and working (eg, debridement, anchor placement), peripheral compartment viewing and working (Fig. 30-5)
- Risks: iatrogenic chondral and/or labral injury, superior gluteal nerve injury

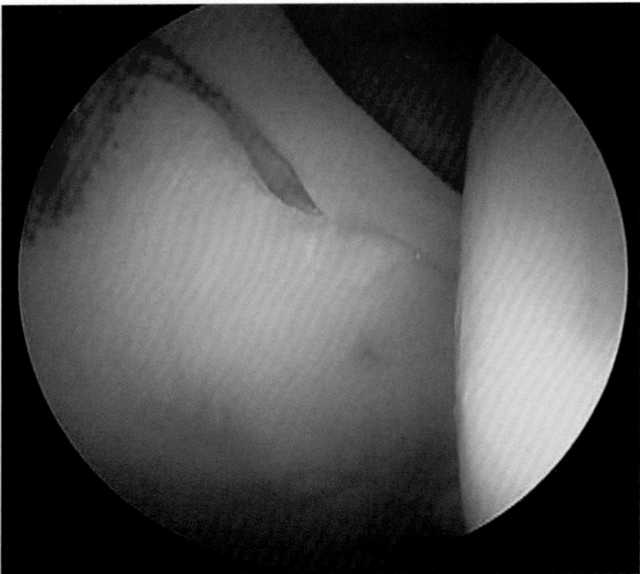

Figure 30-5 | Arthroscopic image with a 70-degree arthroscope through the anterolateral portal showing the anterosuperior labrum on the left, the femoral head on the right, and capsule straight up, between the femoral head and labrum (V shaped).

Anterior Portal

- Location: 1-2 cm lateral to intersection of line going distal from ASIS and line going transverse at the tip of the greater trochanter. Trajectory for spinal needle localization is ~40-45 degrees cephalad and 25-30 toward the midline.
- Uses: central compartment viewing and working (labral takedown, retraction, and debridement) (Fig. 30-6)
- Risks: lateral femoral cutaneous nerve injury (a knife is used to cut skin only and not deeper)

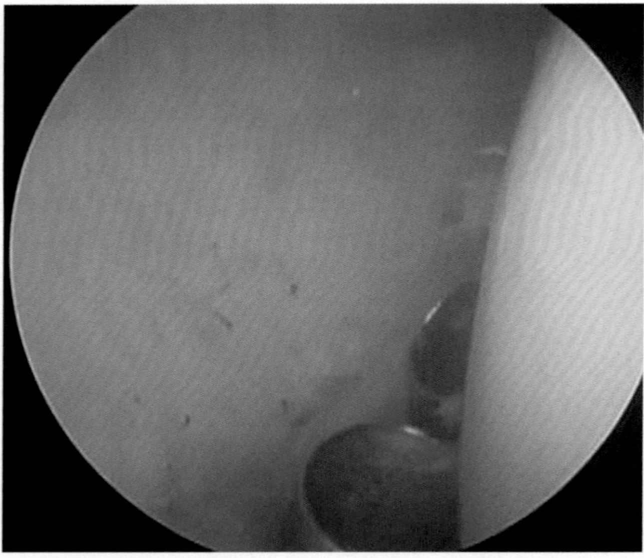

Figure 30-6 | Arthroscopic image with a 70-degree arthroscope through the anterior portal looking posteriorly showing the acetabular cartilage and labrum on the left, the femoral head on the right, and the anterolateral and posterolateral cannulas.

Modified/Mid-Anterior Portal

- Location: 4-6 cm anterior and distal to anterolateral portal. Trajectory for spinal needle localization is ~30 degrees posterior and 30 degrees superior.
- Uses: central compartment viewing and working (labral takedown and debridement), anchor placement (especially anterior and anterolateral acetabulum)

Distal Anterolateral Portal

- Location: 3-5 cm distal to anterolateral portal
- Uses: anchor placement (especially lateral and posterolateral acetabulum), peripheral compartment work

Proximal Anterolateral Portal

- Location: 3-4 cm proximal and slightly posterior to anterolateral portal
- Uses: peripheral compartment work

Posterolateral Portal

- Location: 1 cm posterior to the superior-posterior tip of the greater trochanter
- Uses: central compartment viewing, posterior labral repair (Fig. 30-7)
- Risks: sciatic nerve injury (portal is placed with hip in neutral rotation), deep branch of medial femoral circumflex artery injury

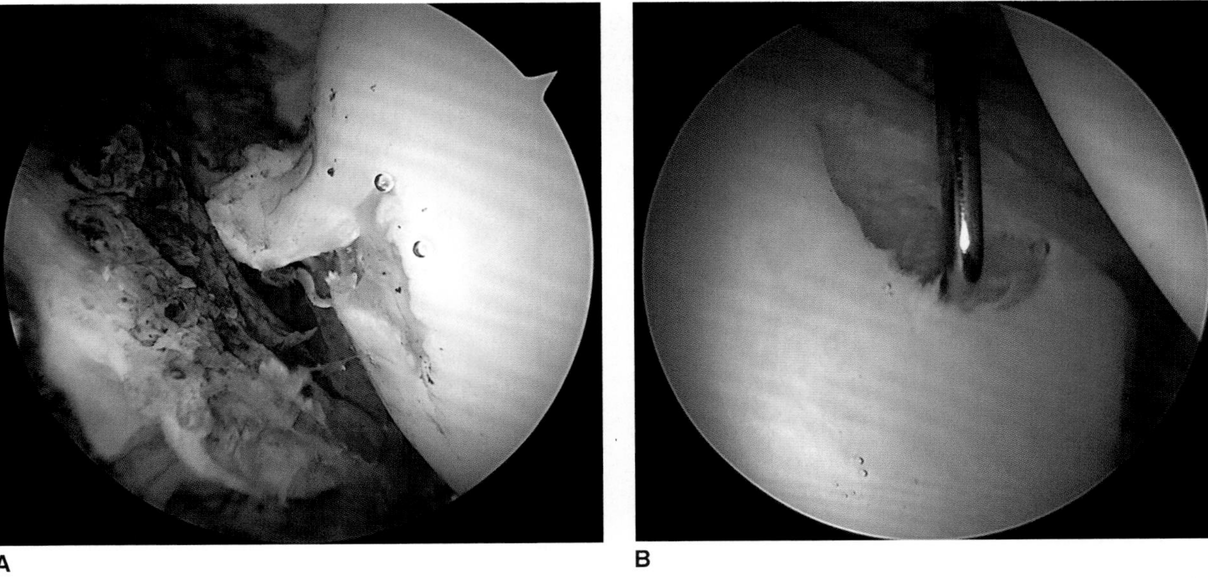

Figure 30-7 | **A.** Arthroscopic image with a 70-degree arthroscope through the posterolateral portal showing the cotyloid fossa on the left and the femoral head with chondral flap on the right. **B.** Arthroscopic image with a 70-degree arthroscope through the posterolateral portal showing the arthroscopic probe entering the mid-anterior portal, an acetabular articular cartilage defect on the left with the intact labrum above it, and the femoral head on the right.

Indications for Hip Arthroscopy

- Femoroacetabular impingement (pincer, cam, subspine, ischiofemoral, combined type)
- Labral pathology
- Chondral pathology
- Ligamentum teres injuries
- Iliopsoas pathology
- Hip instability or capsular laxity or insufficiency
- Snapping hip (internal or external)
- Loose bodies or heterotopic ossification
- Synovial disorders
- Septic arthritis
- Gluteus medius and/or minimus repair
- Peritrochanteric conditions

- Proximal hamstring repair
- Expanding indications
  - Acetabular rim fractures
  - Femoral head fractures
  - In conjunction with treatment of osteonecrosis
  - Sciatic nerve endoscopy/deep gluteal space

Diagnostic Arthroscopy

- Femoral head and acetabular articular cartilage
- Labrum
- Ligamentum teres/cotyloid fossa
- Capsule

Postoperative Protocols

- 20 lb foot flat weight bearing with crutches is allowed for 2 weeks after chielectomy/femoral head osteoplasty. An additional week is used per decade for women over 39 years of age, and men over 49 years of age. An abduction brace is used if there is a concomitant labral repair and/or capsular plication. Crutches are used for 6 weeks if microfracture was done.
- Naproxen 500 mg PO bid is given for 4 weeks for heterotopic ossification prophylaxis (as well as for pain control and to reduce the risk of deep venous thrombosis).

Chapter 31
Arthroscopic Hip Labral Repair

MARC J. PHILIPPON
IOANNA K. BOLIA
KAREN K. BRIGGS

The greatly increased prevalence of hip injuries over the past 15 years is mainly due to the improved description and diagnosis of femoroacetabular impingement (FAI), which is the most common indication for hip arthroscopy today. The damage caused by FAI includes chondrolabral dysfunction, where impingement causes damage to the labrum and the adjacent cartilage (Fig. 31-1). Treatment of labral tears has evolved since early in the decade, and extensive research has been done on the advantages of labral repair over labral debridement.

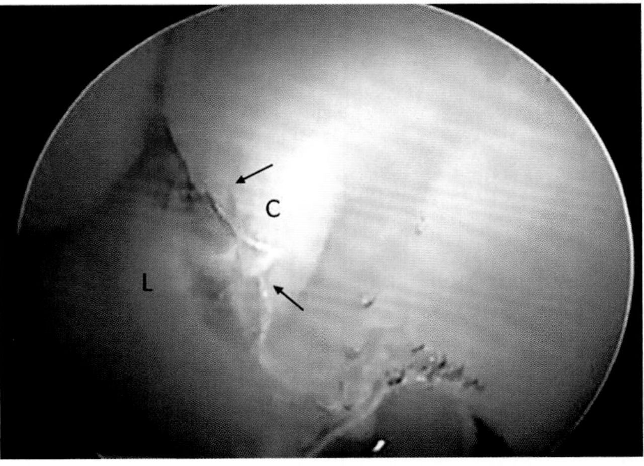

Figure 31-1 | A labral tear involving the chondrolabral junction. The cartilage has separated from the labrum and the acetabulum (*arrows*). L, labrum; C, cartilage.

The acetabular labrum is a dense, fibrocartilage connective tissue ring attached to the bony rim of the acetabulum, which deepens the acetabulum and extends the coverage of the femoral head.[1] The labrum has been shown to enhance hip stability and also provides a fluid seal with the femoral neck.[2,3] Anatomical, biomechanical, and outcomes studies have led to arthroscopic labral repair being the preferred treatment of labral tears in selected patients (Table 31-1).

Table 31-1 | Tips for patient selection for hip arthroscopy

- Positive physical examination indicating hip pathology
- Well-defined pathology on MRI and radiographs
- Outcome score not too low
- Patient willing to comply with rehabilitation
- Good presurgical muscle strength
- Condition (BMI)

Diagnosis and Preoperative Planning

- The patient should be evaluated to determine duration and type of symptoms, history of trauma, prior surgeries, level of physical activity, impact of the injury on the patient's quality of life, patient's knowledge of his or her condition, and the patient's expectation of treatment.[4]
- Specific tests included in the clinical examination include the following:
  - Anterior and posterior impingement test
  - FABER (Flexion, ABduction, and External Rotation) distance test
  - Dial test
  - Trendelenburg test
  - Dynamic motion evaluation to recreate symptoms
    - The most common complaint of patients with labral pathology resulting in hip dysfunction is anterior groin pain exacerbated by hip flexion.
- **Additional testing includes the following:**
  - Gait analysis
  - Muscle strength testing
  - Range-of-motion measurement
  - Maneuvers to rule out distracting pathology such as athletic pubalgia and lumbar radiculopathy
- **Radiographic evaluation**
  - Identify cam, pincer, or mixed-type FAI
  - High-quality supine AP pelvic radiograph to measure joint space, acetabular version, lateral center edge angle, and weight-bearing surface angle (Fig. 31-2)

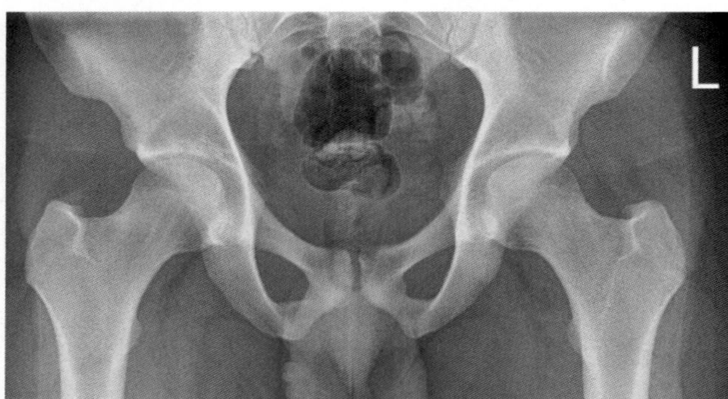

Figure 31-2 | High-quality supine AP pelvic radiograph to measure joint space, acetabular version, lateral center-edge angle, and weight-bearing surface angle.

  - Dunn view to measure the alpha angle to assess the offset of the anterior femoral head-neck junction for a CAM lesion (Fig. 31-3)

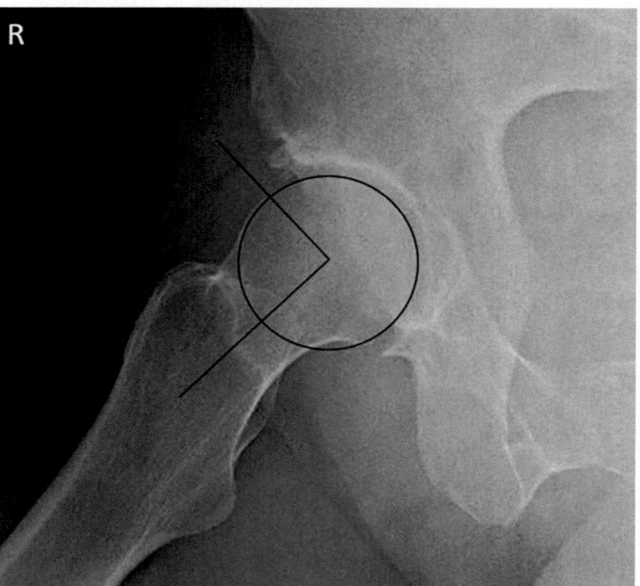

Figure 31-3 | Dunn view to measure the alpha angle to assess the offset of the anterior femoral head-neck junction for a CAM lesion.

- 3T noncontrast MRI to evaluate the quality of the labral tissue and chondral surfaces, rule out concomitant intra- and extra-articular impingement lesions and pathology, and identify periarticular muscle pathology around the hip (Fig. 31-4)

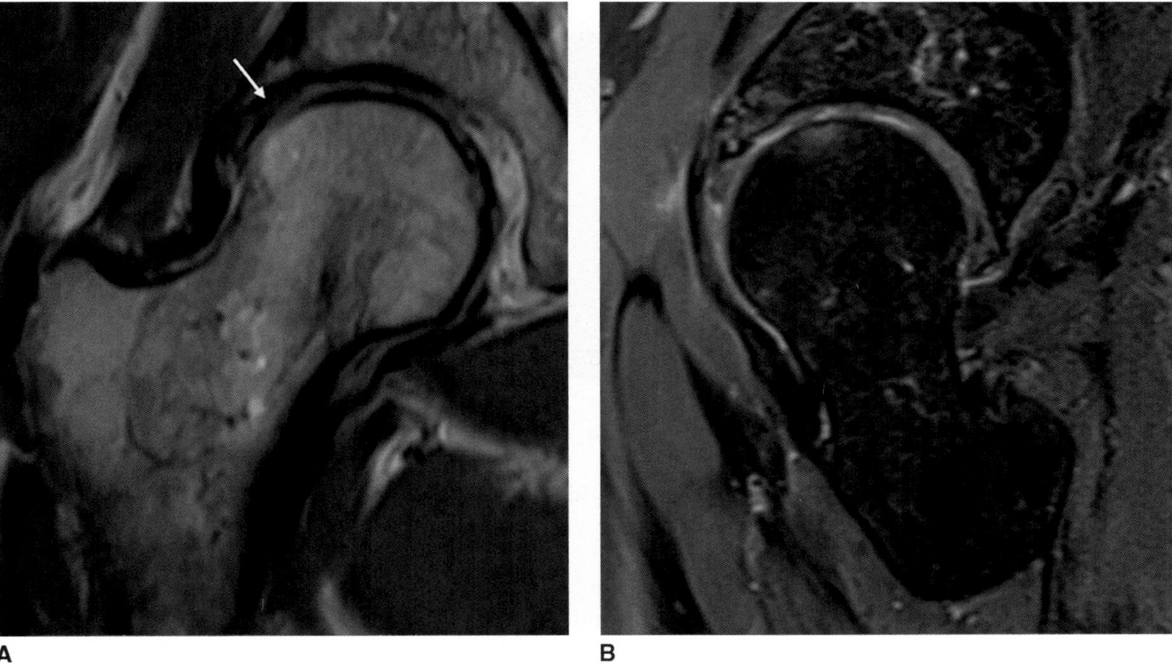

Figure 31-4 | 3T noncontrast MRI evaluating the quality of labral tissue on the coronal plane **(A)** and the articular cartilage on the oblique-sagittal plane where the alpha angle can also be measured **(B)**. The *arrow* indicates a labral tear at 12 o'clock on the acetabular rim.

- **Relative contraindications for arthroscopic labral repair**
  - Joint space narrowing
  - Low center-edge angle (<20 degrees)
  - Advanced osteoarthritic changes
  - High body mass index (BMI)
  - Femoral neck-shaft angle of more than 140 degrees

Surgical Technique

- The patient is placed in a modified supine position.
- Conscious anesthesia in combination with spinal-epidural injection is used.
- Distraction is applied to the hip using a fracture table and ~50 lb of traction. The amount of traction is dependent on achieving 10 mm of joint distraction (Fig. 31-5).

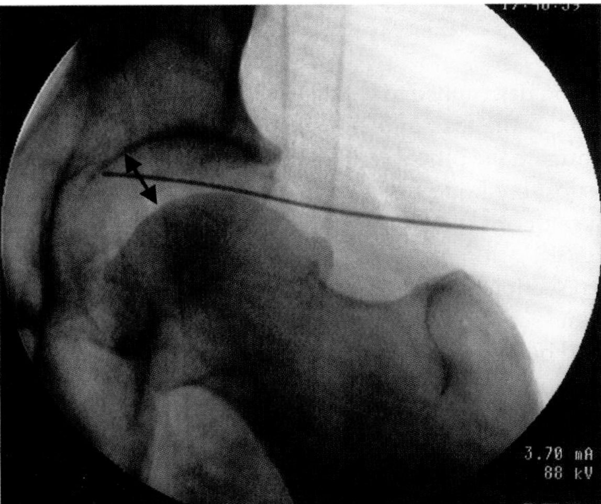

Figure 31-5 | Distraction is applied to the hip using a fracture table and ~50 lb of traction. The amount of traction is dependent on achieving 10 mm (*arrow*) of joint distraction.

- Two portals are used: a mid-anterior (MA) portal and an anterolateral (AL) portal (Fig. 31-6).
  - The AL portal is established first, and the arthroscope is used to identify the anterior triangle, and the MA portal is established.
  - The MA portal is used as the primary viewing portal.

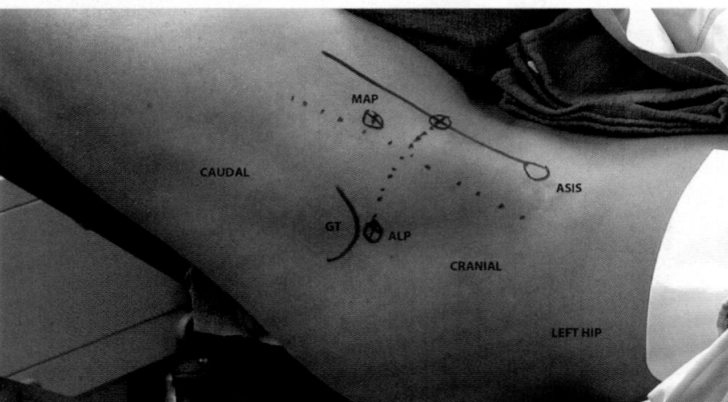

Figure 31-6 | The two portals used: a mid-anterior (MA) portal and an anterolateral (AL) portal. ALP, anterolateral portal; ASIS, anterior superior iliac spine; GT, greater trochanter; MAP, mid-anterior portal.

- A capsulotomy parallel to the labrum is made ~12 mm from the labral tip, most often connecting the MA and AL portals.
- A diagnostic arthroscopy is done to identify pathology of the labrum, cartilage, ligamentum teres, capsule, and bone abnormalities.
- Landmarks are identified.
  - The superior extent of the anterior labral sulcus (psoas-u) is the most consistent landmark of the acetabulum. It is situated in the antero-superior hemisphere of the acetabulum and is a reliable landmark for the 3:00 position on the face of the acetabulum for orientation and description of pathology (Fig. 31-7).

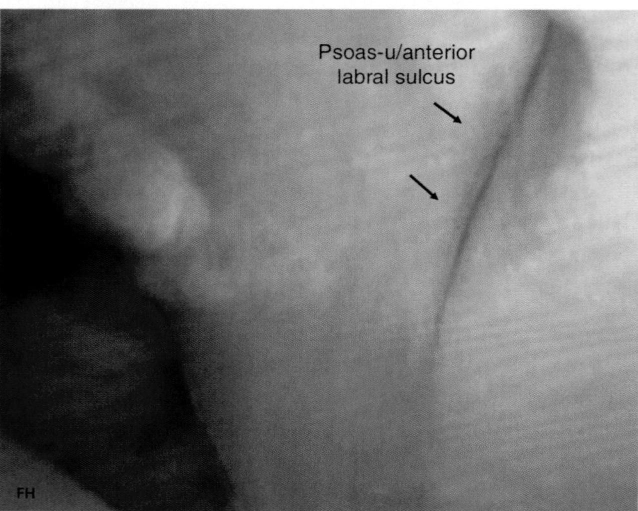

Figure 31-7 | Anterior labral sulcus (psoas-u) is the most consistent landmark of the acetabulum. It is situated in the antero-superior hemisphere of the acetabulum and is a reliable landmark for the 3:00 position on the face of the acetabulum for orientation and description of pathology.

- Once the tear is identified and determined to be suitable for repair, the rim of the acetabulum is prepared.
  - The rim is exposed next to the tear, and an acetabuloplasty is performed with a curved 4.5-mm burr to completely eliminate the pincer lesion (Fig. 31-8).
  - When needed, focal subspine bone resection is performed to decompress the area between the acetabular rim and the anterior inferior iliac spine (ASIS). Care must be taken to protect the tendons attaching to the ASIS.
  - The amount of bone resection should be guided by the preoperative center-edge angle and the depth of the acetabulum.[5]
    - Rim trimming should be limited to avoid creating undercoverage, which carries the risk of postoperative dislocation.
    - If no pincer impingement is present or the patient has a low center-edge angle, the bony rim should just be "roughed up" enough to create a healing bed.
  - The cartilage near the rim trimming should be stabilized (Fig. 31-9).

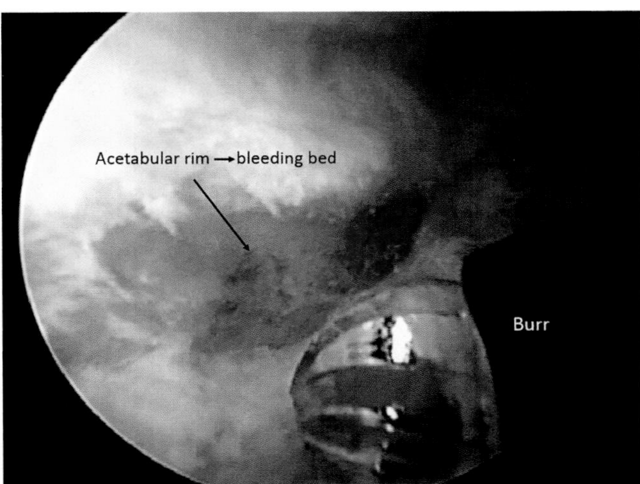

Figure 31-8 | The rim is exposed next to the tear, and an acetabuloplasty is performed with a curved 4.5-mm burr to completely eliminate the pincer lesion.

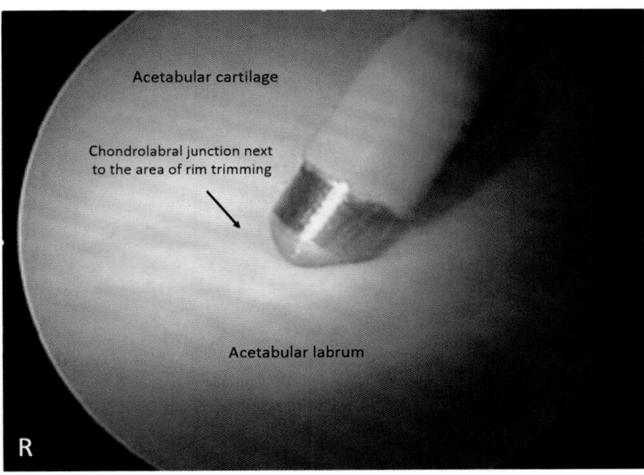

Figure 31-9 | The cartilage near the rim trimming should be stabilized.

- For a labral repair, the size of the anchor is based on the anatomic location.
  - For tears involving the 12 o'clock position, a 2.3-mm anchor and a loop stitch are used.
  - For 1-2 o'clock, a 2.3-mm anchor and a loop stitch are used.
  - At the 3 o'clock position, a 1.7-mm anchor is used with a through stitch, if enough labral tissue is present, or a loop stitch.
- Outcomes are not different based on the type of stitch; however, the loop stitch tends to evert the labrum and the through stitch tends to invert the labrum. The stitches should be used in combination to anatomically reduce the labrum to the acetabulum without significant eversion or inversion.
- The labrum must sit properly on the acetabulum to ensure recreation of the seal with the femoral head (Fig. 31-10).

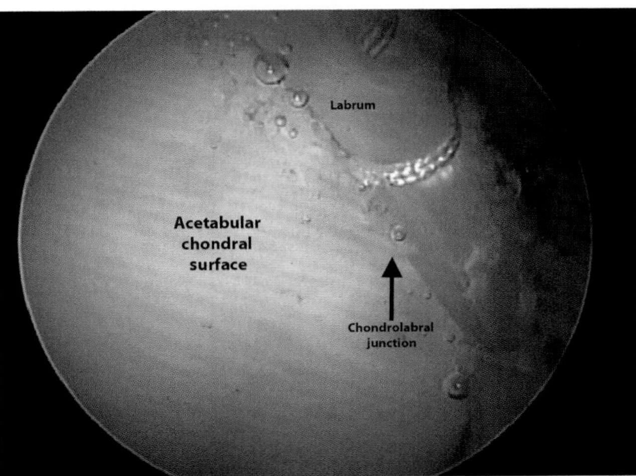

Figure 31-10 | The labrum must sit properly on the acetabulum to ensure recreation of the seal with the femoral head.

- The acetabular rim angle is an anatomic measurement of the safety margin for inserting anchors.[5]
  - To ensure that neither the drill bit nor the anchor penetrate the articular suture, this angle should be considered when placing any anchor around the rim.
    - The angle is formed by two straight lines from the acetabular rim to the subchondral bone margin on one side and the outer cortex on the other side.
    - The larger the angle, the more safety, which reduces the risk of the anchor penetrating the acetabular surface.

- Arthroscopic knots are tied on the capsular side of the labrum and seeded in the anchor hole to avoid the development of post-operative adhesions (Fig. 31-11).

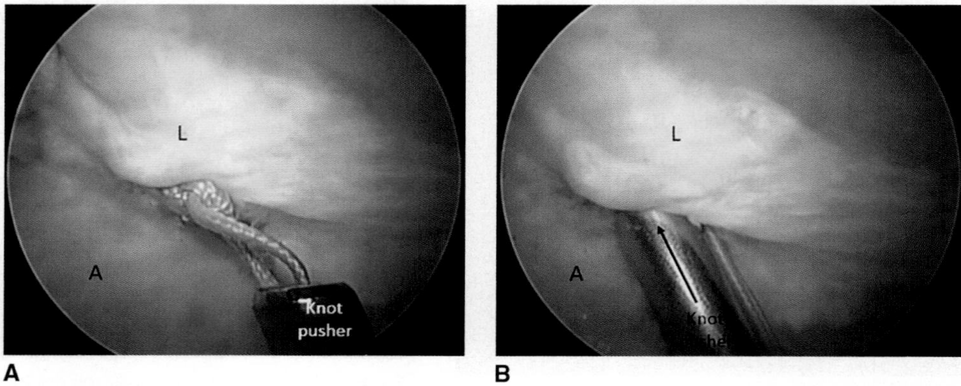

Figure 31-11 | Arthroscopic knots are tied on the capsular side of the labrum **(A)** and seeded in the anchor hole **(B)**. A, acetabulum; L, labrum.

- Anchors are placed ~1.0-1.5 cm apart, depending on the stability of the repair (Video 31-1).
- After all anchors are placed, traction is released and a dynamic examination is performed.
  - The hip is moved through a range of motions, including those identified on preoperative examinations causing symptoms.
- The labral stability and the suction seal are assessed, especially in abduction and flexion (Fig. 31-12). If the labrum is unstable or does not maintain the seal, additional sutures or revision of the sutures must be performed until the labrum is stable and the suction seal is maintained through the range of motion.
- At the end of the case, the capsulotomy is repaired with two absorbable sutures (Vicryl 2.0).

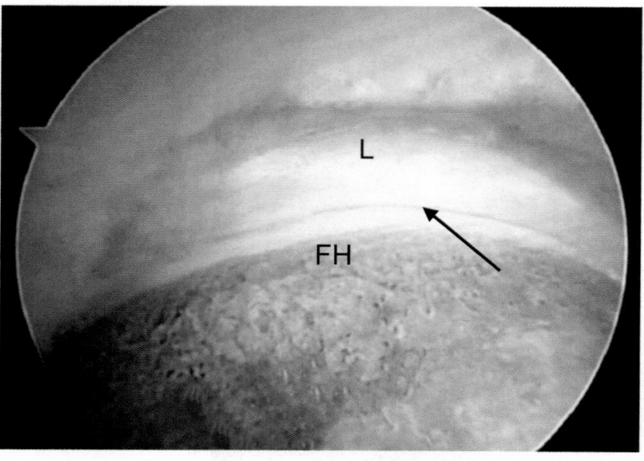

Figure 31-12 | The labral stability and the suction seal (*arrow*) are assessed during the intra-operative dynamic hip examination, especially with the hip flexed and abducted. FH, femoral head; L, labrum.

Rehabilitation

- Postoperatively, patients are limited to 10 kg (20 lb) of flatfoot weight bearing with crutches for 2-3 weeks depending on when they can walk without a limp. If microfracture was done at arthroscopy, this is increased to 6-8 weeks.
- In addition, a continuous passive motion machine, hip abduction brace, and antirotation bolsters are used during the first 2 weeks following the procedure.

- Physical therapy is started immediately, focusing on restoring passive and active motion.
  - The patient is started on a stationary bike, with no resistance, within 4 hours after surgery.
  - Hip circumduction is emphasized to avoid development of adhesions (Fig. 31-13).

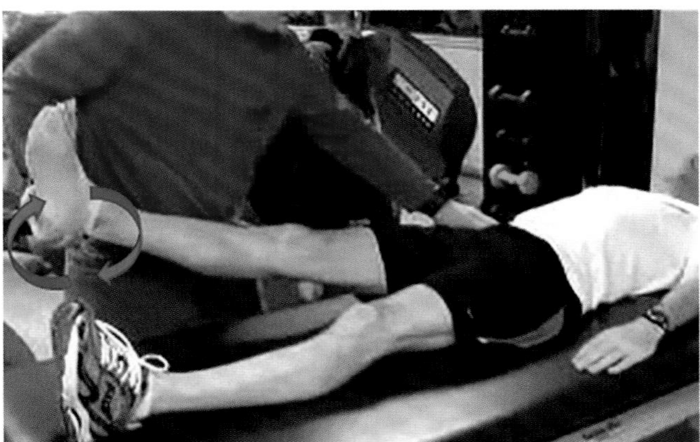

Figure 31-13 | Hip circumduction is emphasized to avoid development of adhesions.

- After range of motion has been re-established and the patient is pain-free, focus is placed on strengthening the muscles around the joint with functional rehabilitation exercises to allow faster return to daily activities or sports.
- The hip sports test (exercise performance evaluation tool) is used in our institution to assess the patient's ability to return to activity after hip arthroscopy.
- The Vail Hip Sport Test is used to determine whether the patient is ready to return to sport-specific training. This test consists of four components that assess patient strength, endurance, and motor control. Patients usually pass the Vail Hip Sport Test between 8 and 12 weeks postoperatively.

References

1. Crawford MJ, Dy CD, Alexander JW, et al. The 2007 Frank Stinchfield Award. The biomechanics of the hip labrum and the stability of the hip. *Clin Orthop Relat Res.* 2007;465:16-22.
2. Nepple JJ, Philippon MJ, Campbell KJ, et al. The hip fluid seal—Part II: the effect of an acetabular labral tear, repair, resection, and reconstruction on hip stability to distraction. *Knee Surg Sports Traumatol Arthrosc.* 2014;22:730-736.
3. Philippon MJ, Nepple JJ, Campbell KJ, et al. The hip fluid seal—Part I: the effect of an acetabular labral tear, repair, resection, and reconstruction on hip fluid pressurization. *Knee Surg Sports Traumatol Arthrosc.* 2014;22:722-729.
4. Philippon MJ, Maxwell RB, Johnston TL, Schenker M, Briggs KK. Clinical presentation of femoroacetabular impingement. *Knee Surg Sports Traumatol Arthrosc.* 2007;15(8):1041-1047.
5. Philippon MJ, Wolff AB, Briggs KK, Zehms CT, Kuppersmith DA. Acetabular rim reduction for the treatment of femoroacetabular impingement correlates with preoperative and postoperative center-edge angle. *Arthroscopy.* 2010;26(6):757-761.

Chapter 32
Arthroscopic Treatment of Femoroacetabular Impingement

J. W. THOMAS BYRD

Understanding and Planning for Treatment of Femoroacetabular Impingement (FAI)

- Distinguishing FAI morphology from FAI pathology
  - FAI may be present as an asymptomatic, incidental finding.[1,2]
- The etiology of pathologic FAI often is multifactorial ("perfect storm").
  - FAI may explain why damage occurs, but how are some individuals lifelong compensators?
  - Numerous factors coming together just wrong lead to joint damage.
  - All factors may never be identified, but enough factors should be treated with both surgical and nonsurgical means to achieve symptomatic improvement.
  - Pelvic orientation influences over- or undercoverage from the anterior acetabulum.[3]
    - This can be significantly influenced by lumbar kyphosis or lordosis.
    - Coverage can be partly altered with a pelvic stabilization program.
  - It is essential to know femoral version.[4]
    - This can be calculated with the addition of images through the femoral condyles with either MRI or CT (Fig. 32-1).

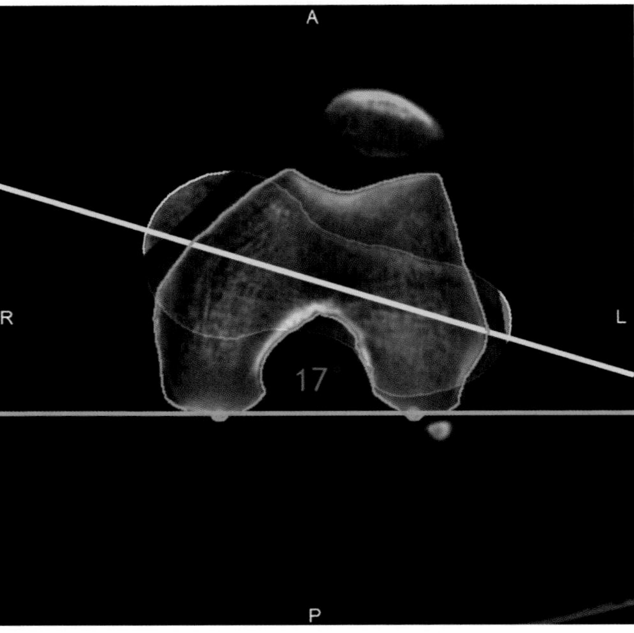

Figure 32-1 Superimposed CT images illustrate determination of the femoral version as the angle formed from a line approximating the axis of the femoral neck and a line across the posterior femoral condyles.

- Increased femoral version may make modest cam lesions tolerable but may also increase concerns of instability.
- Reduced femoral version can make small cam lesions clinically relevant or result in pincer-type labral failure, even in the presence of normal acetabular morphology.

- Radiographs are two-dimensional images attempting to interpret complex three-dimensional anatomy.[5-7]
  - 3-D CT scans are helpful at precisely discerning bony architecture (Fig. 32-2A-C).
    - Lower radiation dose protocols are now equivalent to a five-radiograph hip series.
  - Software systems are available for dynamic analysis discerning areas of bony collision between the acetabulum and proximal femur.[8]

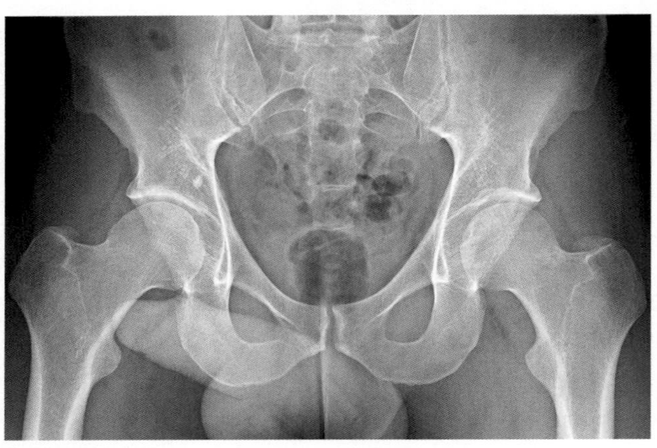

A

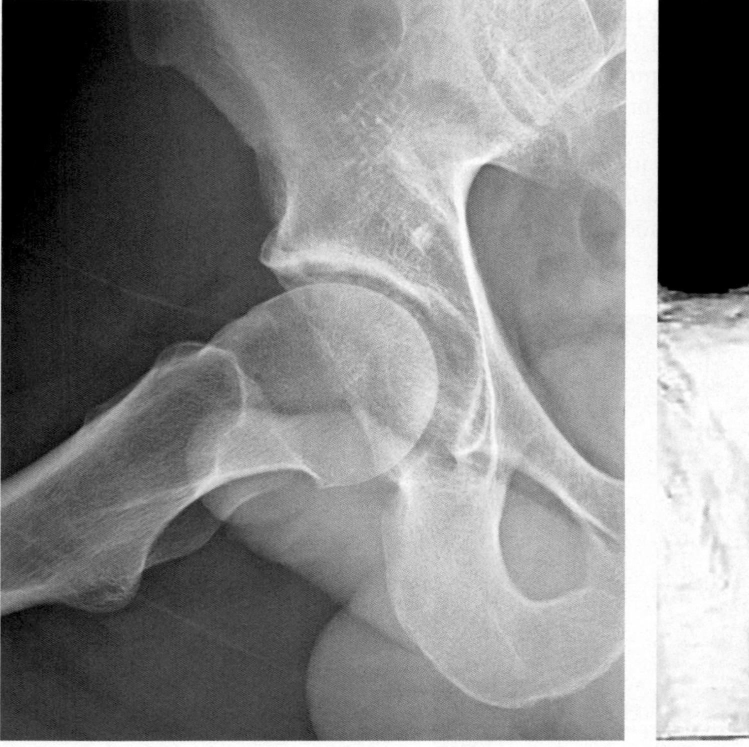

B

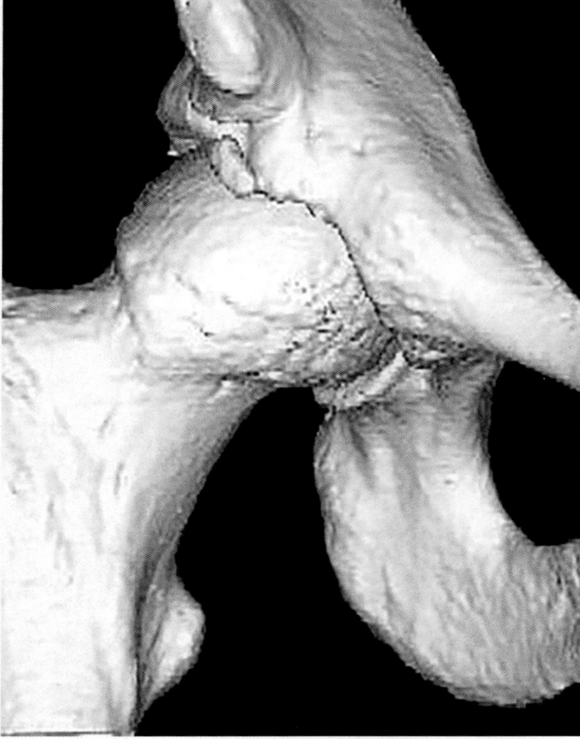

C

Figure 32-2 | AP **(A)** and lateral **(B)** radiographs illustrate the presence of FAI, especially cam type. 3-D CT scan **(C)** more clearly delineates the presence of a pincer lesion with accompanying os acetabulum.

Portal Positions (Fig. 32-3A and B)[9]

- The anterolateral portal is the most consistent workhorse portal for viewing.
  - This portal is used by most surgeons with just slight variations.

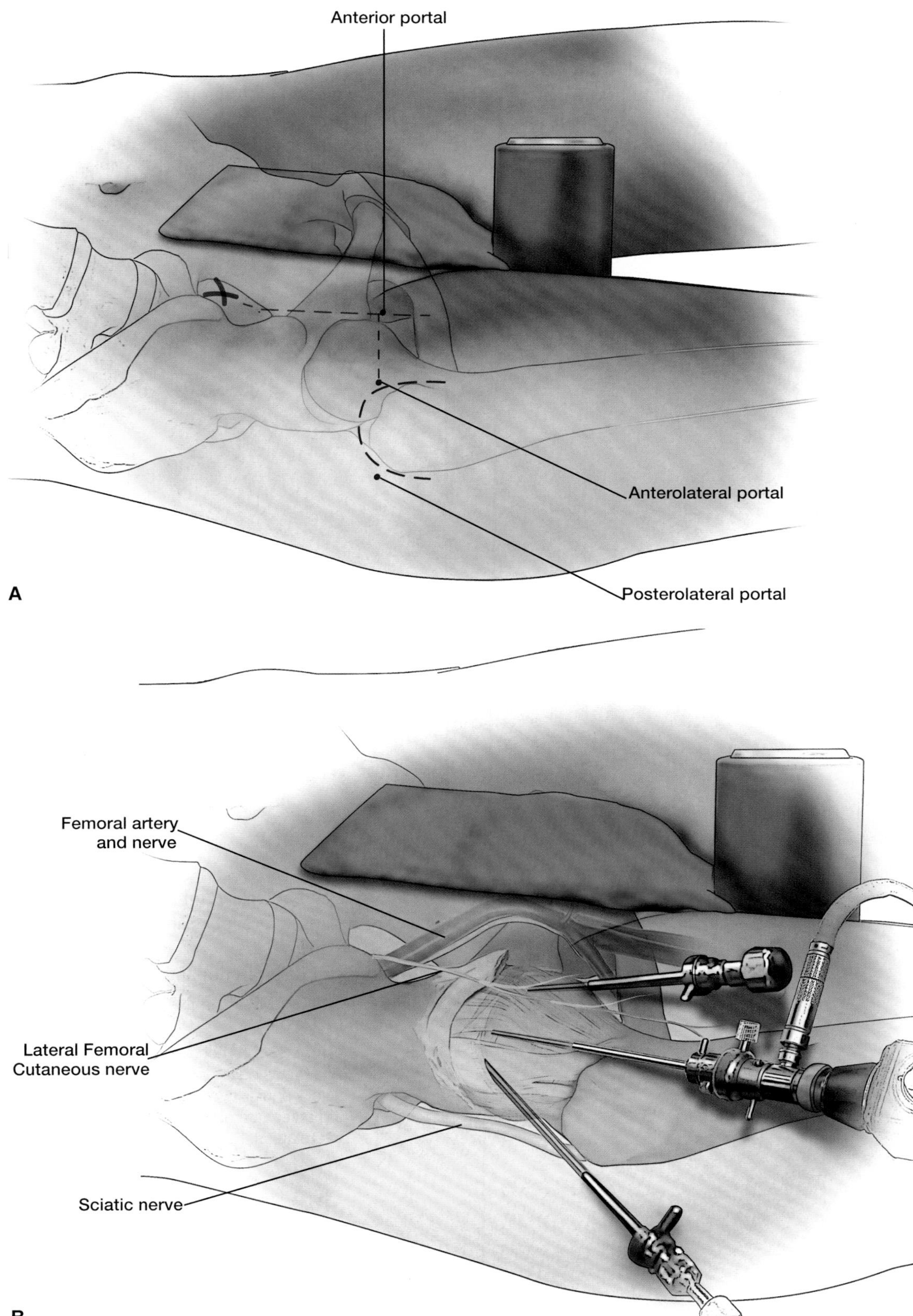

Figure 32-3 | **A.** The anterior portal roughly coincides with the intersection of a sagittal line drawn distally from the anterosuperior iliac spine and a transverse line across the superior margin of the greater trochanter. Generally, it is directed ~45 degrees cephalad and 30 degrees toward the mid-line. Depending on the patient's anatomy, this may be placed slightly more lateral and distal to properly intersect the joint. The anterolateral and posterolateral portals are positioned at the anterior and posterior borders of the trochanteric tip, converging slightly as they enter the joint. **B.** The relationship of the major neurovascular structures to the three standard portals is demonstrated. The femoral artery and nerve lie well medial to the anterior portal. The sciatic nerve lies posterior to the posterolateral portal. Small branches of the lateral femoral cutaneous nerve lie close to the anterior portal. Injury to these is avoided by using proper technique in portal placement. The anterolateral portal is established first because it lies most centrally in the safe zone for arthroscopy.

- The anterior working portal is the most often modified.
  - It often is modified laterally and distally to optimize triangulation within joint.
  - Modifications for anchor placement are not necessary because anchors can be placed percutaneously.
  - An anterior portal often is useful for placement of far-medial anchors, avoiding perforation of the medial pelvic cortex because of a more anterior-to-posterior direction of placement (Fig. 32-4).
    - Avoiding perforation of the acetabulum is of paramount importance.

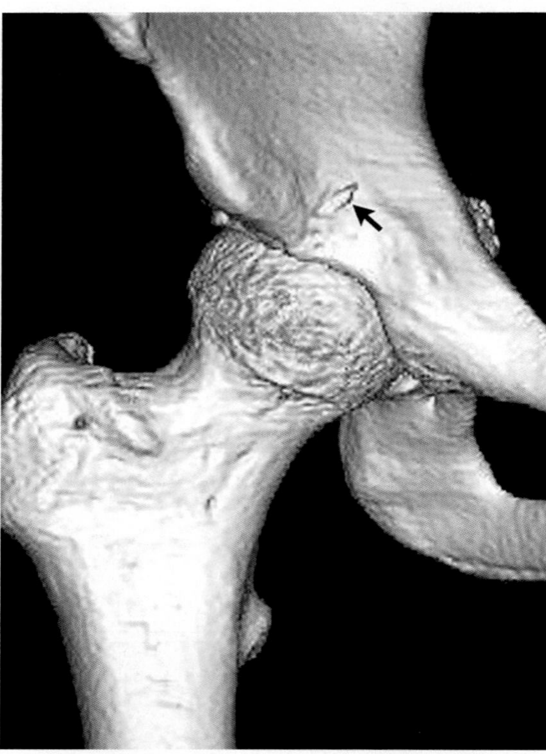

Figure 32-4 | 3-D CT image illustrates an anchor perforating the medial cortex at the psoas groove (*arrow*).

- A percutaneous distal site equidistant between the anterior and anterolateral portals allows more divergence of anchors from the acetabular surface, providing a broader safe zone for placing anchors close to the acetabular rim (Fig. 32-5).[10]
  - Placing anchors away from the rim to avoid perforation can result in nonanatomic approximation of the labrum and is less likely to properly restore a labral seal.

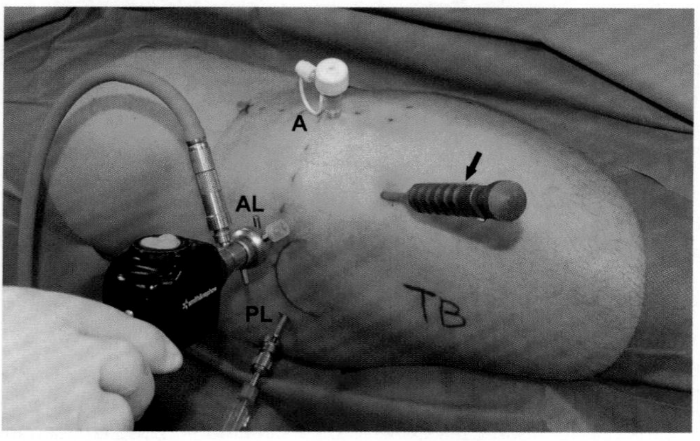

Figure 32-5 | Anchor delivery system (*arrow*) has been positioned percutaneously, distally equidistant between the anterior and anterolateral portals. A, anterior; AL, anterolateral; PL, posterolateral.

- The posterolateral portal is most often neglected.
  - It is the portal that can most often be skipped.
  - It may be a helpful adjunct for posteriorly based pathology and for accessing the acetabular fossa.
  - Using this portal for separate inflow allows smaller diameter scope cannula.

- Peripheral compartment
  - Hip flexion is titrated to expose the cam lesion (~35 degrees).
  - A cephalad anterolateral portal is made in addition to the anterolateral portal (Fig. 32-6).
    - This allows two portals centered on the cam lesion.
    - With the hip flexed, the distal portal allows access to the anterior portion of cam, while the proximal portal can be used for lateral or posterolateral cam lesions.

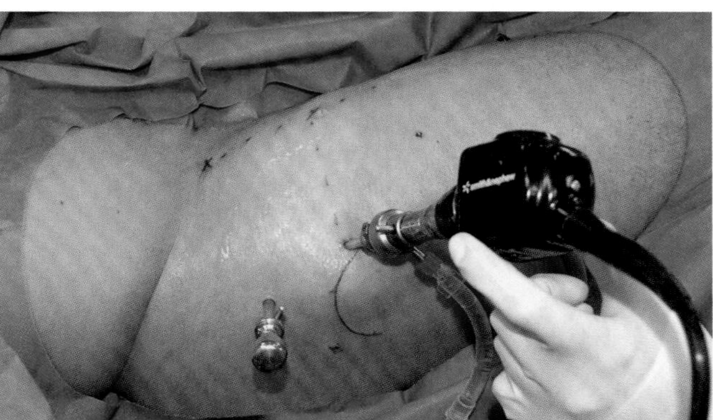

Figure 32-6 | Proximal and distal anterolateral portals have been created by adding a cephalad portal in addition to the original anterolateral portal.

  - This provides a broad safe zone in which to work.
  - There are numerous portal options.
  - Portal placement should be consistent.
    - This is important for optimizing orientation to the three-dimensional anatomy of a cam lesion.

Interportal Capsulotomy (Fig. 32-7)

- Capsulotomy commonly is performed to optimize exposure in correcting FAI.
- The capsulotomy is created by connecting the anterior and anterolateral portals and extending as far medial and posterior as necessary for exposure and access.

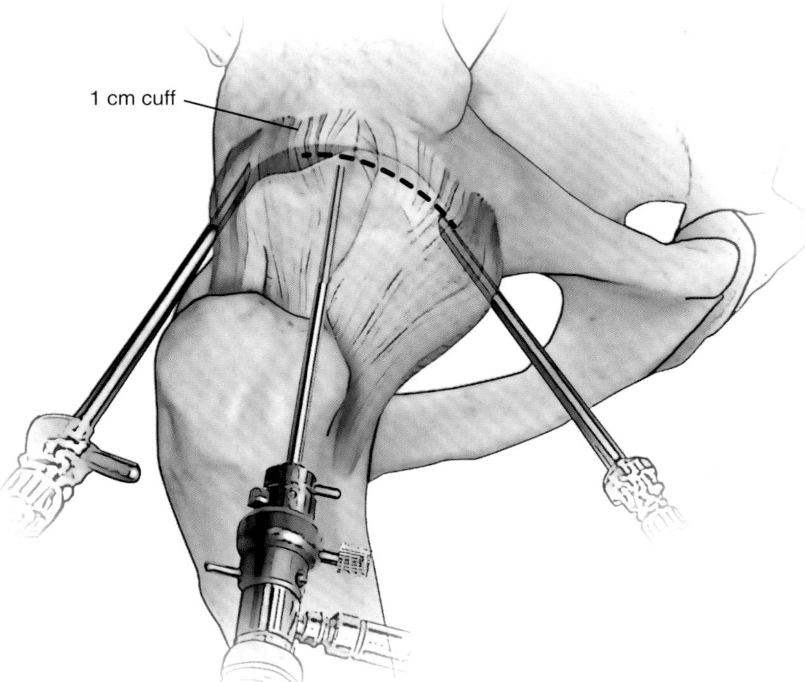

Figure 32-7 | A capsulotomy is performed by connecting the anterior and anterolateral portals (*dotted line*). This is geographically located adjacent to the area of the cam lesion. This capsulotomy is necessary for the instruments to pass freely from the central to the peripheral compartment as the traction is released and the hip flexed.

- At least 1 cm of cuff should be left on the acetabular side when planning on closure.
- Exposure in the periphery for treating a cam lesion can be facilitated by retraction sutures in the inferior leaf or a T-capsulotomy.
- Capsular management.
  - Many authors advocate routine capsular closure,[11,12] because of concerns about iatrogenic instability and possibly better outcomes.
  - The capsulotomy should definitely be closed in the following circumstances.
    - Bony geometry susceptible to instability (eg, reduced anterior or lateral CE angle, excessive femoral anteversion)
    - Extreme physiological laxity
    - Returning to activities that require extremes of motion (eg, gymnastics, figure skating, ballet, wrestling)
  - In some circumstances, capsulectomy may be therapeutic.
    - Stiff hips
    - Modest degenerative disease

Soft Tissue Preparation

- This often is the most time-consuming portion of the procedure.
- It is best to fully expose the pincer and/or cam lesion, visualizing exactly where the resection will start and where it will stop.
- The labrum is mobilized only as necessary to expose the pincer lesion.
  - Formal labral takedown usually is not necessary.
- Cam lesions often are covered in fibrocartilage.
  - Clearance of overlying soft tissue often is necessary to precisely discern the bony component.

How Much to Resect?

- When to address the cam, the pincer, or both?
  - This is influenced by the pattern of joint damage found at arthroscopy.
  - Labral pathology most commonly is associated with a pincer lesion.
  - Articular delamination is associated with cam lesions (Fig. 32-8).

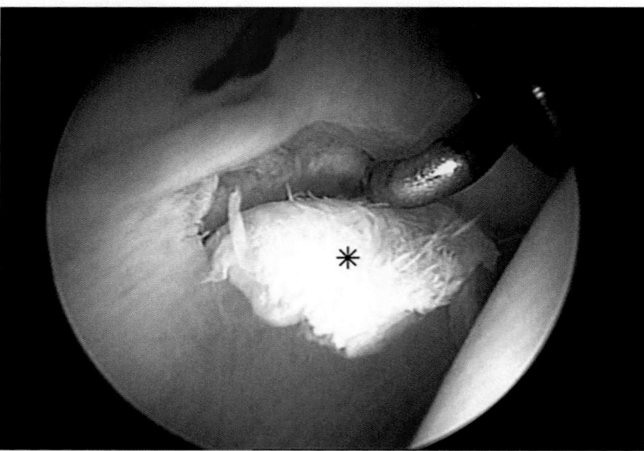

Figure 32-8 | Acetabular articular surface delaminating away from the chondrolabral junction, indicative of pathologic cam impingement (*asterisk*).

  - Closed grade I chondral blistering ("wave sign") most often is associated with sheer forces of a cam lesion (Fig. 32-9).
    - Sometimes it is associated with pure pincer impingement where the articular surface is failing in continuity with the adjacent labrum.
- The extent of a pincer lesion is determined by preoperative imaging, and its pathologic relevance is substantiated by arthroscopic findings.
  - Caution is required when relying solely on two-dimensional radiographic images.
    - The crossover sign and posterior wall sign often are nonspecific for pathologic FAI.

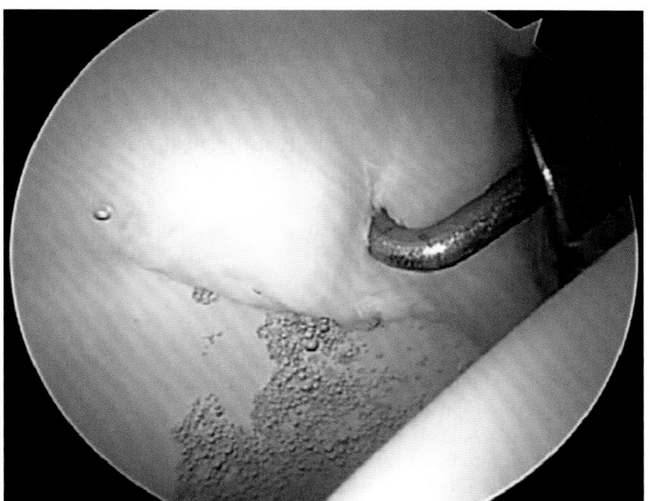

Figure 32-9 | Ballotable closed grade I chondral blistering ("wave sign") is being probed.

- 3-D imaging provides more precise geometric determination.
  - It also can help in assessing acetabular volume.
  - Excessive rim resection can make the hip vulnerable to iatrogenic instability, but simply reducing the acetabular surface volume also can increase the risk of subsequent degenerative disease.
- The goal of cam resection is restoration of the normal sphericity of the femoral head.
  - The epicenter of cam lesions is variable from anterior to lateral, and thus, no single radiographic view is ideal for all cases.
  - 3-D CT scanning precisely discerns cam morphology.[8]
  - The goal of arthroscopy is first to fully expose the cam lesion recognized on preoperative imaging.
  - Reshaping includes restoring the circumferential sphericity of the femoral head and the concave relationship at the head/neck junction.
  - Excessive resection should be avoided.
    - Excessive proximal resection eliminates coaptation with the adjacent labrum and compromises the labral seal.
    - Excessive distal resection can create a stress riser and a risk of femoral neck fracture.
  - Dynamic intraoperative assessment is used by many surgeons.[13]
    - Visualization may be limited with the hip in the impingement position.
    - This method lends itself to more piecemeal resection of the cam lesion and can make it more difficult to keep track of how much resection has occurred.
  - Intraoperative fluoroscopy is helpful but caution must be exercised in using this as a sole guide.
    - Various intraoperative imaging positions are necessary to achieve proper three-dimensional recontouring.[14]
    - Sometimes a compromise in proximal resection must be reached if the femoral head is not perfectly spherical, but more resection to normalize sphericity could result in the labrum no longer having the articular surface against which to coapt and achieve the labral seal.

Chondral Damage

- In the presence of FAI, most damage is on the acetabular side.
  - The femoral surface typically is well preserved until late in the disease course.
    - Femoral-sided changes are indicative of more advanced disease and less successful outcomes.
- Results of microfracture in the hip are highly favorable compared to other joints, possibly because of more constrained architecture and less sheer forces.[15]
  - This still is an imperfect solution for young people, but it has successful outcomes and little morbidity.
  - Accessing the lesion for microfracture can be challenging, requiring the use of various portals.
    - New devices have been developed for getting better angles on creating subchondral perforations.

- What to do with the wave sign?
  - The articular surface is firmly probed and, if it remains patent, it can be left alone.
    - If it breaks open, it should be treated with chondroplasty for partial-depth lesions and microfracture for full-thickness loss to subchondral bone.
  - Accessing the depth of the wave sign peripherally underneath the labrum has been advocated with in situ microfracture, fibrin glue, and even chondral sutures.[16,17]
    - This may be ill-advised because many of these wave signs are relatively innocuous and are partial-thickness lesions that do not need more aggressive preparation of the subchondral surface.

References

1. Frank JM, Harris JD, Erickson BJ, et al. Prevalence of femoroacetabular impingement imaging findings in asymptomatic volunteers: a systematic review. *Arthroscopy.* 2015;31(6):1199-1204.
2. Anderson LA, Anderson MB, Kapron A, et al. The 2015 Frank Stinchfield Award: radiographic abnormalities common in senior athletes with well-functioning hips but not associated with osteoarthritis. *Clin Orthop Relat Res.* 2016;474(2):342-352.
3. Ross JR, Tannenbaum EP, Nepple JJ, Kelly BT, Larson CM, Bedi A. Functional acetabular orientation varies between supine and standing radiographs: implications for treatment of femoroacetabular impingement. *Clin Orthop Relat Res.* 2015;473(4):1267-1273.
4. Fabricant PD, Fields KG, Taylor SA, Magennis E, Bedi A, Kelly BT. The effect of femoral and acetabular version on clinical outcomes after arthroscopic femoroacetabular impingement surgery. *J Bone Joint Surg Am.* 2015;97(7):537-543.
5. Zaltz I, Kelly BT, Hetsroni I, Bedi A. The crossover sign overestimates acetabular retroversion. *Clin Orthop Relat Res.* 2013;471(8):2463-2470.
6. Dolan MM, Heyworth BE, Bedi A, Duke G, Kelly BT. CT reveals a high incidence of osseous abnormalities in hips with labral tears. *Clin Orthop Relat Res.* 2011;469(3):831-838.
7. Heyworth BE, Dolan MM, Nguyen JT, Chen NC, Kelly BT. Preoperative three-dimensional CT predicts intraoperative findings in hip arthroscopy. *Clin Orthop Relat Res.* 2012;470(7):1950-1957.
8. Milone MT, Bedi A, Poultsides L, et al. Novel CT-based three-dimensional software improves the characterization of cam morphology. *Clin Orthop Relat Res.* 2013;471(8):2484-2491.
9. Byrd JWT. Routine arthroscopy and access: central and peripheral compartments, iliopsoas bursa, peritrochanteric, and subgluteal spaces. In: Byrd JWT, ed. *Operative Hip Arthroscopy.* 3rd ed. New York: Springer; 2012:131-160.
10. Byrd JWT. Modified anterior portal for hip arthroscopy. *Arthrosc Tech.* 2013;2(4):e337-e339.
11. Domb BG, Philippon MJ, Giordano BD. Arthroscopic capsulotomy, capsular repair, and capsular plication of the hip: relation to atraumatic instability. *Arthroscopy.* 2013;29(1):162-173.
12. Frank RM, Lee S, Bush-Joseph CA, Kelly BT, Salata MJ, Nho SJ. Improved outcomes after hip arthroscopic surgery in patients undergoing T-Capsulotomy with complete repair versus partial repair for femoroacetabular impingement: a comparative matched-pair analysis. *Am J Sports Med.* 2014;42(11):2634-2642.
13. Locks R, Chahla J, Mitchell JJ, Soares E, Philippon MJ. Dynamic hip examination for assessment of impingement during hip arthroscopy. *Arthrosc Tech.* 2016;5(6):e1367-e1372.
14. Larson CM, Wulf CA. Intraoperative fluoroscopy for evaluation of bony resection during arthroscopic management of femoroacetabular impingement in the supine position. *Arthroscopy.* 2009;25(10):1183-1192.
15. MacDonald AE, Bedi A, Horner NS, et al. Indications and outcomes for microfracture as an adjunct to hip arthroscopy for treatment of chondral defects in patients with femoroacetabular impingement: a systematic review. *Arthroscopy.* 2016;32(1):190.e2-200.e2.
16. Stafford GH, Bunn JR, Villar RN. Arthroscopic repair of delaminated acetabular articular cartilage using fibrin adhesive. Results at one to three years. *Hip Int.* 2011;21(6):744-750.
17. Kaya M, Hirose T, Yamashita T. Bridging suture repair for acetabular chondral carpet delamination. *Arthrosc Tech.* 2015;4(4):e345-e348.

Chapter 33
Principles of Knee Arthroscopy

MATTHEW C. BESSETTE
KURT P. SPINDLER

Preoperative Planning

- Knee arthroscopy can be performed safely on an outpatient basis with general, spinal, regional, or local anesthesia.
- Preoperative antibiotics are commonly administered but have not been shown to be more effective than no antibiotics at preventing infection after uncomplicated knee arthroscopy.[1]
- A recent randomized controlled study showed no benefit when chemoprophylaxis was used to prevent thromboembolic events in otherwise healthy patients.[2]
- Although basic science studies have demonstrated deleterious effects of local anesthetics on cartilage in vitro, human studies have failed to recreate these findings.[3] Intra-articular or portal site injections of local anesthetics, epinephrine, opioids, and nonsteroidal anti-inflammatory drugs before or after arthroscopy are effective analgesic and hemostatic adjuvants.[4] Preoperative portal site injections can help verify correct portal placement when patients are obese or have difficult anatomy.

Instruments and Equipment

- 4.0-mm arthroscope with 30-degree lens and light source (Fig. 33-1)
  - A 70-degree lens should be available if posterior compartment pathology or instrumentation is expected.
  - Inflow through the camera obturator can improve visualization directly adjacent to the camera lens by increasing fluid pressures in the immediate vicinity.

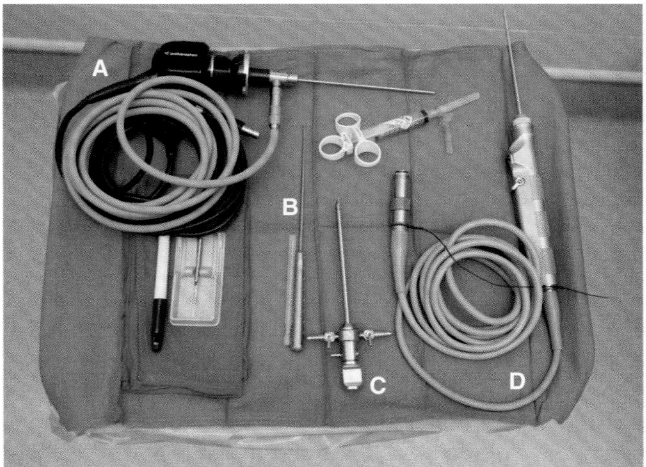

Figure 33-1 | Equipment for basic knee arthroscopy, including an arthroscopic camera attached to a 30-degree 4.0-mm arthroscopic lens and a cord for a light source (Smith & Nephew, Andover, MA) (*A*), an arthroscopic probe (*B*), a camera sheath with an indwelling trochar (*C*), and a motorized arthroscopic shaver (*D*).

- Arthroscopy fluid
  - Lactated Ringer or normal saline
    - Adding diluted epinephrine can improve visualization (1 mg/L).[5]
  - Fluid management
    - Most contemporary pumps can independently control fluid pressures and flow rates, aiding in visualization. Pressures between 40 and 80 mm Hg are commonly used for knee arthroscopy.
    - Arthroscopic fluid bags can alternatively be suspended above the field to use gravity to generate positive intra-articular fluid pressures. Less equipment is necessary, but pressures and flows may be too low or too inconsistent for optimal visualization.
    - Outflow or suction can either be attached to the camera obturator or through a separate obturator placed in the superomedial or superolateral portals. Use of a separate outflow cannula can aid in visualization by clearing blood and debris away from the camera.
- Tourniquet
  - The tourniquet is not routinely inflated, though it is commonly placed on the patient. While its use has deleterious effects on muscle function and physiology, short-term use during knee arthroscopy does not seem to impact outcomes.[6]
- Motorized shaver with suction
- Instruments
  - Scalpel
  - Arthroscopic probe
  - Arthroscopic punches or biters

Positioning

- Supine
  - Patient may either have both legs supported by the bed or positioned so that the knees bend freely over a break in the bed.
    - While dropping the end of the bed offers better access to the posterior compartments and better control over the operative leg, this requires additional steps before surgery and care must be taken to flex the nonoperative leg at the hip to avoid a femoral nerve traction palsy.
  - A lateral post or leg holder should be used to provide a fulcrum for opening the medial or lateral compartments (Fig. 33-2).

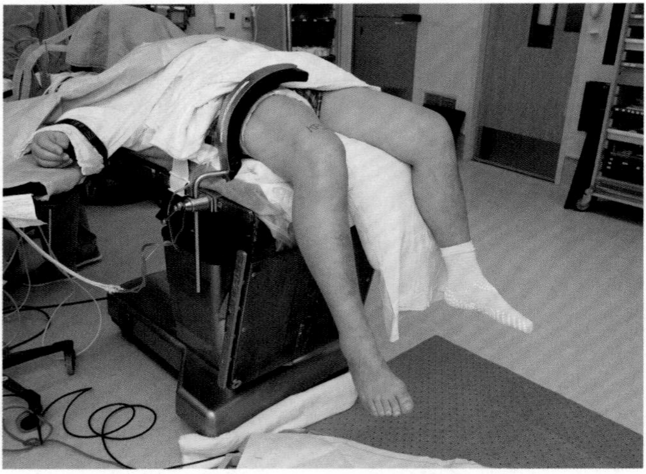

Figure 33-2 | Patient positioning for a right knee arthroscopy. The right leg has been marked by the surgeon and has a tourniquet in place. A well-padded post is in position to provide counterforce when applying valgus stress to the leg. The nonoperative leg is partially flexed over a pillow to prevent excessive stretch on the femoral nerve. The end of the table has been dropped to allow flexion and to provide easy access to the posterior portals if necessary.

Approach

- The tibiofemoral joint line, inferior pole of the patella, and patella tendon are important landmarks for portal site identification (Fig. 33-3).
- The anteromedial and anterolateral are the two most commonly used portals. They are the only portals necessary for many procedures. These are located at the soft spots just medially and laterally to the patellar tendon ~1 cm above the level of the joint line and below the level of the inferior patellar pole.

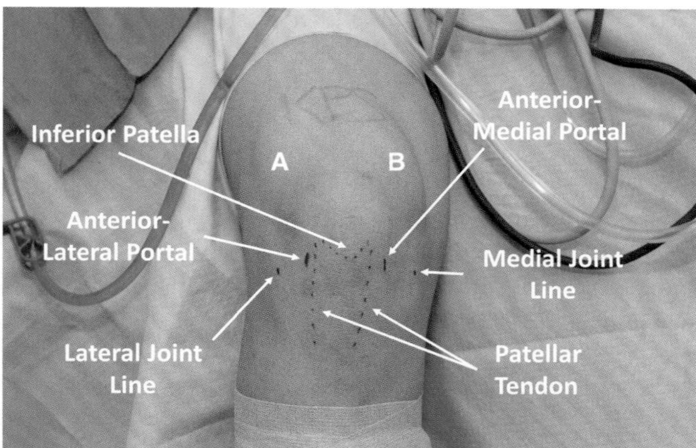

Figure 33-3 | Common reference points and portal placement on a right knee. The sites for superolateral (*A*) and superomedial (*B*) portals are noted if needed for fluid management or evaluation of patellofemoral alignment.

- Skin incisions are ~1 cm and can be vertical, which allows easy extension for removal of large objects or creation of formal arthrotomies, or horizontal, which are more cosmetic and have a lower chance of saphenous nerve injury.
- Superomedial and superolateral portals are commonly used for an outflow portal or to assess patellofemoral pathology. While the use of an independent outflow portal can improve visualization and fluid management, superomedial portals have been associated with quadriceps muscle dysfunction postoperatively. These portals are placed several centimeters proximal to the patella and either medial or lateral to the quadriceps tendon.[7]
- A central trans-patellar tendon portal can improve access to a narrow intercondylar notch.
- Far medial or lateral portals can improve access to the posterior aspects of the medial or lateral compartments.
- Posteromedial and posterolateral portals, created in an outside-in fashion under direct visualization, provide access to the posterior compartment.

Techniques

- With the knee flexed 90 degrees, an incision for an anterolateral portal is made and the camera obturator with a blunt trochar is introduced into the joint capsule, aiming at the intercondylar notch. The obturator is withdrawn slightly, the knee is extended, and the obturator is introduced into the suprapatellar pouch. Plunging into the quadriceps muscle, which will create bleeding and may allow fluid extravasation into the thigh, should be avoided.
- The suprapatellar pouch, patellofemoral joint, and lateral and medial gutters are examined with the knee in extension. The lens is aimed proximally to the view the patellofemoral joint and distally to visualize the gutters (Figs. 33-4 and 33-5).

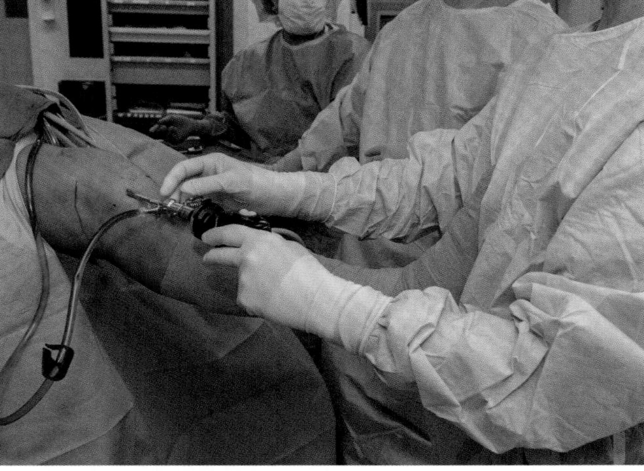

Figure 33-4 | Examination of the patellofemoral joint with the knee in extension supported by surgeon's abdomen and the camera in the anterolateral portal.

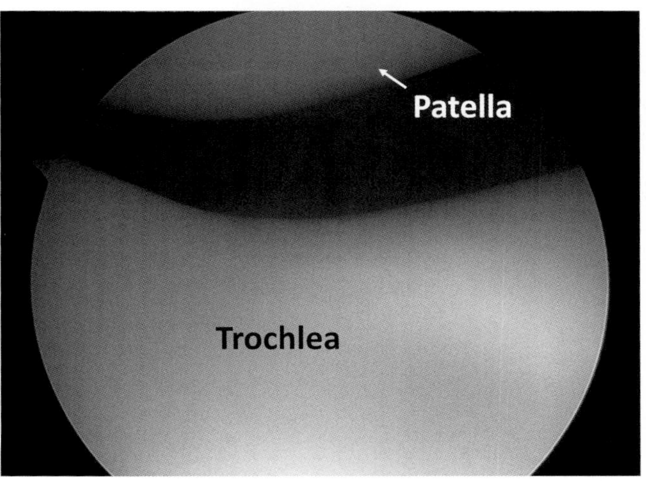

Figure 33-5 | Arthroscopic view of patellofemoral joint with the knee brought into slight flexion to assess patellofemoral tracking.

- The medial compartment is best seen with the knee in slight flexion with a valgus force applied to the knee.
  - Curved instruments facilitate instrumentation of the posterior medial meniscus while avoiding iatrogenic cartilage injury to the medial femoral condyle.
  - In the case of tight medial compartments, the medial collateral ligament can safely be percutaneously "pie crusted" with a needle without any effect on postoperative rehabilitation or outcomes.[8]
  - In most cases, the anteromedial portal is created at this step to facilitate easy passage of instruments into the medial compartment. Localization of the correct trajectory with a spinal needle decreases the chances of iatrogenic cartilage injury or multiple passages through the fat pad and capsule (Figs. 33-6 and 33-7).

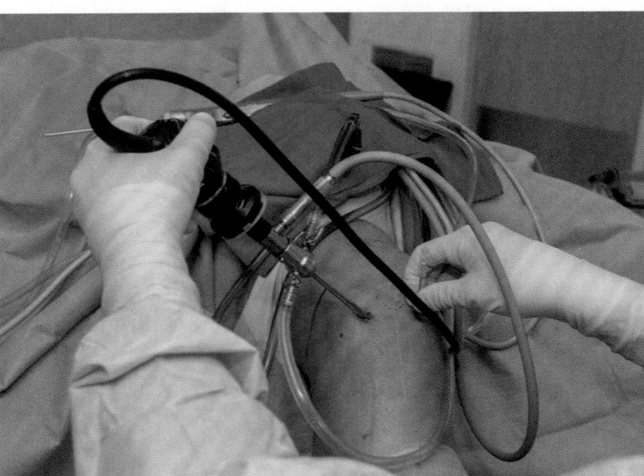

Figure 33-6 | With the knee in 30 degrees of flexion and a valgus force applied, a spinal needle is used to confirm the correct trajectory of the anteromedial portal under direct visualization. Once the portal is made, this position is held to establish easy access to the medial compartment.

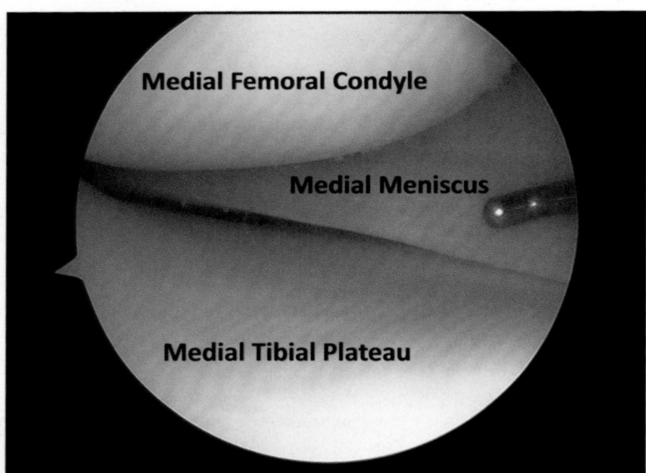

Figure 33-7 | Arthroscopic view of the medial compartment.

- The intercondylar notch is best seen with the knee in 90 degrees of flexion.
  - The probe is placed through the lateral portion of the notch over the posterior root of the lateral meniscus before the leg is moved to a figure-four position to facilitate faster access to the compartment (Figs. 33-8 and 33-9).
- The lateral compartment is best seen with the leg in a figure-four position with the knee bent around 90 degrees and a varus force applied (Fig. 33-10).

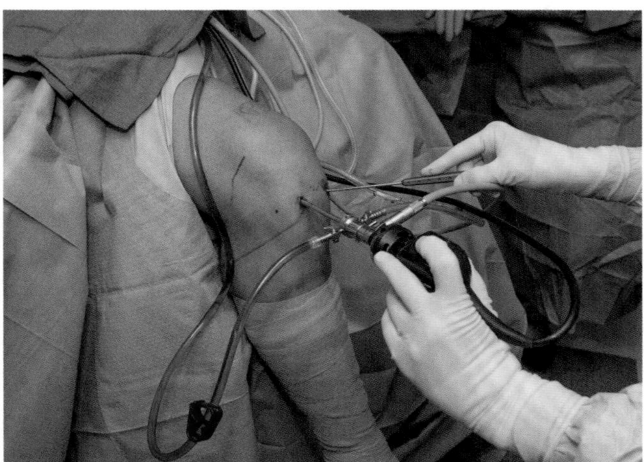

Figure 33-8 | Access to the intercondylar notch with the right knee in 90 degrees of flexion.

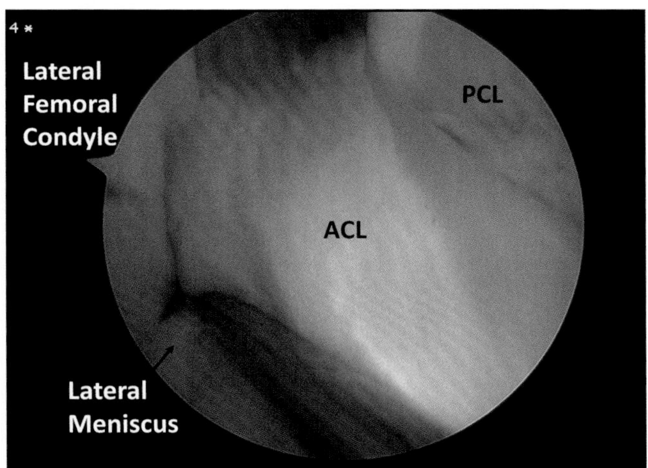

Figure 33-9 | Arthroscopic view of the intercondylar notch of the right knee. The arthroscopic probe is placed over the posterior horn of the lateral meniscus so that the instrument is already in the lateral compartment when the knee is brought into the figure-four position. This maneuver saves time re-instrumenting the lateral compartment from the anteromedial portal, which can be blocked by the fat pad. ACL, anterior cruciate ligament; PCL, posterior cruciate ligament.

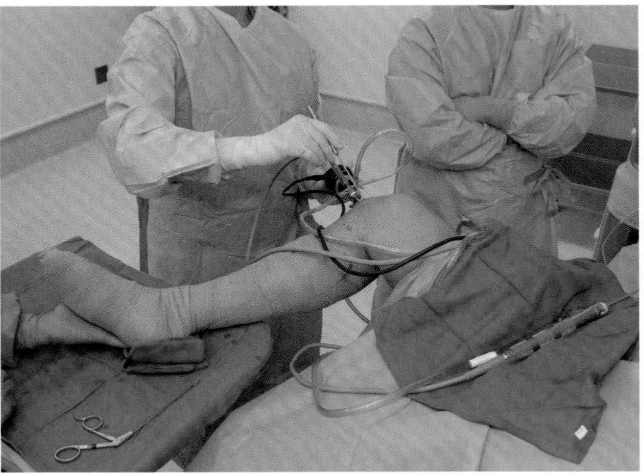

Figure 33-10 | The right knee is placed in the figure-four position with heel on a padded Mayo stand (alternatively, this can be supported by an assistant or on the surgeon's thigh) for easy access to lateral compartment.

- The tip of the camera is kept on the anterior horn of the lateral meniscus to keep the fat pad from obscuring the view (Fig. 33-11).

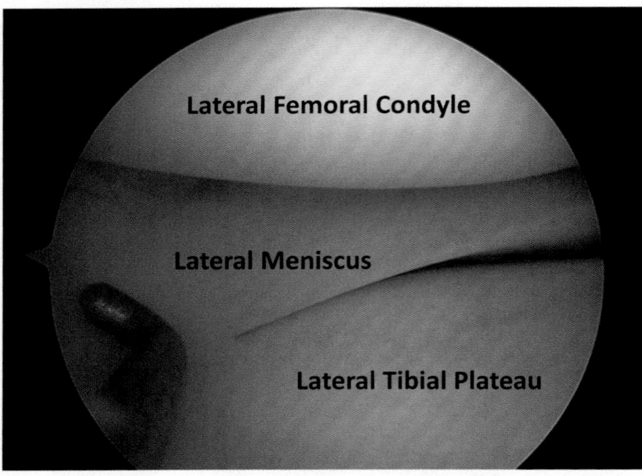

Figure 33-11 | Arthroscopic view of lateral compartment.

- If the planned procedure involves mostly laterally sided work, waiting to create an anteromedial portal until in this position can help ease the passage of instruments by creating a single pathway in the correct orientation.
- The modified Gillquist maneuver involves viewing the posterior compartments through the anterior portals. A 70-degree arthroscopic lens will further improve visualization posteriorly.
  - The posteromedial compartment is viewed by advancing the arthroscope with a blunt obturator from the anterolateral portal through the intercondylar notch and under the posterior cruciate ligament (PCL).
  - The posterolateral compartment is viewed by advancing the arthroscope from the anteromedial portal through the intercondylar notch and under the anterior cruciate ligament (ACL).
- A posteromedial portal is established under direct vision with a modified Gillquist maneuver, which also allows for trans-illumination.
  - Bending the knee to 90 degrees optimally protects nearby branches of the saphenous nerve[9] (Fig. 33-12).

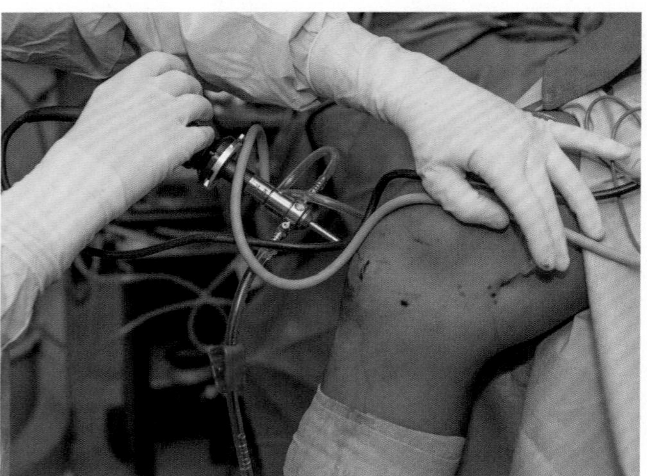

Figure 33-12 | With the knee flexed to 90 degrees and the camera advanced from the anterolateral portal through the notch via the modified Gillquist maneuver, the posteromedial compartment is visualized. A spinal needle is introduced proximal and posterior to the posteromedial joint line to identify the trajectory of the posteromedial portal. To aide in guidance, the lights can be dimmed to allow for trans-illumination of the posteromedial compartment.

- A spinal needle is used to assess the proposed trajectory (Fig. 33-13).
- An incision is made several centimeters posterior and superior to the posteromedial joint line.
- A blunt instrument is used to establish the portal in an outside-in fashion to avoid injury to the saphenous nerve, and a cannula is used to prevent fluid extravasation.

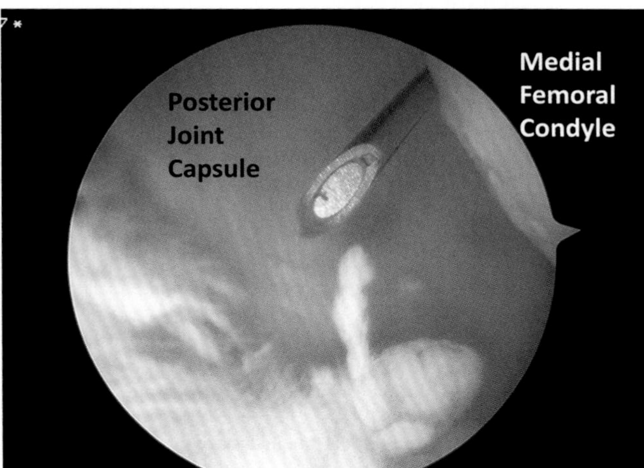

Figure 33-13 | Arthroscopic view of posteromedial compartment from the anterolateral portal with a spinal needle showing the proposed positioning and trajectory for a posteromedial portal.

- A posterolateral portal can be established in a similar fashion.
  - The knee is flexed to 90 degrees, and the portal is made anterior to the biceps tendon to avoid injury to the common peroneal nerve.

Postoperative Care

- Portals can be left open, covered with adhesive dressings, or sutured with either buried absorbable or nonabsorbable simple sutures.[10]
- Wounds should be covered with a compressive dressing (Fig. 33-14).
- Cryotherapy has short-term benefits for pain control and rehabilitation after surgery.[11]
- Complication rates are low and mostly related to infection and thromboembolic events. In the absence of risk factors, there is no clear indications for chemoprophylaxis for the prevention of deep vein thrombosis or pulmonary embolism.[12,13]

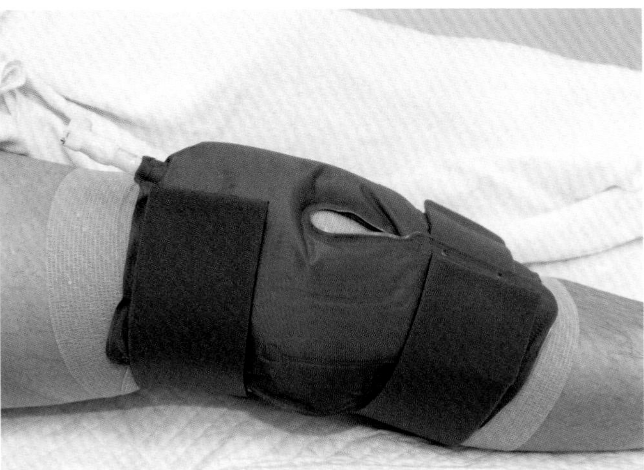

Figure 33-14 | Postoperatively, the knee is dressed with a compressive dressing (Coban, 3M, St. Paul, MN) and a cryotherapy device. (Cryo/Cuff, DJO Global, Vista, CA.)

References

1. Bert JM, Giannini D, Nace L. Antibiotic prophylaxis for arthroscopy of the knee: is it necessary? *Arthroscopy.* 2007;23(1):4-6.
2. van Adrichem RA, Nemeth B, Algra A, et al. Thromboprophylaxis after knee arthroscopy and lower-leg casting. *N Engl J Med.* 2017;376(6):515-525.
3. Piper SL, Kramer JD, Kim HT, et al. Effects of local anesthetics on articular cartilage. *Am J Sports Med.* 2011;39(10):2245-2253.
4. Mitra S, Kaushal H, Gupta RK. Evaluation of analgesic efficacy of intra-articular bupivacaine, bupivacaine plus fentanyl, and bupivacaine plus tramadol after arthroscopic knee surgery. *Arthroscopy.* 2011;27(12):1637-1643.
5. Olszewski AD, Jones R, Farrell R, et al. The effects of dilute epinephrine saline irrigation on the need for tourniquet use in routine arthroscopic knee surgery. *Am J Sports Med.* 1999;27(3):354-356.
6. Tsarouhas A, Hantes ME, Tsougias G, et al. Tourniquet use does not affect rehabilitation, return to activities, and muscle damage after arthroscopic meniscectomy: a prospective randomized clinical study. *Arthroscopy.* 2012;28(12):1812-1818.
7. Stetson WB, Templin K. Two-versus three-portal technique for routine knee arthroscopy. *Am J Sports Med.* 2002;30(1):108-111.
8. Claret G, Montanana J, Rios J, et al. The effect of percutaneous release of the medial collateral ligament in arthroscopic medial meniscectomy on functional outcome. *Knee.* 2016;23(2):251-255.
9. Ahn JH, Lee SH, Jung HJ, et al. The relationship of neural structures to arthroscopic posterior portals according to knee positioning. *Knee Surg Sports Traumatol Arthrosc.* 2011;19(4):646-652.
10. Sikand M, Murtaza A, Desai VV. Healing of arthroscopic portals: a randomised trial comparing three methods of portal closure. *Acta Orthop Belg.* 2006;72(5):583-586.
11. Lessard LA, Scudds RA, Amendola A, et al. The efficacy of cryotherapy following arthroscopic knee surgery. *J Orthop Sports Phys Ther.* 1997;26(1):14-22.
12. Sun Y, Chen D, Xu Z, et al. Deep venous thrombosis after knee arthroscopy: a systematic review and meta-analysis. *Arthroscopy.* 2014;30(3):406-412.
13. Krych AJ, Sousa PL, Morgan JA, et al. Incidence and risk factor analysis of symptomatic venous thromboembolism after knee arthroscopy. *Arthroscopy.* 2015;31(11):2112-2118.

Chapter 34
Arthroscopic Meniscectomy

JOSEPH D. LAMPLOT
MATTHEW J. MATAVA

Sterile Instruments and Equipment

- Nonsterile tourniquet
- Thigh holder or lateral post (surgeon preference)
- 30- and 70-degree arthroscopes
- High-definition video camera
- Lactated Ringer solution or normal saline (3-L bags)
  - Epinephrine (1 mg epinephrine/3-L bag [0.33 mg/L]) may improve hemostasis
- Arthroscopic pump
  - Ideally, the arthroscopic pump has independent controls for both flow and pressure
- Arthroscopic pump tubing
- Arthroscopic cannulae
- Blunt arthroscopic trocar
- No. 11 scalpel
- 4-mm probe
- Arthroscopic basket punches (Fig. 34-1)
  - Straight
  - Up-biting
  - Left-angled
  - Right-angled
  - Back-biting

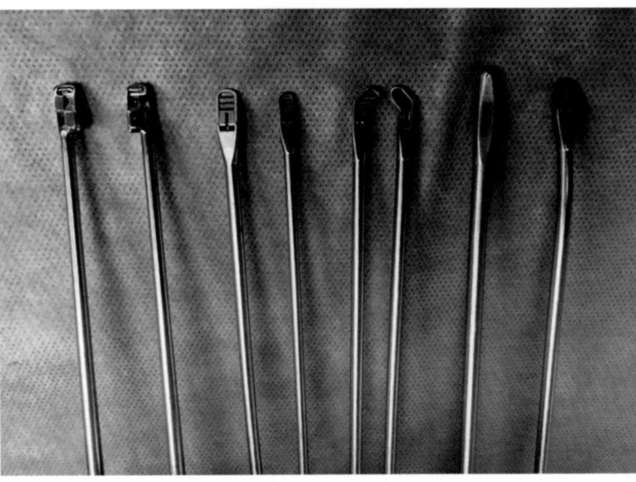

Figure 34-1 | Arthroscopic basket punches include straight, up-biting, left- and right-angled, and back-biting.

- Tissue graspers
- Rotary shavers (toothed and nontoothed) (Fig. 34-2)
  - Straight (4.0 mm, 5.0 mm)
  - Curved
  - Tapered

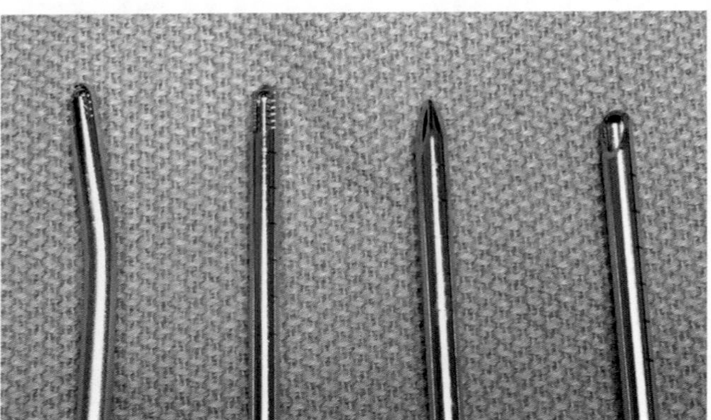

Figure 34-2 | Rotary shavers commonly used including straight (4.0 mm, 5.0 mm), curved, and tapered.

Patient Positioning

- The procedure can be done with the foot of the operating room (OR) table flexed downward 90 degrees or kept straight based on surgeon preference.
  - If the foot of the OR table is flexed 90 degrees, the lower extremity can be flexed over the edge of the table with the thigh placed in a padded holder proximal to the table break and the tourniquet (if used) applied proximal to the thigh holder.
  - If the lower extremity is kept in full extension, a nonsterile post should be placed lateral to the distal thigh.
- The contralateral lower extremity is flexed at the hip and supported by a padded well-leg holder, "butterfly" stirrup, and/or blanket(s) to relieve tension on the femoral nerve (Fig. 34-3).

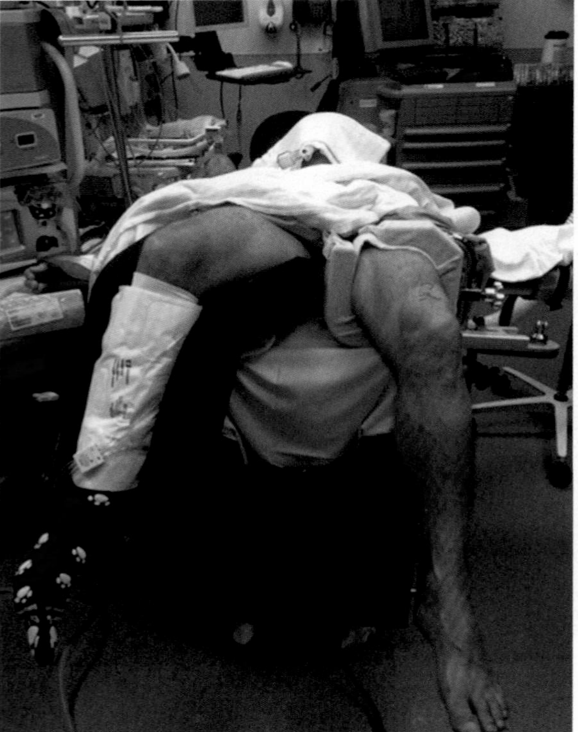

Figure 34-3 | The contralateral (right) lower extremity should be abducted, flexed at the hip, and supported to relieve tension on the femoral nerve.

- If the surgeon prefers the operative knee flexed to 90 degrees, the OR table can be placed in a Trendelenburg position to elevate the operative knee to the level of the surgeon's waist to optimize arthroscopic manipulation.

Portal Placement

- Basic portals (Fig. 34-4)
  - Superomedial (SM): used for the outflow cannula
  - Anterolateral (AL): used for initial arthroscope placement
  - Anteromedial (AM): used for instrumentation (ie, shaver, basket punches)

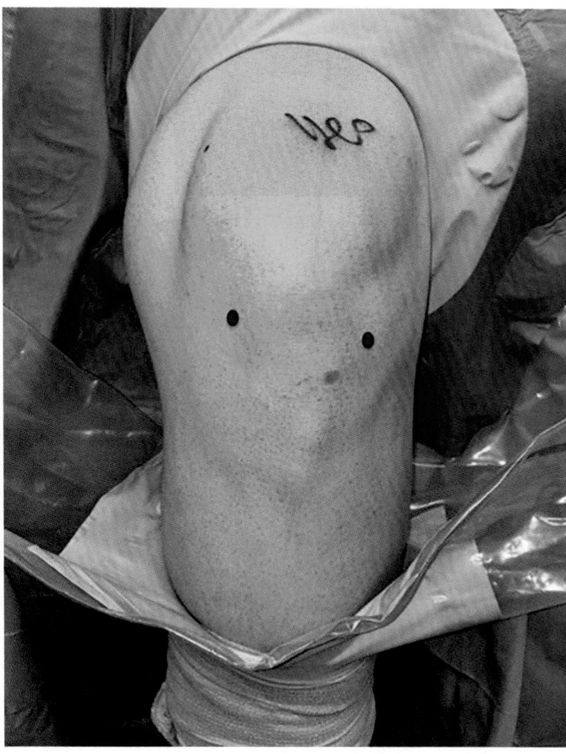

Figure 34-4 | Basic anterior arthroscopy portals. The anteromedial portal is typically more proximal than the anterolateral portal.

- All portals are created with a no. 11 scalpel.
  - The scalpel should be angled 45 degrees to the coronal plane for the AL and AM portals with the sharp edge upward to avoid inadvertent laceration of the anterior horn of the menisci.
- Some surgeons prefer to place the AM portal under direct arthroscopic visualization, whereas others prefer to create all three portals in a "blind" fashion.
- Accessory posterior portals occasionally are necessary to remove a displaced meniscal fragment or loose body in the posterior compartments (see below).
  - Posteromedial (PM)
  - Posterolateral (PL)

Diagnostic Arthroscopy

- The medial and lateral gutters are inspected to locate any displaced meniscal tissue (Fig. 34-5).
- Medial compartment
  - The medial meniscus is viewed and sequentially probed starting at the posterior root and moving anteriorly along the superior and inferior surfaces to identify any displaced meniscal flap between the meniscal body and tibial plateau (Fig. 34-6).
  - If a tear is identified, it is probed to assess its stability.

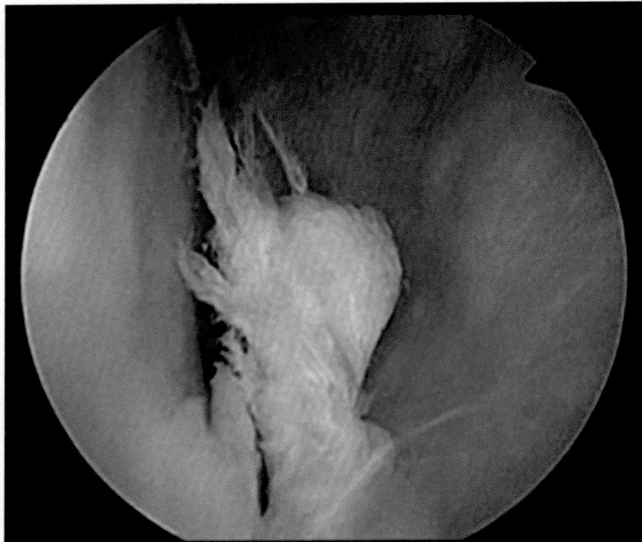

Figure 34-5 | A displaced fragment of meniscal tissue in the medial gutter.

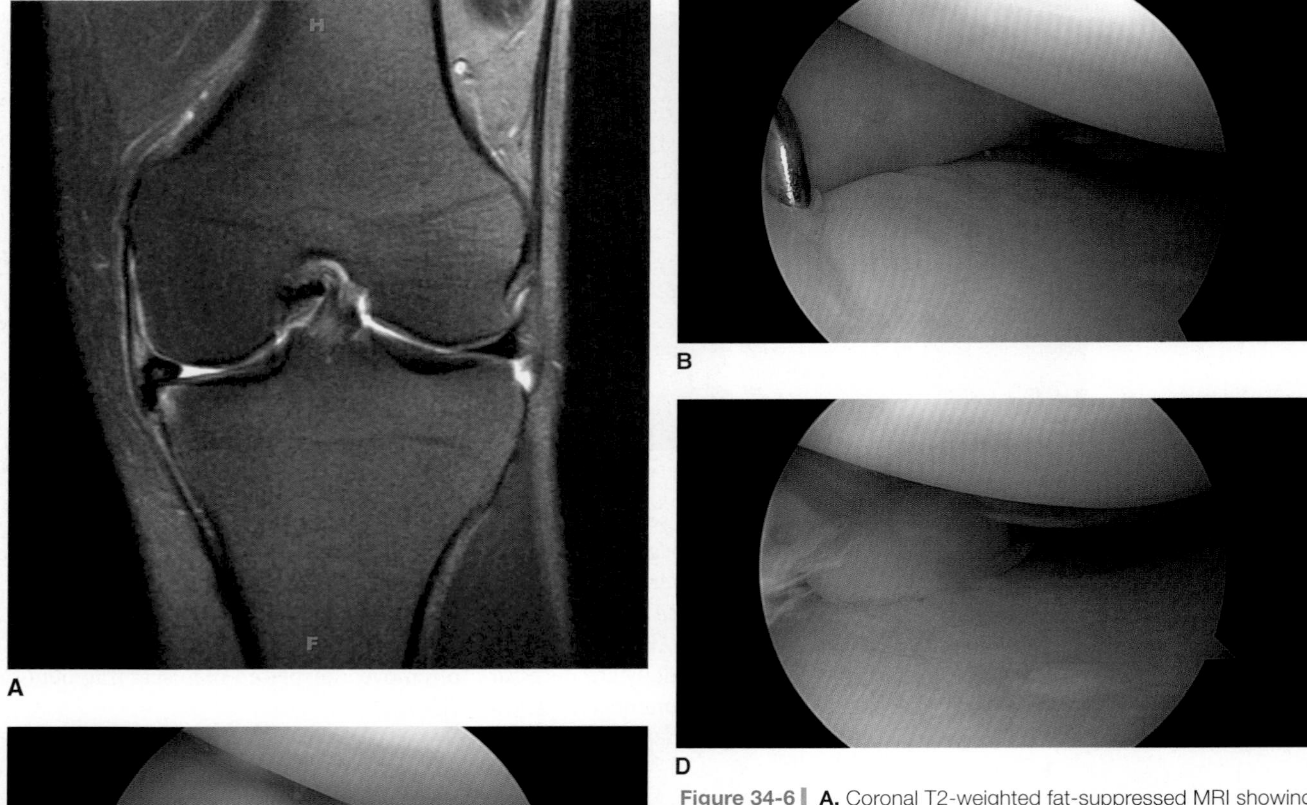

Figure 34-6 | **A.** Coronal T2-weighted fat-suppressed MRI showing a displaced flap of medial meniscus entrapped between the medial tibial plateau and meniscus. **B.** Arthroscopic image of entrapped meniscal flap folded under itself corresponding to the MRI. **C.** A probe is used to reduce the displaced meniscal fragment into view. **D.** The meniscal flap reduced in its entirety.

- If the medial meniscus can be pulled anteriorly past the "equator" of the medial femoral condyle, it is considered unstable and likely torn (Fig. 34-7).
- External pressure on the PM knee can help deliver the posterior horn into view.

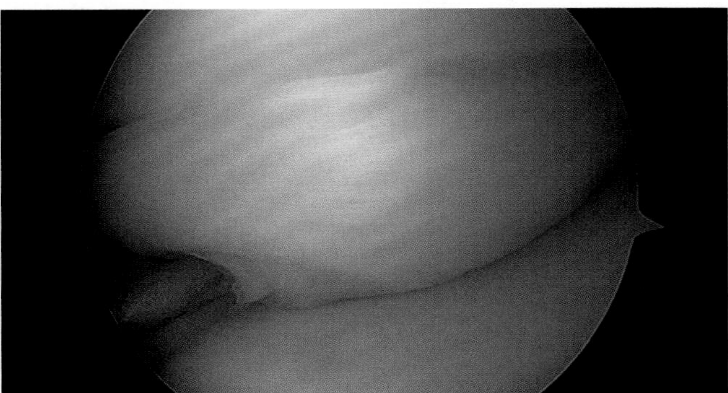

Figure 34-7 | The torn medial meniscus is pulled anteriorly past the "equator" of the medial femoral condyle, indicating a peripheral tear.

- Lateral compartment
  - The knee is placed in 20 degrees of flexion with internal rotation and a varus load applied.
  - If the arthroscopy is performed with the lower extremity extended, placing the knee in the "figure-four" position can facilitate examination of the lateral compartment.
  - Systematic evaluation begins at the posterior horn of the lateral meniscus, including the root insertion.
  - The midbody of the lateral meniscus is evaluated around the popliteal hiatus by sweeping the arthroscope laterally and viewing inferiorly (Fig. 34-8).
  - The anterior horn is evaluated by retracting the arthroscope and viewing inferiorly.

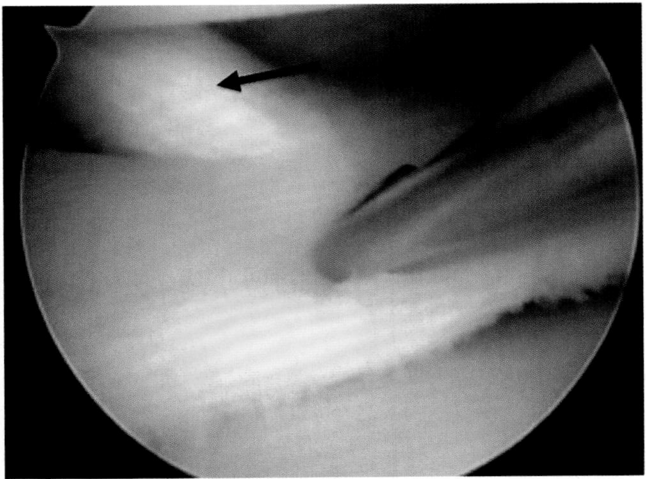

Figure 34-8 | The midbody of the lateral meniscus is evaluated and probed around the popliteus tendon (*arrow*) by aiming the arthroscope laterally and viewing inferiorly.

- Posteromedial compartment
  - To view the PM compartment, the cannula, with blunt trocar, is introduced through the AL portal, directed posteriorly and inferiorly along the medial wall of the intercondylar notch under the posterior cruciate ligament.[1]
  - An accessory PM portal is created by trans-illuminating the skin over the PM corner of the knee. An 18-gauge spinal needle is inserted into the compartment 1 cm above the medial joint line, posterior to the medial femoral condyle. A longitudinal stab incision is made with a no. 11 scalpel, with care to avoid the saphenous nerve and vein, which can occasionally be seen by trans-illumination. A blunt trocar is then advanced through the incision, puncturing the capsule under direct vision (Fig. 34-9).

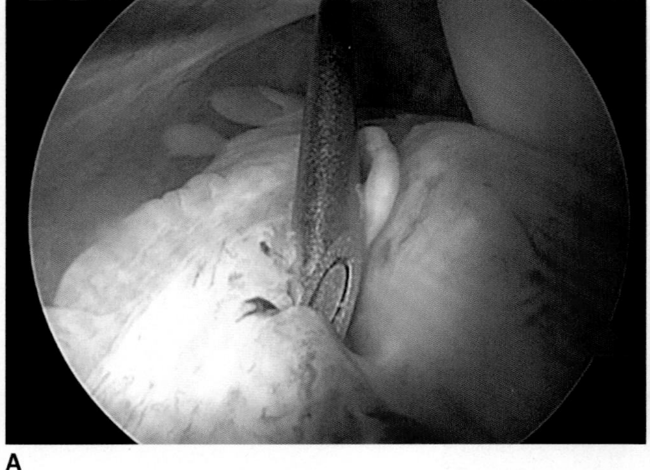
A

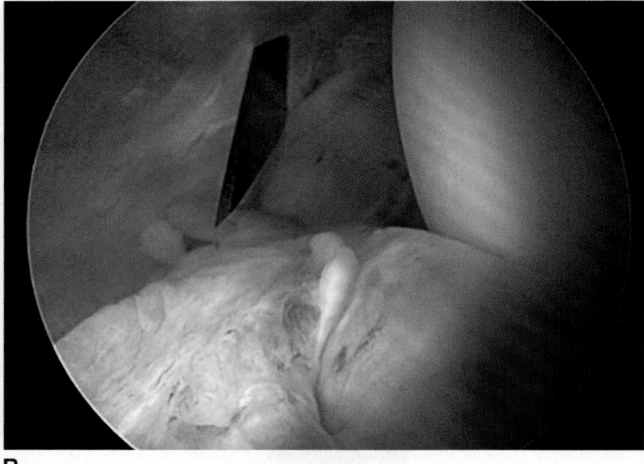
B

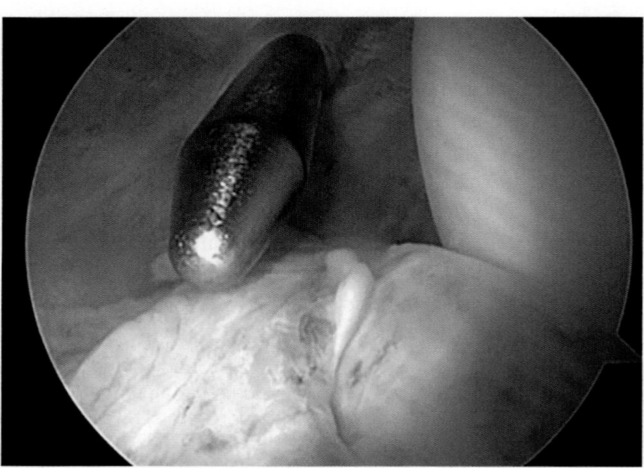
C

Figure 34-9 | Placement of a posteromedial portal by viewing with a 70-degree arthroscope through the intercondylar notch from an anterolateral portal. **A.** An 18-gauge needle is used to localize the portal in relation to a meniscal tear. **B.** A no. 11 scalpel is used to make a longitudinal incision to avoid injury to the saphenous vein or nerve. **C.** A blunt trocar is used to dilate the posteromedial portal.

- Posterolateral compartment
  - The PL compartment is examined by inserting the 70-degree arthroscope through the AM portal, over the anterior cruciate ligament (ACL), through the intercondylar notch, and past the lateral femoral condyle (Fig. 34-10).

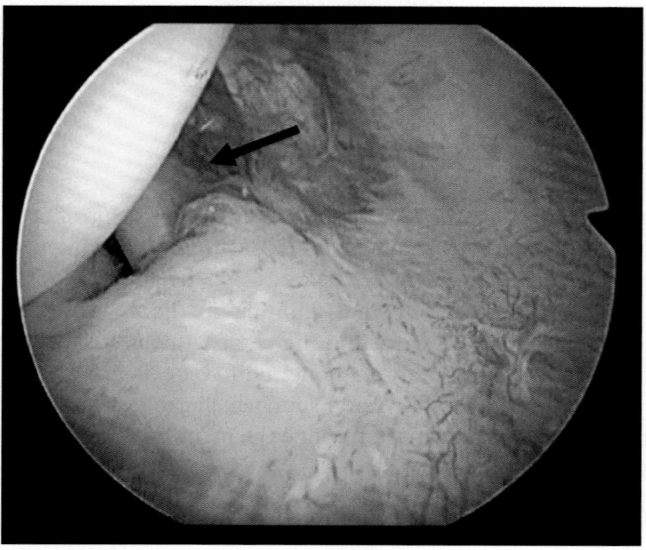

Figure 34-10 | The posterolateral compartment is examined with a 70-degree arthroscope through the intercondylar notch from the anteromedial portal. The popliteus tendon is visualized (*arrow*).

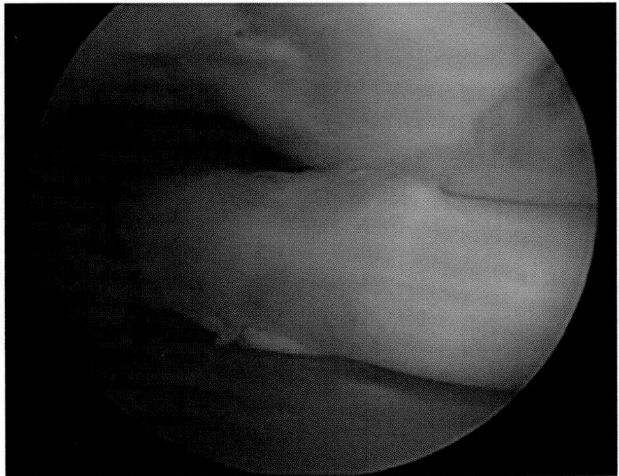

A

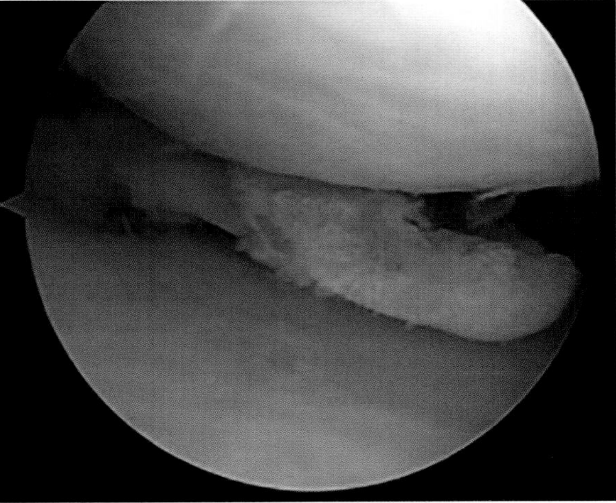

B

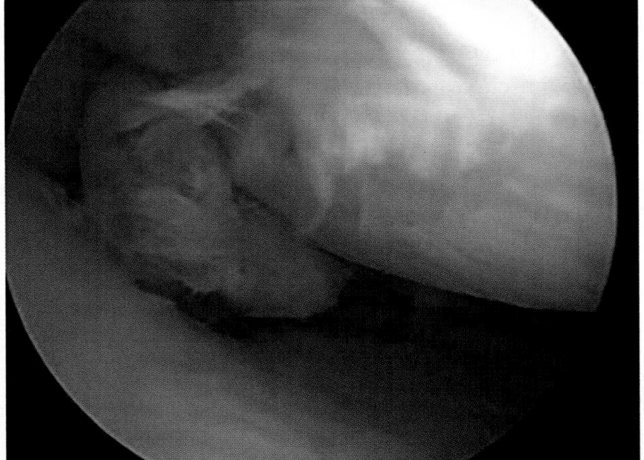

C

Figure 34-21 | **A.** An irreparable bucket-handle medial meniscal tear. **B.** The anterior horn attachment was released before the posterior horn. **C.** The bucket-handle fragment is displaced into the posterior compartment making removal difficult. It is important that the posterior horn attachment be released first to prevent this displacement.

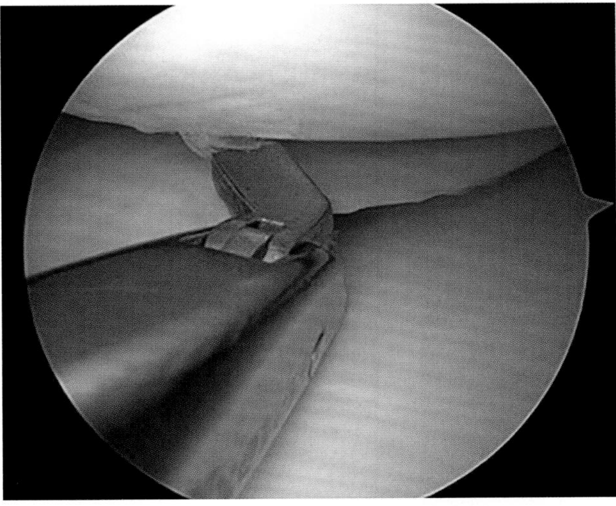

Figure 34-22 | A left-angled basket punch is used to resect the anterior horn of the left medial meniscus.

- Posterior root tears
  - Oblique lateral root tears often occur in association with an ACL tear (Fig. 34-23).
    - Nonreparable lateral root tears in conjunction with an ACL tear often are easier to resect after the torn ACL is debrided.

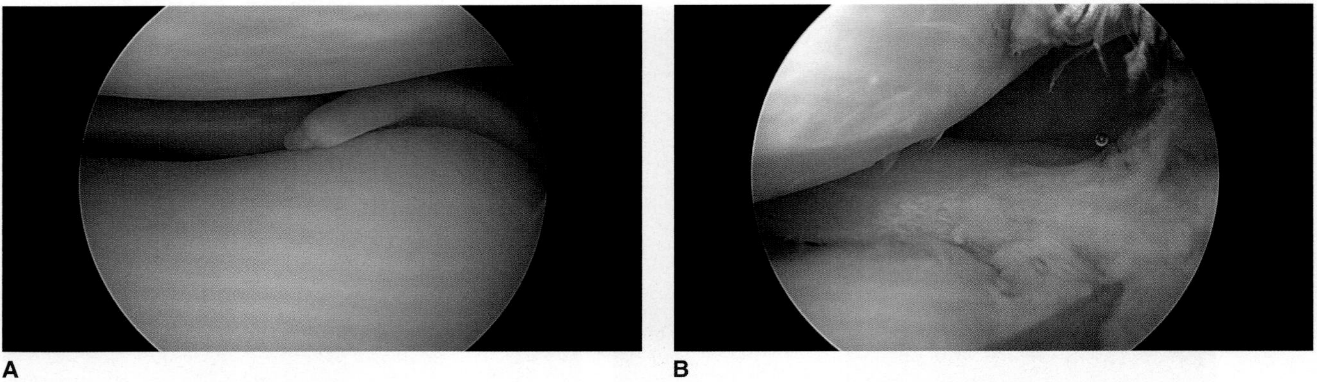

A B

Figure 34-23 | **A.** An oblique lateral meniscal root tear in association with an ACL tear. **B.** The lateral meniscal root remains intact following tear debridement from the anterolateral portal to avoid interference from the tibial spines.

- Switching the arthroscope to the ipsilateral portal may facilitate debridement of a posterior root tear that may be difficult to reach because of the tibial spines.
- It is crucial not to blindly "resect" the posterior meniscal root, because this may cause iatrogenic damage to the posterior neurovascular structures and/or the root attachment.

- Posterior root tears, in association with chondrosis of the femoral condyle, are common in the medial meniscus in middle-aged females (Fig. 34-24).

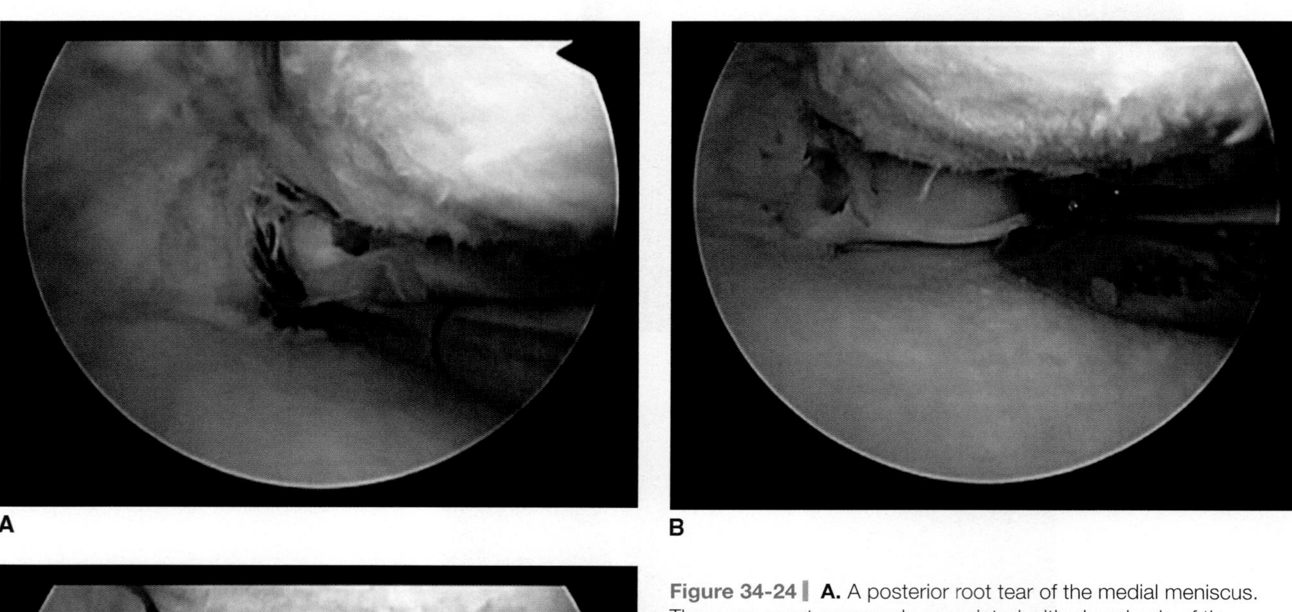

A B

C

Figure 34-24 | **A.** A posterior root tear of the medial meniscus. These are most commonly associated with chondrosis of the medial femoral condyle in middle-aged females. **B.** Debridement of the posterior root is limited to the unstable flap of tissue. **C.** The posterior root following tear debridement.

- Horizontal cleavage tears
  - It can be difficult to determine the most functional and least symptomatic "leaf" of meniscal tissue in the setting of a horizontal cleavage tear (Fig. 34-25).

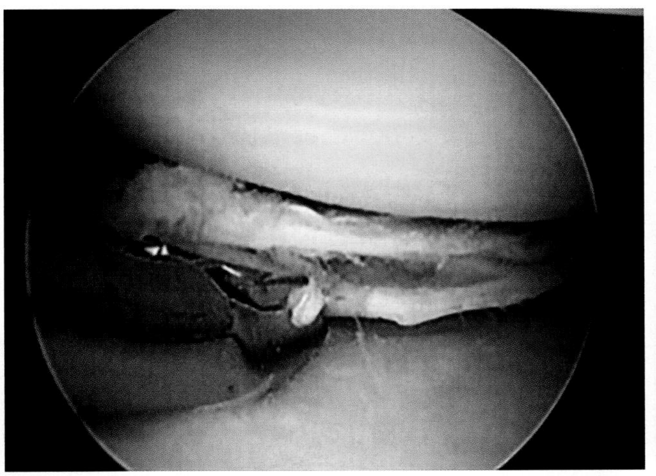
A

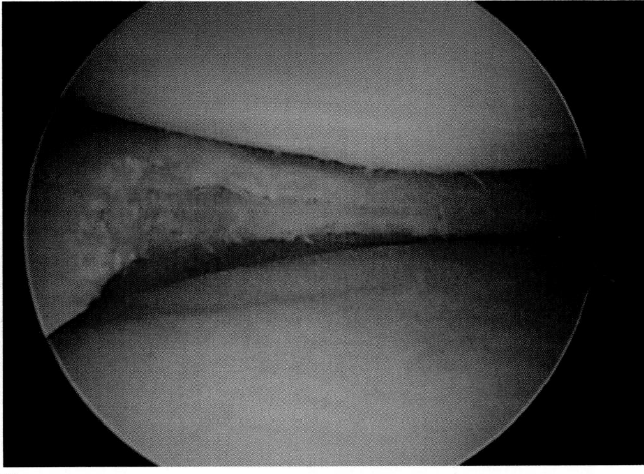
B

Figure 34-25 | **A.** A horizontal cleavage tear of the medial meniscus. **B.** Debridement should consist of the unstable tissue or least functional meniscal leaf.

  - The meniscal leaf that possesses the most meniscal tissue should be preserved.
  - Debridement can be facilitated with either a left- or right-angled basket punch.
  - Horizontal cleavage tears often are associated with meniscal cysts.
    - The cyst can be debrided through the tear, as evidenced by gelatinous fluid emanating from the tear as the cyst is entered (Fig. 34-26).
- Discoid meniscus
  - Discoid menisci occur in 3%-5% of the U.S. population and in ~15% of the Japanese population, though the true incidence of asymptomatic discoid menisci is unknown.[5]
  - Most discoid menisci involve the lateral meniscus (Fig. 34-27).
  - The Watanabe classification is based on the degree of coverage of the tibial plateau:
    - Type I: complete
    - Type II: incomplete
    - Type III (Wrisberg variant): the posterior horn is attached solely by the meniscofemoral (Wrisberg) ligament

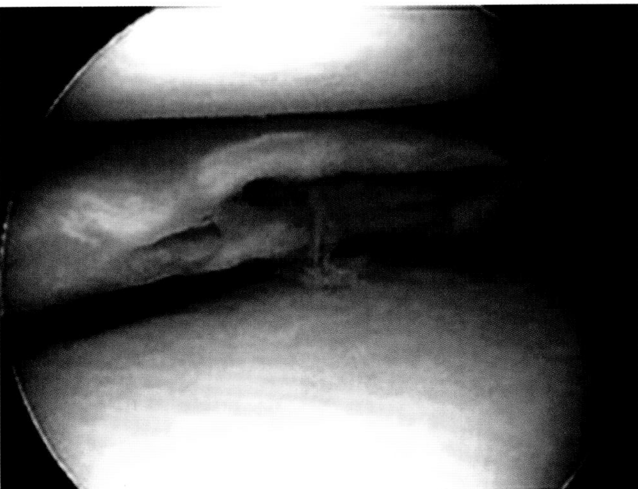

Figure 34-26 | A meniscal cyst associated with a horizontal cleavage tear. The cyst can be debrided through the tear, as evidenced by gelatinous fluid emanating from the tear as the cyst is entered.

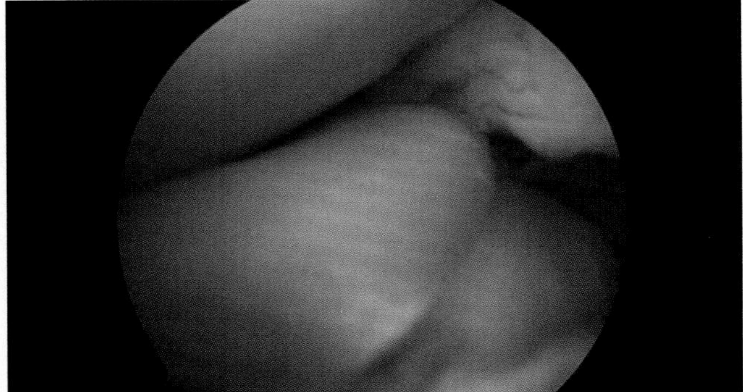

Figure 34-27 | A "complete" discoid lateral meniscus in which the lateral tibial plateau is completely covered by the misshapen meniscus.

- Treatment of a symptomatic, torn discoid meniscus is arthroscopic saucerization.
  - The torn central segment is debrided to recreate the normal C-shaped configuration with a 6- to 8-mm peripheral rim (Fig. 34-28).
  - Angled or back-biting punches or an electrocautery ablation device can be used.
  - The 30-degree arthroscope through the AM portal or the 70-degree arthroscope through the AL portal can facilitate viewing of the entire lateral meniscus.
  - Caution must be taken not to completely excise the entire meniscus unless necessitated by the extent of the tear.
- For Wrisberg variants, stabilization of the posterior horn can be done similar to a standard meniscal repair.

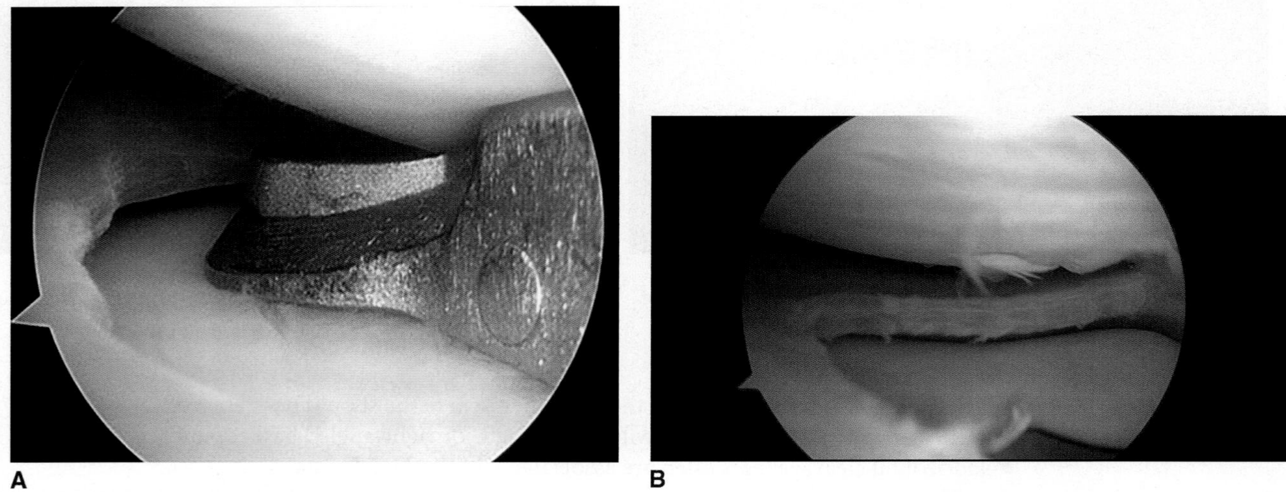

Figure 34-28 | **A.** "Saucerization" of the torn central segment of a discoid lateral meniscus. **B.** The meniscus should be debrided to recreate its normal C-shaped configuration.

Pearls and Pitfalls

- Accurate portal placement is key to a successful meniscectomy.
- The intact medial meniscus has a typical fold ("flounce") at the junction of the posterior horn and midbody (Fig. 34-29).
  - Absence of "flounce" is highly associated with a medial meniscal tear.[6]

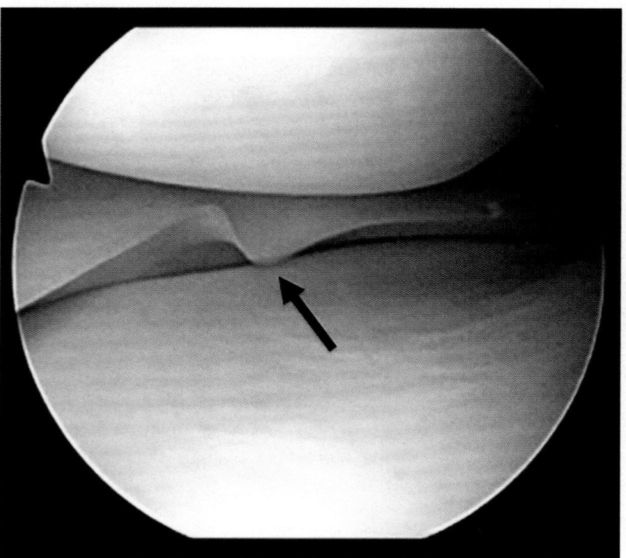

Figure 34-29 | The intact medial meniscus has a typical fold ("flounce") at the junction of the posterior horn and midbody (*arrow*).

- Older male patients with associated osteoarthritis often have a tight medial compartment, making posterior horn visualization difficult.
  - Overly aggressive valgus force can cause rupture of the medial collateral ligament (MCL) or iatrogenic fracture of the distal femur.
  - "Pie crusting" of the deep MCL can be done by inserting an 18-gauge needle just above the joint line to allow incremental opening of the medial joint space and visualization of the entire posterior horn (Fig. 34-30).

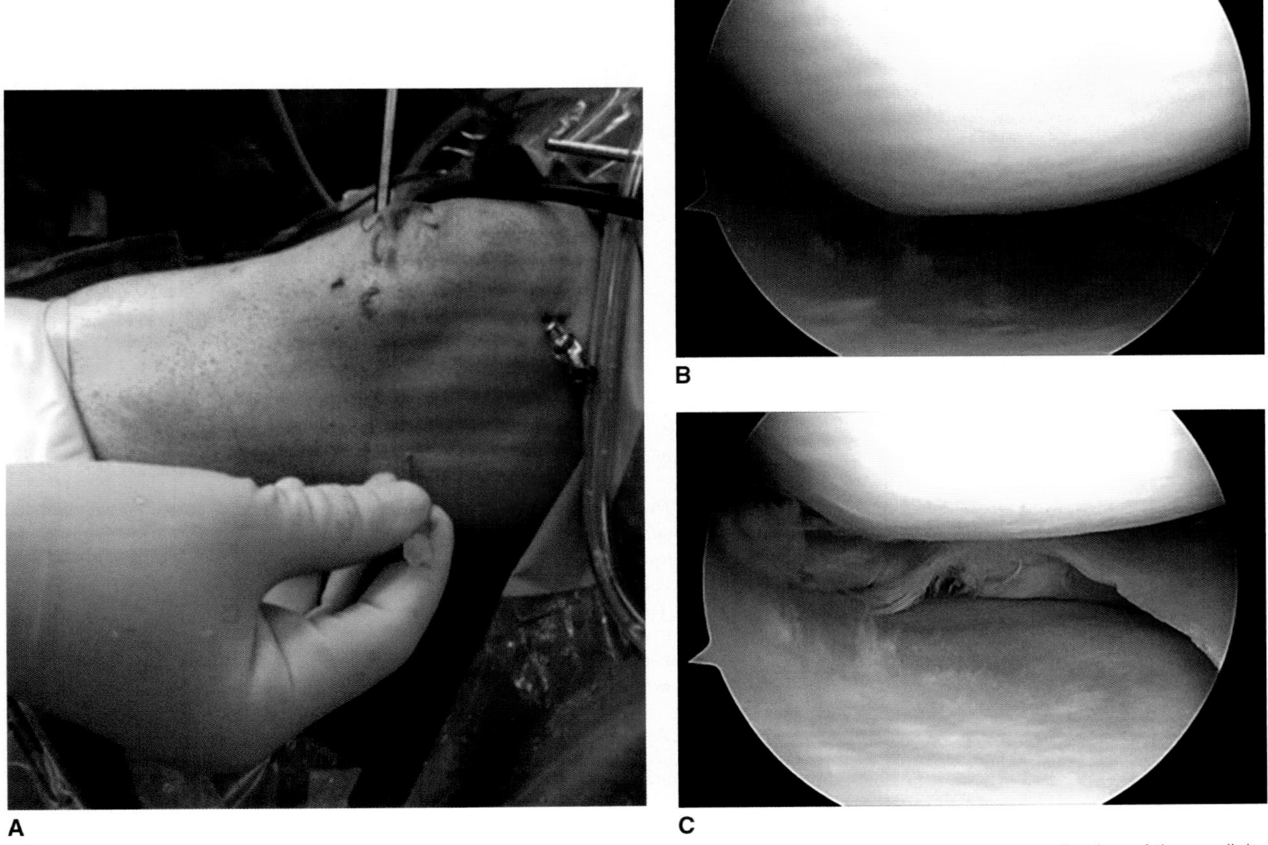

Figure 34-30 | **A.** "Pie crusting" of the medial collateral ligament with an 18-gauge spinal needle to improve visualization of the medial meniscus. **B.** A tight medial compartment makes visualization of the posterior horn of the medial meniscus difficult. **C.** Improved visualization of the medial meniscus following the "pie-crusting" procedure in the same knee.

- Medial meniscocapsular tears ("ramp" lesions) may not be identified with a 30-degree arthroscope from standard anterior portals in "tight" knees.
  - Visualization is facilitated with a 70-degree arthroscope through the intercondylar notch (Fig. 34-31).
- An asymptomatic discoid meniscus found incidentally during knee arthroscopy should *not* be surgically excised, because this may lead to a symptomatic tear.
- Saucerization of a discoid meniscus in children may require a 2.7-mm arthroscope.
- An accessory trans-patellar tendon portal can be used to access various parts of the meniscus if this cannot be done with standard portals.
- A perfectly smooth inner meniscal rim is not necessary, because the edge will "smooth out" over time (Fig. 34-32).

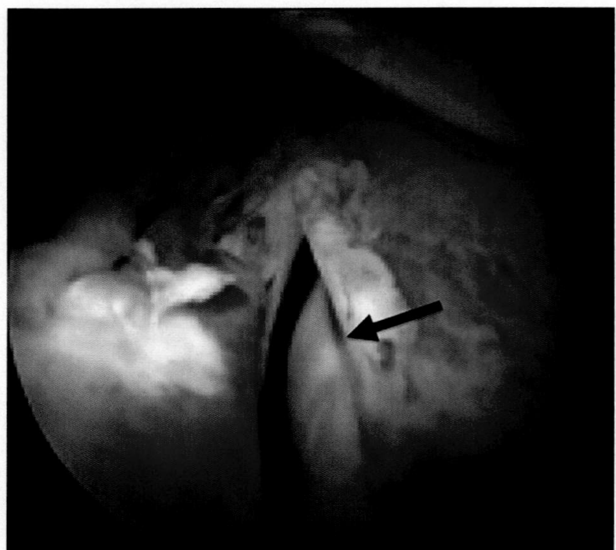

Figure 34-31 | A medial meniscocapsular tear ("ramp lesion") (*arrow*) may be best identified with a 70-degree arthroscope through the intercondylar notch. Visualization often is not possible with a 30-degree arthroscope from standard anterior portals.

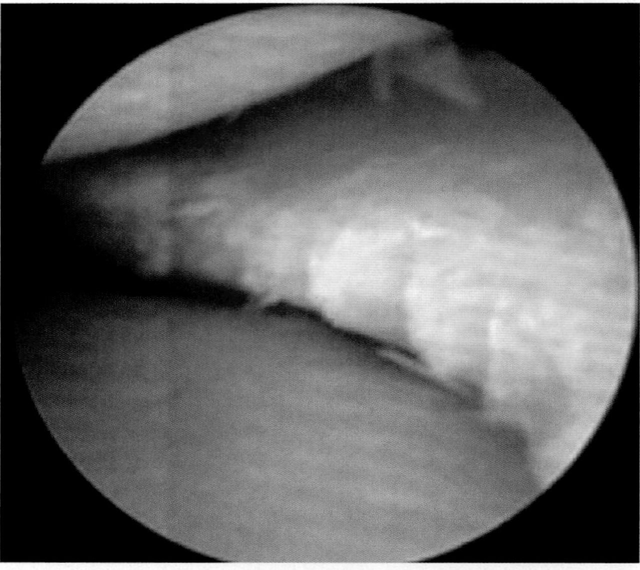

Figure 34-32 | A perfectly smooth inner meniscal rim is not necessary when performing a partial meniscectomy.

References

1. Gillquist J, Hagberg G, Oretorp N. Arthroscopic visualization of the posteromedial compartment of the knee joint. *Orthop Clin North Am.* 1979;10:545-547.
2. Hoser C, Fink C, Brown C, Reichkendler M, Hackl W, Bartlett J. Long-term results of arthroscopic partial lateral meniscectomy in knees without associated damage. *J Bone Joint Surg Br.* 2001;83:513-516.
3. Binnet MS, Gurkan I, Cetin C. Arthroscopic resection of bucket-handle tears with the help of a suture punch: a simple technique to shorten operating time. *Arthroscopy.* 2000;16:665-669.
4. Paksima N, Ceccarelli B, Vitols A. A new technique for arthroscopic resection of a bucket handle tear. *Arthroscopy.* 1998;14:537-539.
5. Jordan M. Lateral meniscal variants: evaluation and treatment. *J Am Acad Orthop Surg.* 1996;4:91-200.
6. Wright RW, Boyer DS. Significance of the arthroscopic meniscal flounce sign: a prospective study. *Am J Sports Med.* 2007;35:242-244.

Chapter 35
Arthroscopic All-Inside Meniscal Repair

MATTHEW H. BLAKE
DARREN L. JOHNSON

Indications

- Timing
  - Acute traumatic meniscal tear
  - Chronic tear without complex geometry
- Tear patterns
  - Vertical longitudinal tears >1 cm
  - Horizontal tears
  - Bucket-handle tears (may be best repaired using inside-out techniques)
  - Radial tears are difficult to repair with an all-inside technique
- Location
  - Posterior horn
  - Body
  - Anterior horn best repaired by outside-in technique
  - Red-red zone
  - Red-white zone in patients younger than 40 years
- Stability
  - Must be done in a ligamentously stable knee
  - Can be done with concomitant ligament reconstruction

Equipment

- Tower
  - Light source
  - Monitor and recording device
  - 4-mm 30- and 70-degree arthroscope with cannula
  - Shaver system
- Irrigation
  - Gravity or high-pressure pump system
  - Suction
- Draping
  - Knee arthroscopy pack with sterile drapes
  - Impervious stockinette and 6-in elastic bandage wrap for the leg and foot
- Accessory
  - Well-leg holder or lateral post
  - ±Tourniquet
    - Performing surgery without a tourniquet may allow better visualization of bleeding from the prepared meniscal tissue.

- Instruments
  - All-inside suture passing device of surgeon's choosing
  - Various angled meniscal graspers and biters
  - Meniscal shaver
  - Probe
  - Rasp
  - 18-gauge spinal needle
  - Microfracture awls

Anesthesia

- General with laryngeal mask airway (LMA) or sedation and local anesthesia
- 0.5% ropivacaine at the portal sites
- ±Regional block
- Weight-based dose of third-generation cephalosporin
- ±Anticoagulation: stratified by risk factors such as prior deep venous thrombosis (DVT) or clotting disorder

Positioning

- The patient is positioned supine.
- A bump can be placed underneath operative hip.
- Leg support must allow the knee to achieve full range of motion including application of varus and valgus stress and should be positioned to allow circumferential access to the knee.
  - *Leg holder:*
    - Placed perpendicular to the femur at mid- to upper thigh to allow placement of varus and valgus forces on the knee.
    - The leg should be internally rotated before the holder is secured so that the patella is en face.
    - The end of the table is lowered past 90 degrees from horizontal to allow the leg to hang freely (Fig. 35-1).

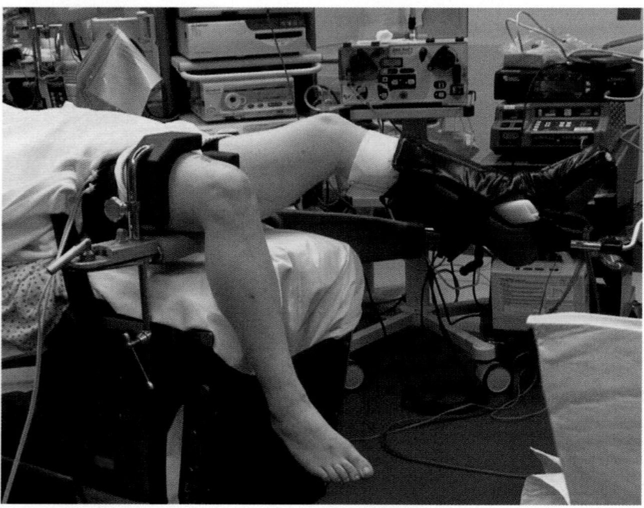

Figure 35-1 | Patient positioned with a leg holder to allow circumferential access to the knee.

  - *Lateral post:*
    - Placed midthigh and angled to allow a valgus force on the knee.
    - The surgeon may leave the end of the table up or drop the end of the table.
- The contralateral leg with a sequential compression device (SCD) is placed in a padded well-leg holder of surgeon's choosing.

Surgical Approach

- Overview
  - Portals are created using no. 11 blade.
  - Standard portals are the anterolateral and anteromedial portals.
  - Accessory portals can be used depending on tear patterns and repair strategies (Fig. 35-2).

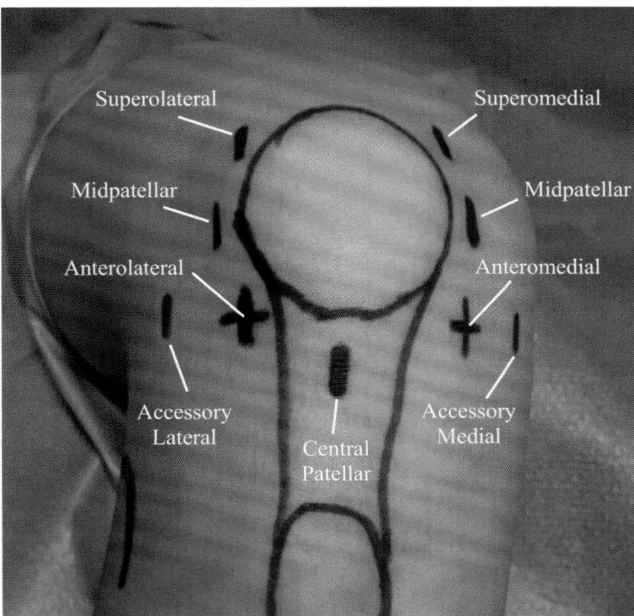

Figure 35-2 | Standard anterolateral and anteromedial portals shown with possible accessory portals (right knee).

- Portals
  - The anterolateral portal is created 5-10 mm lateral to and at the level of the inferior pole of the patella in the anatomic "soft spot."
  - The arthroscope is introduced to the notch, and the fat pad is swept anteriorly.
  - The anteromedial portal is established under direct vision by localizing the entry point with a spinal needle.
    - If the lateral meniscus is to be repaired, then the portal should be 3-5 mm superior to the anteromedial horn of the meniscus so that the suture passage device can be advanced over the tibial eminence and underneath the femoral condyle (Fig. 35-3).

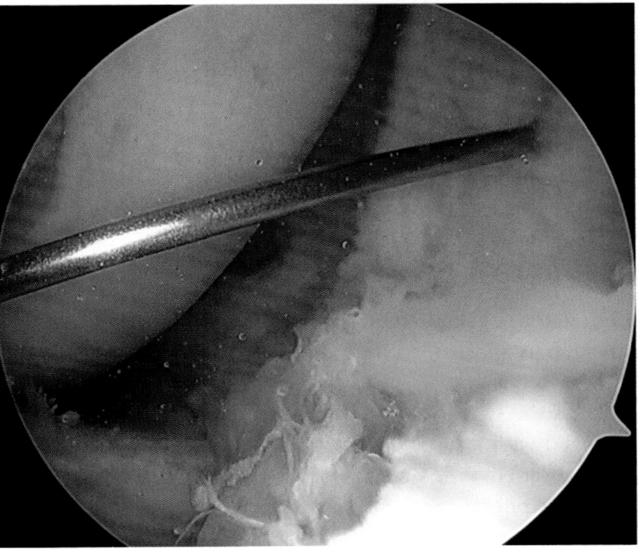

Figure 35-3 | Medial portal localization 5 mm above the anteromedial horn of the medial meniscus.

        - An anteromedial portal adjacent to the patellar tendon will facilitate repair of the posterior horn of the lateral meniscus.
        - An anteromedial portal placed more medially will facilitate repair of the body of the lateral meniscus.
        - If the posterior horn of the medial meniscus is to be repaired, it should be confirmed that a needle passes easily to the posterior horn of the medial meniscus without touching the medial femoral condyle.
    - Accessory working portals can be created to facilitate easier passage of suture.
    - Placement of the arthroscope can be changed for better visualization.

Visualization

- A diagnostic arthroscopy is performed.
- Instruments should not be forced to avoid damage to the articular cartilage.
- A varus stress with the knee flexed to ~70 degrees increases the visualization and working space of the lateral joint.
    - The flexion angle can be adjusted and/or the varus load can be increased by lowering the table to increase the lateral joint working space.
- A valgus force with knee flexed at ~20 degrees increases the visualization and working space of the medial joint.
    - Adjusting the flexion angle and/or increasing the valgus load (by lowering the table) will increase the medial joint working joint space.
    - "Pie crusting" the medial collateral ligament (MCL) with an 18-gauge needle can increase the medial working space.
        - The MCL beneath the medial meniscus is repeatedly punctured with an 18-gauge needle while a valgus stress is applied (Fig. 35-4).
        - After surgery, the patient is placed into a hinged brace until the ligament tightens.

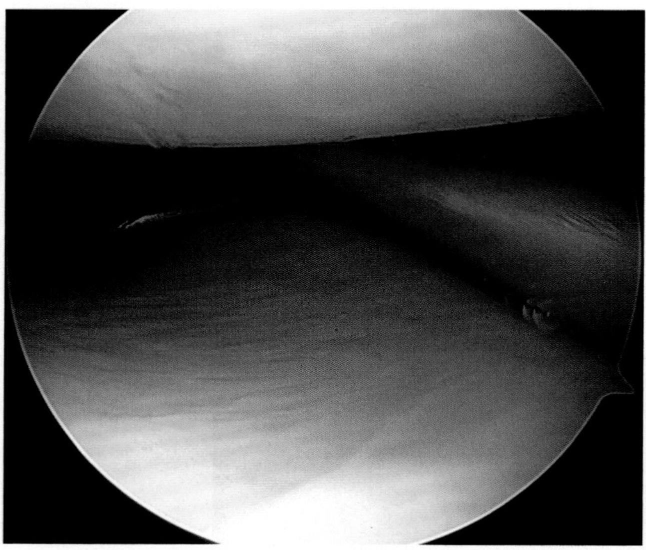

Figure 35-4 | Puncturing the MCL underneath the medial meniscus to increase medial working space.

Meniscal Preparation

- The tourniquet is deflated to evaluate meniscal vascularity.
- A blunt instrument, such as an arthroscopic trocar or probe, is used to reduce a bucket-handle tear (Fig. 35-5).
- A probe is used to assess the size, location, and shape of the tear.
- Fibrous tissue is removed with a rasp or shaver (no suction) to improve vascularity.
    - Synovial fringes are abraded with a rasp (Fig. 35-6).
    - Trephination of the peripheral meniscal rim is done with an 18-gauge needle from inside out or outside in.

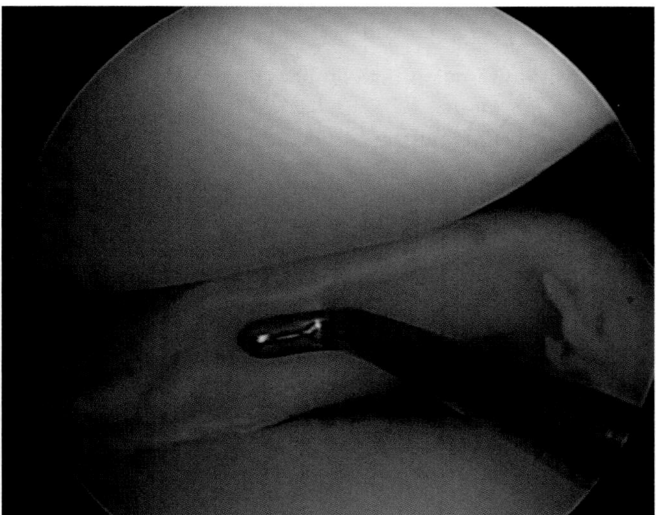

Figure 35-5 | Reducing a bucket-handle meniscus with probe. The probe can also be used to hold reduction while the repair is performed.

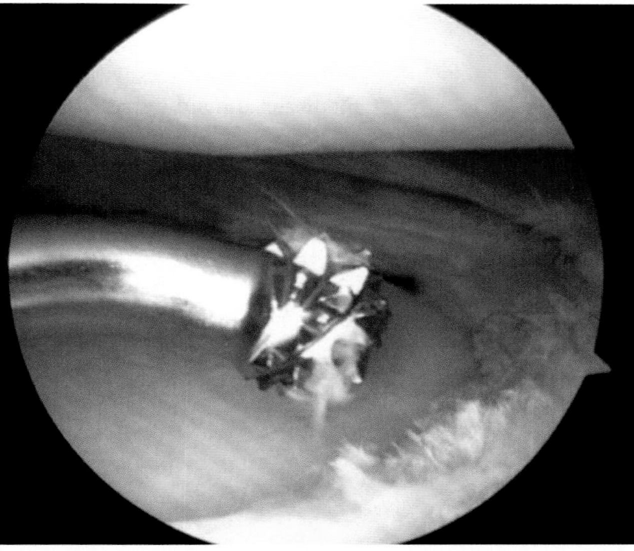

Figure 35-6 | Rasping to remove fibrous tissue and increase vascularity to promote healing.

- Temporary fixation
  - A probe is used to reduce and hold the inner portion to the peripheral rim.
  - A small needle is introduced from outside in across the tear.
  - A mulberry knot is made.
    - No. 0-Prolene suture with passed with an 18-gauge needle from outside in and retrieved through a working portal. Multiple knots are tied and pulled back into the joint. The meniscus will then reduce to the periphery with continued traction.

Repair

- Viewing through an ipsilateral portal with instrumentation through the contralateral portal.
- A larger capsular incision may aid in passage of the suture device.
- Fixation should be perpendicular to the tear to increase compressive forces (Fig. 35-7).

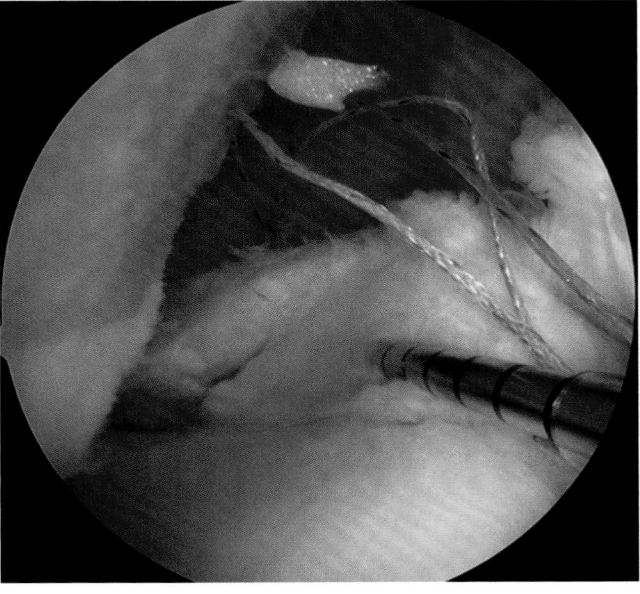

Figure 35-7 | Fixation perpendicular to tear.

- Vertical mattress suture orientation provides the strongest repair construct. Accessory portals can be used for a better trajectory. Horizontal mattress sutures also can be used.

- A skid, sheath, or insertion cannula can be used to insert suturing devices into the knee and to protect the chondral surface (Fig. 35-8).
- Suture repair devices with a curved tip better fit underneath the condyles and may help reduce the meniscus and aid in passing and positioning of the sutures.
- The repair is begun from the center of the tear, working outward to decrease the incidence of "dog ears."
- Sutures are spaced ~5 mm apart to avoid gapping, puckering, and incongruence (Fig. 35-9).

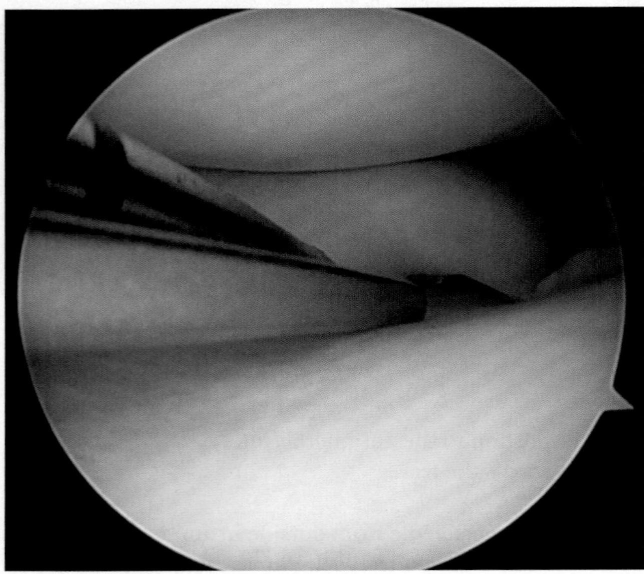

Figure 35-8 | Introduction of suture device with aid of a skid.

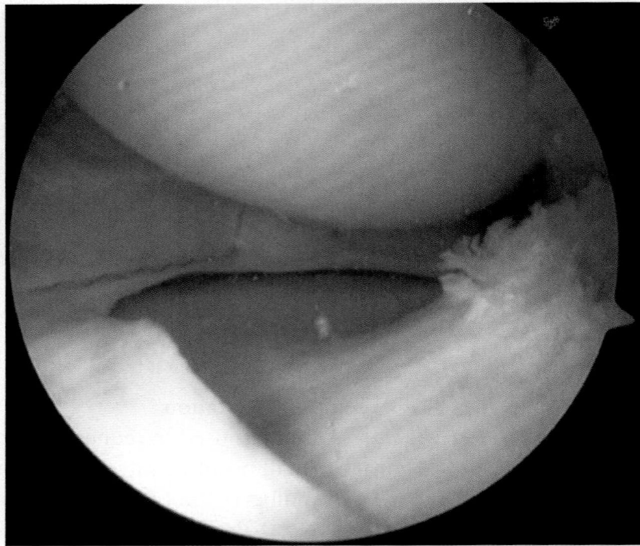

Figure 35-9 | Repaired meniscus with sutures spaced ~5 mm apart.

- Placement of the sutures can be alternated between the undersurface of the meniscus and the top of the meniscus to help the meniscus lie flat on the tibia.
- The sutures are placed in accordance with manufacturer's protocol.
  - Sutures can be arthroscopically tied, may come pre-tied, or may be a knotless design.
  - A knot pusher can be used to slide and cinch the knot.
  - The repair should not be overtightened to avoid puckering of the meniscus.

Caution

- The repair device or anchor should not pierce the iliotibial band, MCL, or the skin (Fig. 35-10).

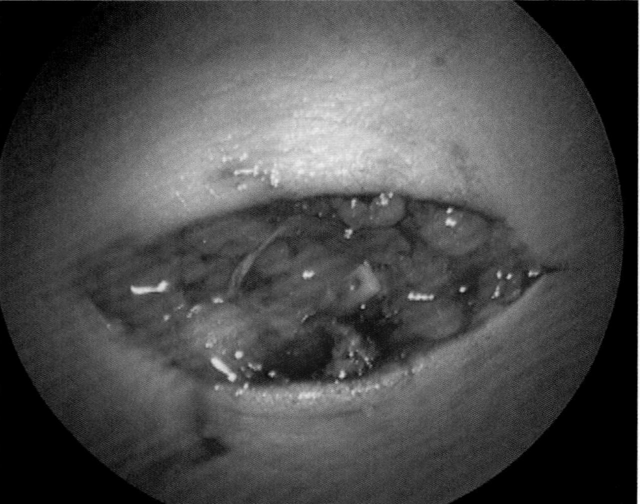

Figure 35-10 | Prominent anchor that has pierced the MCL lying in subcutaneous fat.

- The repair device should not be aimed directly posterior to the lateral meniscal root because of its proximity to the popliteal artery and tibial nerve.
- If there is a misfire or if the suture pulls out, all foreign objects are removed from the knee before leaving the OR.

Biological Augmentation

- A fibrin clot can be created, inserted, and incorporated into the repair to enhance healing of the meniscus (Fig. 35-11).

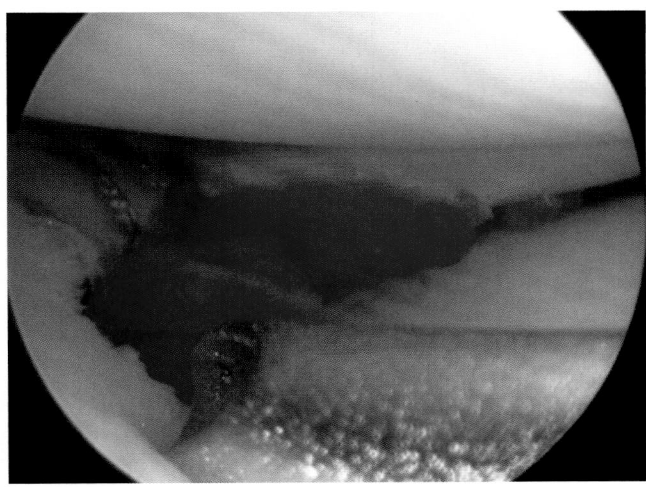

Figure 35-11 | Fibrin clot incorporated into a meniscal repair.

- Alternatively, a microfracture of the anterior intracondylar lateral wall can be performed to create bleeding to enhance meniscal repair (Fig. 35-12).
- Protein-rich plasma (PRP) also has been suggested as a biological augment but has not yet proven efficacious.

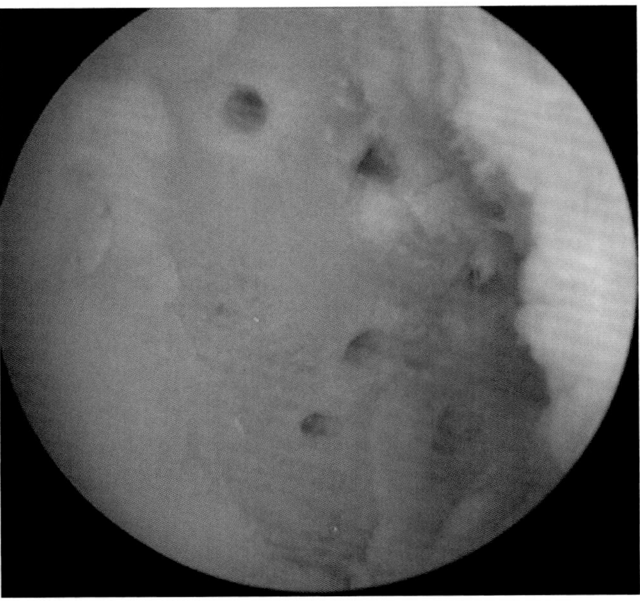

Figure 35-12 | Limited notchplasty and microfracture of the anterior intracondylar lateral wall.

Postoperative Rehabilitation

- Rehabilitation is individualized based on tear geometry, repair construct strength, associated surgical procedures, and surgeon preference.
- We often place patients in an I-ROM brace locked at 30 degrees of flexion. Patients are toe-touch weight bearing with crutches for 4-6 weeks with full active and passive range of motion.
- At 4-6 weeks after surgery, the patient may begin weight bearing. No pivoting is allowed.
- Return to sports is anticipated at 4-6 months. The patient must have no effusion and be able to show full extension and full painless terminal flexion.

Chapter 36
Arthroscopic Inside-Out Meniscal Repair

DAVID C. FLANIGAN
CHRISTOPHER C. KAEDING

Why Repair vs Resection[1]

- Restore meniscal function
  - Peak force dissipation
  - Increased congruity of articulating surfaces
  - Increased nutrition to chondrocytes
  - Increased knee stability
  - Increased lubrication function in the knee
- Repair results in
  - Decreased risk of chondral degeneration in the future
  - Decreased discomfort from peak contact overload
  - Decreased risk of increased knee instability
- Resection indicated
  - Risk of failure of repair and need for repeat surgery outweighs potential for successful repair and its subsequent benefit

Reparable Tears[1]

- Tear pattern
  - Vertical longitudinal—ideal
  - Horizontal cleavage—perhaps with newer techniques
  - Radial—challenging, perhaps repair if tear propagates into peripheral third of meniscus
  - Complex—perhaps, depending on location and status of unstable fragment and age of patient
- Condition of unstable fragment
  - Intact and undamaged—ideal.
  - The more the unstable fragment is damaged and compromised, the less desirable it is to repair, because the strength of the repair and the ultimate function of the meniscal fragment are questionable if it were salvaged.
- Location of tear[2]
  - The more peripheral, the better. Repair site needs access to the vascularity along the periphery (meniscal-capsular junction).
  - The more the tear involves the avascular central portion of the meniscus, the less healing potential it has unless combined with techniques such as vascular channeling or biologics to improve healing potential.

Why Use Inside/Out Technique[3]

- Considered historically to be the strongest type of repair.
- Needle puncture into meniscus has less impact than all-inside devices and outside-in systems.

Patient Indications/Contraindications

- Age
  - Must consider the risk vs the benefit of attempting meniscal repair in older patient.
  - The younger the patient, the greater the benefit of "saving the meniscus."
  - Younger patient also may have greater healing potential.
- Activity demands
  - The higher the activity demands of the patient, the greater the benefit of saving the meniscus.
- Body mass index (BMI)[4]
  - Likely does not have an effect on the success of a repair.
- Laxity
  - Knee instability may increase the risk of repair failure and is considered by many to be a contraindication to repair unless corrected at time of repair or as a staged procedure.
- Chondral status
  - The more severe the arthritis in the knee, the lower the risk/benefit ratio for the patient.
- Prior failed repair
  - Repeat attempt at stabilizing a peripheral meniscal tear can be done, but often the unstable fragment is significantly damaged from the previous sutures or implants during the mechanism of the new injury, making the success and benefit of a repeat repair attempt less attractive.
- Smoking[5]
  - Has been shown to increase risk of repair failure

Equipment Needed (Figs. 36-1 and 36-2)[3]

- Zone-specific cannulas
- Retractors to protect neurovascular structures and aid in retrieval of needles
  - Options include Army-Navy, a spoon, Henning retractor, bottom portion of a small or medium speculum
- Long flexible needles
- Suture: nonabsorbable typically preferred
- Rasp or shaver to abrade tear edges and synovium
- Standard arthroscopic equipment
- Standard open exposure tray
  - Multiple hemostats to snap each individual suture pairs for tying
  - Extra needle forceps for retrieval of meniscal needles
- Stool for surgical team member retrieving the needles
- Thigh tourniquet (inflate only if needed)

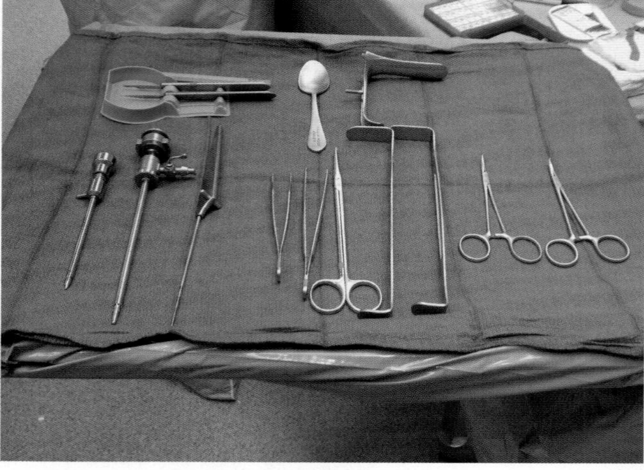

Figure 36-1 | Instruments required for successful inside-out repair.

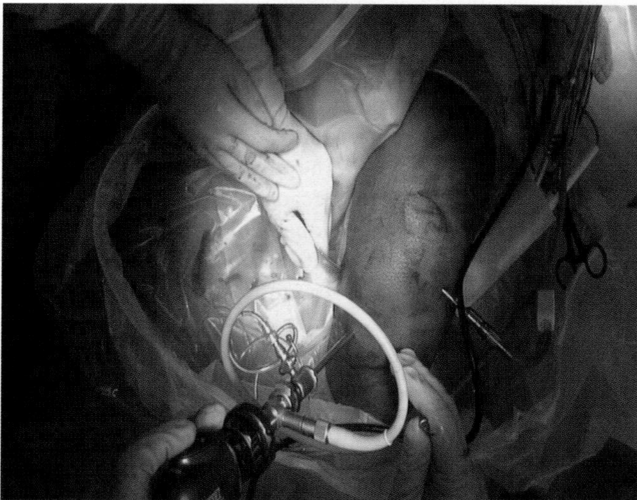

Figure 36-2 | Arthroscopic setup.

Positioning (Fig. 36-3)

- Typically supine, using the surgeon's preferred knee arthroscopy setup
- If using a thigh holder or lateral post, enough exposure of thigh above the knee should be ensured, as well as circumferential access to the knee for posterolateral or posteromedial incisions.

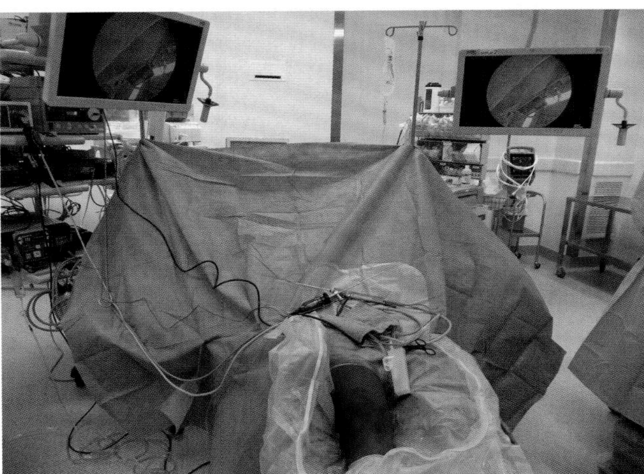

Figure 36-3 | Overview of help needed for successful inside-out meniscal repair. Surgeon is holding arthroscope and positioning zone-specific cannula, assistant is retrieving needles from posterior incision, and scrub tech is helping load and push needles.

Diagnostic Arthroscopy

- A complete diagnostic arthroscopy should be performed before treatment of the meniscal pathology (Fig. 36-4; Video 36-1).

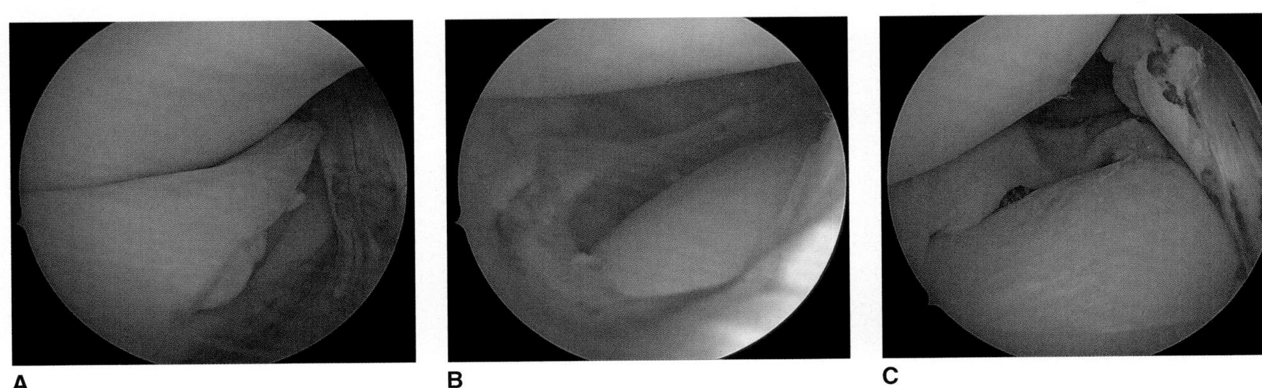

Figure 36-4 | Arthroscopic evaluation of bucket-handle lateral meniscus **(A)** and evaluation behind meniscus revealing tear at meniscal-capsular junction **(B)**. Meniscus reducible and appropriate for repair **(C)**.

- The status/condition of the entire knee should be verified.
- Meniscal repair should be part of a master plan for the entire knee (Fig. 36-5).

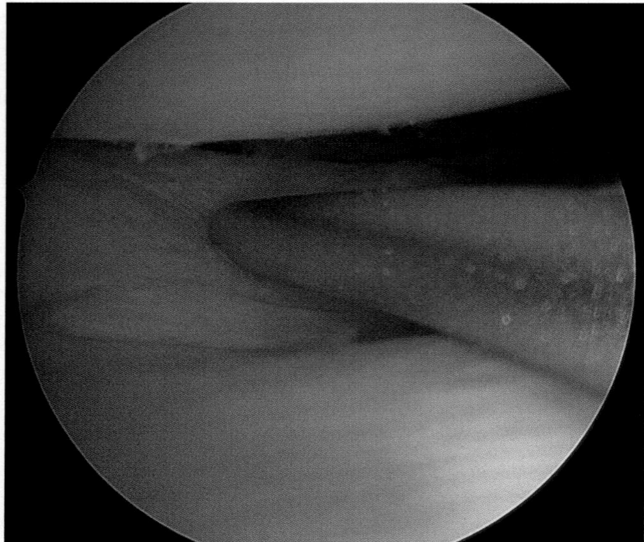

Figure 36-5 | Arthroscopic view of placement of zone-specific cannula. We recommend starting posterior and coming from the contralateral portal to direct needles away from neurovascular structures.

Lateral Meniscal Repair Exposure (Figs. 36-6 and 36-7)

- A 3- to 5-cm longitudinal incision is made over the posterolateral corner of the knee, just behind the lateral collateral ligament (LCL).
  - The incision is made with one-third above the joint line and two-thirds below the joint line.

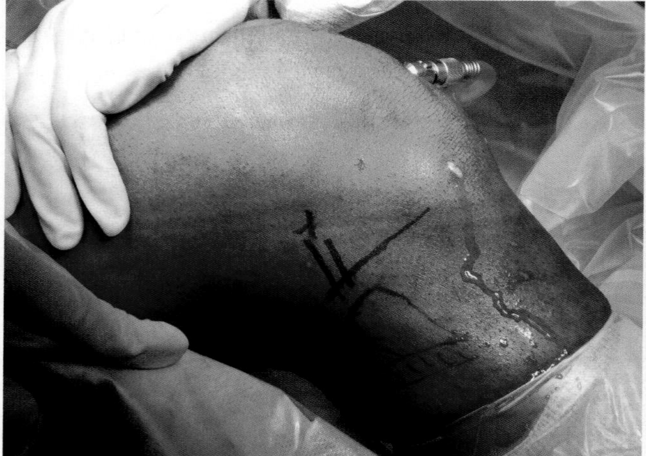

Figure 36-6 | Anatomic landmarks for incision.

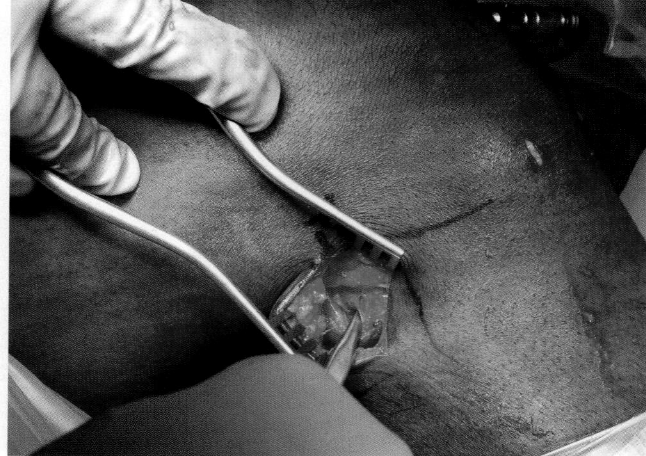

Figure 36-7 | Interval between the posterolateral capsule and the lateral head of the gastrocnemius is developed after the split between the iliotibial (IT) band and biceps.

- The deep fascia is exposed and the interval between the iliotibial (IT) band and biceps femoris is identified.
- The plane between the IT band and biceps femoris is developed to expose the posterolateral capsule behind the LCL.
- The plane between the posterolateral capsule and the lateral head of gastrocnemius is developed.
- A retractor is placed between the capsule and lateral head of gastrocnemius to protect the biceps femoris, peroneal nerve, and posterior knee neurovascular structures and to enable needle retrieval.

Lateral Complication Risks

- Peroneal nerve injury. Dissection and retraction should stay anterior to the biceps femoris and lateral head of gastrocnemius.

- Popliteal neurovascular injury. Needles should be captured by the retractor.
  - Zone-specific cannulas inserted through the contralateral (medial) portal are recommended for the posterior and most aspects of the lateral knee.

Medial Exposure

- A 3- to 4-cm longitudinal incision is made over the posteromedial joint, just behind the medial collateral ligament (MCL).
  - One-third of the incision is above the joint line and two-thirds below the joint line.
- The fascia over pes tendons is exposed and incised along the anterior margin of the sartorius.
- The pes tendons are bluntly dissected free, and the interval between the medial head of the gastrocnemius and the posteromedial tibia is located to expose the posteromedial capsule.
- A retractor is placed to protect the pes tendons and saphenous nerve and to allow needle retrieval.

Medial Complications Risks

- Saphenous nerve injury. The nerve should be posterior to the incision and protected by a retractor.
- Popliteal neurovascular injury. Needles must be captured by the retractor.
  - Approaching the medial meniscus from the contralateral (lateral) portal with zone-specific cannulas is recommended.

Personnel Needs

- Typically requires three sets of hands.
  - One to hold arthroscope and cannula
  - One to pass the needles
  - One to retrieve the needles

Repair Technique Principles

- Anatomic reduction of the tear.
- Vertical mattress sutures are preferred.
  - Oblique-oriented sutures have excellent strength as well.
- Sutures are placed every 3-5 mm (Fig. 36-8).
  - Sutures can be placed on both the superior and inferior aspects of the meniscus for appropriate compression of the repair site.

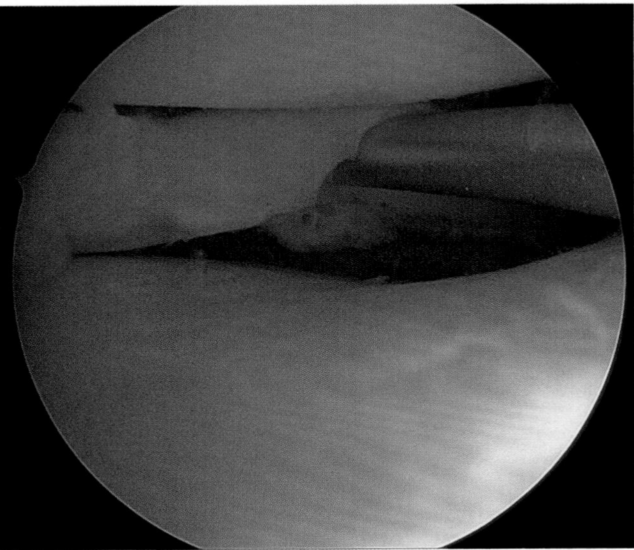

Figure 36-8 | Sutures placed on superior and inferior aspects of meniscus to balance repair.

- Meniscal tear edges and surrounding synovium are abraded to stimulate bleeding and initiate a healing response. This can be done with a rasp or a shaver (Fig. 36-9; Video 36-2).

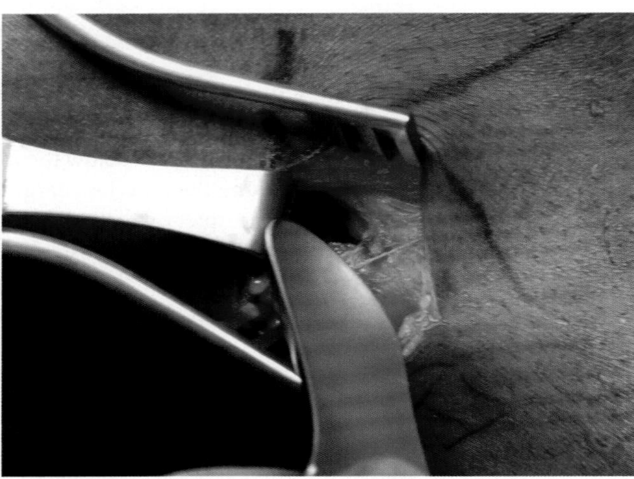

Figure 36-9 | After initial development of the plane between the lateral head of the gastrocnemius and the posterolateral capsule, a speculum or spoon can slide over an Army-Navy retractor.

- Chondral scuffing should be avoided.
- Enough sutures are placed to ensure strong repair and minimize gaping at the repair site (Videos 36-3 and 36-4).
- Needles are directed away from the midline of the knee and toward the retractor to avoid inadvertent passage of a needle through the posterior knee structures uncaptured by the retractor (Fig. 36-10).
- Tying sutures with the knee in extension can minimize the risk of capturing significant posterior capsule in the repair and producing a postoperative knee flexion contracture (Figs. 36-11 to 36-14; Video 36-5).
- If a biological enhancement to healing is used, it can be placed in the tear site before the sutures are tied.
- A thigh tourniquet is applied but is inflated only as needed.

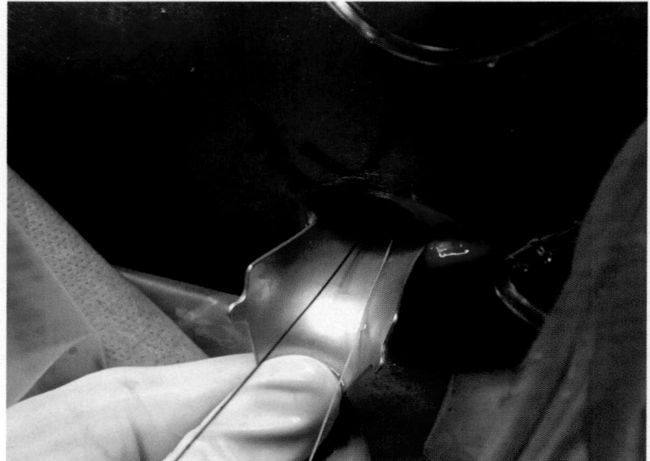

Figure 36-10 | Needles are retrieved by an assistant. Communication is paramount, and care must be taken to prevent iatrogenic needle sticks.

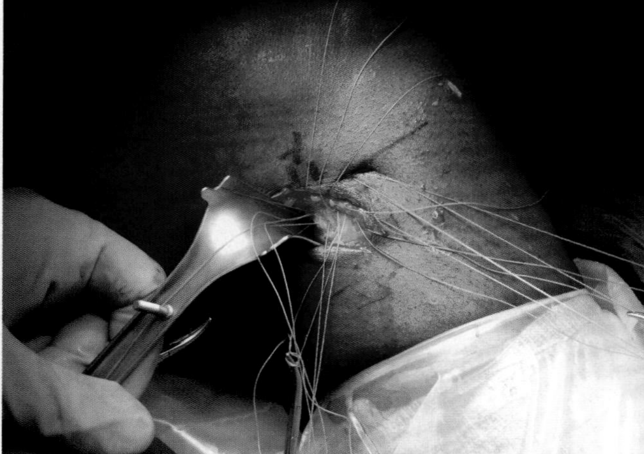

Figure 36-11 | Attempting to arrange and order paired sutures can prevent aggravation later when tying.

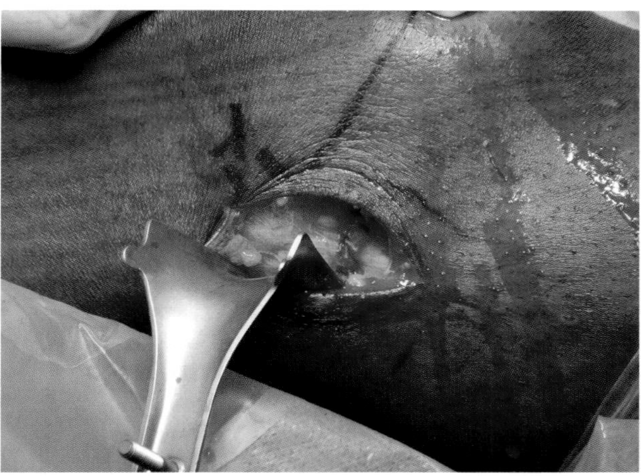

Figure 36-12 | Tying knots from posterior to anterior with the knee bent about 30 degrees.

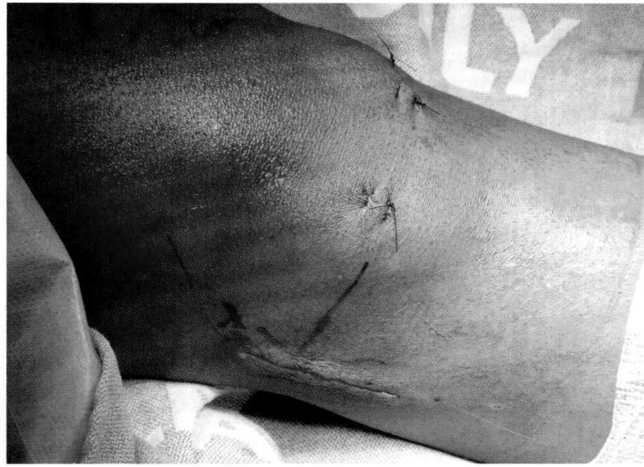

Figure 36-13 | Final closure.

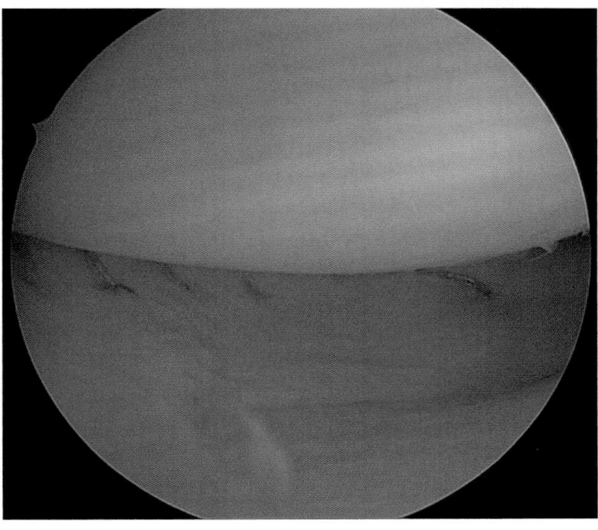

Figure 36-14 | Repaired meniscus.

Biological Enhancement

- Fibrin clot, whole blood, and platelet-rich plasma have been used to enhance the biological healing potential at the repair site. Efficacy of these efforts is still being investigated.
- A limited notchplasty or microfracture of the notch also has been described to create an environment similar to that of anterior cruciate ligament (ACL) reconstruction for meniscal healing (Fig. 36-15).

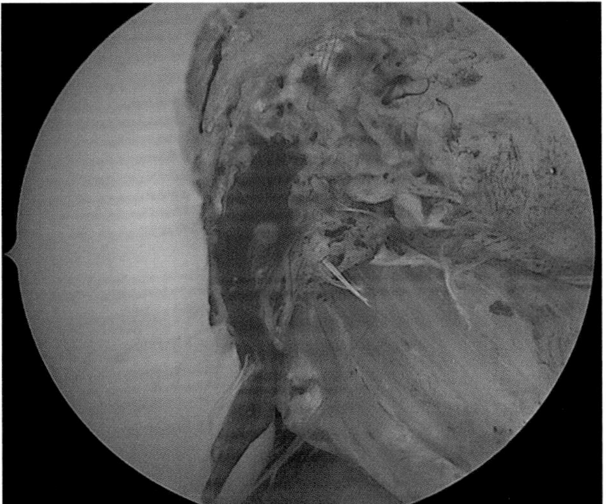

Figure 36-15 | Small notchplasty performed to help with healing.

Postoperative Care (Fig. 36-16)

- Most meniscal repairs involve the posterior one-third of the meniscus. The greater the knee flexion, the more the posterior portion of the meniscus is pinched and the repair is placed under tension. Avoiding weight-bearing knee flexion for several months after a meniscal repair is typically recommended.
- Many believe that, after a posterior repair, weight bearing in full extension does not stress the repair.
- Traditionally, most surgeons have recommended a period of nonweight bearing after a meniscal repair.

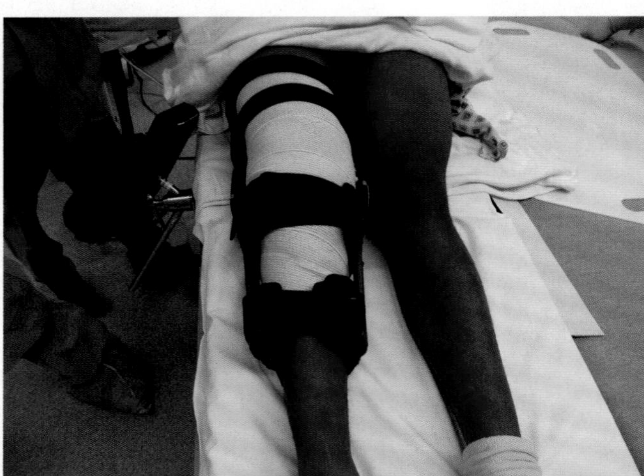

Figure 36-16 | Patient braced for initial postoperative care.

Results[5–7]

- Repair of peripheral meniscal tears has an ~85% success rate.
- Early evidence showed that repairs are more likely to be successful when done in conjunction with an ACL reconstruction; however, more recent reports are less supportive of this concept.
- Smoking has a detrimental effect on outcome.

References

1. Sgaglione NA, Steadman J, Shaffer B, et al. Current concepts in meniscus surgery: resection to replacement. *Arthroscopy.* 2003;19:161-188.
2. Rubman MH, Noyes FR, Barber-Westin SD. Arthroscopic repair of meniscal tears that extend into the avascular zone: a review of 198 single and complex tears. *Am J Sports Med.* 1998;26:87-95.
3. Bottoni CR, Arciero RA. Conventional meniscal repair techniques. *Oper Tech Orthop.* 2000;10:194-208.
4. Sommerfeldt MF, Magnussen RA, Randall KL, et al. The relationship between body mass index and risk of failure following meniscus repair. *J Knee Surg.* 2016;29(8):645-648.
5. Blackwell R, Schmitt LC, Flanigan DC, Magnussen RA. Smoking increases the risk of early meniscus repair failure. *Knee Surg Sports Traumatol Arthrosc.* 2016;24(5):1540-1543.
6. Johnson MJ, Lucas GL, Dusek JK, et al. Isolated arthroscopic meniscal repair: a long-term outcome study (more than 10 years). *Am J Sports Med.* 1999;27:44-49.
7. Westermann RW, Wright RW, Spindler KP, Huston LJ; MOON Knee Group, Wolf BR. Meniscal repair with concurrent anterior cruciate ligament reconstruction: operative success and patient outcomes at 6-year follow-up. *Am J Sports Med.* 2014;42(9):2184-2192.

Chapter 37
Arthroscopic Meniscal Root Repair

ANDREW G. GEESLIN
JORGE A. CHAHLA
ROBERT F. LAPRADE

Preoperative Workup

- Anteroposterior, Rosenberg, sunrise, long-leg alignment, and lateral knee radiographs are obtained in all patients.
- Magnetic resonance imaging is routinely obtained in the evaluation of meniscal root tears (77% sensitive, 72% specific, positive predictive value 22%, and negative predictive value 97%). The following are signs of root tears (Fig. 37-1):
  - Meniscal extrusion (>3 mm) and edema of the femoral condyle on a coronal section.
  - Sagittal view demonstrating the absence of the posterior horn of the meniscus ("ghost sign") or a thin fluid interposition at the native root attachment location.
  - If obtained at the correct height, the axial view may also demonstrate a displaced root tear with fluid interposition between the root and the native attachment location.

Indications/Contraindications

- Indications
  - Acute, traumatic root tears (Figs. 37-2 and 37-3) in patients with normal or nearly normal cartilage (Outerbridge <3) and minimal joint space narrowing (Kellgren-Lawrence <3).
  - Chronic symptomatic root tears in physiologically young or middle-aged patients with normal or nearly normal cartilage (Outerbridge <3) and minimal joint space narrowing (Kellgren-Lawrence <3).
- Contraindications
  - Poor surgical candidates (multiple comorbidities or advanced age), those with advanced osteoarthritis (grade 3 or 4 chondromalacia of the ipsilateral compartment), and those with asymptomatic chronic meniscal root tears are excluded from surgical repair.
  - Patients with significant mechanical axis malalignment involving the affected compartment may have inferior outcomes; consideration should be given to correction of the mechanical axis concurrently or before the meniscal root repair.

Sterile Instruments, Equipment

- Arthroscopy monitor, light source, fluid pump
- Arthroscope, shaver, radio-frequency probe
- Arthroscopic probe, grasper, arthroscopic scissors

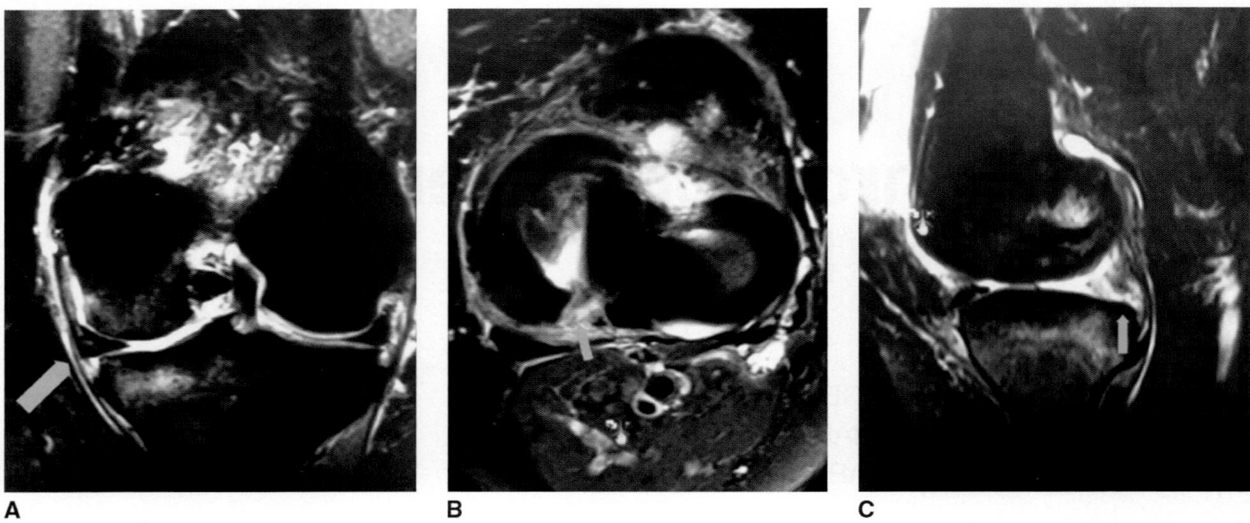

Figure 37-1 | Visualization of meniscal root tears in three planes via magnetic resonance imaging. **A.** Coronal T2-weighted section demonstrating medial meniscal extrusion (*arrow*) (left knee). **B.** Axial image demonstrating fluid interposition in the region of meniscus root and posterior horn at the location of a radial root tear (*arrow*) (right knee). **C.** Sagittal image demonstrating ghost sign (*arrow*) (right knee). (Reproduced from Bhatia S, LaPrade CM, Ellman MB, LaPrade RF. Meniscal root tears: significance, diagnosis, and treatment. *Am J Sports Med*. 2014;42(12):3016-3030, with permission.)

- Aiming device, drill sleeve, drill
- Cannula for suture passing
- Cannula for possible accessory posteromedial or posterolateral portal
- Arthroscopic suture passer
- Implants
  - High-strength, nonabsorbable no. 2 suture
  - Suture button

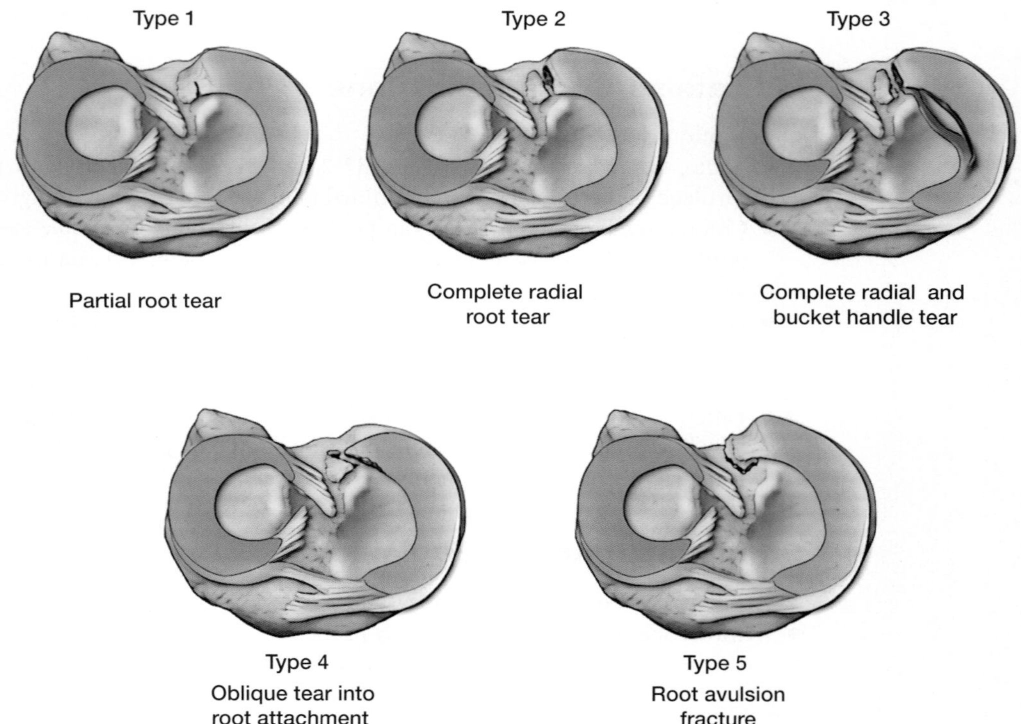

Figure 37-2 | Root tear classification including partial tear, complete tear (at varying distance and obliquity relative to the anatomic root attachment), combined meniscal tear patterns, and bony avulsions. (Reproduced from LaPrade CM, James EW, Cram TR, Feagin JA, Engebretsen L, LaPrade RF. Meniscal root tears: a classification system based on tear morphology. *Am J Sports Med*. 2015;43(2):363-369, with permission.)

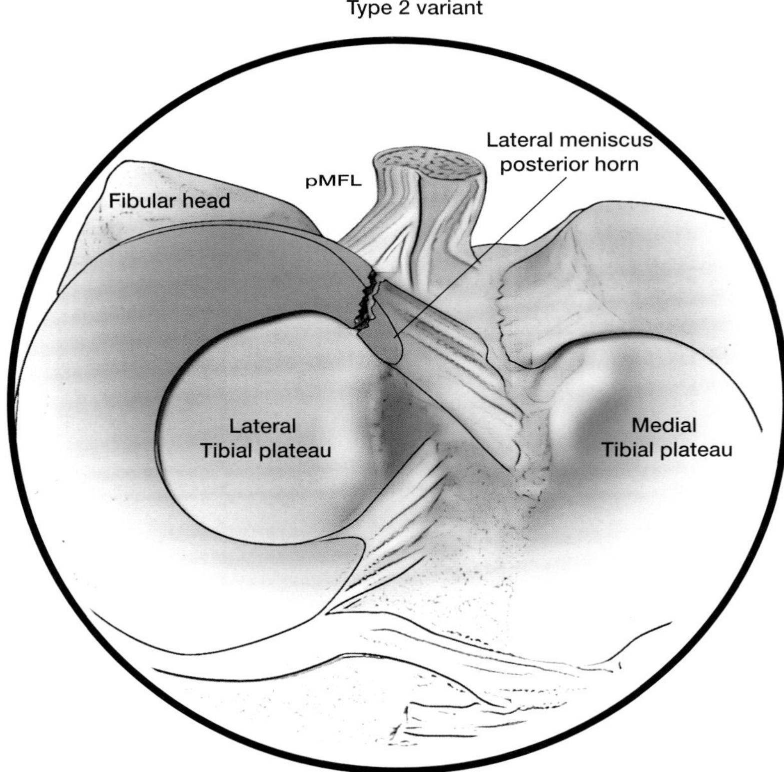

Figure 37-3 | Illustration of a left knee lateral meniscal posterior root tear with an intact posterior meniscofemoral ligament (pMFL). Lateral meniscal posterior root tears may also occur in the setting of a torn or absent pMFL. (Reproduced from LaPrade CM, James EW, Cram TR, Feagin JA, Engebretsen L, LaPrade RF. Meniscal root tears: a classification system based on tear morphology. *Am J Sports Med*. 2015;43(2):363-369, with permission.)

Positioning (Fig. 37-4)

- The patient is positioned supine with the foot of the bed dropped.
- The surgical extremity is placed in a thigh holder with a well-padded thigh tourniquet.
- Contralateral extremity is placed in a well-leg holder with the bony prominences well padded.

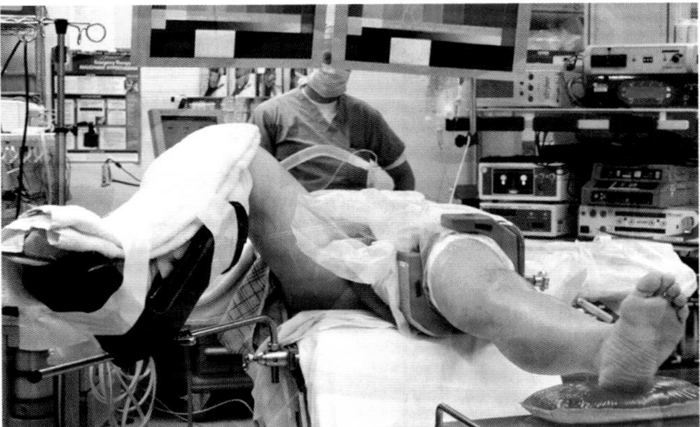

Figure 37-4 | Patient positioning on the operating table is shown. The surgical limb (*left*) is placed into a leg holder, allowing the surgeon to freely manipulate the knee during the procedure. The nonoperative limb is kept on a well-padded abduction stirrup.

Surgical Approach

- Standard anterolateral and anteromedial parapatellar portals and possibly posteromedial or posterolateral accessory portal are used.
- A diagnostic arthroscopy is performed to identify concomitant meniscal, chondral, and ligamentous pathology.

- Complete root tear is confirmed, and tear pattern (ie, avulsion, radial tear adjacent to root) is identified (Figs. 37-2, 37-3, and 37-5).

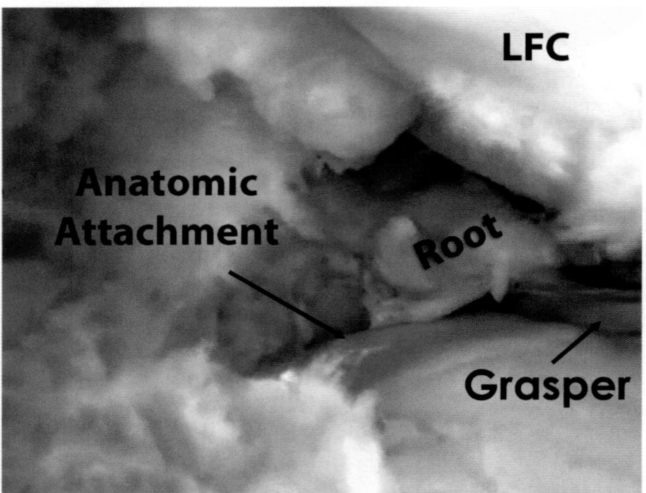

Figure 37-5 | Left knee arthroscopic image demonstrating a displaced lateral meniscal posterior root tear in a patient with a concomitant ACL tear. The root is shown displaced from its anatomic attachment location. LFC, lateral femoral condyle.

Medial Meniscus Posterior Root Repair Technique

- Through the anteromedial portal, a grasper is used to reduce the root to the anatomic attachment site. The most reproducible landmark for the medial meniscus root attachment is the apex of the medial tibial eminence (MTE). The distance between the MTE apex to the center of the root attachment is 9.6 mm posterior and 0.7 mm lateral (Fig. 37-6).
  - In chronic tears, arthroscopic scissors are required to release the scarred root from the posterior capsule and allow for an anatomic reduction.

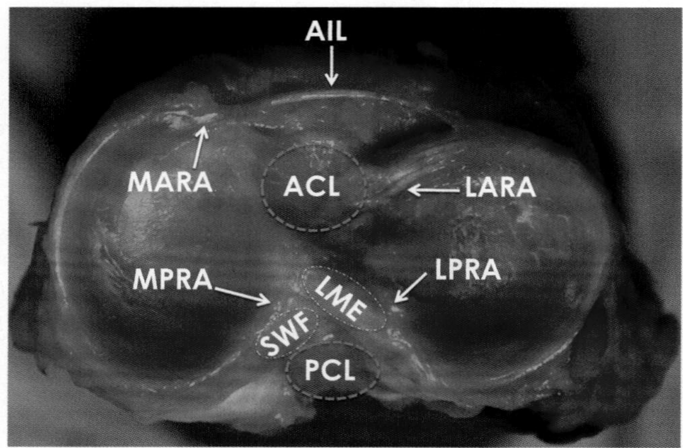

Figure 37-6 | Cadaver knee dissection (superior view) demonstrating the anatomic landmarks to identify posterior meniscal root attachment in a right knee. AIL, anterior intermeniscal ligament; ACL, anterior cruciate ligament; PCL, posterior cruciate ligament; MARA, medial meniscus anterior root attachment; LARA, lateral meniscus anterior root attachment; MPRA, medial meniscus posterior root attachment; LPRA, lateral meniscus posterior root attachment; SWF, shiny white fibers; LME, lateral meniscal expansion.

- The arthroscopic shaver and radio-frequency probe are used to debride the root attachment site and prepare a bony surface for healing.

- An incision is made slightly medial to the tibial tubercle, and the aiming guide is used to place the first tibial tunnel guide pin and cannulated sleeve along the posterior aspect of the root insertion. The guide pin and cannulated sleeve for a second tunnel are placed slightly anterior to the first tunnel using a 5-mm offset guide. Appropriate placement is verified arthroscopically (Fig. 37-7), and the guide pins are then removed, leaving the sleeves in place.

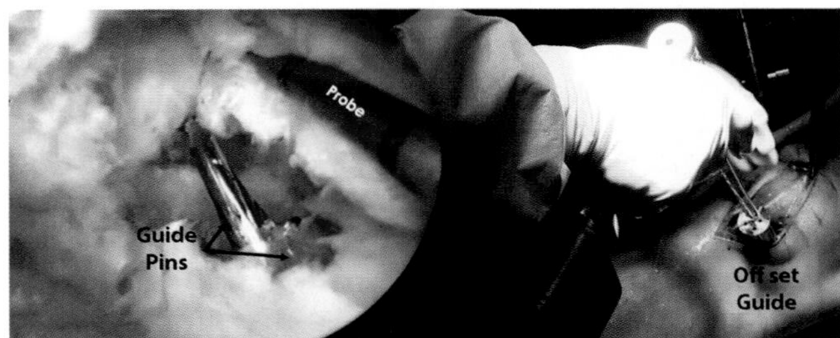

Figure 37-7 | Two transtibial tunnels are created at the location of the lateral meniscal root attachment (*left*, *inset*) with the use of an aiming device. The posterior tunnel is drilled first and a sheath is left in place. Using an offset guide (*right photograph*), the second tunnel is created approximately 5 mm anterior to the first.

- Suture passage (two simple sutures) is completed with a self-delivery device through the anteromedial portal. An accessory portal is created to allow grasping of the root during suture passage. The first suture is passed at the posterior aspect of the root, and the second is passed at the anterior aspect. A cannula is used to ensure that there are no soft tissue bridges formed anteriorly in the retropatellar fat pad during suture passage.
  - An accessory posterior portal may be required if the sutures cannot be passed through standard anterior portals because of a narrow notch, intact cruciate ligaments, or tight compartments.
- A looped passing wire is advanced up the posterior tunnel, and the posterior sutures are shuttled through the tunnel (Fig. 37-8). This process is repeated for the anterior tunnel.
  - The guide sleeves are recessed 1-2 mm before suture shuttling to avoid fraying/damaging the suture limbs.

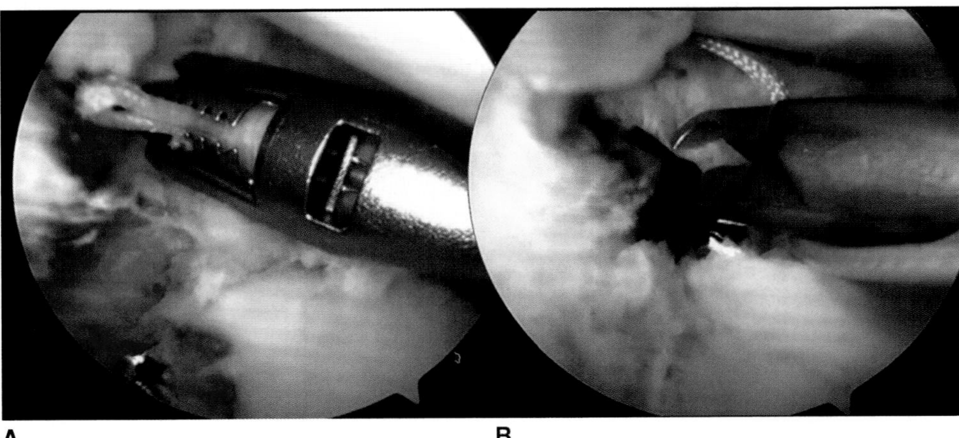

Figure 37-8 | Arthroscopic view through the anteromedial portal of the lateral posterior root. **A.** Suture passage through the meniscal root using an arthroscopic passing device. **B.** A nitinol wire is inserted through the posterior transtibial tunnel and retrieved through the anterolateral portal for subsequent suture shuttling.

- The sutures are tied over a metallic button at the anteromedial tibia (Fig. 37-9)

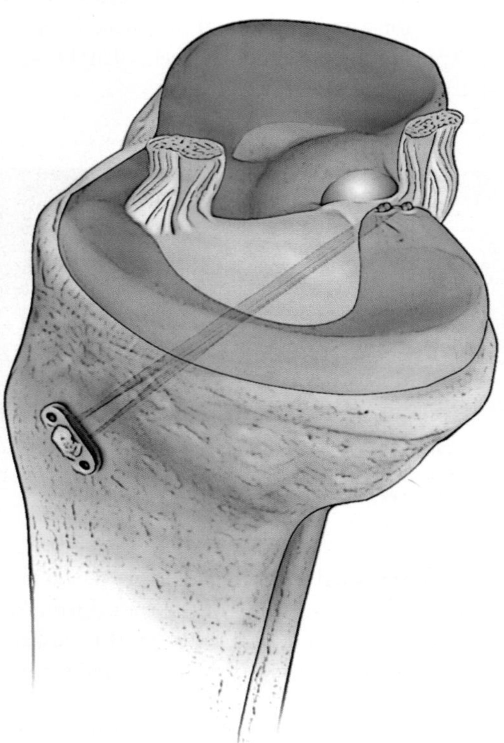

Figure 37-9 | An illustration of a two-tunnel transtibial posterior medial meniscal root tear is shown. The sutures are tied over a button at the anteromedial tibia. (Reproduced from Padalecki JR, Jansson KS, Smith SD, et al. Biomechanical consequences of a complete radial tear adjacent to the medial meniscus posterior root attachment site: in situ pull-out repair restores derangement of joint mechanics. *Am J Sports Med*. 2014;42(3):699-707, with permission.)

Lateral Meniscus Posterior Root Repair Technique

- Most commonly, lateral meniscal root tears occur concurrently with an anterior cruciate ligament (ACL) tear, which facilitates access and visualization through the notch, with the knee in the figure-of-four position.
- Through the anterolateral portal, a grasper is used to reduce the root to the anatomic attachment site (Fig. 37-10). The most consistent landmark for the lateral meniscus posterior root attachment is the apex of the lateral tibial eminence (LTE). The center of the lateral meniscus posterior root is consistently located 1.5 mm posterior and 4.2 mm medial to the LTE.

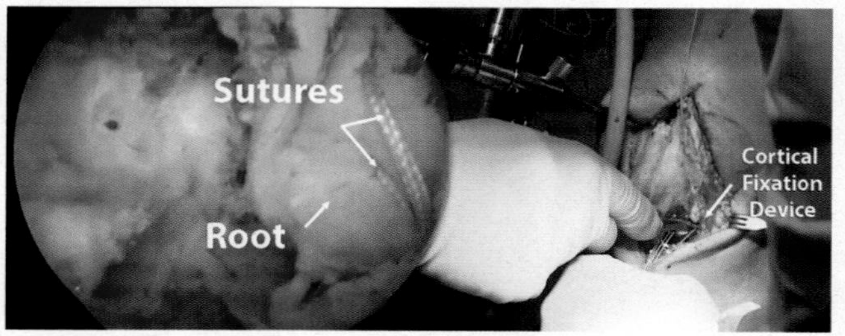

Figure 37-10 | Anatomic lateral posterior meniscal root repair visualized through the arthroscope (*inset, left*) and during suture knot tying over a cortical button (*right*).

  - In chronic tears, arthroscopic scissors are required to release the scarred root from the posterior capsule and allow for an anatomic reduction.
- The arthroscopic shaver and radio-frequency probe are used to debride the root attachment site and expose a bony surface.
- An incision is made at the anterolateral tibia, distal to the medial aspect of Gerdy tubercle. The anterior compartment musculature is elevated off the tibia extending ~1 cm distally. The aiming guide is used to place the first tibial tunnel guide pin and cannulated sleeve along the posterior aspect of the root insertion. The guide pin and cannulated sleeve for a second tunnel are placed slightly anterior to the first tunnel using a 5-mm offset guide. Appropriate placement is verified arthroscopically, and the guide pins are then removed, leaving the sleeves in place.

- Suture passage (two simple sutures) is completed through the anteromedial portal. If necessary, an accessory portal is created to allow grasping of the root during suture passage. The first suture is passed at the posterior aspect of the root, and the second is passed at the anterior aspect. A cannula is used to ensure that there are no soft tissue bridges formed anterior during suture passage.
  - An accessory posterior portal may be required if the sutures cannot be passed through standard anterior portals because of a narrow notch, intact cruciate ligaments, or tight compartments.
- A looped passing wire is advanced up the posterior transtibial tunnel, and the posterior sutures are shuttled through the tunnel. This process is repeated for the anterior tunnel.
  - The guide sleeves are recessed 1-2 mm before suture shuttling to avoid fraying/damaging the suture limbs.
- Sutures are tied over a button with the knee in 90 degrees of flexion and neutral rotation.

Rehabilitation

- Patients are restricted to non–weight bearing for 6 weeks.
- Immediate postoperative physical therapy includes early passive range of motion exercises in a safe zone of 0-90 degrees of flexion for the initial 2 weeks.
- After 2 weeks, further increases in knee flexion are allowed as tolerated.
- Progressive advancement to full weight bearing begins at 6 weeks.
- Deep leg presses and squats >70 degrees of knee flexion should be avoided for at least 4 months after surgery.

Suggested Readings

Bhatia S, LaPrade CM, Ellman MB, LaPrade RF. Meniscal root tears: significance, diagnosis, and treatment. *Am J Sports Med.* 2014;42(12):3016-3030.

Chahla J, Moulton SG, LaPrade CM, Dean CS, LaPrade RF. Posterior meniscal root repair: the transtibial double tunnel pullout technique. *Arthrosc Tech.* 2016;5(2):e291-e296.

Ellman MB, LaPrade CM, Smith SD, et al. Structural properties of the meniscal roots. *Am J Sports Med.* 2014;42(8):1881-1887.

Geeslin AG, Civitarese D, Turnbull TL, Dornan GJ, Fuso FA, LaPrade RF. Influence of lateral meniscal posterior root avulsions and the meniscofemoral ligaments on tibiofemoral contact mechanics. *Knee Surg Sports Traumatol Arthrosc.* 2016;24(5):1469-1477.

Johannsen AM, Civitarese DM, Padalecki JR, Goldsmith MT, Wijdicks CA, LaPrade RF. Qualitative and quantitative anatomic analysis of the posterior root attachments of the medial and lateral menisci. *Am J Sports Med.* 2012;40(10):2342-2347.

LaPrade CM, Foad A, Smith SD, et al. Biomechanical consequences of a nonanatomic posterior medial meniscal root repair. *Am J Sports Med.* 2015;43(4):912-920.

LaPrade CM, James EW, Cram TR, Feagin JA, Engebretsen L, LaPrade RF. Meniscal root tears: a classification system based on tear morphology. *Am J Sports Med.* 2015;43(2):363-369.

LaPrade CM, Jisa KA, Cram TR, LaPrade RF. Posterior lateral meniscal root tear due to a malpositioned double-bundle anterior cruciate ligament reconstruction tibial tunnel. *Knee Surg Sports Traumatol Arthrosc.* 2015;23(12):3670-3673.

LaPrade CM, Smith SD, Rasmussen MT, et al. Consequences of tibial tunnel reaming on the meniscal roots during cruciate ligament reconstruction in a cadaveric model, Part 2: the posterior cruciate ligament. *Am J Sports Med.* 2015;43(1):207-212.

LaPrade RF, Ho CP, James E, Crespo B, LaPrade CM, Matheny LM. Diagnostic accuracy of 3.0 T magnetic resonance imaging for the detection of meniscus posterior root pathology. *Knee Surg Sports Traumatol Arthrosc.* 2015;23(1):152-157.

Moatshe G, Chahla J, Slette E, Engebretsen L, LaPrade RF. Posterior meniscal root injuries. *Acta Orthop.* 2016;87(5):452-458.

Padalecki JR, Jansson KS, Smith SD, et al. Biomechanical consequences of a complete radial tear adjacent to the medial meniscus posterior root attachment site: in situ pull-out repair restores derangement of joint mechanics. *Am J Sports Med.* 2014;42(3):699-707.

Chapter 38
Arthroscopic Medial Meniscal Allograft

JAMES D. McDERMOTT
RYAN J. WARTH
CHRISTOPHER D. HARNER

Selection Criteria

- Age (relative) 14-55 years
- Pain localized to joint line
- Previous surgery
- Status of articular cartilage
  - 45-degree posterior-anterior weight-bearing radiograph
  - MRI
  - Arthroscopic findings
- Alignment (long cassette)
  - Within 3 degrees of normal knee.
  - If >3 degrees, osteotomy should be considered.

Sterile Instruments/Equipment

- Graft choice
  - Fresh frozen allografts
  - Donor age 15-35 years
  - Size matched
    - Radiographs vs MRI
  - *Nonirradiated*
- 2-0 synthetic, nonabsorbable braided suture on a 10-in straight-cutting needle
- No. 2 synthetic, nonabsorbable braided suture
- No. 0 synthetic, nonabsorbable braided suture
- Specific cannulas, various flexion angles
- Popliteal retractor
- Anterior cruciate ligament (ACL) guide, tip-to-tip
- 3/32-in (or 2.4-mm) guide wires
- Standard arthroscopic equipment/setup
- Standard arthroscopic rasp
- 30- and 70-degree arthroscopes

Positioning

- Supine.
- Pneumatic leg holder (Fig. 38-1).
  - As an alternative, sandbags attached to the bed at multiple flexion angles can be used.

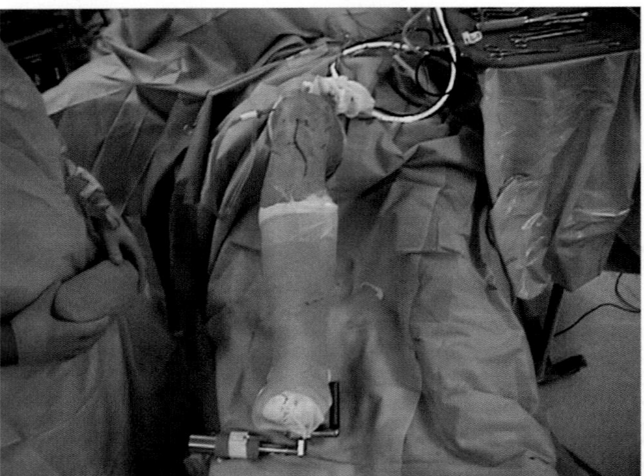

Figure 38-1 | Pneumatic leg holder.

- No tourniquet is used.
- All planned incisions are marked.
  - This may be difficult if there are multiple prior incisions.
  - The goal is to have 6-cm skin bridges between adjacent incisions.
  - This sometimes requires using a less than ideal prior incision and creating a skin flap.

Meniscal Allograft Preparation

- The meniscus is detached from bone.
- Soft tissue is debrided from the meniscal rim.
- A no. 2 nonabsorbable suture is secured to the anterior and posterior roots.
- Graft passage/fixation.
- Three or four no. 2 nonabsorbable sutures are placed in the posterior horn (vertical mattress stitch).
- The anterior and posterior horns and top of the meniscus are marked with a marking pen (Fig. 38-2).
  - The anterior horn is marked with a "T."

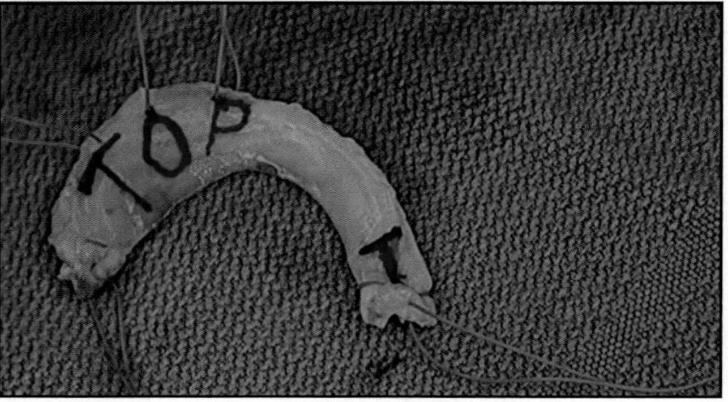

Figure 38-2 | The anterior and posterior horns on top of the meniscus are marked with a marking pen.

Surgical Approach/Technique

- Transosseous fixation using combined arthroscopic and open approach
- Arthroscopy
  - Diagnostic arthroscopy
    - Standard anteromedial/anterolateral arthroscopy portals are used.
    - The articular cartilage of the medial compartment is assessed to reconfirm that the patient is a candidate for a meniscal allograft.
      - If the above criteria are met, the meniscal allograft is thawed.
    - The degree of meniscal deficiency is documented.

- Anterior-to-posterior measurement of the medial compartment is made to confirm that the allograft is appropriately sized and matched to the patient (Fig. 38-3A and B).

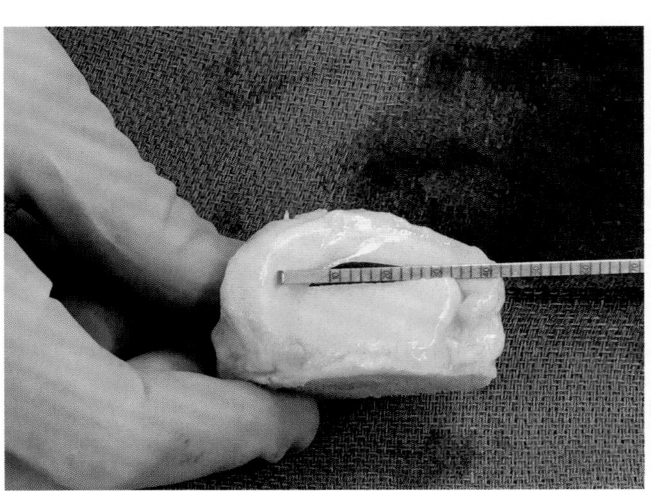
A

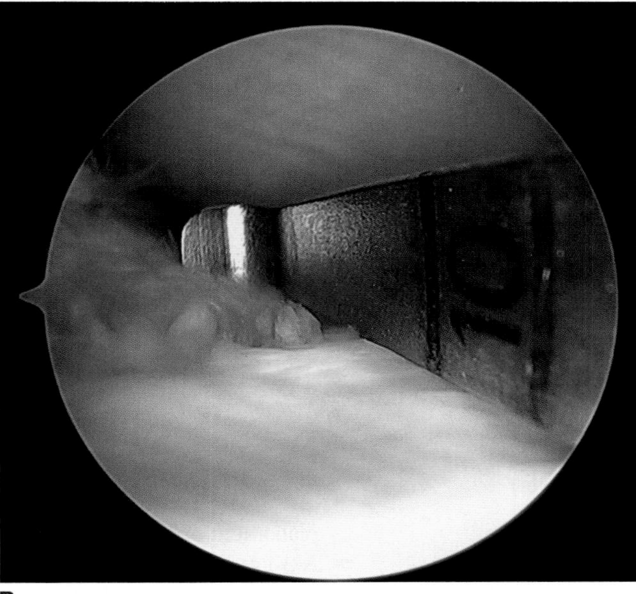
B

Figure 38-3 | A and B. Anterior-to-posterior measurement of medial compartment to confirm allograft is appropriately sized and matched to the patient.

- If appropriately sized/matched, the medial meniscal rim is prepared and preserved.
  - Insertion sites are preserved.
  - Excellent tissue is needed to anatomically/biomechanically secure the transplant.
- Posterior tunnel placement
  - A reverse notchplasty can be done with an osteotome if overgrown osteophytes are present anteriorly (Fig. 38-4).

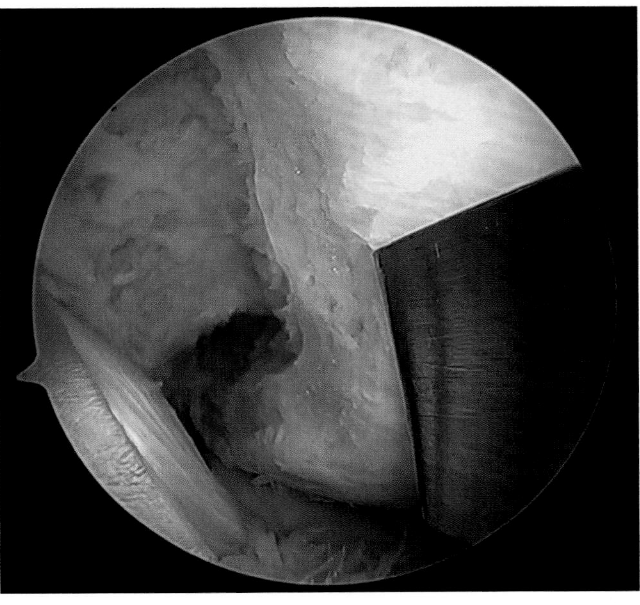

Figure 38-4 | Reverse notchplasty with the use of an osteotome if overgrown osteophytes are present.

  - A posteromedial portal is created for identification of the tibial insertion of the meniscus.
  - An ACL tip-to-tip guide through the anterolateral (AL) portal is placed directly on the native posterior root medial meniscal insertion site (Fig. 38-5).

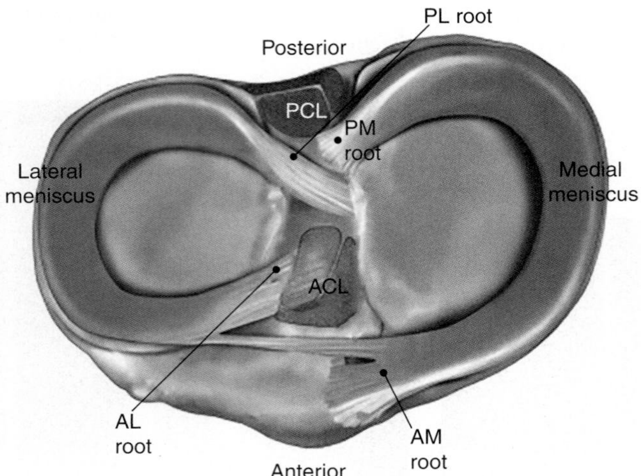

Figure 38-5 | ACL tip-to-tip guide, through the AL portal is placed place directly on the native posterior root medial meniscus insertion site.

- The arthroscope is placed in the anteromedial (AM) portal to confirm placement of the guide underneath the posterior cruciate ligament (PCL).
- The arthroscope is then switched to the posteromedial (PM) portal to directly observe guide placement on the root insertion.
- A 3-cm incision is made on the contralateral side of knee through which the ACL guide is positioned and a guidewire is drilled (Fig. 38-6).
- The guidewire is exchanged with a Hewson suture passer.

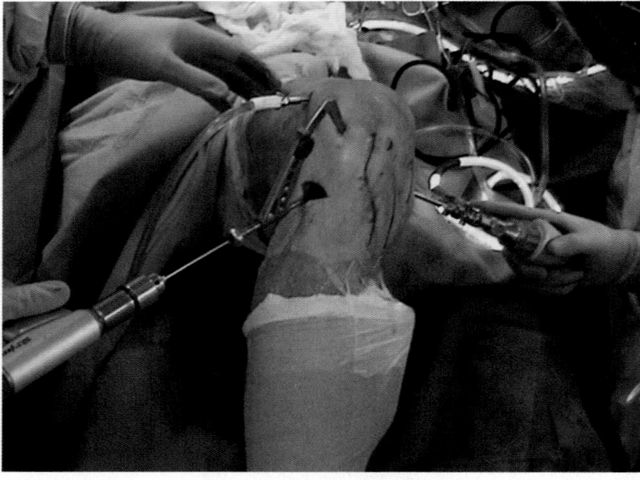

Figure 38-6 | Three-centimeter incision made on contralateral side of the knee: ACL guide positioned, guidewire drilled.

- Medial parapatellar arthrotomy
  - The anterior capsule is opened through the AM portal.
  - The anterior rim of the meniscus is identified and the inner two-thirds is removed.
  - The rim of the anterior horn of the meniscus is tagged with several no. 0 braided, nonabsorbable sutures.
    - "Meniscal" needle
    - Vertical mattress stitch
  - Anterior tunnel placement
    - The ACL tip-to-tip guide is placed through an arthrotomy directly on the native medial meniscal anterior root insertion site, which is identified arthroscopically.
    - A 1-cm bone bridge is created between the tunnels on the contralateral side of the knee.
      - The ACL guide is positioned, and the guidewire is drilled 1 cm medial from the posterior tunnel.
      - Sutures will be tied over the top after graft passage.
    - The guidewire is exchanged with the Hewson suture passer.

- Posteromedial arthrotomy
  - The interval between the posterior oblique ligament (POL) and the medial collateral ligament (MCL) "window" is opened (Fig. 38-7).

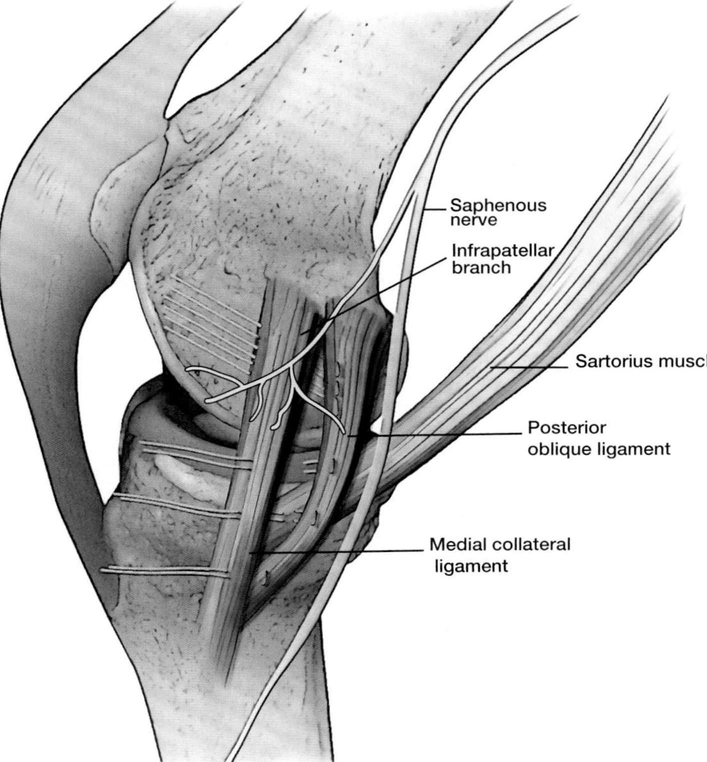

Figure 38-7 | Open interval between posterior oblique ligament and medial collateral ligament "window."

  - The posterior border of the superficial MCL is identified.
  - The infrapatellar branch of the saphenous nerve (proximal aspect of incision) is identified and carefully protected with a vessel loop (Fig. 38-8).
  - The capsule is incised in the MCL/POL interval ("window"), creating a posteromedial arthrotomy for graft passage.
  - The insertion of the POL is detached and tagged with horizontal mattress no. 2 nonabsorbable suture.
  - The meniscal rim is identified and painted blue with a marking pen.
- Graft passage
  - With the knee in 90 degrees of flexion, the graft is passed through the posteromedial arthrotomy "window" (Fig. 38-8).

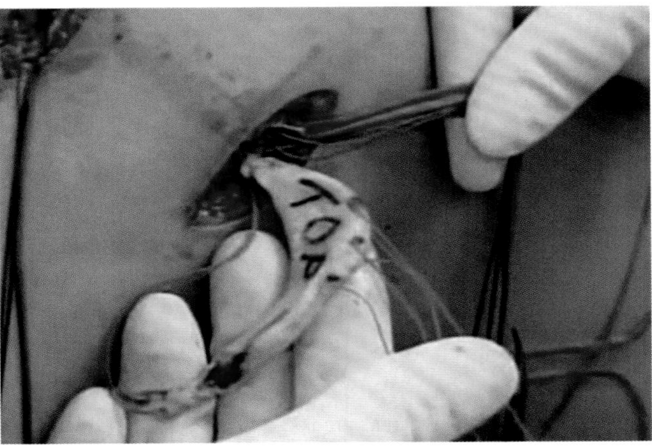

Figure 38-8 | Graft is passed through posteromedial arthrotomy.

- The posterior horn is passed first, then the anterior horn is passed intra-articularly under the superficial medial collateral ligament (Fig. 38-9).

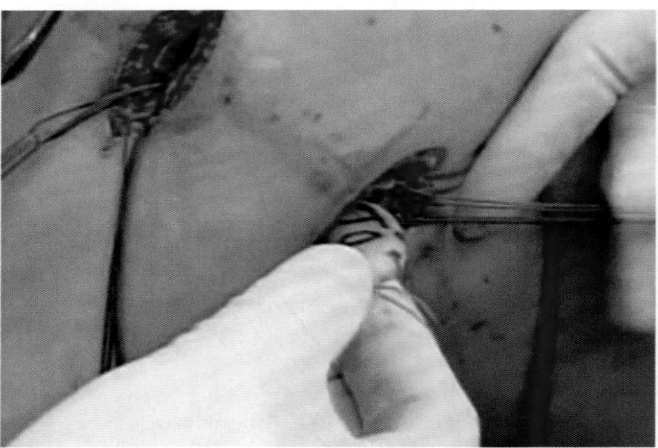

Figure 38-9 | The posterior horn is passed first, then the anterior horn.

  - A Hewson suture passer or shuttling sutures are used.
  - After the anterior/posterior horns are passed, a gentle valgus force with flexion and extension of the knee will aid in seating the meniscus.
- Once the graft is reduced, the knee is cycled 5-10 times from 0-90 degrees making sure that the posterior horn is reduced first, then the anterior horn is reduced second.
- The sutures are tied over the bone bridge, securing the anterior and posterior horns within the transosseous tunnels (Fig. 38-10).

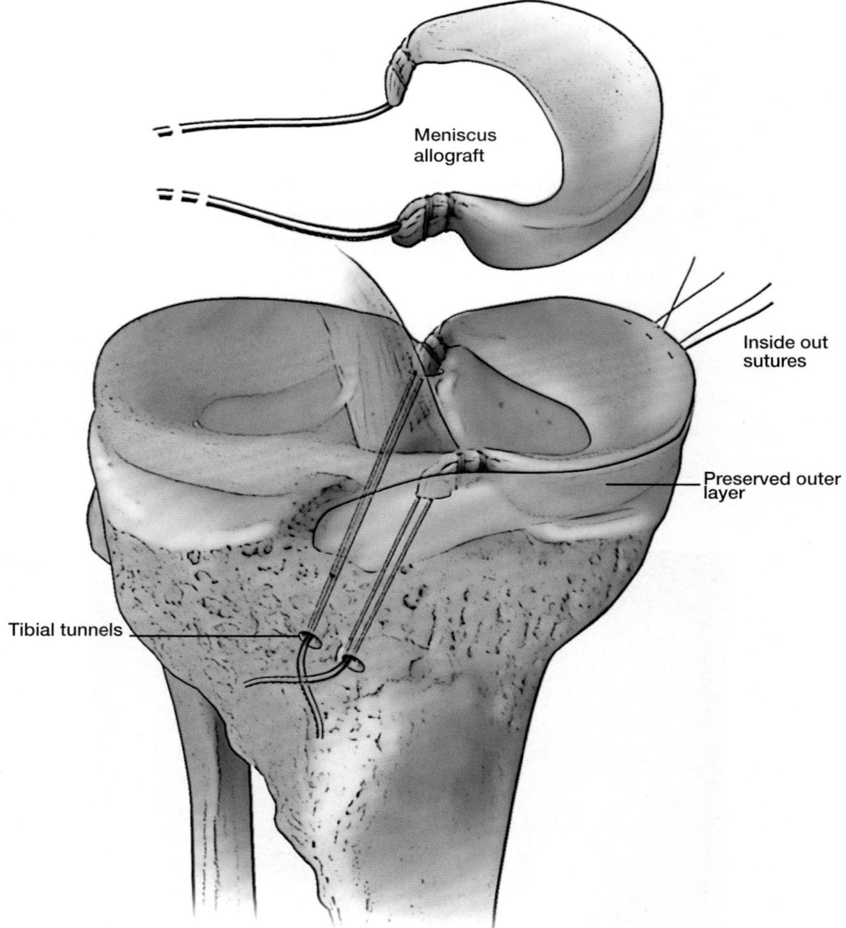

Figure 38-10 | Once the graft is reduced, the sutures are tied over a bone bridge, securing the anterior and posterior horns within the tunnels.

- The meniscal allograft is sutured to the remaining rim of the native meniscal tissue (Fig. 38-11).

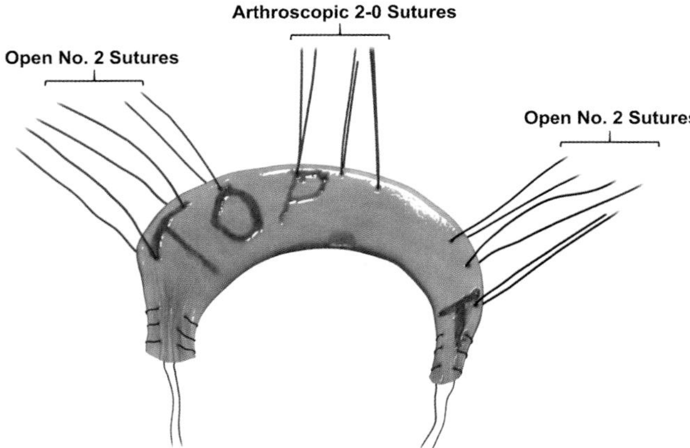

Figure 38-11 | Meniscal allograft is then sutured to the remaining rim of the native meniscal tissue.

  - An inside-out technique, using combined open and arthroscopic techniques, is used.
  - At the anterior horn, open vertical mattress sutures are placed with the previously passed no. 0 braided, nonabsorbable Dacron sutures.
  - At the posterior horn, open vertical mattress sutures are placed with the previously passed no. 2 nonabsorbable suture.
  - In the meniscal midbody, arthroscopic vertical mattress sutures are placed using 2-0 nonabsorbable meniscal repair sutures (Fig. 38-12).

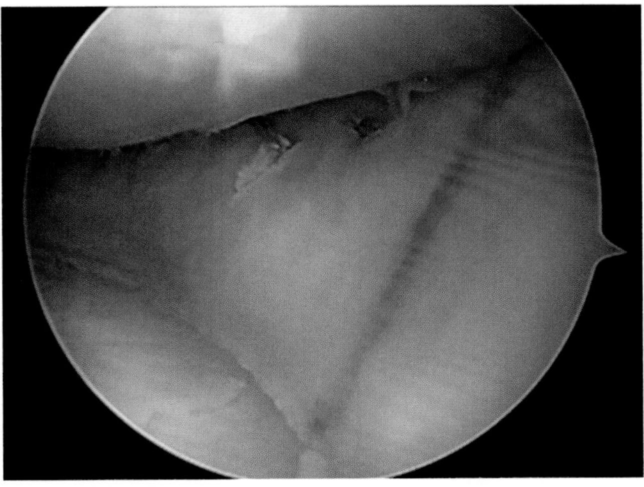

Figure 38-12 | Midbody meniscal allograft sutured to native meniscal rim: arthroscopic vertical mattress sutures using no. 2-0 nonabsorbable meniscus repair sutures.

- The POL is closed to the posterior border of the medial collateral ligament ("window") with no. 2 nonabsorbable suture in a horizontal mattress configuration with the knee in 20 degrees of flexion to prevent a flexion contracture.

Postoperative Protocol

- Partial weight bearing with crutches and a range-of-motion brace.
- Continuous passive motion (CPM) machine started 24 hours after surgery.
- Continued until 90 degrees of passive flexion is obtained.

- Postoperative ROM goal.
  - Full extension equal to contralateral knee at 1 week
  - 90 degrees of flexion at 4-6 weeks
- Crutches are discontinued at ~6 weeks.
  - Full knee extension without quadriceps lag
  - Minimal swelling
  - Flexion to 90 degrees
  - Ability to walk without a bent-knee gait
- Physical therapy is continued for 2-3 months.
  - Emphasis is on full ROM and strength.
  - Quadriceps sets, straight leg raises, heel slides, calf pumps are begun immediately.
  - At 6 weeks, closed-chain exercises from 0 to 45 degrees are begun, then slowly increased to 75 degrees.
  - At 8 weeks, low-impact aerobic exercises (stationary bike) are begun.
  - At 6 months, patient may return to running.

Suggested Readings

Ellingson CI, Sekiya JK, Harner CD. Meniscal allograft transplantation. In: ElAttrache NS, Harner CD, Mirzayan R, Sekiya JK, eds. *Surgical Techniques in Sports Medicine.* Philadelphia, PA: Lippincott Williams & Wilkins; 2006.

Griffith CJ, Kalawadia JV, Harner CD. Meniscus allograft transplantation with bony fixation. In: Hulet C, Pereira H, Peretti G, Denti M, eds. *Surgery of the Meniscus.* Berlin, Germany: Springer-Verlag Berlin Heidelberg; 2016.

Johannsen AM, Civitarese DM, Padalecki JR, Goldsmith MT, Wijdicks CA, LaPrade RF. Qualitative and quantitative anatomic analysis of the posterior root attachments of the medial and lateral menisci. *Am J Sports Med.* 2012;40(10):2342-2347.

Johnson DL, Swenson TM, Livesay GA, Aizawa H, Fu FH, Harner CD. Insertion-site anatomy of the human menisci: gross, arthroscopic and topographical anatomy as a basis for meniscal transplantation. *Arthroscopy.* 1995;11(4):386-394.

Kang RW, Lattermann C, Cole BJ. Allograft meniscus transplantation: background, indications, techniques, and outcomes. *J Knee Surg.* 2006;19(3):220-230.

Kohn D, Moreno B. Meniscus insertion anatomy as a basis for meniscus replacement: a morphological cadaveric study. *Arthroscopy.* 1995;11(1):96-103.

LaPrade RF, Wills NJ, Spiridonov SI, Perkinson S. A prospective outcomes study of meniscal allograft transplantation. *Am J Sports Med.* 2010;38(9):1804-1812.

Shaffer B, Kennedy S, Klimkiewicz J, Yao L. Preoperative sizing of meniscal allografts in meniscus transplantation. *Am J Sports Med.* 2000;28:524-533.

Chapter 39
Arthroscopic Lateral Meniscal Allograft

SCOTT A. RODEO

Background

- The function of the menisci in load transmission across the tibiofemoral joint is well established.
- Meniscal deficiency leads to increased articular cartilage contact stress, which predisposes to progressive joint degeneration.
- Numerous clinical studies demonstrate the relationship between meniscal deficiency and progressive articular cartilage degeneration.
- The lateral meniscus plays a greater role in load transmission in the lateral compartment than does the medial meniscus in the medial compartment.[1]
  - Medial meniscus transmits 50% of compartment load.
  - Lateral meniscus transmits 70% of compartment load.
  - The menisci transmit 50% of load in extension, 85% of load in flexion.[2]
- Degenerative changes typically progress more rapidly in the lateral compartment following lateral meniscectomy than in the medial compartment following medial meniscectomy.
- There is a subgroup of patients in whom degenerative changes can proceed very rapidly following lateral meniscectomy.
  - This occurs most commonly in adolescent females.
  - Valgus alignment may play a role.
- More rapid progression of degenerative changes likely occurs in younger patients due to acute meniscal loss following traumatic injury, in contrast to patients in whom a degenerative tear develops gradually over time, thus allowing the joint to accommodate to the gradual loss of meniscal function.
- The menisci also play a role in knee stability.
- The lateral meniscus has a role in controlling lateral compartment translations during the pivot shift in the anterior cruciate ligament (ACL)-deficient knee.[3]

Indications: Subtotal Lateral Meniscectomy

- Specific tear patterns in the lateral compartment that may require subtotal meniscectomy:
  - Bucket-handle tear.
  - Radial tear that extends to the capsule. This tear pattern typically occurs at the junction of the anterior horn and mid-third of the meniscus and almost exclusively occurs in the lateral compartment.
- Pain and swelling are the typical symptoms following meniscal loss.
- Concomitant lateral meniscal transplantation should be considered during revision ACL reconstruction in patients with prior lateral meniscectomy to replace the role of the lateral meniscus as a secondary stabilizer.

Contraindications

- Extensive, full-thickness cartilage loss on the lateral femoral condyle or lateral tibial plateau.
- In contrast, a focal chondral lesion may be appropriate for concomitant cartilage repair/resurfacing.
- The threshold for acceptable size and location of a cartilage defect that can still allow meniscal transplantation is unknown.
- Erosive cartilage loss on the posterior margin of the lateral tibial plateau is harder to treat and may be considered a relative contraindication.
- Remodeling of the architecture of the lateral femoral condyle, with flattening, is a contraindication.
- A valgus mechanical axis, with the weight-bearing line displaced lateral to the lateral tibial spine, should be corrected with concomitant or prior realignment osteotomy.

Is There a Role for Prophylactic Meniscal Transplantation in the Asymptomatic Knee?

- Patients usually are asymptomatic in the early time period following meniscectomy; however, given the well-established natural history of lateral meniscal deficiency in young patients, the question often arises about doing early lateral meniscal transplantation to prevent progressive degenerative changes.
- The rationale for early or "prophylactic" transplantation is to prevent the known morbid sequelae of lateral meniscectomy.
- Because the results of meniscal transplantation are superior when performed in the setting of minimal chondral degeneration, a case can be made for early transplantation.
- I recommend monitoring of these knees with serial physical examinations and surveillance MRIs. If a patient develops an effusion, or MRI scan begins to demonstrate progressive degenerative changes, then a case can be made for transplantation, even in the absence of overt symptoms.
- Quantitative MRI using measurement of T2 relaxation time (as a measure of collagen organization) and T1rho (as a measure of proteoglycan content) may be helpful to monitor for development of cartilage changes before such changes are evident on standard morphologic MRI.
- In the future, sensitive serum and synovial fluid biomarkers may allow early detection before development of structural changes in MRI.

Patient Evaluation for Meniscus Transplantation

- Careful history and examination
- Understanding of the patient's goals and expectations
- Review of prior operative reports
- Careful physical examination with particular attention to standing alignment, prior incisions, presence of an effusion, range of motion, ligament stability, and presence of joint line tenderness
- Standing (weight-bearing) radiographs, including posterior-anterior view in flexion to show posterior aspect of the joint
- Long films from hip to ankle to measure mechanical axis
- MRI to evaluate articular cartilage, subchondral bone architecture, remaining meniscus, and status of medial and patellofemoral compartments (Fig. 39-1)

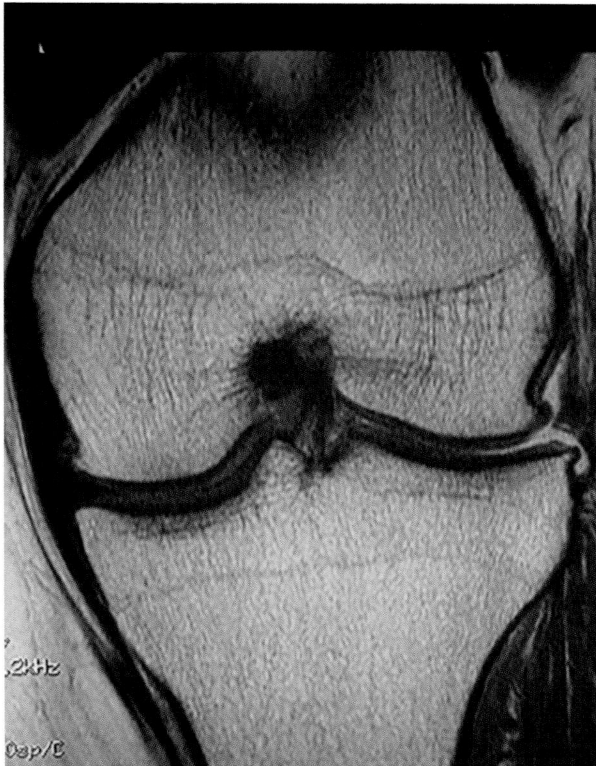

Figure 39-1 | MRI is used to evaluate articular cartilage, subchondral bone architecture, remaining meniscus, and status of the medial and patellofemoral compartments. MRI images depict absence of the lateral meniscus with intact articular cartilage and subchondral bone architecture.

Graft Sizing and Procurement

- Graft is sized relative to bony dimensions.
- Tissue banks generally use plain radiographs to measure length and width of the tibial plateau.
- MRI also can be used for measurement of length and width of the tibial plateau.
- If the tissue bank supplies the meniscus with no attached bone, there are formulae to allow prediction of meniscal dimensions.[4]
  - Meniscal "width" on anterior-posterior (AP) radiograph
    - Respective midpoint of tibial eminence to bony periphery
    - 1:1 ratio
  - Meniscal "length" on lateral radiograph
    - Medial = 80% of sagittal diameter of plateau
    - Lateral = 70% of sagittal diameter of plateau
- The tolerance of the compartment for meniscal size mismatch is not known.
- Undersized grafts should be avoided because of the potential difficulty in achieving anatomic bone attachment of the horns centrally and reaching the capsular periphery.

Surgical Technique—General Considerations

- Biomechanical studies demonstrate superior graft fixation strength with bone fixation compared to sutures alone attached to the horns.[5]
- Options for bone fixation are individual bone plugs attached to the anterior and posterior horns or a common bone slot that connects both anterior and posterior horns ("keyhole" technique) (Fig. 39-2).
- The advantage of a common bone slot is that it maintains the anatomic relationship between the anterior and posterior horns and their attachment sites to bone.
- A potential pitfall with the bone-slot technique is that the slot may be made too much into the lateral compartment in an effort to avoid injury to the ACL in making the central slot.
- An advantage of individual bone plugs attached to the anterior and posterior horns is that these can be placed anterior and posterior to the ACL, allowing anatomic placement.
- Secure suture fixation of the graft to the capsule is critical; the posterolateral capsule is looser than the medial side.
- Native lateral meniscus is more mobile than the medial meniscus.

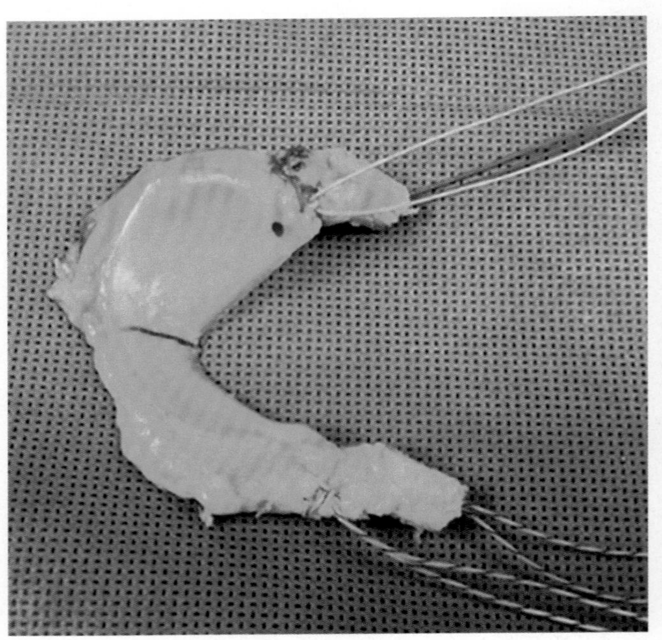

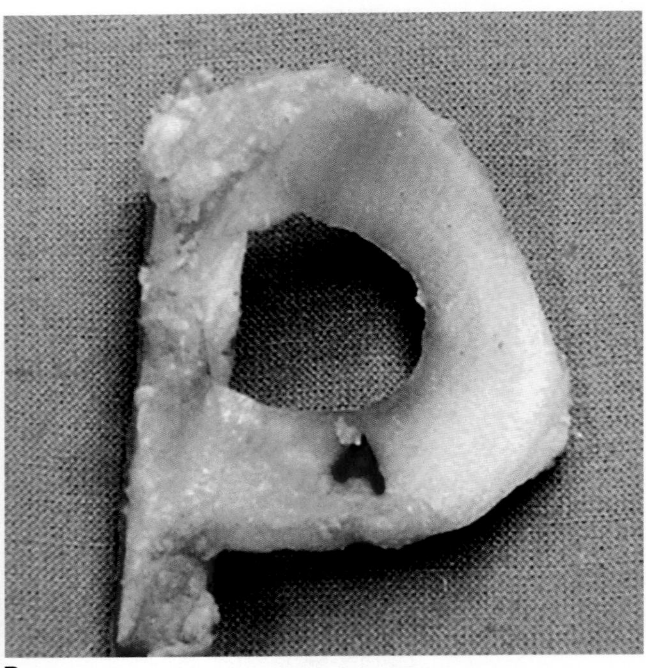

A B

Figure 39-2 | **A.** Meniscal allograft prepared with individual bone plugs attached to anterior and posterior horns. **B.** Meniscal allograft prepared with common bone slot connecting the anterior and posterior horns.

Detailed Surgical Steps for Lateral Meniscus Transplantation

- Standard anteromedial and anterolateral viewing portals are established.
- The medial portal should be placed a bit higher to allow instruments through this portal to pass over the intercondylar eminence to work in the lateral compartment.
- The knee is placed in the "figure-four" position, at 90 degrees of flexion with varus stress to open the lateral compartment.
- The lateral compartment normally has more opening than the medial side, so there typically is ample working room with varus stress.
- In a tight lateral compartment, "pie crusting" of the iliotibial band and/or lateral capsule can be done with an 18-gauge spinal needle from outside-in, although this is rarely required.
- The capsular rim is prepared with a standard shaver. A small remnant of the red zone of the native meniscus (2-3 mm) can be left to suture into (Fig. 39-3).

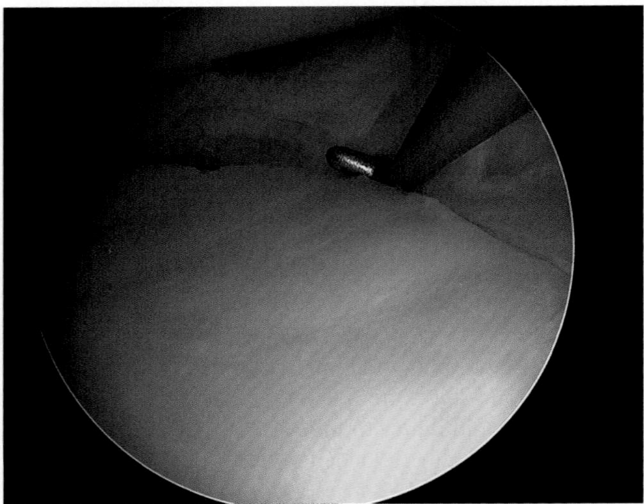

Figure 39-3 | The capsular rim is prepared, leaving a small remnant of the red zone of the native meniscus (2-3 mm) to suture into.

Separate Bone Tunnel Technique

- A standard ACL vector guide is used for tunnel placement (Fig. 39-4).
- I recommend 9-mm tunnels.
- A blind-ended tunnel can be created for the posterior horn with a RetroDrill (Arthrex Inc., Naples, FL) (Fig. 39-5).

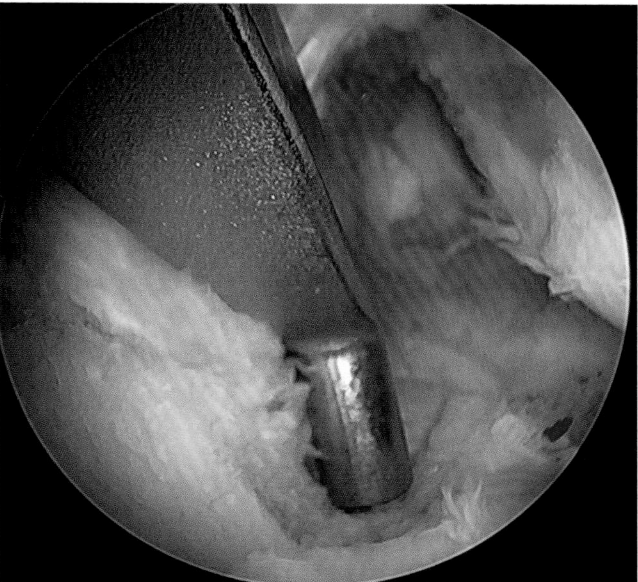

Figure 39-4 | A standard ACL vector guide is used for tunnel placement.

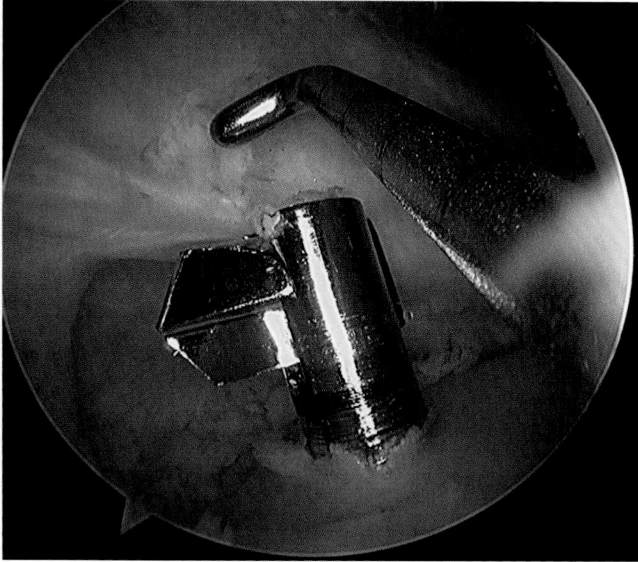

Figure 39-5 | A "Flip cutter" or "RetroDrill" can be used to make a blind-ended tunnel for the posterior horn.

- The anterior horn tunnel is drilled antegrade through the mini-incision used for graft insertion (Fig. 39-6).
- It is critical to identify the anatomic attachment point of the posterior horn. There usually is some remaining meniscus that guides localization of the posterior horn attachment site.

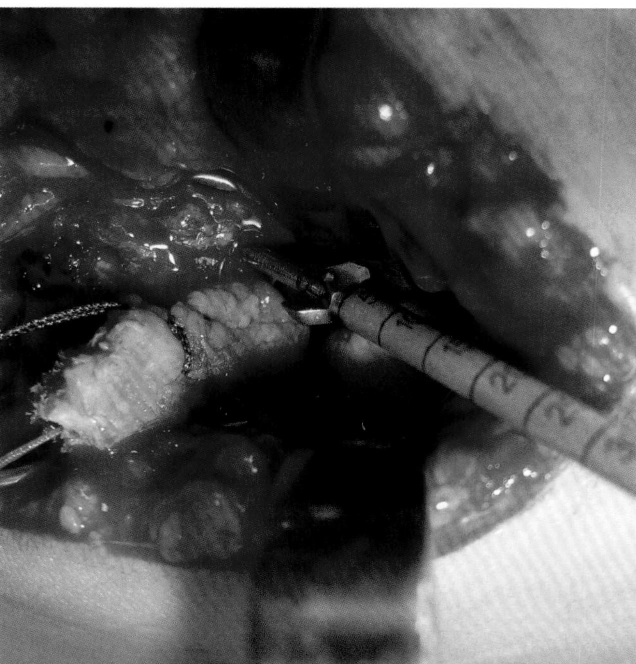

Figure 39-6 | The anterior horn tunnel is drilled antegrade through the mini-incision used for graft insertion.

- Intraoperative fluoroscopy can be used to verify the posterior horn tunnel site.
- If the lateral intercondylar eminence is prominent, a small amount can be removed to achieve good viewing and access to the posterior horn attachment site.
- A minimal notchplasty also can be done, removing some bone from the lateral femoral condyle below the ACL insertion to aid visualization. This also aids in passage of the posterior horn and attached bone plug into the posterior tunnel (Fig. 39-7).

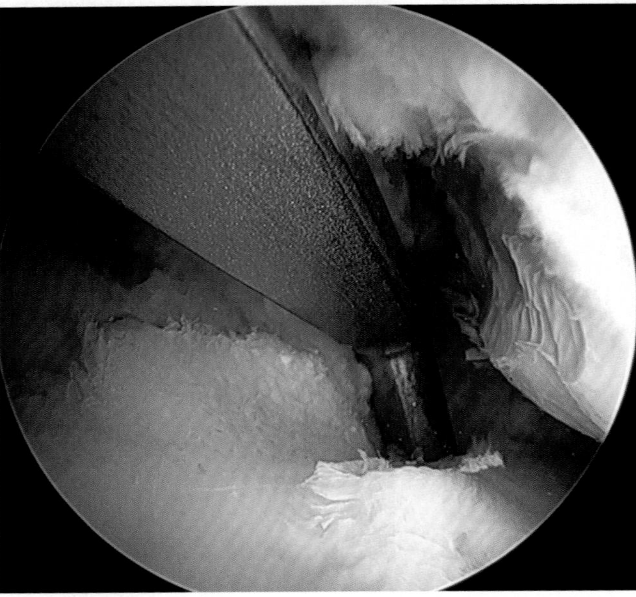

Figure 39-7 | A small amount of the lateral intercondylar eminence may be removed and a minimal notchplasty may also be done, removing some bone from the lateral femoral condyle below the ACL insertion, in order to achieve good visualization and to aid in passage of the posterior horn and attached bone plug into the posterior tunnel.

- A 70-degree arthroscope is helpful to view posteriorly.
- The ACL vector guide is used to begin guide pin insertion. The pin is drilled very carefully, taking care not to plunge posteriorly, which would endanger posterior neurovascular structures.
- Once the guide pin is started, the vector guide is removed and a curette is placed at the planned pin entrance site. The curette acts as a "back stop" to capture the pin as it enters posteriorly, so as to protect the posterior neurovascular structures (Fig. 39-8).
- A 9-mm reamer is used to drill the tunnel, with care taken not to plunge posteriorly.

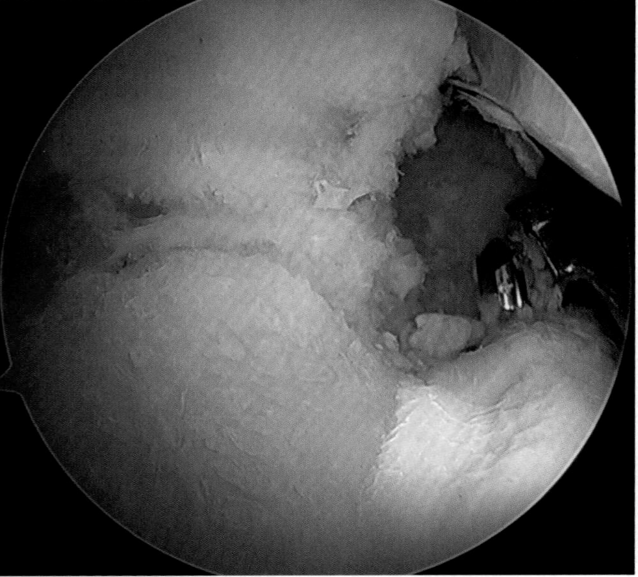

Figure 39-8 | A curette is placed at the planned pin entrance site to act as a "back stop" to capture the pin as it enters posteriorly, protecting the posterior neurovascular structures.

- A small lateral parapatellar incision is made along the lateral border of the patellar tendon. This needs to be just big enough to insert the graft (Fig. 39-9). The anterior horn tunnel also can be drilled antegrade through this small incision.
- A passing suture through the posterior horn tunnel is used to shuttle the sutures attached to the posterior horn bone block into the posterior tunnel (Fig. 39-10).
- A finger can be inserted through the small anterior incision to aid in reducing the graft to the back of the knee, into anatomic position.

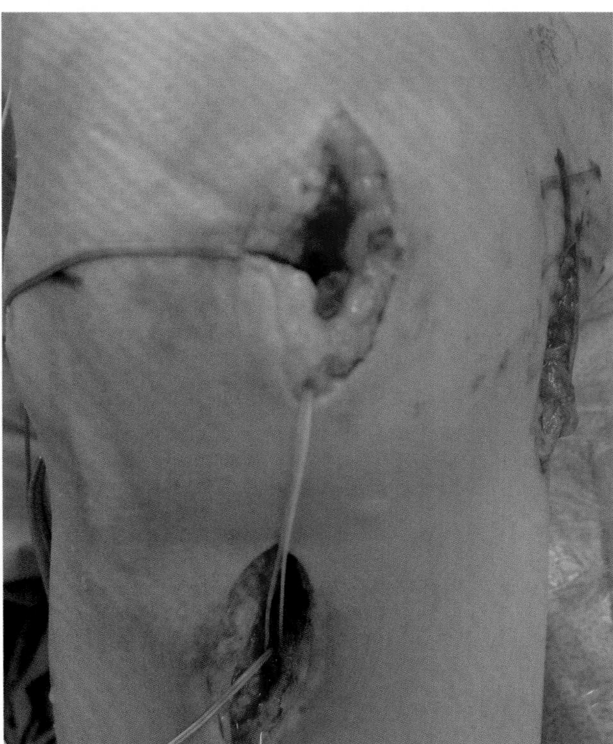

Figure 39-9 | A small lateral parapatellar incision is made along the lateral border of the patellar tendon for graft insertion. In this figure, there is also a distal incision for the tunnel drilling and a posterolateral incision for the inside-out meniscal suturing.

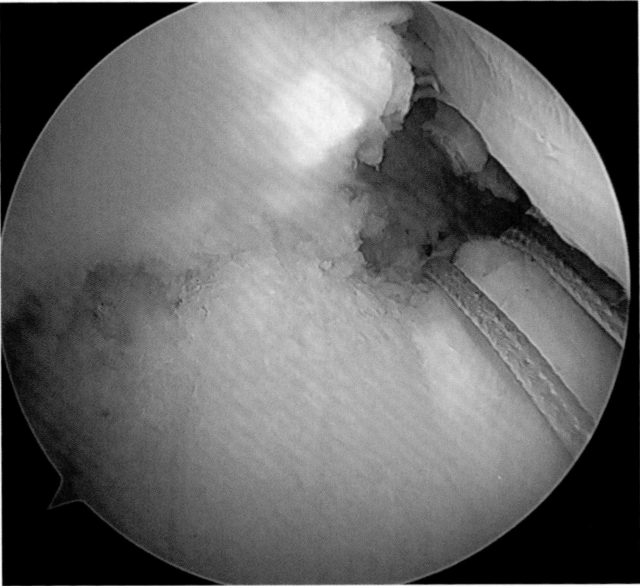

Figure 39-10 | A passing suture through the posterior horn tunnel is used to shuttle the sutures attached to the posterior horn bone block into the posterior tunnel.

- Graft insertion also is aided by a suture placed through the meniscus at the junction of the posterior and middle thirds. This suture is then passed through the posterior lateral capsule and through the posterior lateral incision that was made for the inside-out meniscal repair. This suture aids in pulling the graft into the knee (Fig. 39-11).

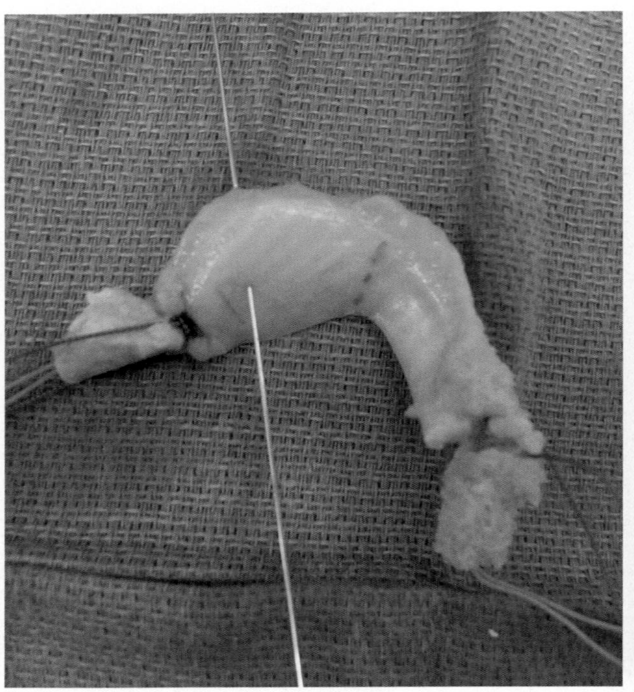

A

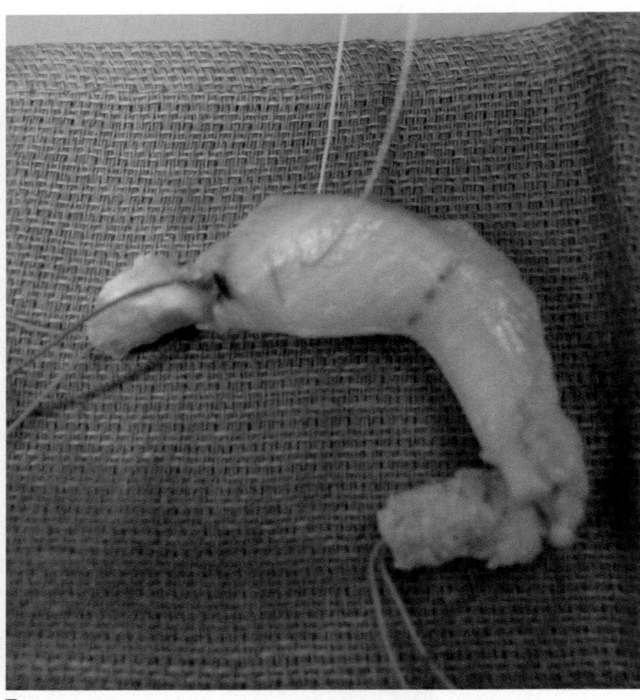

B

Figure 39-11 | Graft insertion is aided by a suture place through the meniscus at the junction of the posterior and middle thirds to aid in pulling the graft into the knee. **A.** The long meniscus repair needle placed through the allograft. **B.** The suture placed at junction of the posterior and middle thirds.

- It can be difficult to "dock" the bone plug in the posterior horn tunnel because of the "killer turn." A probe and the traction suture as noted above are helpful in this step (Fig. 39-12).
- I prefer standard inside-out suturing to attach the meniscus to the capsule.

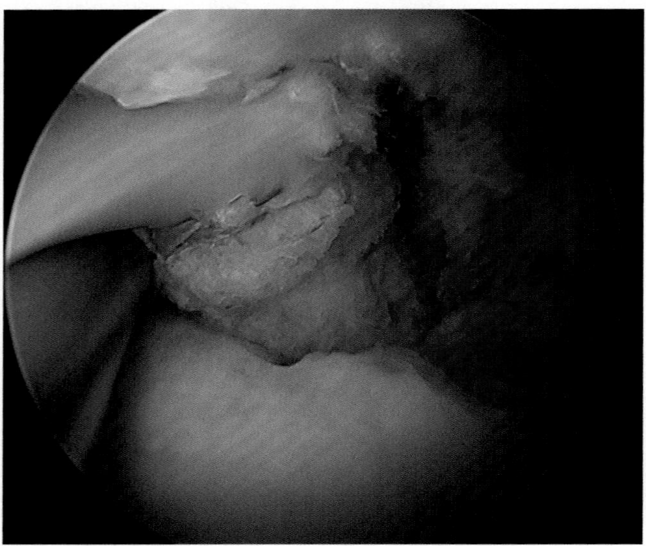

Figure 39-12 | The bone plug attached to the posterior horn is "docked" into the posterior tunnel.

- Braided, nonabsorbable 2-0 suture is used. Sutures are placed on both the femoral and tibial sides of the meniscus. A vertical mattress pattern best captures the circumferential collagen fibers of the meniscus (Fig. 39-13).
- A retractor is placed posterolaterally to retrieve the needles as they exit the capsule and to protect the posterior neurovascular structures.

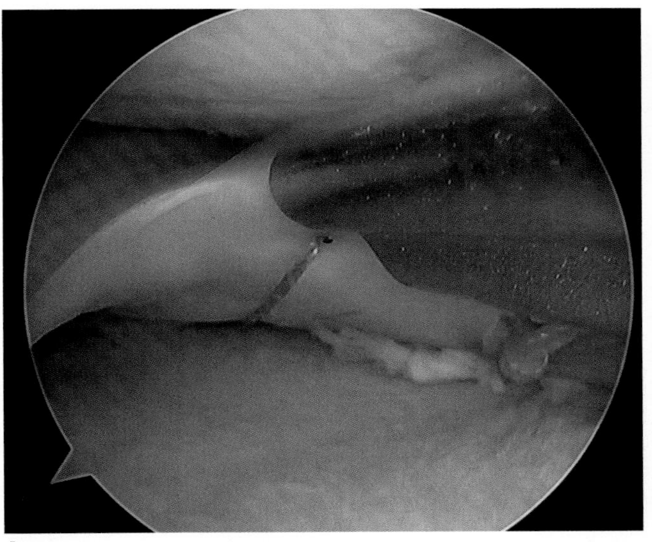

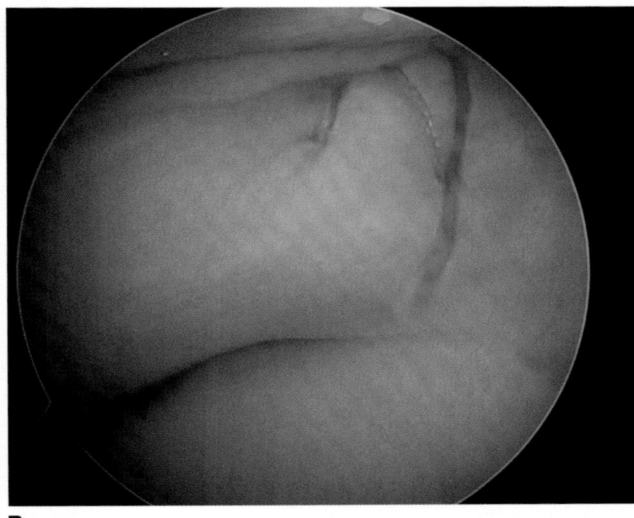

A B

Figure 39-13 | Braided, nonabsorbable 2-0 suture is placed on both the tibial **(A)** and femoral **(B)** sides of the meniscus, ideally in a vertical mattress pattern.

- I recommend first suturing the posterior aspect of the meniscus to the capsule, before drilling the anterior horn tunnel. This allows the position of the anterior horn tunnel to be adjusted as needed, allowing accommodation if the graft is under sized.
- Typically, 9-10 sutures are placed all around the periphery of the meniscus.
- The most anterior aspect of the graft can easily be sutured through the small open incision. A braided, nonabsorbable suture on a small needle (OS-2) works well through the small open incision to suture the anterior horn of the graft (Fig. 39-14).
- The sutures attached to the horns are tied together over the anterior tibial cortex (Fig. 39-15).

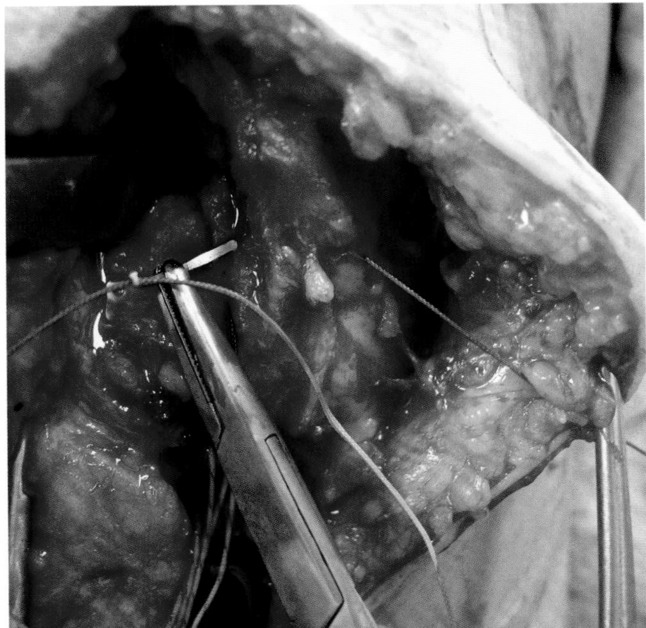

Figure 39-14 | The most anterior aspect of the graft is sutured via the small open incision.

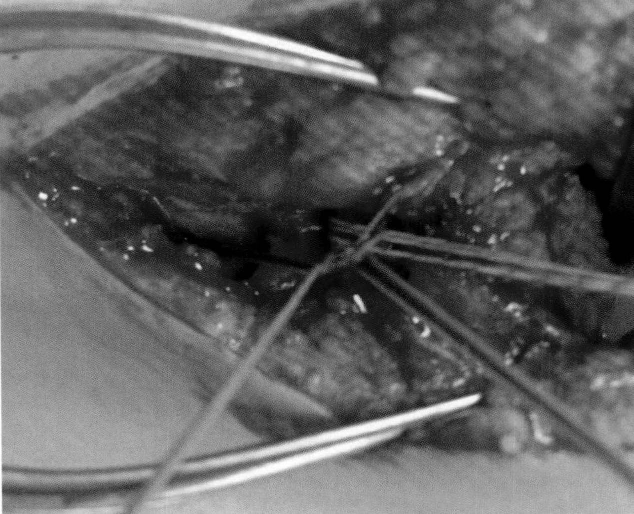

Figure 39-15 | The sutures attached to the horns are tied together over the anterior tibial cortex.

Bone Slot (Keyhole) Technique

- A lateral parapatellar incision is required.
- It is important to be as central (medial) as possible and to avoid the tendency to be pushed into the lateral compartment in an effort to avoid injuring the ACL (Fig. 39-16).

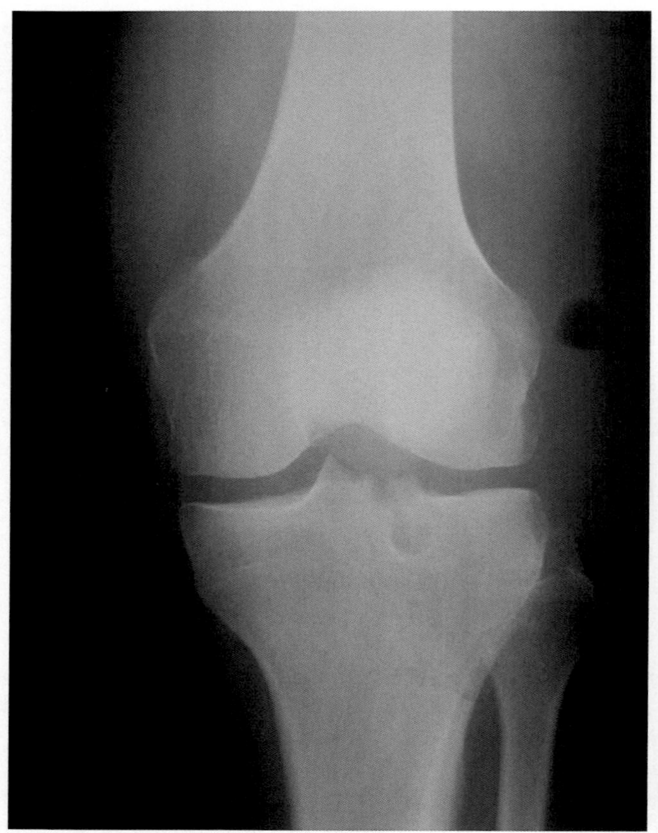

A

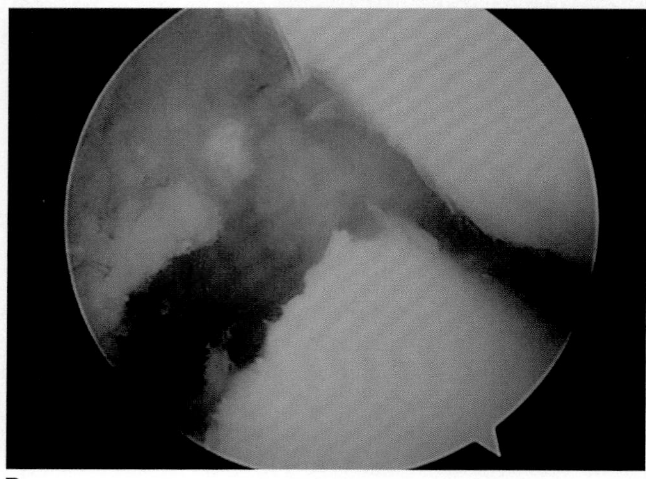

B

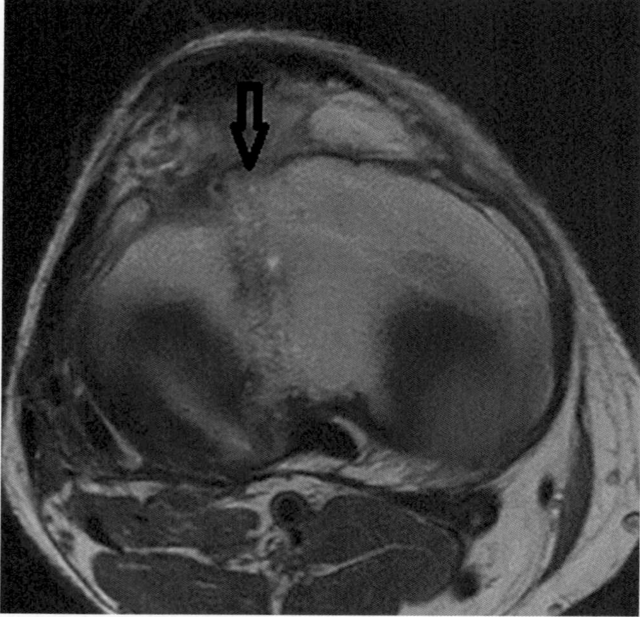

C

Figure 39-16 | The recipient slot for the bone bridge. **A.** Plain radiograph. **B.** Arthroscopic view. **C.** Axial MR image showing slot in lateral compartment (*arrow*).

- Commercially available instruments are available to aid in making a dovetail-shaped (Fig. 39-17) or keyhole-shaped (Fig. 39-18) bone bridge and recipient slot in the tibia.

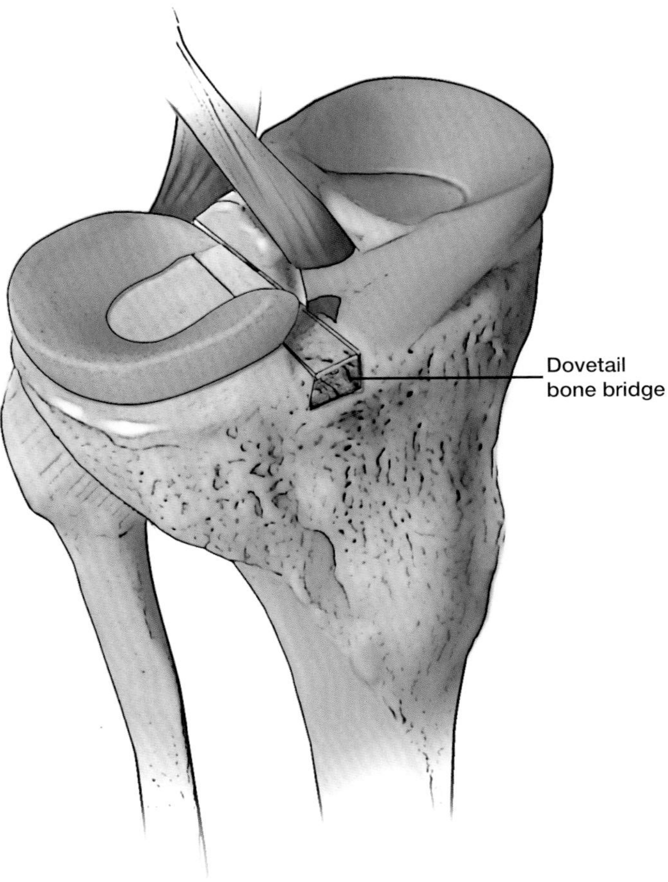

Figure 39-17 | Meniscal allograft being prepared with common bone bridge. This figure shows the "dovetail" technique.

- Alternatively, a guide pin can be placed across the tibia, ~8-10 mm below the surface. Intraoperative fluoroscopy can be used to verify appropriate position of the guide pin. This is followed by reaming over the guide pin with an 8- or 9-mm reamer (Fig. 39-19). A small rongeur or curette can be used to further fashion the opening of the slot at the joint surface.
- A 70-degree arthroscope can be used to view posteriorly, so that the guide pin and reamer are inserted under direct observation to prevent injury to the posterior neurovascular structures.
- The graft is inserted by gently tamping the bone into the recipient slot. A suture attached to the posterior horn of the meniscus can be passed out the posterior lateral incision to provide a vector to pull the meniscus into the joint while the bone block is pushed into the slot.
- The graft typically is stable with press-fit fixation, and no direct bony fixation is required. If there are concerns about stability of the bone block in the recipient slot, an interference screw can be placed at the interface of the bone plug and the slot.

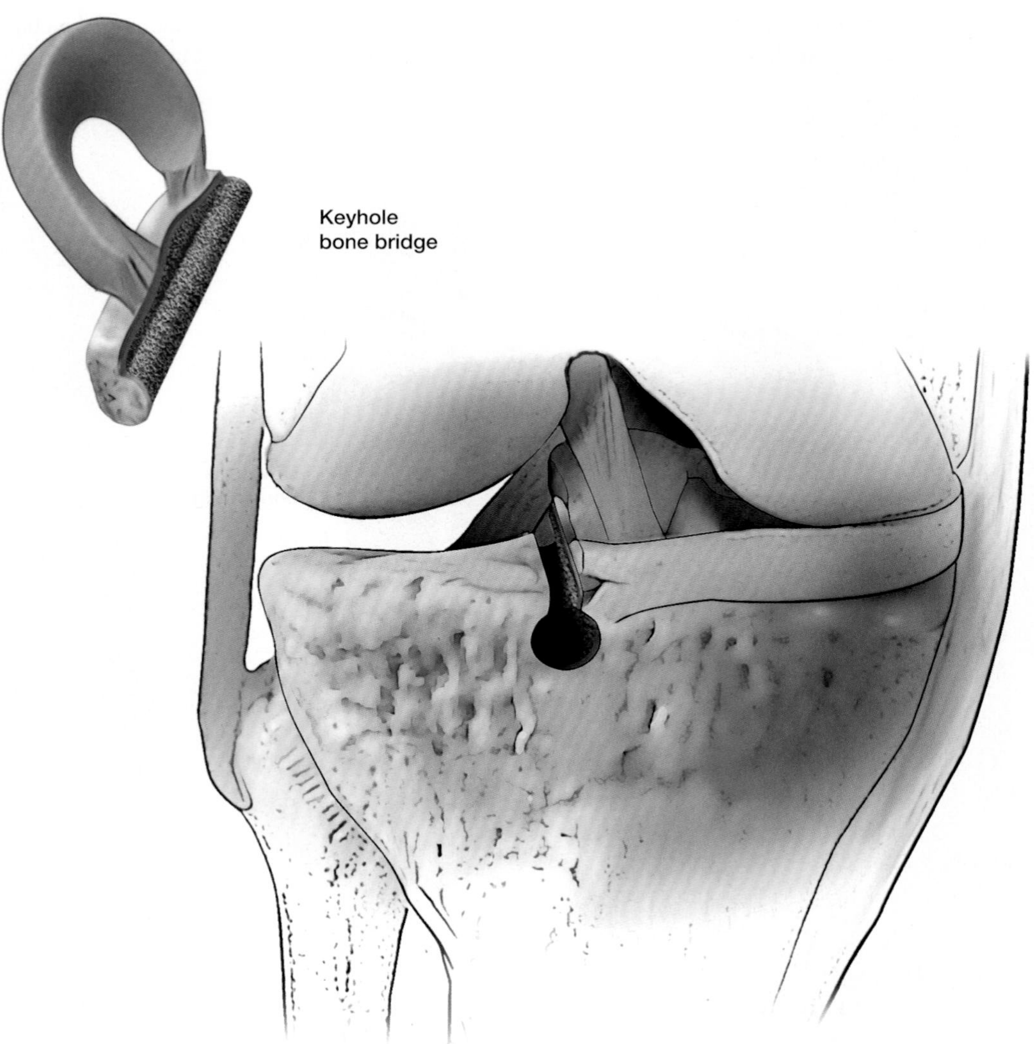

Figure 39-18 | Meniscal allograft being prepared with "keyhole" technique.

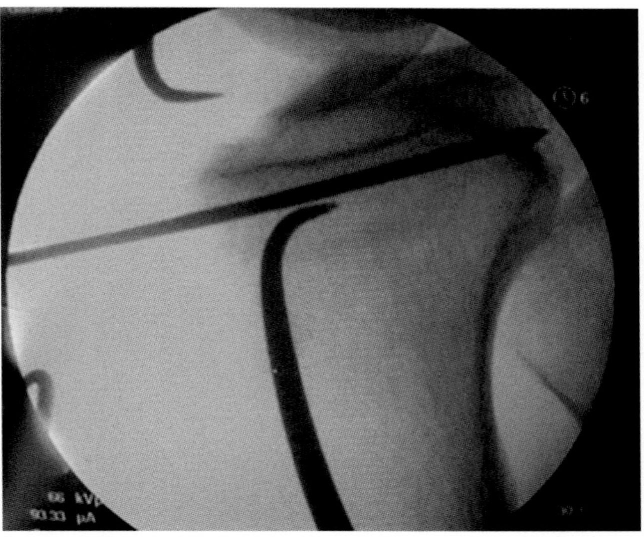
A

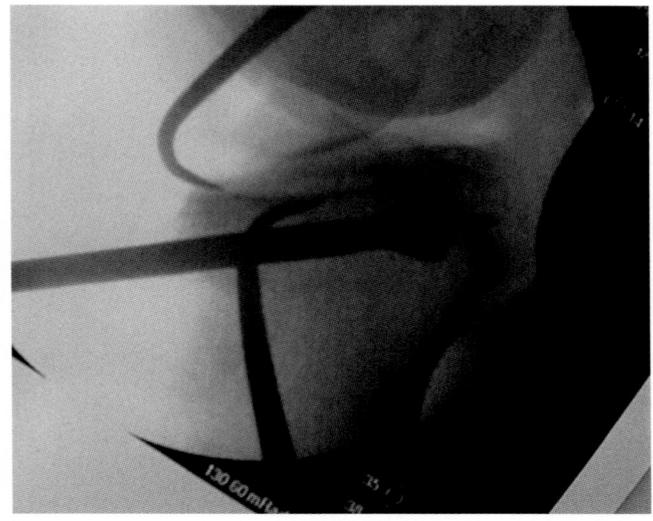
B

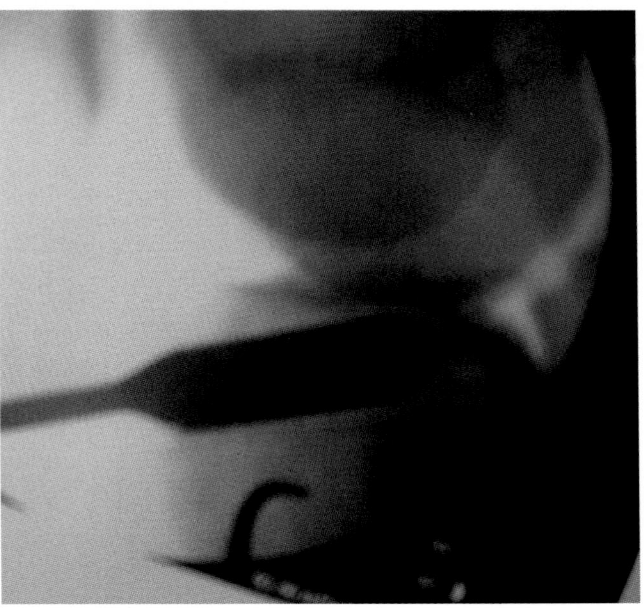
C

Figure 39-19 | **A.** The recipient bone slot can be made by first placing a guide pin across the tibia, ~8-10 mm below the surface. Intraoperative fluoroscopy can be used to verify appropriate position of the guide pin. **B.** This is followed by reaming over the guide pin with an 8- or 9-mm reamer. **C.** A rasp is used to further fashion the opening of the slot at the joint surface.

Tibial Hemiplateau Osteochondral Allograft With Attached Meniscus

- In the uncommon situation where there is damage to the lateral tibial plateau and lateral meniscus, a combined tibial hemiplateau osteochondral allograft with attached lateral meniscus can be considered (Fig. 39-20).
- The advantage of this approach is that it maintains the native horn attachment sites.
- This approach also allows replacement of a damaged tibial plateau, which is an area where standard cartilage repair techniques are difficult to use because of the inability to access posterior tibia.
- This technique requires an exposure similar to that used for unicompartmental arthroplasty.
- The graft is fixed to the tibia with compression screws.
- The thickness of the bone portion should be no more than 10-12 mm because of the prolonged period of time required for revascularization and "creeping substitution" of the transplanted bone.
- A prolonged period of protected weight bearing is required following this procedure to allow progress of revascularization. Early or excessive weight bearing may lead to accumulation of "microdamage" and possible bony collapse before revascularization and creeping substitution of the bone segment. Revascularization is required to repair and remodel the trabecular bone in the osteochondral graft.

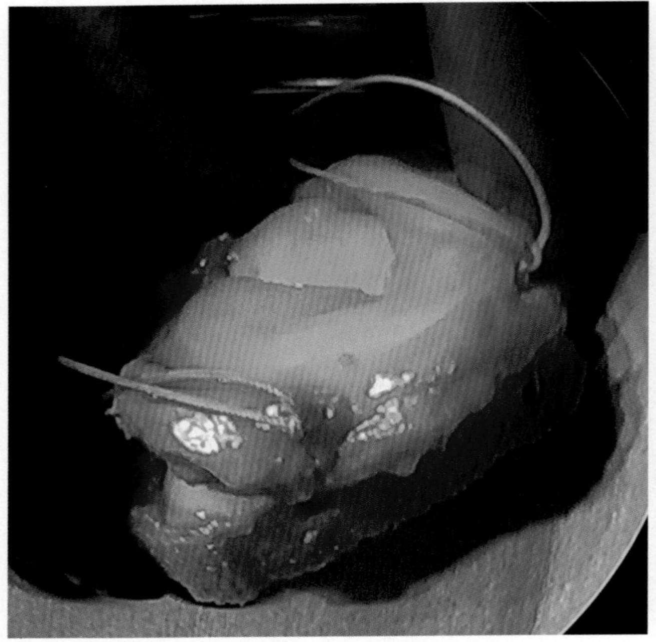

A

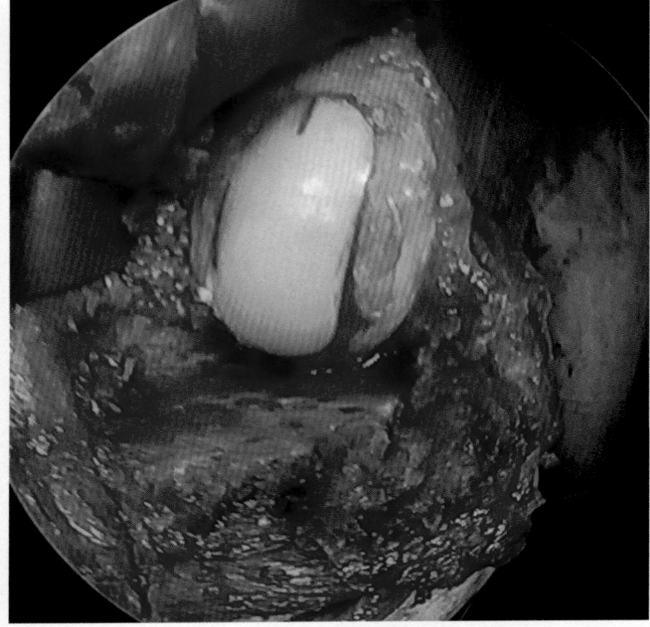

B

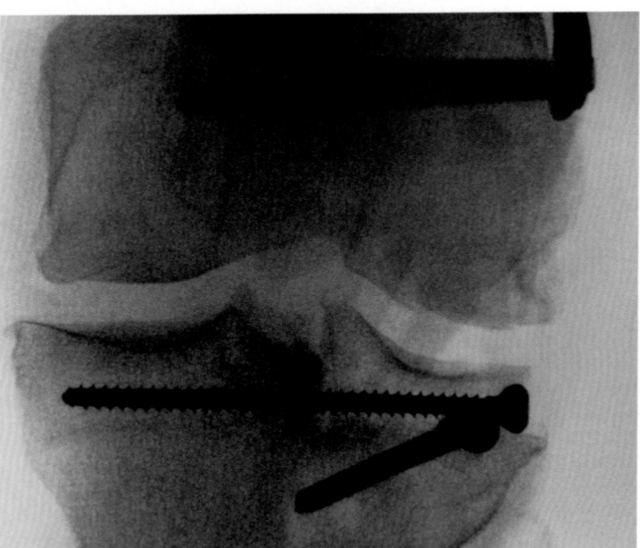

C

Figure 39-20 | A. A lateral tibial hemiplateau osteochondral allograft with attached meniscus. **B.** The recipient site in the lateral tibial plateau. This patient has also undergone placement of an osteochondral allograft to resurface the lateral femoral condyle. **C.** Radiograph showing screw fixation of the lateral tibial hemiplateau osteochondral allograft.

Graft Preparation

Meniscal Graft With Individual Bone Plugs

- I recommend bone plugs that are 10 mm in length and 9 mm in diameter.
- A small oscillating saw and rongeur are used to fashion the bone plugs.
- The orientation of the bone plug relative to its attachment to the posterior horn should be made such that it is in line with the orientation of the bone tunnel (Fig. 39-21).
- A small hole is drilled longitudinally through each bone plug. A suture is placed through this drill hole (Fig. 39-22). The sutures are used for passage of the bone block into the tunnel, and then, the sutures attached to the anterior and posterior horn bone plugs are tied together over the anterior tibial cortex.

Chapter 40
Endoscopic Bone-Patellar-Tendon-Bone ACL Reconstruction

E. LYLE CAIN JR
MICHAEL K. RYAN

Setup/Equipment

- A 10-mm double-10 blade scalpel facilitates an even tendon cut and prevents tendon splitting.
- A small saggital saw with a 10-mm blade and ¼-in curved osteotomes facilitate optimal graft harvest.
- PEEK interference screws (Arthrex, Naples, FL) are inert, do not cause cysts, do not disintegrate, will not break during insertion, and produce minimal artifact if subsequent MRI is needed.
- A 5.5-mm arthroscopic burr facilitates adequate notchplasty.
- A tibial drill guide (tip-aiming guide set at 53 degrees).
- Acorn reamers (10 mm) optimize femoral tunnel drilling with a transtibial technique and allow variable transtibial placement of the femoral tunnel.

Positioning/Draping

- Placing the patient supine on a flat table allows access to the posteromedial knee if a meniscocapsular junction (ramp lesion) repair is needed.
- High thigh tourniquet.
- The bump is clamped at the end of the table on the operative side (Fig. 40-1A).
  - This is positioned just beneath the Achilles tendon, just proximal to the heel so knee is at 60 degrees with the midfoot on the bump and 90 degrees with the toes on the bump (Fig. 40-1B).
- The kidney post is clamped to the ipsilateral side, about four fingerbreadths above the superior pole of the patella to allow valgus stress to be applied.
- The patient is moved close to the post, so that his thigh easily contacts it when placing a valgus force.

Graft Harvest

- The tourniquet is elevated, and a 6-cm midline incision is made from the inferior pole of the patella to the medial aspect of the tubercle.
- The skin and subcutaneous tissue are incised sharply (Fig. 40-2A).

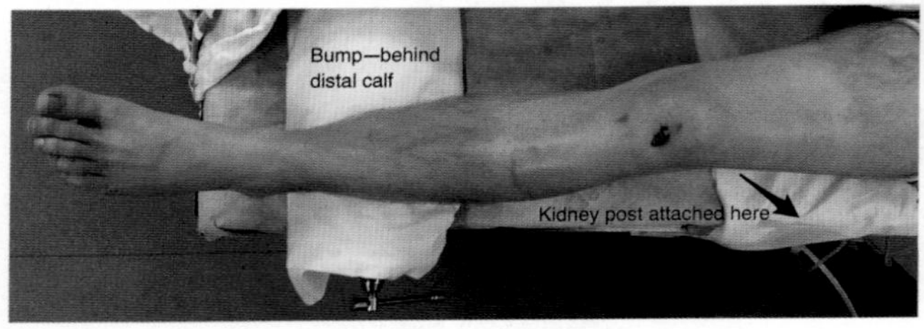

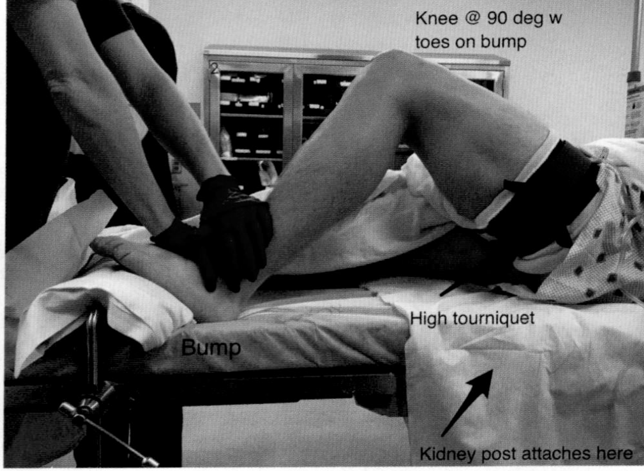

A B

Figure 40-1 | A. Anterior view demonstrating the position of the bump behind the distal calf with the leg fully extended, and the location of the lateral post, which facilitates a valgus force to optimally view the medial compartment. **B.** Lateral view demonstrating the knee at 90 degrees of flexion with the toes on the bump, the location of the tourniquet proximally on the thigh, and the location for the lateral post.

- Dissection with cautery is carried through adipose tissue to the paratenon; then, subcutaneous flaps are developed medially and laterally to allow arthroscopic portal placement (Fig. 40-2B).
- The paratenon is incised in the midline in line with the skin incision.
- Metzenbaum scissors are used to release the paratenon proximally and distally and separate it from the tendon (Fig. 40-2C).
  - The medial and lateral borders of tendon need to be visible for measurement.

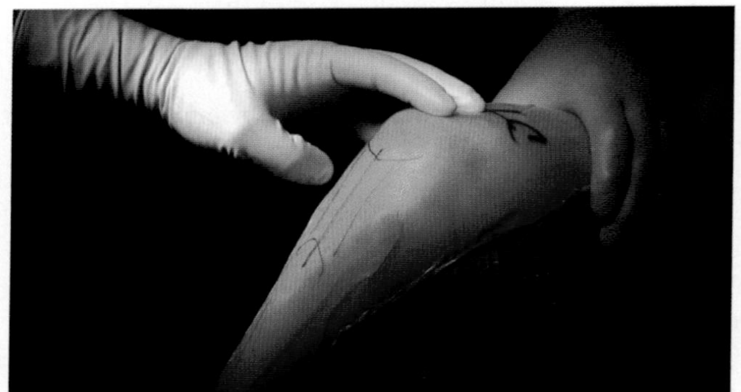
A

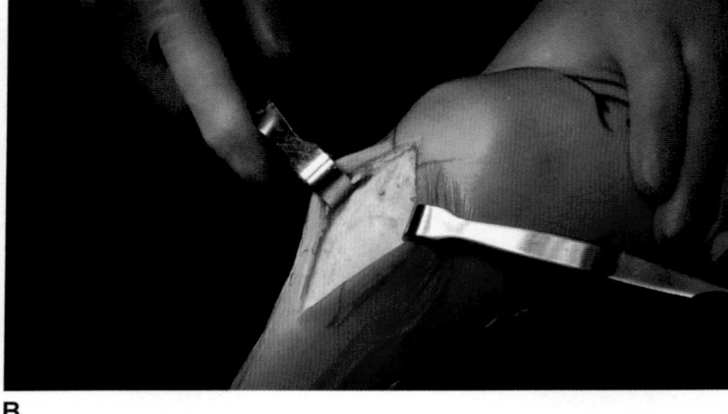
B

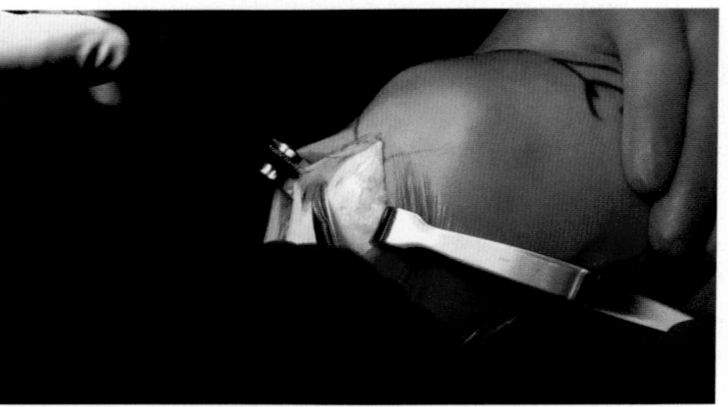
C

Figure 40-2 | Midline approach for graft harvest: **(A)** midline incision from inferior patellar pole to tibial tubercle; **(B)** subcutaneous flaps developed medial and lateral to borders of tendon to allow portal placement and smooth instrument insertion; **(C)** paratenon dissection, medial and lateral flaps created to allow closure over tendon and to prevent soft tissue from blocking portal sites.

- A 10-mm double-blade scalpel is used to incise the middle one-third of the tendon from the inferior pole of the patella down to the tubercle (if tendon width is <30 mm in width, a 9-mm tendon graft is harvested) (Fig. 40-3).

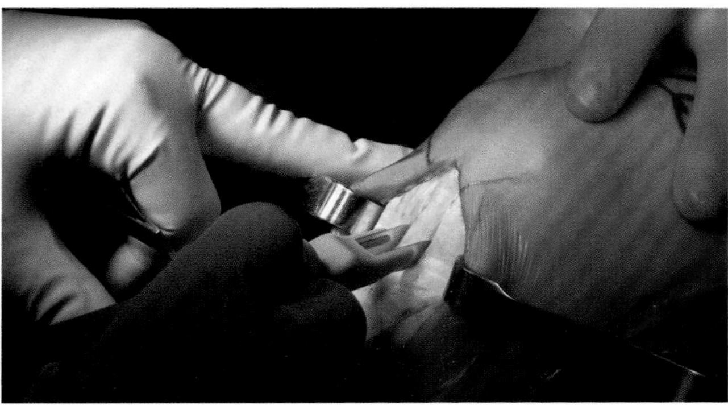

Figure 40-3 | Central third of patellar tendon is incised with a 10-mm-wide double-10 blade. Tendon width of <30 mm requires a 9-mm graft harvest.

- A hemostat clamp is placed behind the graft and pushed down to bone. Measurement is made from the inferior aspect of the hemostat (in cases of Osgood-Schlatter or Sinding-Larsen-Johansson, care should be taken to measure the tendon insertion properly on preoperative radiographs, so as not to inaccurately include the bony ossicle).
- A ruler is used to measure the length of the tibial and patellar plugs.
  - The tibial plug (femur) should be about 25 mm.
  - The patellar plug (tibia) should be about 20 mm (15 mm in very small patients).
- For tibial plug harvest, a small 10 mm wide saggital saw is used to score the tibial cuts (vertical first) and then cuts are made to full depth at an angle of 70-90 degrees on the medial and lateral sides. The transverse cut is made completely through the anterior cortical bone (Fig. 40-4A).
- A ¼-in curved osteotome is used to free the plug from distal cut (Fig. 40-4B).
  - Occasionally, an osteotome may be needed in the medial and lateral cuts if the plug is not freed from the distal cut.

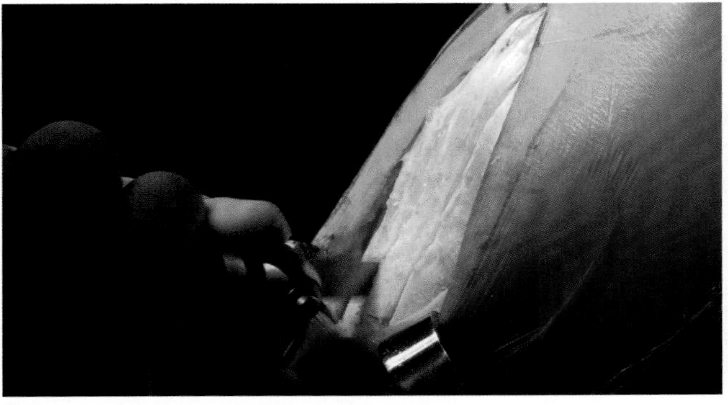

A

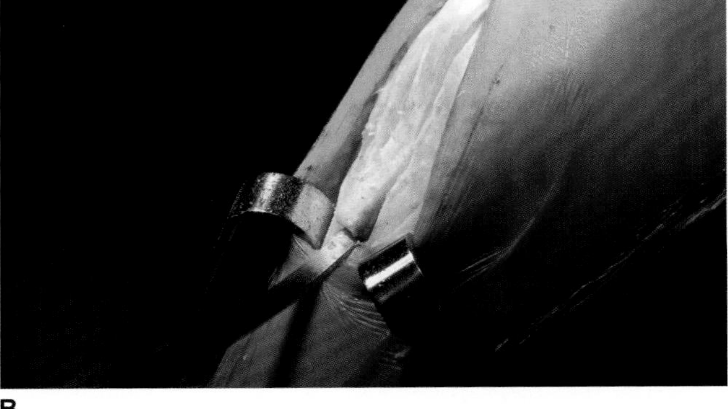

B

Figure 40-4 | Tibial cut: **(A)** small 10 mm wide saggital saw used to make vertical cuts through anterior cortex, followed by distal horizontal cut, making sure to connect the corners; **(B)** a ¼-in curved osteotome frees the plug from its bed easily if cuts were complete.

- Once the bony plug is free, Metzenbaum scissors are used to gently release any soft tissue attachments.
- During cutting of the patellar plug, an assistant holds the graft or the surgeon holds it in his or her noncutting hand, moving it away from the side being cut.
- The patellar plug is cut starting from the distal patellar pole and moving slowly proximally in line with the measured cuts, making sure to keep the blade angled ~30 degrees out of the sagittal plane in each direction (Fig. 40-5A).
  - A 10-mm blade has ~2-mm excursion; so as long as the corner of the blade remains above the anterior surface of the patella, the cut will not be too deep. Angling the blade 30 degrees from the sagittal plane results in a narrow posterior bone plug to prevent a stress riser and subsequent patellar fracture.
- The proximal cut is scored with the corner of the blade, and then a full cut is made to a depth of 10 mm (avoiding a wide transverse patellar cut to prevent patellar fracture).
- An osteotome is used to release the plug proximally, and from medial and lateral if needed (Fig. 40-5B).

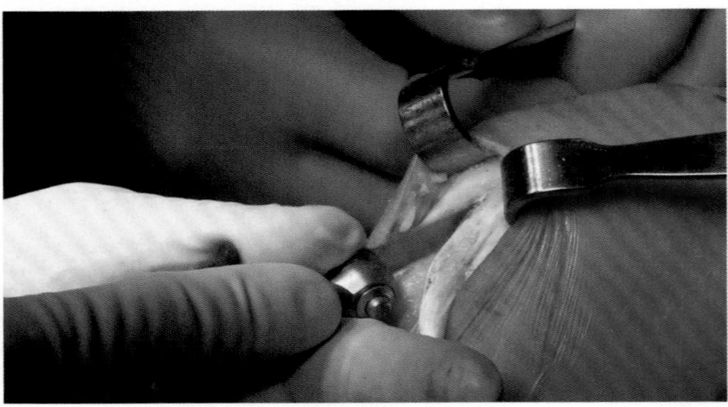
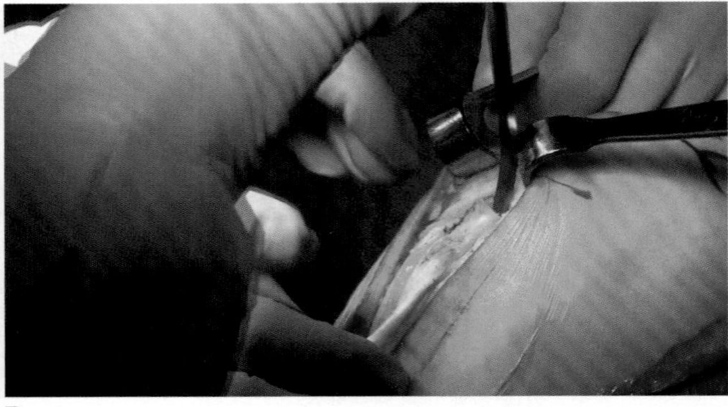

A B

Figure 40-5 | Patellar cut: **(A)** patellar plug is cut from distal to proximal, not anterior to posterior to better control depth. If tip of blade is just above the anterior cortex, depth is no more than 10 mm; **(B)** a ¼-in curved osteotome frees the patellar plug; as with the tibial plug, cuts must be complete and corners must meet.

- The tendon is closed with an interrupted no. 0 braided absorbable suture.
- The bone graft remnants from the patellar and tibial plugs are tamped into the patellar donor site.
- The paratenon is closed with interrupted 2-0 braided absorbable suture.

Graft Preparation

- The bony plugs are trimmed as needed to fit smoothly into a 10-mm tunnel.
  - The end of the femoral (tibial) plug is tapered, and both ends should go easily through the sizing guide.
- A marking pen is used to mark the bone-tendon junctions on each end of the graft and the end of the patellar plug (tibia) to aid determination of the graft position in the tunnels (Fig. 40-6A).
- One hole is drilled in the femoral plug (tibial) 3-5 mm from the bony (nontendinous) end to prevent it from toggling during graft passage.
- Three offset holes are drilled in the patellar plug, evenly spaced in different planes.
- A no. 5 braided nonabsorbable suture is passed through each hole (4 total) with a straight Keith needle, to be used as shuttling sutures (Fig. 40-6B).

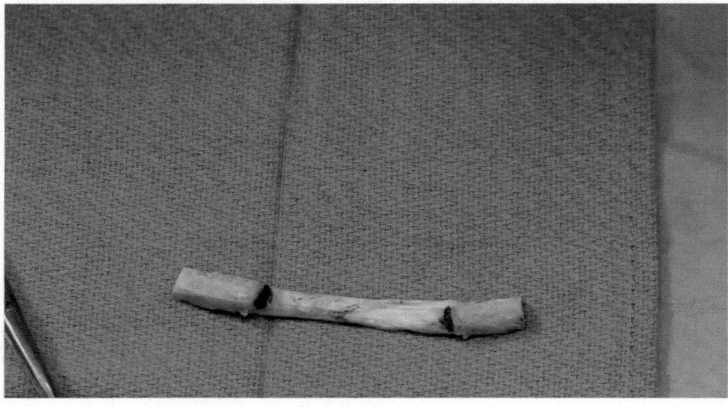
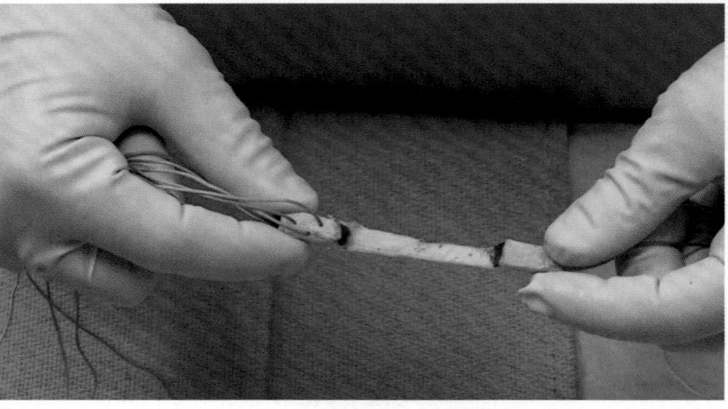

A B

Figure 40-6 | Bone-patellar-tendon-bone graft—**(A)** before and **(B)** after preparation. Both bone plugs should fit easily through a 10-mm sizing guide.

Portals

- A periosteal window (L-shaped) is made with electrocautery, even with the level of the top of the tibial graft harvest site and parallel (but ~2 cm medial) to the medial edge of the graft harvest site (Fig. 40-7).
  - The top should be at the transition point of the tibial plateau from convex to concave.
- The periosteum is elevated with a Key elevator.
  - This allows insertion of the tibial guide down to bone and easy visualization of the tibial tunnel for screw insertion.

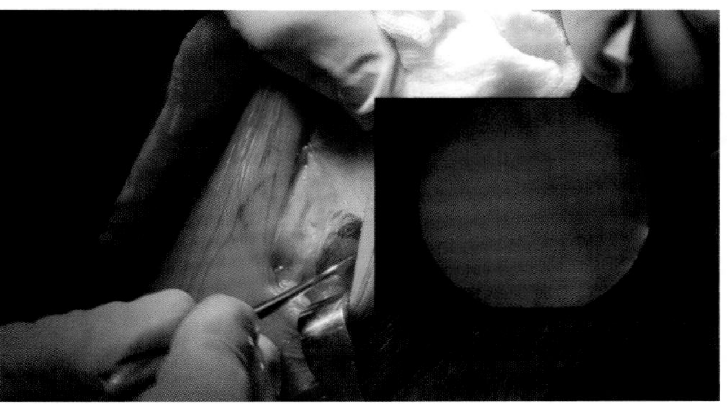

Figure 40-7 | L-shaped periosteal window. Top should be in line with the top of the tibial harvest site, at the transition point of the tibial flare from convex to concave.

- Vertical portals are created through the capsule, under the skin flaps.
- The lateral portal should be high (starting at the inferior pole of the patella) and should hug the tendon.
- The medial portal should be just above the meniscus and should hug the tendon.

Notchplasty

- The anterior cruciate ligament (ACL) remnant is excised with a 5.5-mm shaver (Fig. 40-8A).
- The notchplasty is begun with the knee in about 40 degrees of flexion to evaluate notch anatomy with leg extended; a few millimeters of articular surface are removed. The knee is then gradually flexed to full 90 degrees and beyond, and the notchplasty is continued posteriorly, starting with shaver and then with a burr (Fig. 40-8B and C).
  - The notch should be concave the entire way, from anterior to posterior, when viewed with the knee in 40-90 degrees of flexion.
  - The posterior wall should be visible, but there is no need to raise it.
  - At the end, the notch should resemble the shape of a Roman arch (the surgeon's contralateral thumb should fit into the smooth, concave notch after preparation).

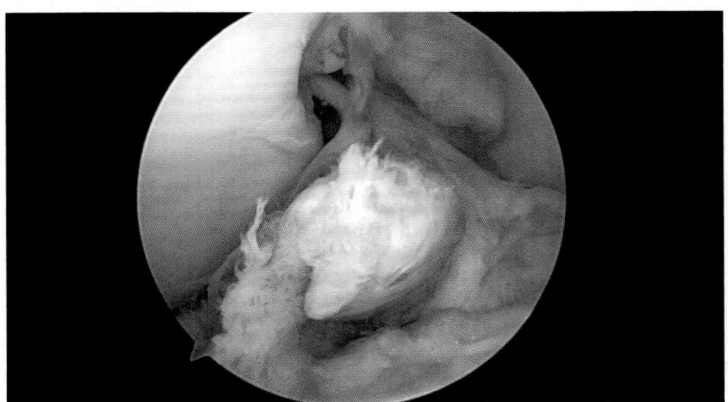

A

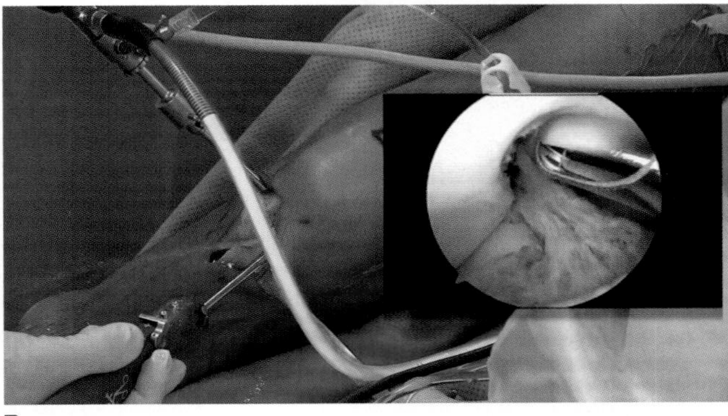

B

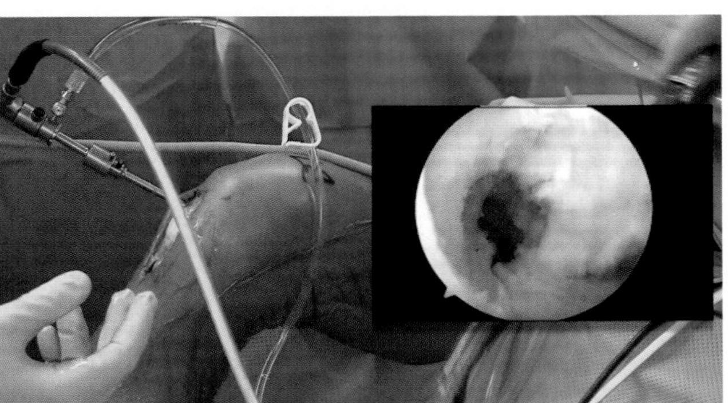

C

Figure 40-8 | The **(A)** remnant ACL stump; **(B)** existing native notch; and **(C)** notch after notchplasty, with trough at ACL footprint to facilitate free-hand, transtibial drilling. Notch is wide enough to allow insertion of a 10-mm-wide graft that does not impinge on the femoral condyle, apex of the notch or the PCL throughout a full range of motion.

- **Key step:** A hemispherical trough is made at the femoral attachment site of the ACL using the 5.5-mm burr to allow the tip of the acorn reamer to engage when beginning femoral tunnel reaming.
- **Pearl:** For short grafts (tendon lengths <40 mm), a major notchplasty should not be done over the attachment site (near posterior wall) because this will increase the intra-articular distance between the attachment sites, potentially making the tendon portion of the graft too short.

Diagnostic Arthroscopy

- The diagnostic examination is done after notchplasty to remove all hematoma and debris from the knee before evaluation.
- A consistent order is used to prevent missing a compartment: lateral compartment, cruciates, medial meniscocapsular junction (Gillquist view), medial compartment, patellofemoral compartment, and medial and lateral gutters.
- The posteromedial capsular junction is assessed for a meniscocapsular junction tear ("ramp lesion") (Fig. 40-9).
  - The leg is allowed to hang off the bed, and the knee is gently flexed to ~30 degrees. The scope is turned to the 6 o'clock position (looking down) and then driven between the medial condyle and posterior cruciate ligament (PCL), pressing into the PCL to avoid scraping articular cartilage of the notch, until scope enters the posteromedial compartment. The knee is then flexed 60-90 degrees.

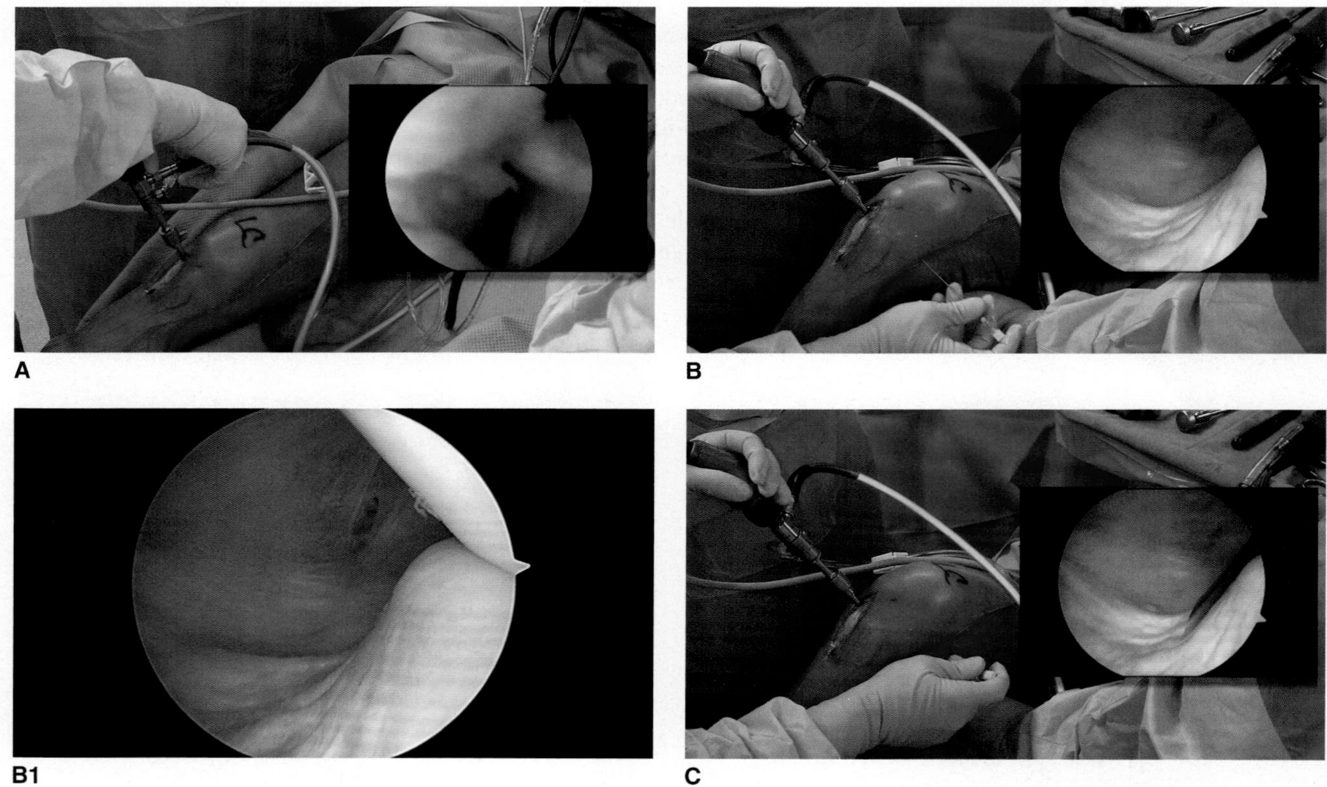

Figure 40-9 | With the scope in the posteromedial knee, **(A)** the knee is flexed off the bed at 30 degrees, and scope looking at 6 o'clock is gently pushed between the PCL and medial condyle into the posteromedial compartment. **B.** The posteromedial capsule, meniscocapsular junction, and the angle and position for creation of a posteromedial portal using an 18-gauge spinal needle. **B1.** View of the posteromedial compartment, meniscocapsular junction, and posteromedial femoral condyle. **C.** Spinal needle indicating the typical location of a meniscocapsular junction tear ("ramp lesion").

Tibial Tunnel

- The tibial tip-aiming guide (53 degrees) is inserted through the medial portal (Fig. 40-10A).
- The tip of the guide is placed on the posterolateral corner of the ACL insertion point (Fig. 40-10B).
- The skin is retracted, and the drill guide is pushed down to bone beneath the periosteal window (entry point should be adjacent to the anterior tibial insertion of the medial collateral ligament [MCL]).

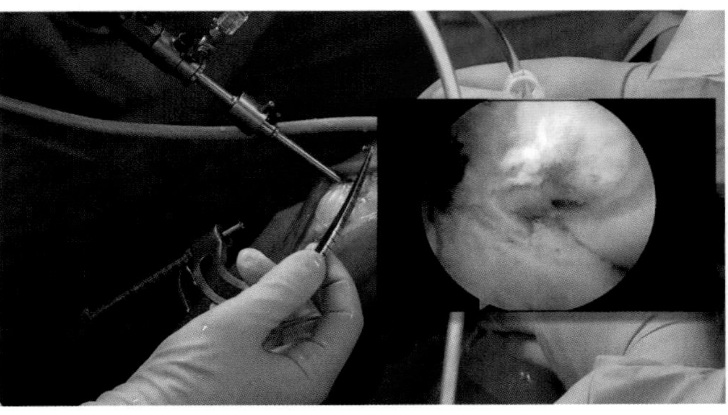
A

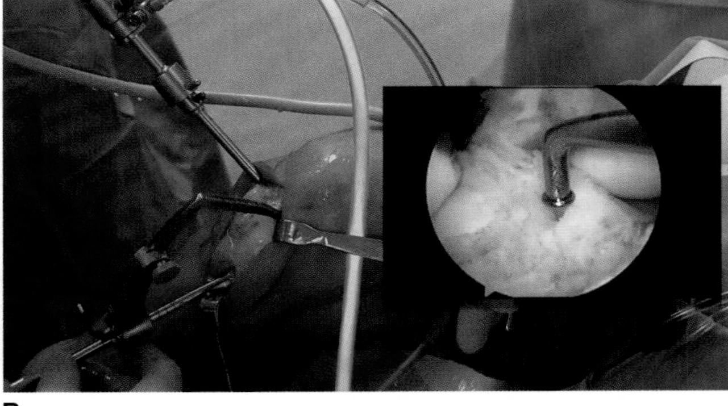
B

Figure 40-10 | Tibial drill guide: **(A)** a tip-aiming guide set at 53 degrees **(B)** placed at the posterolateral aspect of the ACL footprint.

- A guidewire is drilled through the guide into the joint.
  - When viewed from the top (axial view), the angle between the wire and the anterior tibia should be about 30 degrees, and the angle subtended by a line parallel with the tibial surface and the wire should be about 40 degrees.
- The wire is overdrilled with a 10-mm acorn reamer.
- A shaver is used to bevel the edges of the tunnel to prevent graft abrasion and remove any remaining ACL stump and soft tissue to prevent a cyclops lesion.

Femoral Tunnel

- A 10-mm reamer is inserted through the tibial tunnel with the knee in 90 degrees of flexion, and then the leg is extended and internally rotated until the reamer contacts the lateral condyle just superior to the origin of the ACL (generally begins at 45 degrees flexion but varies based on individual notch anatomy) (Fig. 40-11A).
  - The reamer tip should fall into the previously created trough made by the burr at the femoral origin of the ACL stump.
- We use a freehand drilling technique without an over-the-top guide. This allows maximal freedom for femoral tunnel placement through the tibial tunnel without the constraint of a guide.
- The drill is gently advanced 1-2 mm and then checked to ensure correct starting position of the tunnel with a solid 1- to 2-mm posterior wall.
- If correct, the reamer is advanced.
  - An assistant gradually flexes the knee as drilling continues (will end up at 90-120 degrees) to allow drilling to a depth of 25-35 mm (Fig. 40-11B).
  - Knee flexion during passage of the reamer forces the reamer to track along the anterior femoral cortex and prevents posterior wall blowout.

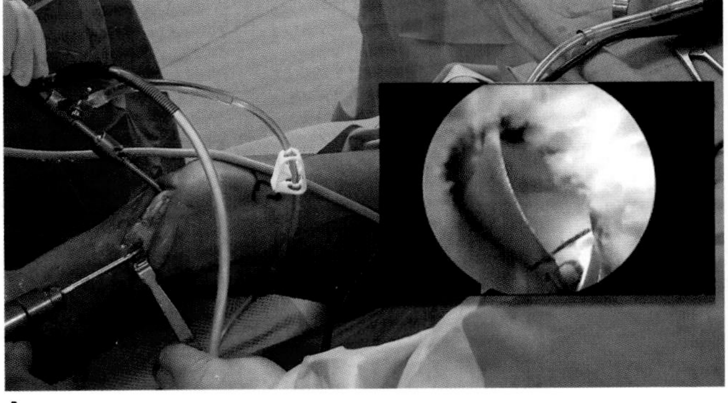
A

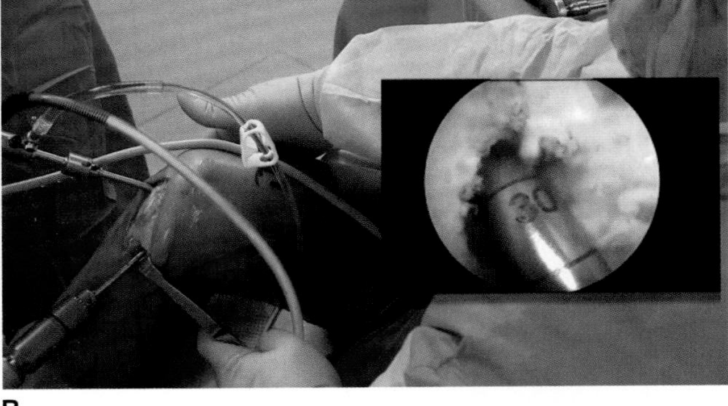

B

Figure 40-11 | Femoral tunnel drilling. **A.** To access the ACL footprint with a transtibial technique, the knee is extended and the leg is internally rotated to allow the tip of the acorn reamer to fall into the trough created during the notchplasty. **B.** The knee is flexed as the reamer is advanced to a depth of 25-35 mm.

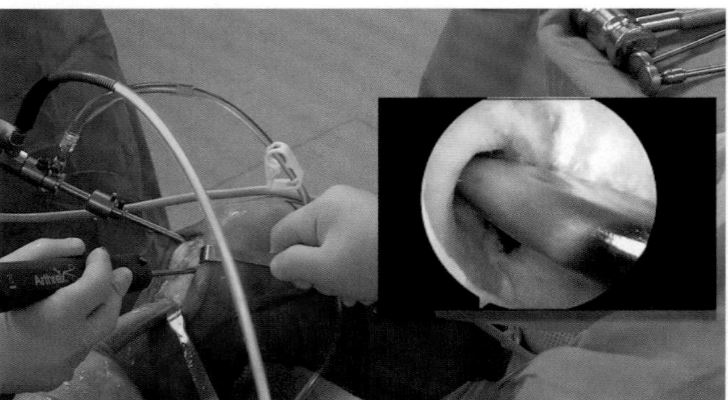

Figure 40-12 | Shaver removing bone debris. Location of the femoral tunnel at the 9:30 to 10 o'clock position (right knee).

- The shaver is used to remove excess bone reamings (Fig. 40-12).
- A Beath pin is inserted through the tibial tunnel and then into the femoral tunnel (the knee is flexed and extended as needed to ensure that the Beath pin is at the proximal apex of the femoral tunnel).
- The pin is drilled through the center of the tunnel and out the lateral cortex of the femur and out the lateral thigh.

Graft Shuttling and Fixation

- The shuttling stitch of the femoral side of the graft is threaded through the eyelet in the Beath pin, and pliers and a mallet are used from above the knee to tap the wire out with the sutures.
- The graft is pulled into the joint, through the tibial tunnel, and into the femoral tunnel so that only the tip of the plug is in the tunnel.
  - The graft is rotated so that the cortical bone is posterior, cancellous bone is anterior, and the widest portion of the graft is facing anterior, not medial or lateral, and no twist is present.
- The tip of a standard AO hex screwdriver is used to make a notch in the anterolateral aspect of the tunnel to allow guidewire insertion (Fig. 40-13A).

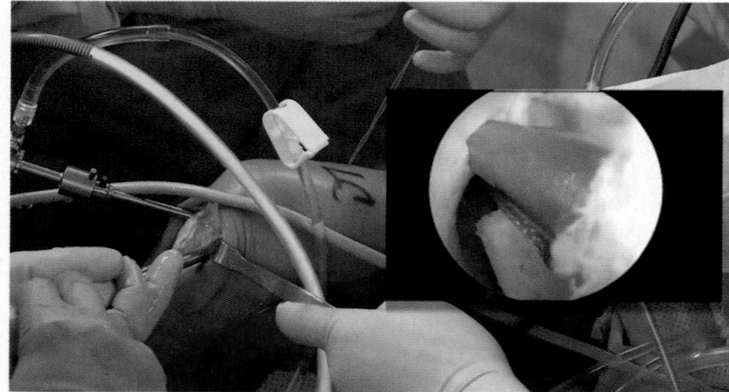

A

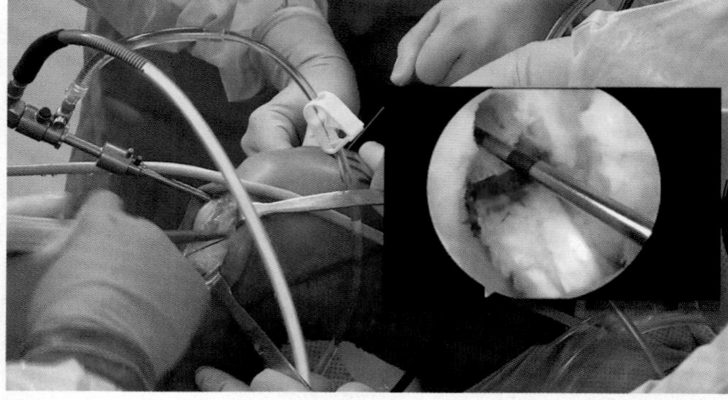

B

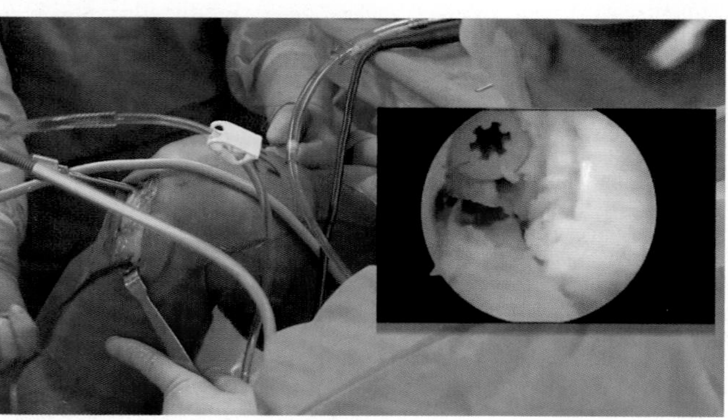

C

Figure 40-13 | **A.** A standard hex-head AO screwdriver is used to create a notch for the guidewire at the anterolateral aspect of the tunnel. **B.** A nitinol wire is inserted into the notch, and then the femoral bone plug is pulled and gently tapped into the tunnel. **C.** The PEEK interference screw sits flush with the condyle and the edge of the bone plug.

- A nitinol guidewire is inserted into the notched portion of the tunnel, and then the graft is pulled completely up into the tunnel (Fig. 40-13B).
  - Normal grafts may be flush, short grafts may be left 1-2 mm proud, and long grafts may be sunk into the tunnel.
- A soft tissue protector is inserted over the nitinol wire to protect the graft, and then an 8-mm tap is used to tap the tunnel to a depth to 25 mm.
- With equal tension on both sets of graft shuttling sutures, a 9 × 23 mm PEEK screw is inserted over the wire until it is flush with the condyle (Fig. 40-13C).
  - Moderate force should be placed on the screwdriver handle, distally and laterally to push the screw anteriorly and medially toward the femoral shaft canal.
- The leg is moved through a range of motion and then placed in full extension for tibial fixation. It is important to assess graft isometry after femoral fixation. Pistoning of the graft into the tibial tunnel with full knee extension (and out of the knee with flexion) indicates graft anisometry, which can cause overconstraint of the knee in flexion. If the graft is found to be anisometric, which is common with a "low" femoral or transmedial portal tunnel placement, the tibial portion of the graft should be fixed with the knee in full extension to prevent capturing the knee in flexion.
- With tension on the graft sutures, the nitinol guidewire is inserted posterolateral to the plug, pushing it anterior.
- An 8-mm tap is used over the wire to tap only the anterior cortex to prevent cutting the shuttling sutures.
- A posterior drawer force is placed on the knee, and then a 9 × 28 mm PEEK screw is inserted while tension is maintained on the graft (Fig. 40-14).

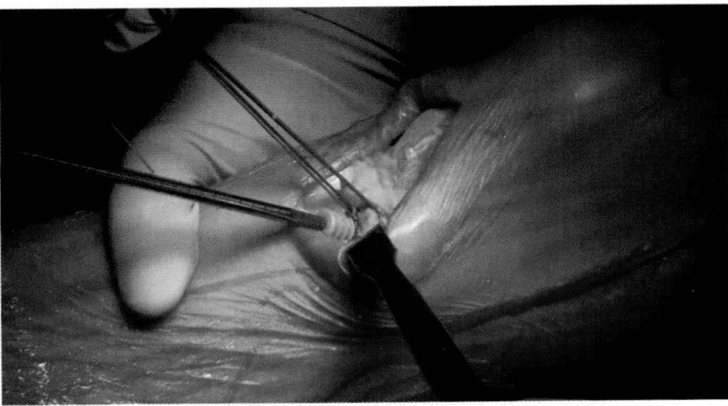

Figure 40-14 | The nitinol wire is inserted posterolateral to the bone plug, pushing it more anterior, and then the screw is inserted over the wire and seated flush with the end of the bone plug or tibial cortex.

- The scope is inserted into the tibial tunnel to check the position of the screw and graft plug—the screw should be flush with the end of the plug.
- The scope is inserted into the joint, and then the ACL is probed. The lateral notch, the apex of the notch, and the PCL are checked for impingement; the notchplasty is enlarged if needed (Fig. 40-15).
- A suction tip is placed into the suprapatellar pouch, and the knee is irrigated to remove any bone debris from tunnel drilling.

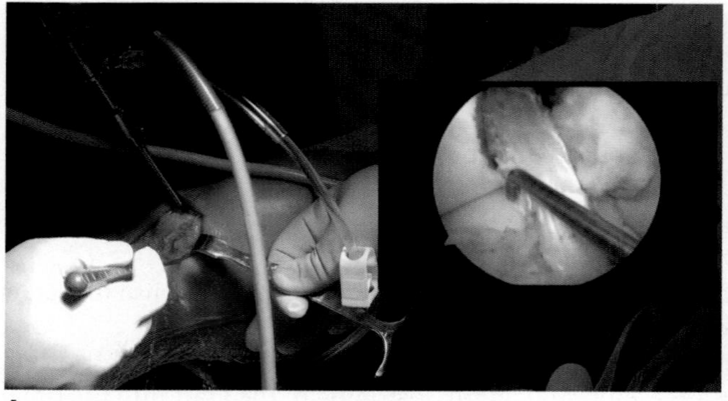
A

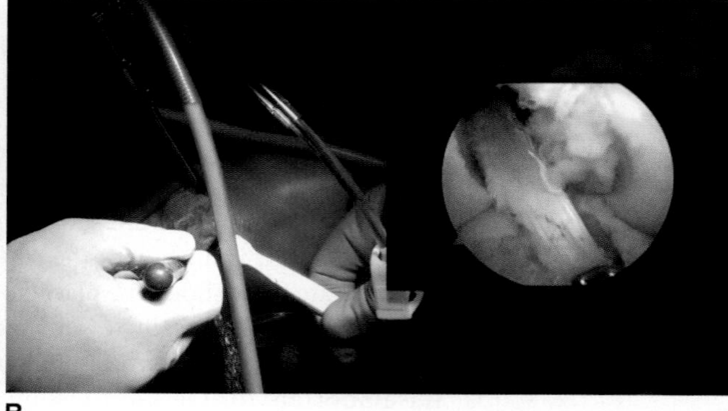
B

C

Figure 40-15 | The final ACL after fixation. **A.** On probing, with appropriate tautness. **B.** The entire graft and both tunnels. **C.** With the leg in full extension and no impingement.

- The sheath is placed in the suprapatellar pouch; the camera is removed and a precut, Hemovac drain (Zimmer, Warsaw, IN) is inserted into the knee; the sheath is removed over the drain; and the trocar is shuttled subcutaneously out the lateral thigh (Fig. 40-16).

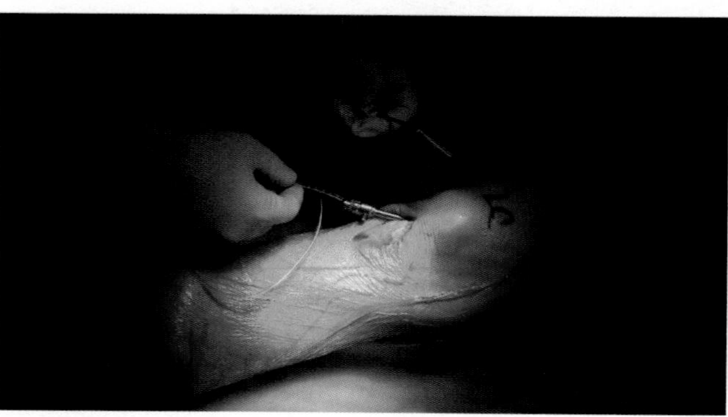

Figure 40-16 | Insertion of the Hemovac drain, retrograde through the arthroscopic sheath (lateral portal), which is then shuttled subcutaneously out the lateral thigh; this is removed in the recovery room before discharge.

- The trocar is left on the drain, and pliers are used to straighten the bend to prevent it from binding in the sheath.
- Cut the drain, leaving five to seven holes on the end opposite the trocar.
- The end with the holes is shuttled into the sheath retrograde.
- The drain will be removed in PACU before the patient is discharged.

Closure

- The portals and periosteal window are closed with a no. 0 absorbable braided suture
- The subcutaneous layer is closed with an interrupted no. 2-0 absorbable, monofilament suture.
- The skin is closed with a running no. 3-0 nonabsorbable, monofilament suture, with tails and an escape stitch.
- Dressings and a hinged postoperative knee brace locked in full extension are applied.

Chapter 41
Endoscopic Hamstring ACL Reconstruction

ROBERT W. WESTERMANN
MIA S. HAGEN
BRIDGET MANSELL
RICHARD D. PARKER

Sterile Instruments/Equipment (Fig. 41-1)

- 4.5-mm arthroscope
- 30-degree lens
- Light source
- Arthroscopy fluid: lactated Ringer solution or normal saline. Dilute epinephrine can be added safely at 1 mg/L.
- Tourniquet
- Verres outflow cannula
- No. 11 and no. 15 blades
- Two right angle munions
- Arthroscopic probe
- Arthroscopic shaver
- Coblation wand
- No. 2 FiberLoop suture × 4 (Arthrex, Naples, FL)
- Graft preparation station (Acufex shown, Smith & Nephew, Memphis, TN)
- Antibiotic solution in graduated cylinder for graft (1 g cefazolin or 80 mg gentamicin in 500 mL normal saline per patient allergy)
- Flexible femoral reaming system (Smith & Nephew, Memphis, TN)
- Tibial reaming system
- Curved curette or posterior cruciate ligament (PCL) protector
- Arthroscopic grasper

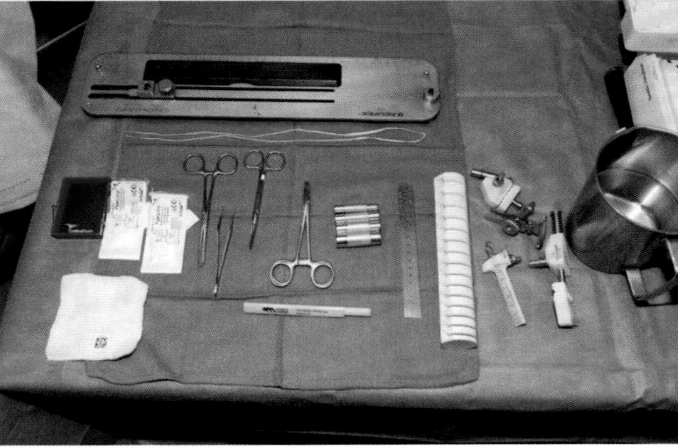

Figure 41-1 | Back table equipment needed for hamstring graft preparation.

- Femoral suspensory fixation (Endobutton, Smith & Nephew, Memphis, TN)
- Tibial fixation: 6.5-mm partially threaded cortical screw with washer

Positioning (Fig. 41-2A and B)

- Before preparation and draping, an intra-articular injection of 50 mg ropivacaine combined with 2 mg of Duramorph is inserted with sterile technique into the knee. This eliminates the need for a femoral nerve block, which can cause quadriceps inhibition.

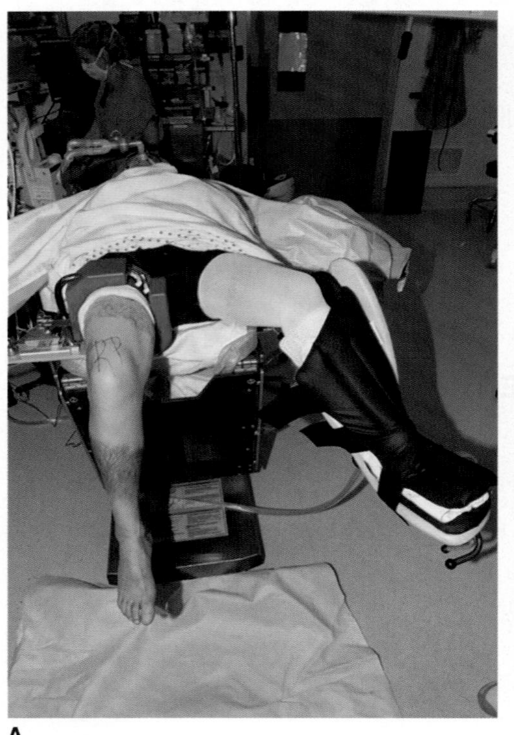
A

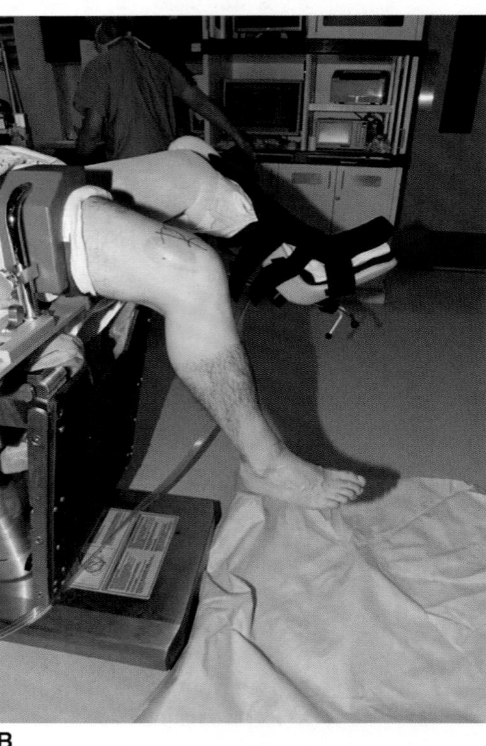
B

Figure 41-2 | A. Our preferred patient positioning for hamstring ACL reconstruction. **B.** Patient positioning with plenty of room for knee flexion.

- Alternatively, regional blockade through the adductor canal also can be administered by the anesthesiologist in the preoperative area.
- A wide area is prepared two hand's breadths above the patella to ensure an adequate sterile field for flexible femoral guidewire passing.
- A tourniquet is placed on the upper thigh; the operative leg is placed in an arthroscopic leg holder and the other leg in a well-leg holder.
- The patient should be distal enough on the bed so that there is room to flex the knee for femoral drilling.
- The table height is raised, and the foot of the bed is dropped. Sterile drapes are applied according to surgeon preference.

Surgical Approach (Fig. 41-3)

Hamstring Harvest

- An Esmarch bandage is used to exsanguinate the limb, and the tourniquet is inflated to 250 mm Hg.

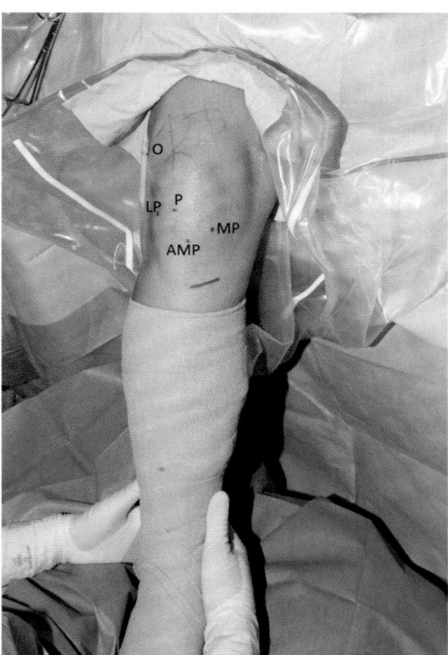

Figure 41-3 | Outflow portal location, deep to the quadriceps tendon, superior lateral. P, inferior pole of the patella; LP, lateral portal just inferior to the inferior pole of the patella adjacent to the patellar tendon; MP, medial portal, mid-medial joint line; AMP, accessory medial portal, medial to the patellar tendon and 1 cm distal to joint line. An oblique incision is made for hamstring harvest to help avoid injury to the infrapatellar branch of the saphenous nerve.

- A half-sheet is placed over the surgeon's lap, and the surgeon sits on a stool with the patient's foot on his or her lap (Fig. 41-4).

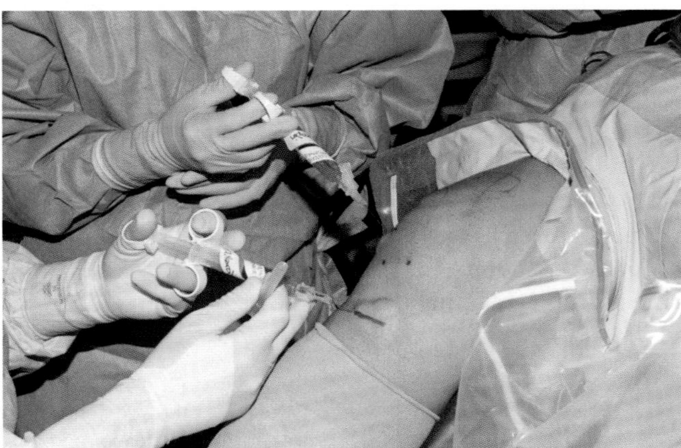

Figure 41-4 | Injection of the hamstring harvest site and arthroscopy portals with local anesthetic and epinephrine prior to incision.

- The hamstring incision is four finger breadths beneath the medial joint line, in Langer lines. The pes anserinus tendons are palpated to locate the correct incision site. The tendency is to be too proximal with this incision.
- The skin over the hamstring harvest and arthroscopy portal sites is injected with local anesthetic and epinephrine prior to incision.
- Sharp dissection with the no. 15 blade is carried down to the level of the sartorial fascia, obtaining hemostasis as necessary. The sartorial fascia is cleared with sponge for manual dissection (Fig. 41-5).

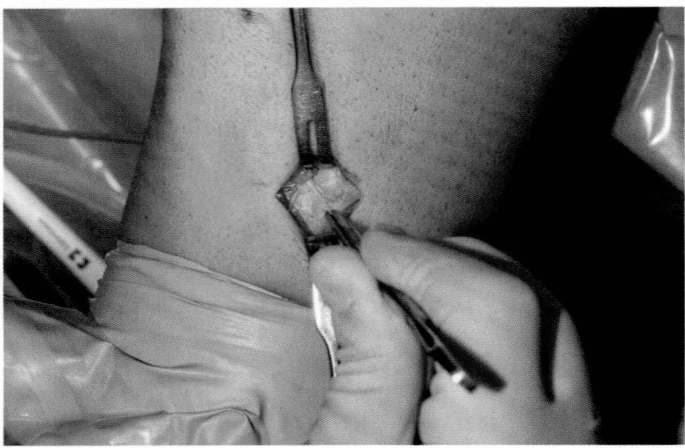

Figure 41-5 | Sartorial fascia overlying hamstring tendons.

- The sartorial fascia is identified and incised in line above the hamstring tendons.
- Once a window is made, the fascia is opened proximally with scissors in line with the tendons, and distally more vertical ("hockey stick" shape) (Fig. 41-6A and B).

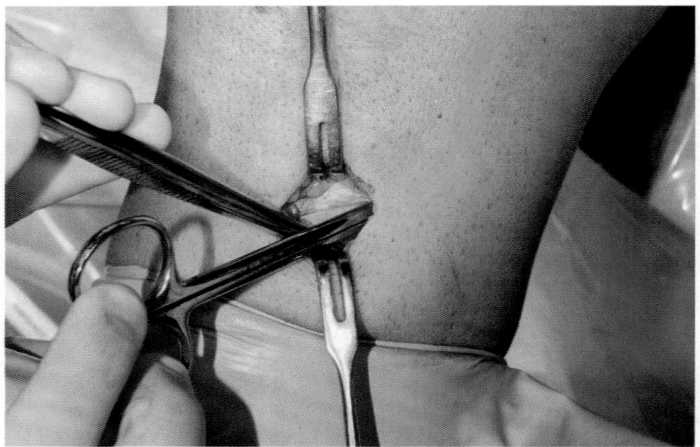

A

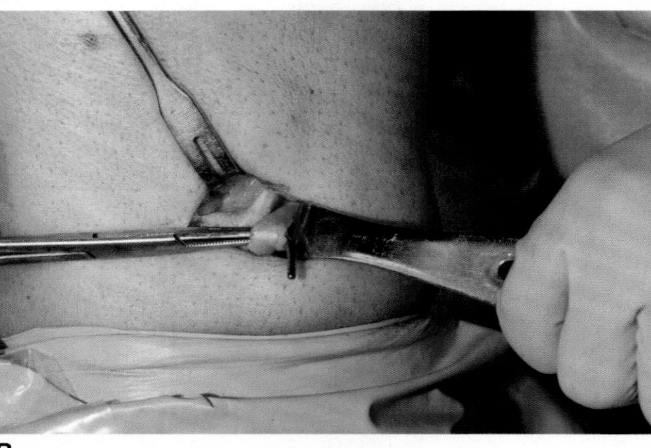

B

Figure 41-6 | A. Release of the sartorial fascia in a hockey stick fashion. **B.** Semitendinosus tendon retrieved with a right-angle device.

- A right-angle instrument is used to retrieve the semitendinosus inferiorly; then, a blue tie from a lap sponge is placed around the tendon.
- More proximally, the gracilis is identified, and a blue tie is placed around it (Fig. 41-7).

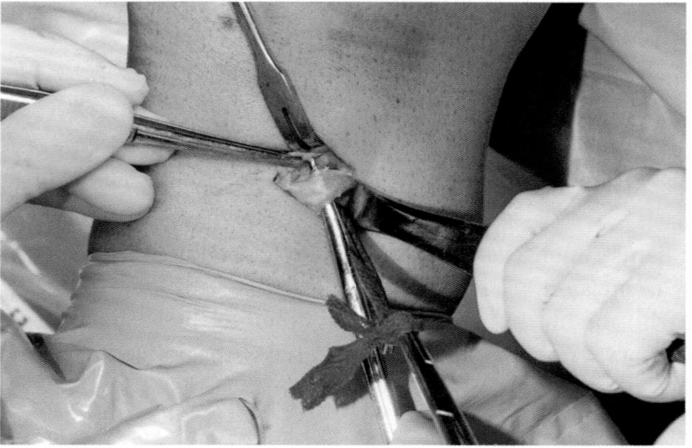

Figure 41-7 | A blue lap tie is placed around the semitendinosus, and the gracilis is identified more proximally.

- With both hamstring tendons identified, the semitendinosus is released from its insertion, and a FiberLoop is placed through the distal 3 cm of the tendon (Fig. 41-8).

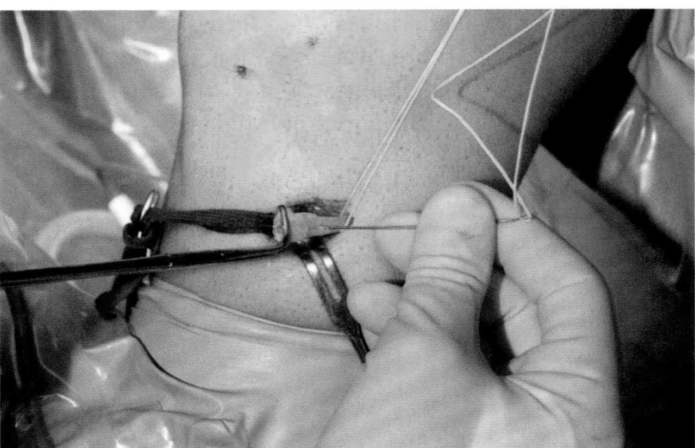

Figure 41-8 | The semitendinosus is released from the tibia, and a FiberLoop is placed through the distal segment of the tendon.

- Adhesions to the tendon, especially the large connection with the medial head of the gastrocnemius, are released.
- When releasing adhesions, we prefer the use of scissors that are opened and pushed proximally rather than repeatedly opened and closed to avoid accidental cutting of the tendon tissue (Fig. 41-9). With excursion of the tendon >10 cm from the incision, a closed end tendon stripper is used to harvest the semitendinosus tendon with the knee flexed.

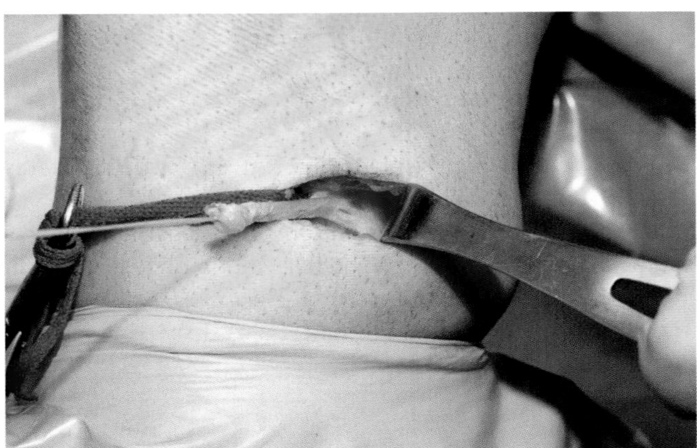

Figure 41-9 | A FiberLoop is placed in the distal semitendinosus tendon, and the adhesion to the gastroc is visualized.

- The gracilis tendon is harvested in the same manner.
- The stripper is passed with slow steady force in line with the tendon's trajectory.
- Each graft is carefully moved from the harvest site to the back table for graft preparation; if handed off to an assistant, this must be done with eye contact over the sterile field so that the graft is not dropped (Fig. 41-10). Muscle is cleared from the tendons on the back table.

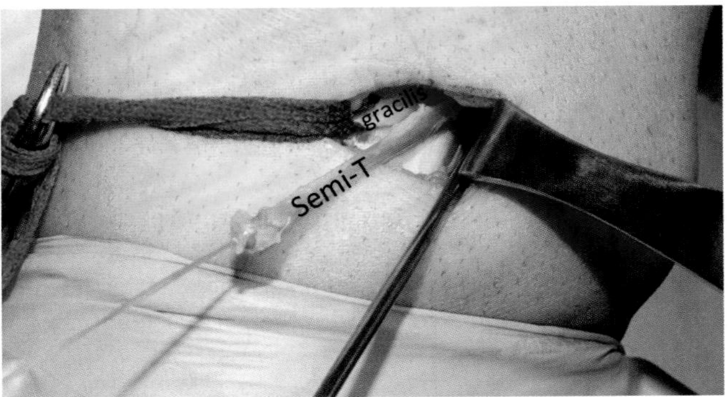

Figure 41-10 | With release of adhesions, and tendon excursion of 10 cm, a tendon stripper is placed over the semitendinosus.

- The graft is briefly soaked in antibiotic solution.
- FiberLoop suture is placed on the proximal end of each tendon.
- The tendons can be folded over once to create a 4-strand graft.
- Often the semitendinosus is folded over 3 times to increase its diameter (Fig. 41-11).
- The graft can be tensioned on the graft preparation station and the diameter and length measured.
- With a 5-strand technique, the graft is typically 8-10 mm in diameter. The length should be at least 70 mm to allow adequate tissue in both the femur and tibia (Fig. 41-12).

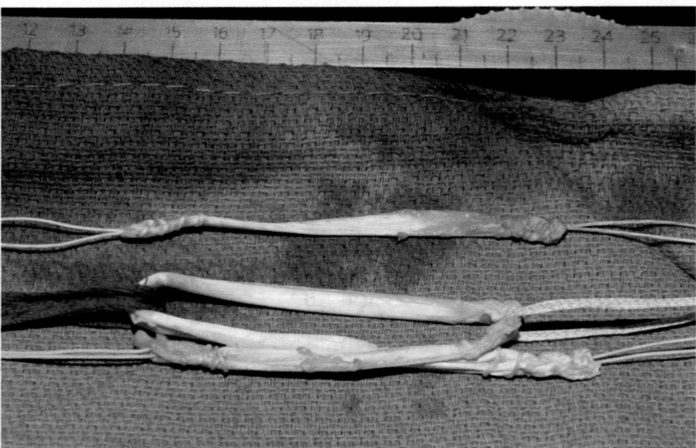

Figure 41-11 | Gracilis (*top*) and semitendinosus (*bottom*) are prepared on the back table.

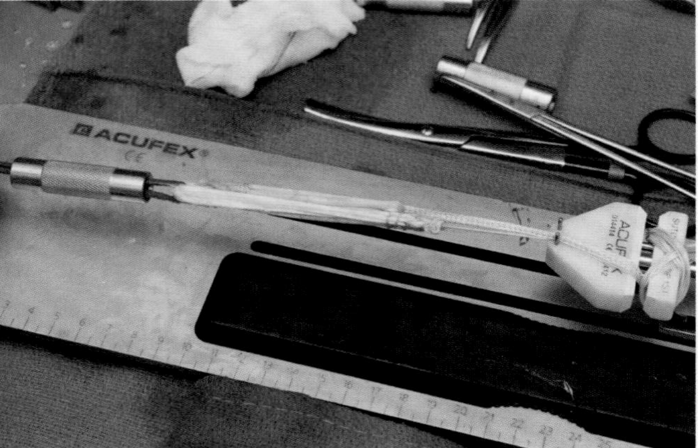

Figure 41-12 | The graft measured for length and diameter on the back table.

Diagnostic Arthroscopy

- The lateral incision should be off the border of the patellar tendon and high near the inferior pole of the patella.
- The incision can be made with the no. 11 blade facing distal, as this portal is high above the lateral meniscal root. The blade should aim straight toward the notch.
  - The skin incision can be small, but the capsulotomy underneath the skin should be larger.
  - We prefer to turn the blade away from the patellar tendon once the capsule has been entered and then cut laterally to widen the capsulotomy.
  - This is done without enlarging the skin incision (Fig. 41-13).

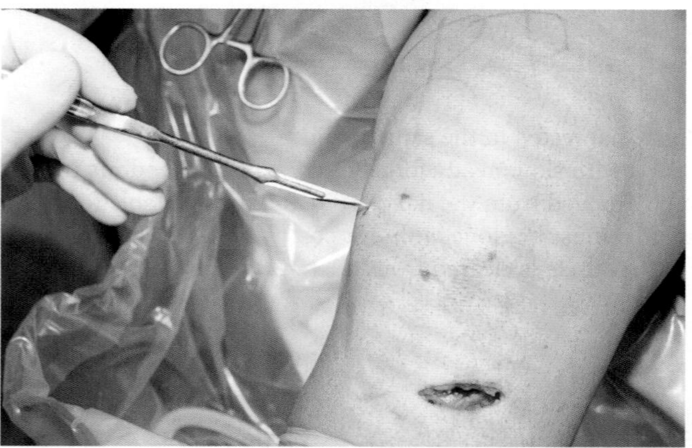

Figure 41-13 | The lateral portal is created adjacent to the inferior pole of the patella off the lateral boarder of the patellar tendon.

- The medial portal should be placed in the center of the joint space, typically 4-5 mm distal to the lateral portal.
  - The no. 11 blade is faced proximal to avoid injury to the anterior horn of the medial meniscus, and then the blade is turned medially away from the patellar tendon to enlarge the capsulotomy (Fig. 41-14A and B).

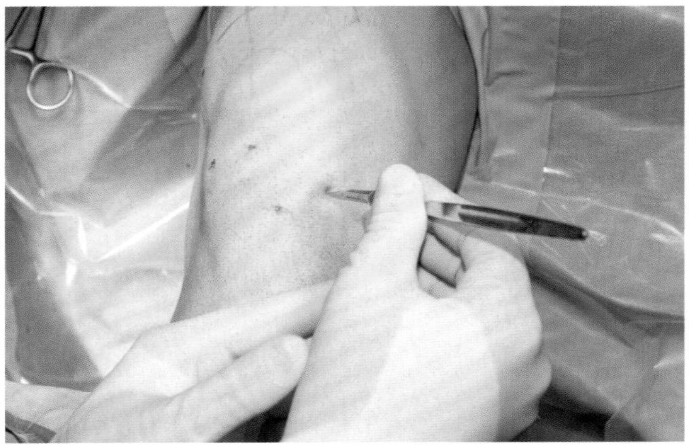

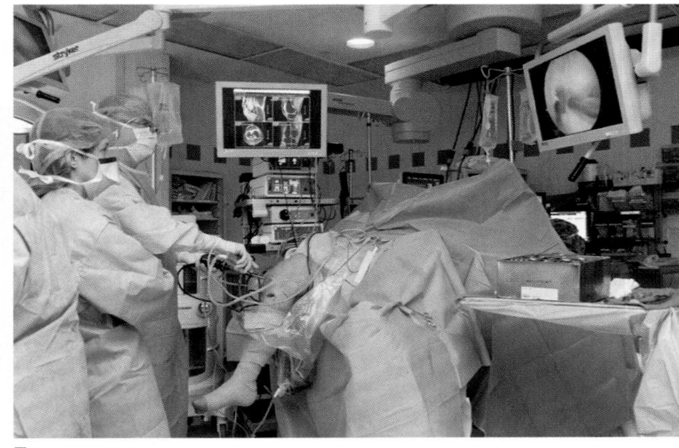

A **B**

Figure 41-14 | A. The lateral portal is created at the inferior margin of the patella, just off the lateral boarder of the patellar tendon. **B.** The medial portal is created with the no. 11 blade aiming up away from the anteromedial meniscal root.

- A superolateral incision is made (as previously shown), and a small outflow cannula is placed.
- A diagnostic arthroscopy of the patellofemoral, lateral, and medial compartments should be performed. Any necessary meniscal or cartilage work can be done at this time.
- Visualization of the notch can be improved by:
  - Taking down the ligamentum mucosum
  - Resecting enough fat pad until the anterior horns of the medial and lateral menisci are seen
  - Looking down to view the intermeniscal ligament, which is not cut
  - Resecting the remaining anterior cruciate ligament (ACL) in the notch down to a tibial stump and identifying the medial tibial spine
- Following diagnostic arthroscopy, meniscal or cartilage treatment, and creation of a visual working space in the center of the knee, the accessory medial portal is created under direct vision.
- A spinal needle is used to confirm trajectory, followed by the no. 11 blade (Fig. 41-15). With the camera moved to the accessory medial portal, there is improved visualization of the ACL femoral footprint.

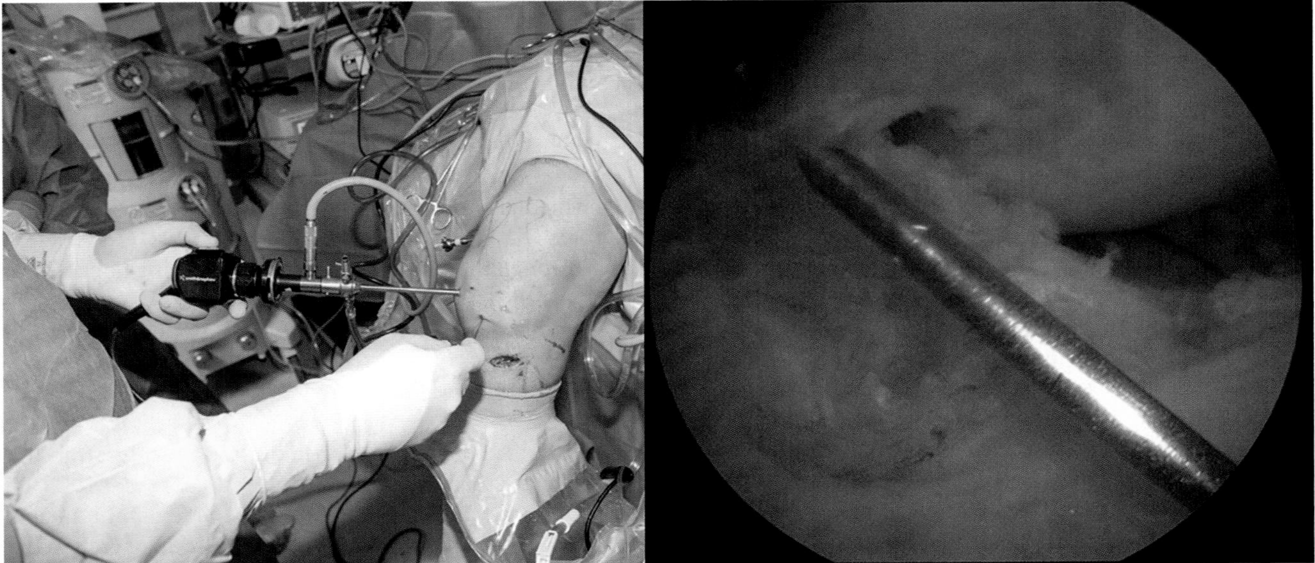

Figure 41-15 | Setup for diagnostic arthroscopy. A spinal needle is introduced to confirm trajectory of the accessory medial portal.

- This area is further cleared with an arthroscopic shaver and coblation wand until the footprint and back wall are clearly seen. Instruments are passed through the medial portal (Fig. 41-16).

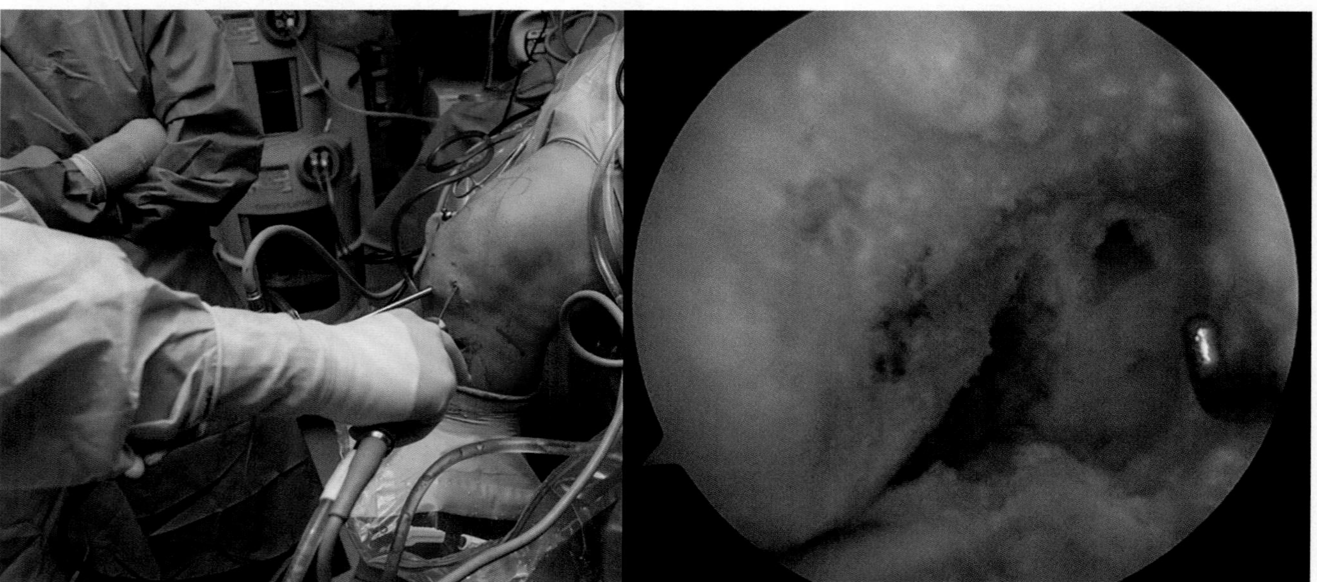

Figure 41-16 | With the camera in the accessory medial portal, the anatomic footprint of the femoral ACL can be easily visualized.

Femoral Reaming

- A microfracture awl can be used to mark the target for the center of the femoral tunnel.
- The femoral tunnel should be below/inferior to the lateral intercondylar ridge ("resident's ridge") but should preserve about 2 mm of back wall after tunnel reaming.
- The flexible reamer guide pin is then introduced to the anatomic footprint of the ACL and is passed with the knee in hyperflexion.
- The guide pin should exit on the anterolateral thigh to avoid damage to neurovascular structures. With the flexible femoral reaming system, the guide pin is advanced to a specific laser mark.
- It is then measured outside-in with a depth gauge on the antero-lateral thigh (the no. 11 blade is used to make an incision around the guide pin). The femoral tunnel length measurement is used to mark on the ACL graft where it is expected to line up with the femoral tunnel in the knee (measuring down from the button) (Fig. 41-17A-C).
- The appropriately sized flexible reamer (matched to graft diameter) is introduced through the medial portal.
  - Care should be taken to avoid damage to the medial femoral condyle when introducing the reamer.
- The camera is still in the accessory medial portal.
  - The shaver can be introduced into the knee through the lateral portal to aid in clearing bone debris to monitor the depth of reaming.
- For Endobutton femoral fixation, the tunnel should be reamed to <6 mm of the total length of the tunnel for the button to have room to flip.
- The outer femoral cortex should not be violated with the reamer.
- The appropriate suture button length is selected.
  - Ideally, there should be at least 15 mm of graft in the femoral tunnel, but too much graft in the femoral tunnel will limit the amount of graft in the tibial tunnel.
  - For example, if the guide pin measures a total tunnel length of 36 mm, and the femoral tunnel is reamed to 31 mm to allow the button to flip, a 15-mm suture button will place 21 mm of graft in the tunnel, while a 10-mm suture button will place 26 mm of graft in the femoral tunnel (Fig. 41-18 A).
- The outer cortex of the femur is drilled to accommodate suspensory fixation (usually a 4.5-mm reamer).
- The flexible guidewire is pulled back but is not removed from the knee (Fig. 41-18B).

- Placement of the posteromedial portal is key for exposure of the tibial footprint and visualization while the femoral tunnel is established.
  - The portal is placed under spinal needle guidance while viewing in the posterior knee from the inferolateral portal (Fig. 42-3).
  - This portal must be positioned behind the medial femoral condyle to allow the appropriate angle to reach the tibial footprint (Fig. 42-4).

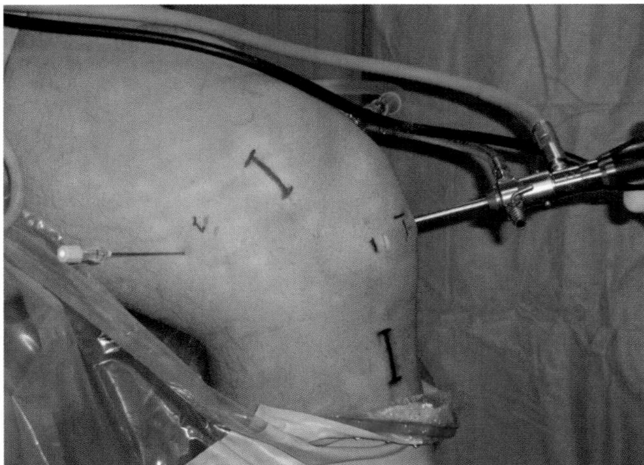

Figure 42-3 | A posteromedial portal is localized with spinal needle guidance while viewing from the inferolateral portal.

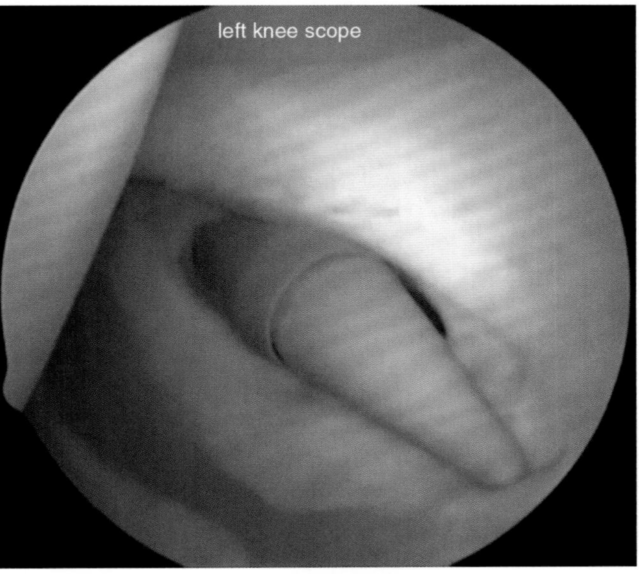

Figure 42-4 | An intra-articular view of cannula placement demonstrates proper positioning of the posteromedial portal behind the condyle to allow free access to the tibial footprint of the PCL.

Preparation

- The PCL stump is resected with a motorized shaver. Soft tissue at the footprints is preserved to allow identification of landmarks for tunnel placement (Fig. 42-5).
- A radiofrequency ablator is used to dissect towards the tibial footprint.
  - The posterior meniscal attachments are in close proximity and must be identified early in this dissection to avoid injury to these structures.
- The posterior capsule is dissected off to identify the tibial ridge to help protect against injury to the popliteal vessels.

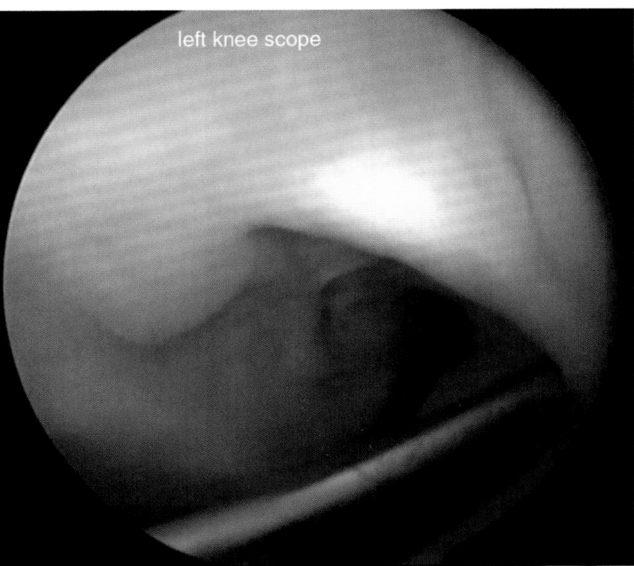

Figure 42-5 | An intra-articular view of an empty medial wall of the intercondylar notch following debridement of the PCL stump.

Tibial Tunnel Placement

- The tibial tunnel is placed first.
- Distally, the starting point is immediately distal to the pes anserine insertion.
- The center of the tibial footprint lies 2-3 mm distal to the posterior articular surface.
- The drill guide is placed through either the inferomedial or mid–patellar tendon portal.
- The pin is advanced at a 45-degree angle to the tibial shaft or parallel to the proximal tibial-fibular joint.
- The guide pin is advanced under fluoroscopic guidance to ensure both the appropriate trajectory and depth of pin placement (Fig. 42-6).

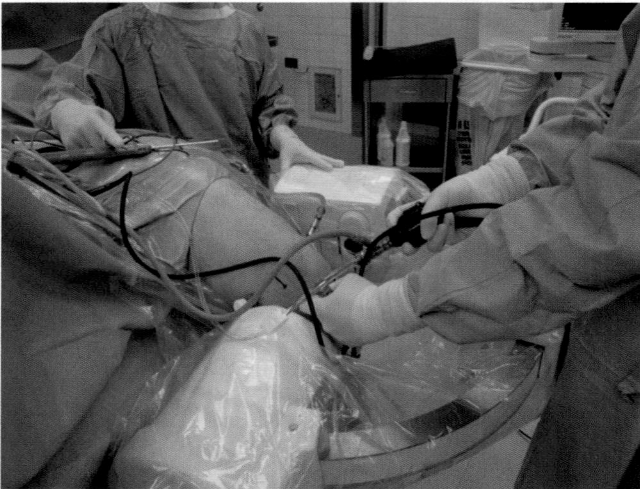

Figure 42-6 | Intraoperative fluoroscopy is used throughout the procedure to ensure proper tunnel positioning and reaming for the tibial side.

- The popliteal vessels lie in close proximity to the posterior tibia, and care is taken to visualize the depth of the guide pin at all times to limit the risk of vascular injury.
- A curette or guide is used while reaming to protect the popliteal vessels (Fig. 42-7).
- The tibial tunnel is reamed with cylindrical reamers to avoid vessel entrapment if there is posterior tibial blowout.

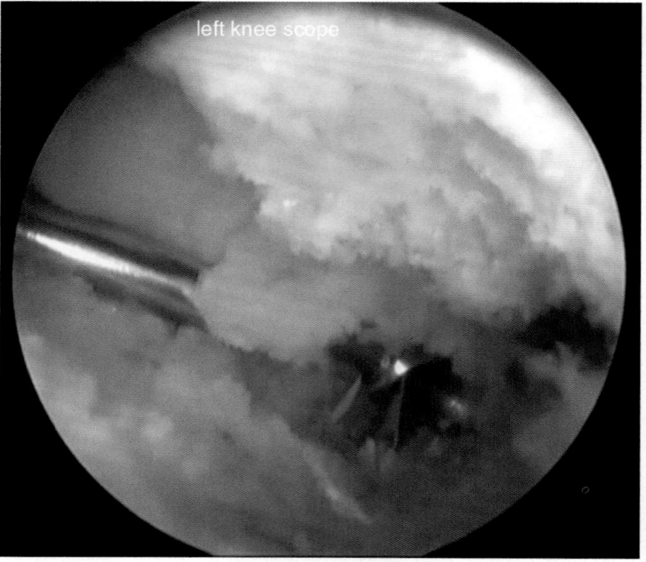

Figure 42-7 | A curette is positioned over the guide pin at the tibial tunnel to decrease the risk of the pin being pushed into the popliteal fossa.

- The tibial tunnel is generally reamed to 11-12 mm.
- Reaming is performed under fluoroscopic guidance to maintain the appropriate trajectory and depth of reaming (Fig. 42-8).

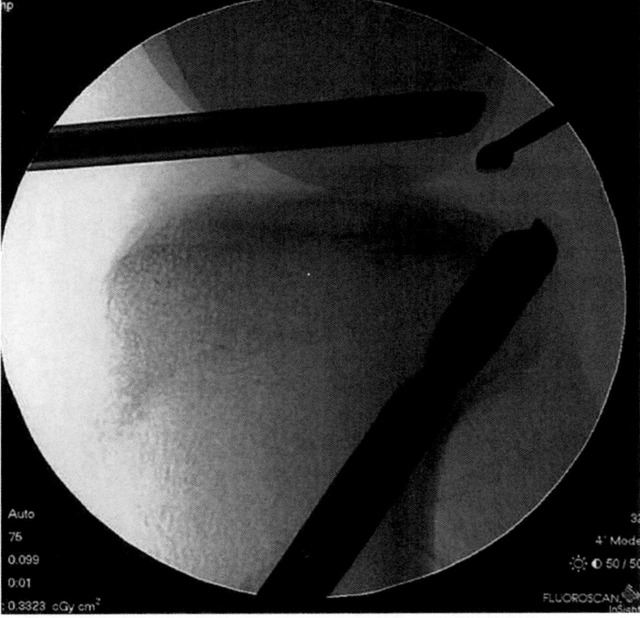

Figure 42-8 | An intraoperative fluoroscopic image shows the arthroscope in place posteriorly, a curette in place over the tibial tunnel, and a cylindrical reamer being advanced in the proper trajectory to establish the tibial tunnel.

Femoral Tunnel Placement

- A subvastus extra-articular approach is used to place the femoral tunnels (Fig. 42-9).
  - A 2- to 3-cm longitudinal incision is made over the distal femur.
  - The vastus medialis obliquis is identified, and its insertion is not disrupted.
  - Dissection is carried down to the anteromedial surface of the femur.

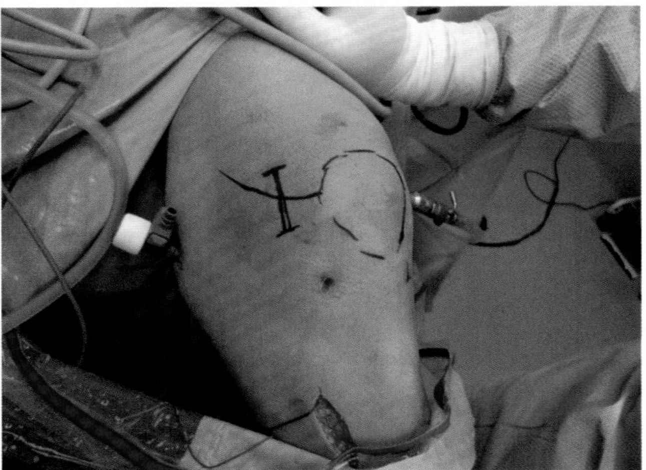

Figure 42-9 | Skin markings demonstrate the approach for femoral tunnel placement.

- Ideally, bony landmarks are used to determine optimal guide pin placement:
  - The medial intercondylar ridge and medial bifurcate ridge can be used as landmarks when positioning the anterolateral (AL) and posteromedial (PM) tunnels.
  - The AL and PM footprints are separated by the medial bifurcate ridge.[3]
  - The proximal extent of the PCL is defined by the medial intercondylar ridge.[3]

- If the bony anatomy is not visible, other prior descriptions are used for tunnel placement.
  - Takahashi et al. reported that the center of the AL bundle is 9.6 mm from the anterior articular cartilage and the center of the PM bundle is 10.6 mm.[4]
  - Edwards et al. described the center of the AL bundle at 7 mm from the 10:20 position on a clock face (left knee) and the PM bundle at 10 mm from the 8:30 position.[5]
- Guide pins are placed for the AL and PM tunnels.
  - We prefer inside-out pin placement to ensure positioning, to protect the integrity of each tunnel, and to preserve at least a 2-mm bone bridge between the tunnels (Fig. 42-10).
  - Outside-in placement can be used as well.
  - Inside-out drilling is performed over the guide pins if closed-end tunnels are planned.
  - Outside-in drilling may be used if bone plugs are planned.
- Our preferred tunnel diameters are 10-11 mm for the AL bundle and 7-8 mm for the PL bundle (Fig. 42-11).
- Closed-end tunnels are placed if intra-articular soft tissue screw fixation is planned.
- A complete tunnel can be placed if using a bone plug.
- Tunnel edges are smoothed to limit the risk of graft abrasion.

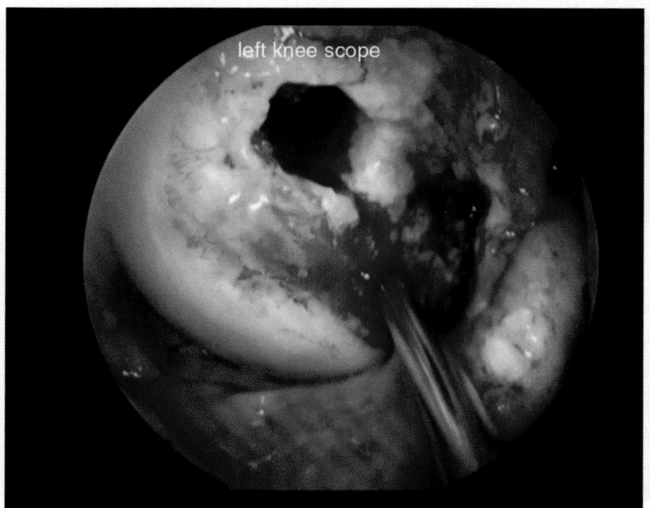

Figure 42-10 | An intra-articular view displays the intercondylar notch after the anterolateral bundle has been reamed with a guide pin in place for the posterolateral bundle.

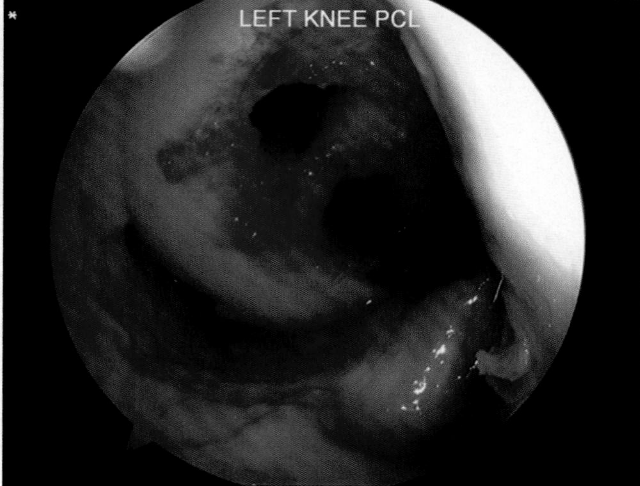

Figure 42-11 | An intra-articular view of the knee shows both femoral tunnels after reaming.

Graft Selection

- Graft choices for double-bundle PCL reconstruction include hamstring autograft, Achilles allograft, patellar tendon allograft, and quadriceps allograft.
- Our preference for double-bundle PCL reconstruction is a bone plug on the tibial side with two soft tissue limbs on the femoral side.
- The bone plug is undersized relative to the diameter of the tibial tunnel to allow easy passage through the tunnel.

Graft Passage

- The graft is passed with the arthroscopic pump off to avoid graft distension.
- A tourniquet is routinely used during graft passage to maintain a dry field of view.
- The graft is passed from distal to proximal (Fig. 42-12).

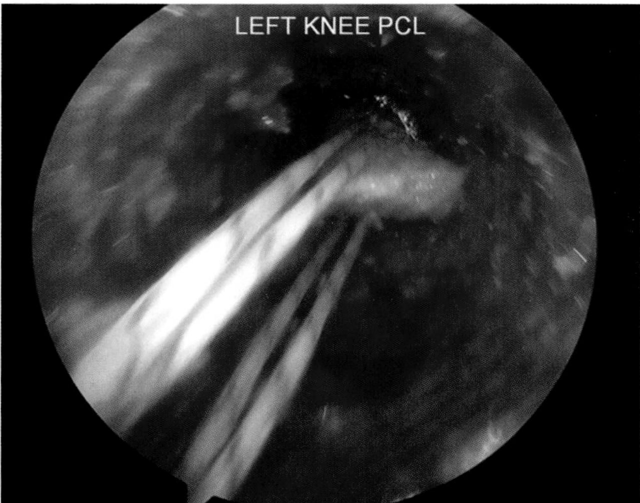

Figure 42-12 | The graft is advanced through the tibial tunnel.

Tensioning and Fixation

- Each bundle is tensioned separately with the knee at 70 degrees of flexion.
- It is imperative to not overconstrain the knee while tensioning the grafts, as this can lead to graft failure.
- The tibia is placed in a reduced position to reestablish the normal tibial-femoral relationship as the graft is tensioned.
- A titanium interference screw is used on the tibial side for interference fixation.
- In addition to bioabsorbable interference screw fixation, backup fixation in the form of a staple or tying over a post is used for all soft tissue grafts.
- The appearance of the final reconstruction is confirmed intra-articularly (Fig. 42-13).

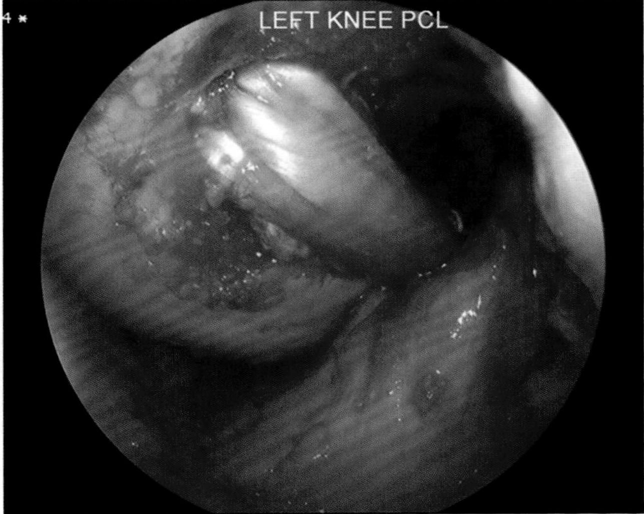

Figure 42-13 | The graft is viewed intra-articularly after final fixation.

Closure

- The tourniquet is deflated before closure to inspect for any evidence of intra-articular or extra-articular bleeding.
- The incisions for the tibial and femoral tunnels are closed in layers, with interrupted, absorbable sutures in the subcutaneous layer and running, subcuticular sutures for the skin.
- The arthroscopic portals are closed with non-absorbable, interrupted sutures.

Immediate Postoperative Care

- The operative knee is placed into a hinged knee brace, locked in extension (Fig. 42-14).

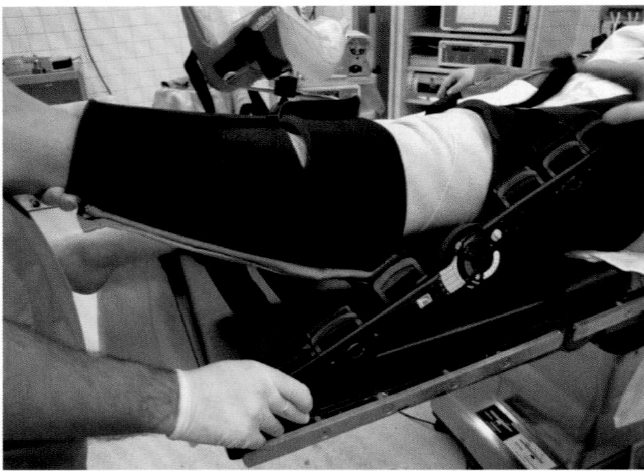

Figure 42-14 | After closure, the patient is placed in a hinged knee brace, locked in extension and with a bolster behind the tibia to prevent posterior sag while in the brace.

- A bolster may be placed behind the tibia to limit initial posterior force.
- Postoperative radiographs are obtained at follow-up to confirm tunnel positioning and restoration of the anatomic tibiofemoral alignment (Fig. 42-15).

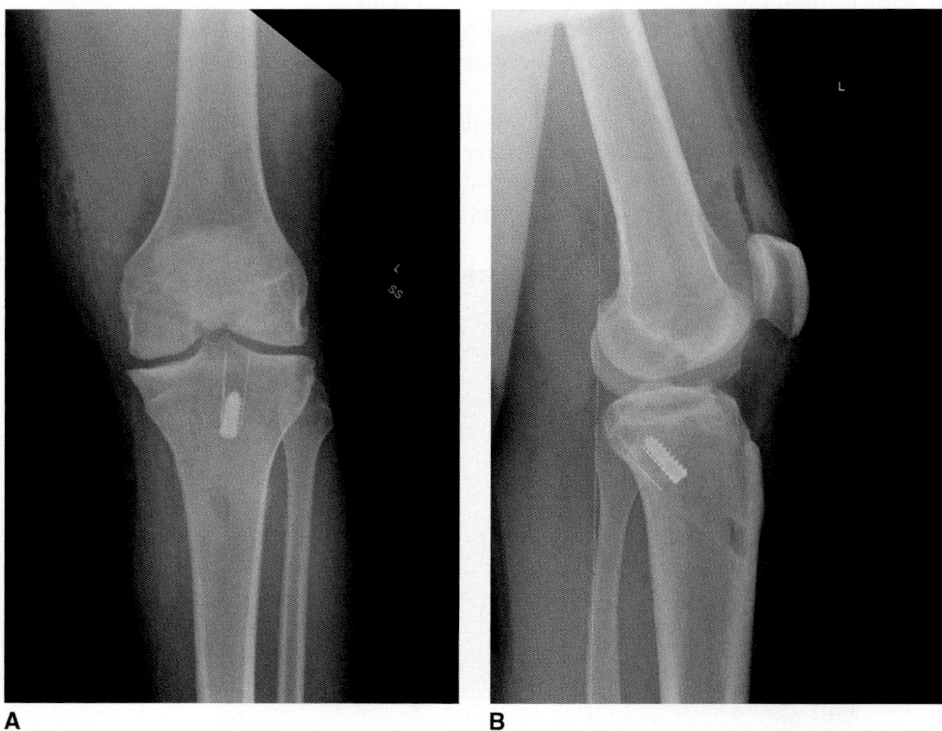

Figure 42-15 | Postoperative **(A)** AP and **(B)** lateral radiographs demonstrate restoration of tibiofemoral alignment, tunnel positioning, and interference screw fixation on the tibial side. The bone plug is outlined in yellow on the tibial side.

References

1. Yoon KH, Bae DK, Song SJ, Cho HJ, Lee JH. A prospective randomized study comparing arthroscopic single-bundle and double-bundle posterior cruciate ligament reconstructions preserving remnant fibers. *Am J Sports Med.* 2011;39(3):474-480.
2. Harner CD, Janaushek MA, Kanamori A, Yagi M, Vogrin TM, Woo SL. Biomechanical analysis of a double-bundle posterior cruciate ligament reconstruction. *Am J Sports Med.* 2000;28(2):144-151. doi:10.1177/03635465000280020201.
3. Lopes OV Jr, Ferretti M, Shen W, Ekdahl M, Smolinski P, Fu FH. Topography of the femoral attachment of the posterior cruciate ligament. *J Bone Joint Surg Am.* 2008;90(2):249-255. doi:10.2106/JBJS.G.00448.
4. Takahashi M, Matsubara T, Doi M, Suzuki D, Nagano A. Anatomical study of the femoral and tibial insertions of the anterolateral and posteromedial bundles of human posterior cruciate ligament. *Knee Surg Sports Traumatol Arthrosc.* 2006;14(11):1055-1059.
5. Edwards A, Bull AM, Amis AA. The attachments of the anteromedial and posterolateral fibre bundles of the anterior cruciate ligament. *Knee Surg Sports Traumatol Arthrosc.* 2008;16(1):29-36.

Chapter 43

ACL Reconstruction in the Skeletally Immature Patient

PETER D. FABRICANT
MININDER S. KOCHER

Sterile Instrument/Equipment

- All cases
  - Tourniquet
  - Knee arthroscopy equipment
- Preadolescents: modified MacIntosh procedure, combined extra- and intra-articular anterior cruciate ligament (ACL) reconstruction using iliotibial (IT) band autograft (Fig. 43-1)
  - Cobb elevator
  - Burr

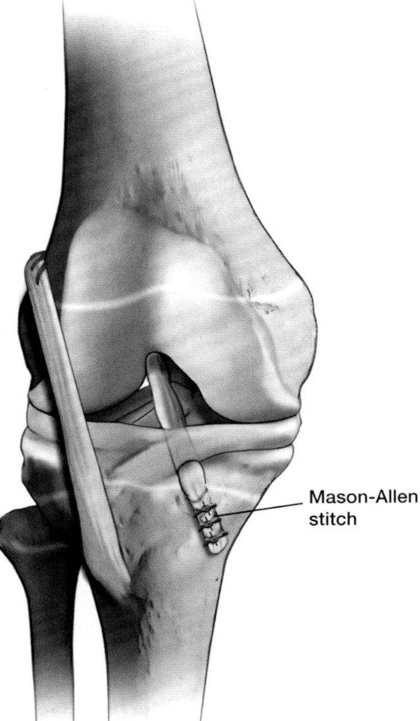

Figure 43-1 | Modified MacIntosh procedure: combined extra- and intra-articular ACL reconstruction using iliotibial (IT) band autograft.

- Periosteal elevator
- Meniscotomes (left, right, and end cutting) (Fig. 43-2A)
- Large curved hemostat/clamp (Fig. 43-2B)
- "Rat-tail" rasp (Fig. 43-2C)
- Heavy nonabsorbable suture

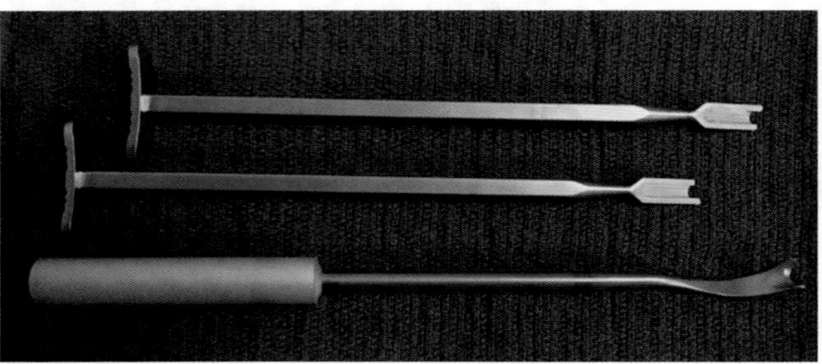

A

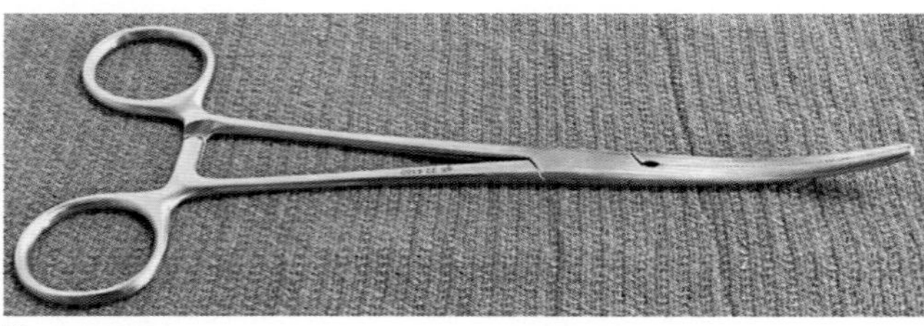

B

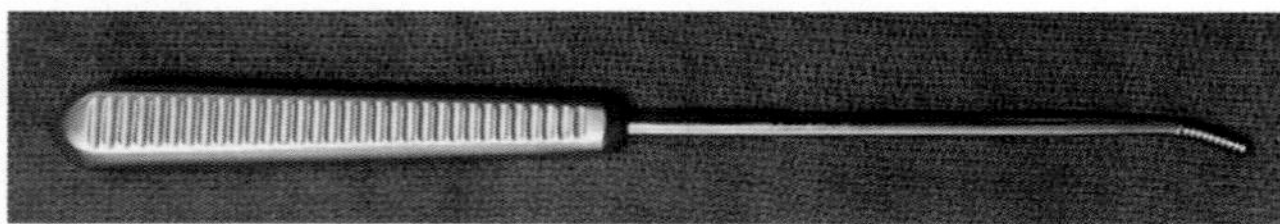

C

Figure 43-2 | Equipment for the modified MacIntosh procedure. Meniscotomes **(A)**, large curved hemostat/clamp **(B)**, and rat-tail rasp **(C)**.

- Adolescents: transphyseal hamstring ACL reconstruction (Fig. 43-3)
  - Graft preparation board
  - Suspensory fixation button (femoral fixation)
  - Nonmetal interference screw (tibial fixation)
  - ACL drill guides based on surgeon preference
  - Open- or closed-ended tendon harvester based on surgeon preference

Positioning

- The patient is placed supine.
  - Bumps can be placed under the hip and at the foot of the table to help with knee flexion.
  - A nonsterile pneumatic tourniquet is placed on the proximal thigh.
  - A lateral post is used based on surgeon preference.

Surgical Technique Considerations

- Minimal (<1 cm in each limb segment) growth remains around the knee after age 12-13 in girls (ie, 1 year after menarche) and 14 in boys.[1]
  - Before this time, reconstruction strategies must respect growing physes.
- Posteroanterior left hand radiograph can be obtained to measure skeletal age for surgical decision-making.

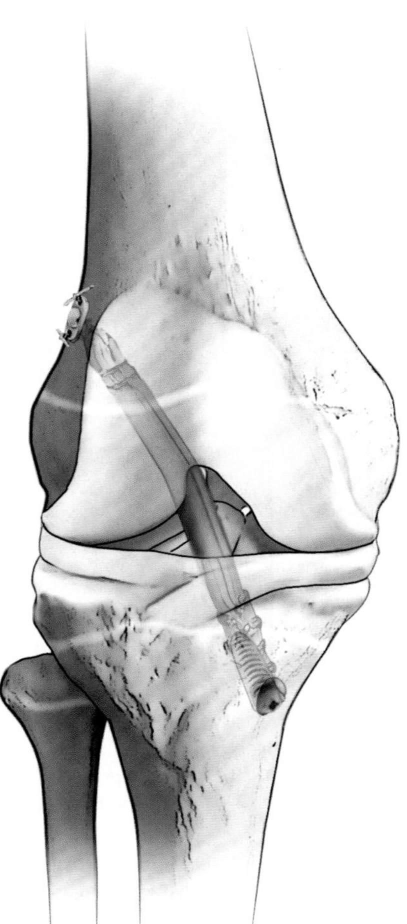

Figure 43-3 | Transphyseal ACL reconstruction using hamstring autograft. (From Fabricant PD, Kocher MS. Management of ACL injuries in children and adolescents. *J Bone Joint Surg*. 2017;99(7):600-612, Ref.[2], with permission.)

Preadolescents: Modified MacIntosh Procedure, Combined Extra- and Intra-articular ACL Reconstruction Using IT Band Autograft[3,4]

- Indicated for children who are Tanner stage 1 or 2; skeletal age ≤11 in females, ≤12 in males.
- The thigh tourniquet is inflated based upon surgeon preference.
- IT band graft harvest
    - An 8- to 10-cm longitudinal oblique incision is centered over the mid-portion of the IT band just proximal to the lateral joint line.
    - The central portion of the IT band is harvested proximally and left attached to Gerdy tubercle distally.
    - A Cobb elevator is used to elevate the subcutaneous tissue off the superficial surface of the IT band a minimum of 15 cm up the thigh.
    - The IT band is incised with a no. 15 scalpel near the border of the fascia of the vastus lateralis anteriorly and the posterior intermuscular septum posteriorly.
        - A few millimeters of intact IT band are left anteriorly and posteriorly.
    - Left and right meniscotomes are used to dissect the IT band proximally in line with its fibers (Fig. 43-4A).
    - A curved meniscotome or an open-ended tendon harvester is used to truncate the graft proximally.
        - If similar instruments are unavailable, a counterincision can be made proximally to detach the graft.
    - The graft is further freed from the lateral joint capsule with a knife or dissecting scissors but is left attached to Gerdy tubercle distally (Fig. 43-4B).
    - The graft is tubularized and whipstitched for 2 cm with a heavy nonabsorbable suture.
    - The stitched graft is placed back in the wound to prevent desiccation.
- Diagnostic knee arthroscopy
    - A diagnostic knee arthroscopy is performed using standard anterolateral and anteromedial portals to treat any concurrent pathology (eg, meniscal tears).

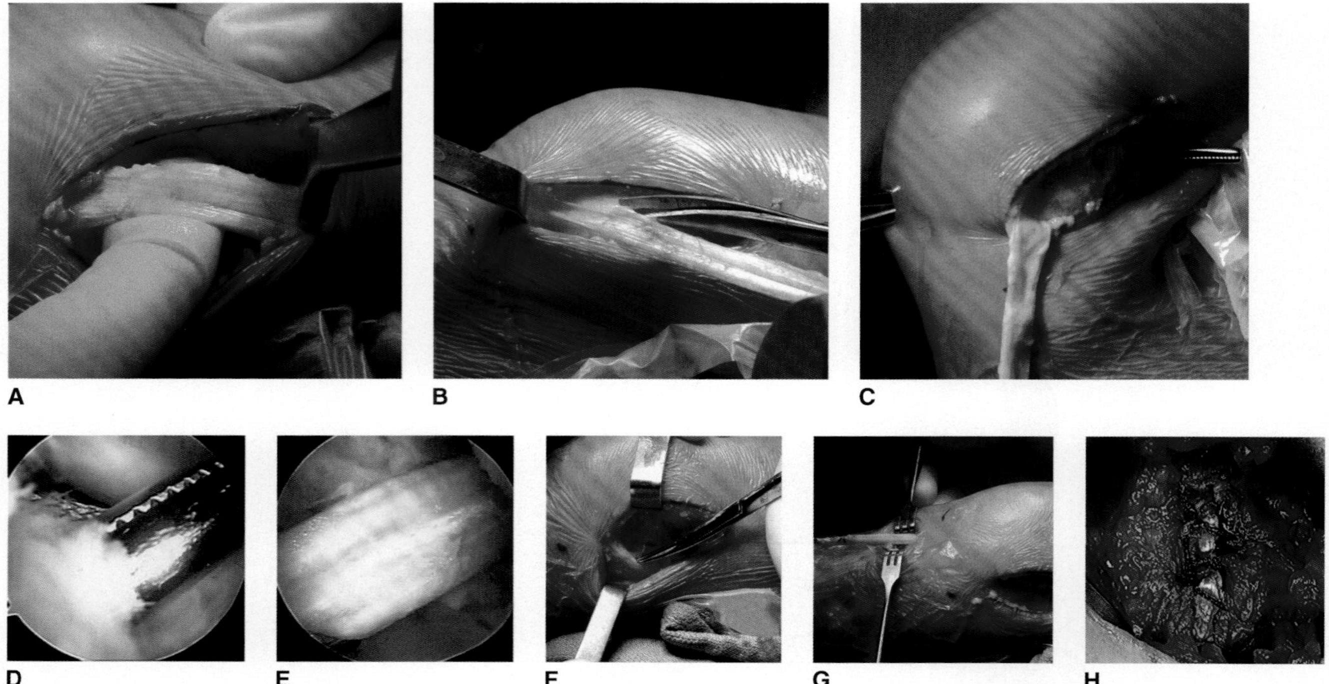

Figure 43-4 | A-H. Modified MacIntosh procedure—combined extra- and intra-articular ACL reconstruction using IT band autograft. (Images for panels A through H from Kocher MS, Garg S, Micheli LJ. Physeal sparing reconstruction of the anterior cruciate ligament in skeletally immature prepubescent children and adolescents. *J Bone Joint Surg Am.* 2005;87:2371-2379 and image H from Fabricant PD, Kocher MS. Management of ACL injuries in children and adolescents. *J Bone Joint Surg.* 2017;99(7):600-612, with permission.)

- The ACL remnant is gently debrided. Intact posterolateral bundle fibers may be left in place.
- Radiofrequency ablation is avoided in the notch because of the close proximity of the distal femoral physis to the over-the-top position.

- Preparation for graft passage
  - The medial portal is widened for easier clamp spreading and a minimized chance of traumatic and irregular enlargement of the portal.
  - A small hemostat (eg, Schnidt tonsil) is used to create a path in the over-the-top position between bone and soft tissue while leaving a sling of soft tissue to prevent graft subluxation.
  - This track is widened with the large clamp and directed proximal to the lateral femoral condyle with bimanual palpation through the lateral graft harvest incision (Fig. 43-4C).
- Graft passage
  - The graft sutures are passed with the large clamp and retrieved through the joint and out the anteromedial portal, parking the graft in the over-the-top position.
  - A longitudinal incision medial to the tibial tubercle is made and dissected down to the periosteum.
    - This is followed by blunt dissection directly proximally into the knee (under the intermeniscal ligament) with a curved clamp (eg, Schnidt tonsil) (Fig. 43-4D).
    - The passageway is dilated to aid with tibial preparation and graft passage.
  - A groove in the tibial ACL footprint is created with a "rat-tail" rasp.
    - This facilitates intra-articular healing of the graft and moves the tibial footprint posteriorly to a more anatomic position that minimizes the chance of impingement in extension.
  - The clamp is reintroduced in the knee, and the intra-articular sutures are brought out through the tibial incision to their final position (Fig. 43-4E).
- Graft fixation
  - The arthroscope is removed, and the knee is allowed to hang in 90 degrees of relaxed flexion with neutral foot rotation.
    - This position prevents overconstraining the knee.[5]
  - Femoral fixation
    - With tension on the graft distally, the extra-articular limb is sewn into the periosteum of the lateral femoral condyle and the intermuscular septum with at least three passes of heavy nonabsorbable suture (Fig. 43-4F).

- Tibial fixation
  - The proximal-medial fixation footprint lies just medial to the tibial tubercle, distal to the proximal tibial physis, and proximal to the pes anserinus.
  - The periosteum in the footprint is incised longitudinally and elevated medially and laterally with a periosteal elevator.
  - The footprint is lightly decorticated with a burr.
  - With firm tension on the graft distally (Fig. 43-4G) and the knee in 30 degrees of flexion with a posterior drawer force applied, the graft is fixed to the tibia with 3 or 4 heavy nonabsorbable sutures in a Mason-Allen (self-locking) stitch and by advancing 1 cm with each pass through the graft and periosteum to further tension the graft (Fig. 43-4H).
- Wound closure
  - Wounds are closed in layers according to the surgeon's preference.

Adolescents: Transphyseal Hamstring ACL Reconstruction[6]

- Indicated for children who are Tanner stage ≥3; skeletal age ≥12 in females, ≥13 in males.
- A thigh tourniquet is inflated based upon surgeon preference.
- Hamstring graft harvest
  - A 3-cm vertical incision is made over the pes anserinus midway between the posteromedial tibial crest and the tibial tubercle.
  - The semitendinosus and gracilis tendons are individually detached distally and whipstitched with heavy nonabsorbable suture.
  - Each tendon is harvested proximally with a closed-ended tendon harvester.
- Graft preparation
  - The proximal end of each tendon is whipstitched with heavy nonabsorbable suture.
  - The tendons are folded through a 15-mm closed loop cortical suspensory button to produce a quadrupled graft.
  - The graft is pretensioned at 20 Nm until graft passage.
- Diagnostic knee arthroscopy
  - A diagnostic knee arthroscopy is performed using standard anterolateral and anteromedial portals to treat any concurrent pathology (eg, meniscal tears).
  - The ACL remnant is debrided. A small tibial stump remnant can be left in place to enhance biologic healing (Fig. 43-5A).
  - A notchplasty is performed if necessary.
  - Radiofrequency ablation is avoided in the notch because of the close proximity of the distal femoral physis to the over-the-top position.
- Tibial tunnel drilling
  - The tibial guide is set to 55 degrees to ensure a long metaphyseal tunnel distal to the physis (Fig. 43-5B).
    - This provides adequate tunnel length for metaphyseal interference screw fixation.
  - A guide pin is started 1 cm anterior to the posteromedial tibial crest (just anterior to the superficial medial collateral ligament [MCL] insertion) to ensure that the tibial tunnel does not violate the tibial tubercle apophysis.
  - The drill guide is placed in the posterior portion of the tibial ACL footprint, allowing easy access to the over-the-top position.
  - A guide pin is drilled, its position is checked, and an appropriate reamer is used to create the tibial tunnel (Fig. 43-5C).
- Femoral tunnel drilling
  - An offset transtibial over-the-top femoral guide is selected to allow a 1- to 2-mm back wall and is positioned through the tibial tunnel.
    - The appropriate femoral guide is selected based on the formula (0.5 × graft diameter +1).
    - The femoral tunnel also can be created with an independent anteromedial portal or retrocutting techniques based on surgeon preference.
  - The femoral guide pin is drilled (Fig. 43-5D).
  - Tunnel length is measured with a depth gauge or directly with the guide pin.
  - The femoral tunnel is reamed to a depth accounting for the length of tunnel required for the fixed loop and flipping of the cortical button.
    - Typically, a 7-mm lateral femoral cortical wall is left for a 15-mm closed loop button.
    - This will support the suspensory fixation construct.

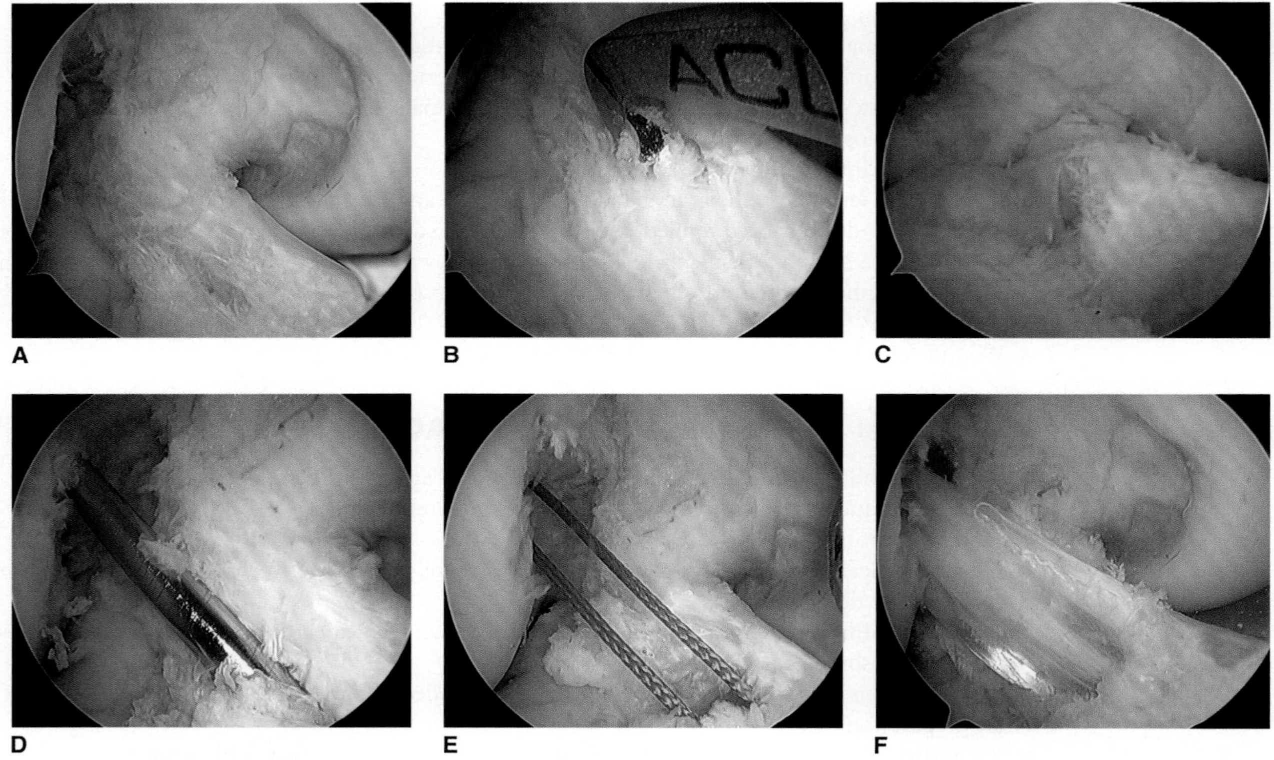

Figure 43-5 | A-F. Transphyseal hamstring ACL reconstruction. (Images for panels A through F from Fabricant PD, Kocher MS. Management of ACL injuries in children and adolescents. *J Bone Joint Surg*. 2017;99(7):600-612, with permission.)

- Graft passage and femoral fixation
  - The guide pin is used to pass sutures for graft passage (Fig. 43-5E).
  - The distal end of the suture is passed out the tibial tunnel.
  - The suspensory button sutures are passed, followed by the graft (Fig. 43-5F).
  - The button is flipped, toggling the sutures to ensure appropriate seating of the button.
    - Fluoroscopy can be used to check the suspensory cortical button position.
  - The graft is viewed arthroscopically to confirm appropriate position and impingement-free motion.
- Tibial fixation
  - The knee is cycled 20-25 times with tension on the graft distally to remove creep from the graft-fixation construct.
  - Tibial fixation is done with the knee in 20-30 degrees of flexion with tension on the graft and a posterior drawer force applied to the tibia. A 20- to 25-mm nonmetal interference screw is placed and remains distal to the physis.
    - Screw diameter typically is line-to-line in hard bone or 1 mm larger than the graft/tunnel in softer bone.
- Wound closure
  - Wounds are closed in layers according to the surgeon's preference.

References

1. Kelly PM, Dimeglio A. Lower-limb growth: how predictable are predictions? *J Child Orthop*. 2008;2(6):407-415.
2. Fabricant *PD*, Kocher MS. Management of ACL injuries in children and adolescents. *J Bone Joint Surg*. 2017;99(7):600-612.
3. Kocher MS, Garg S, Micheli LJ. Physeal sparing reconstruction of the anterior cruciate ligament in skeletally immature prepubescent children and adolescents. *J Bone Joint Surg Am*. 2005;87(11):2371-2379.
4. Micheli LJ, Rask B, Gerberg L. Anterior cruciate ligament reconstruction in patients who are prepubescent. *Clin Orthop Relat Res*. 1999;(364):40-47.
5. Kennedy A, Coughlin DG, Metzger MF, et al. Biomechanical evaluation of pediatric anterior cruciate ligament reconstruction techniques. *Am J Sports Med*. 2011;39(5):964-971.
6. Kocher MS, Smith JT, Zoric BJ, et al. Transphyseal anterior cruciate ligament reconstruction in skeletally immature pubescent adolescents. *J Bone Joint Surg Am*. 2007;89(12):2632-2639.

Chapter 44
Revision ACL Reconstruction

RICK W. WRIGHT

Indications

- Functional instability with desired or daily activities
- Positive pivot shift, Lachman test consistent with anterior cruciate ligament (ACL) insufficiency
- KT 1000 >5 mm
- MRI demonstrating

Preoperative Evaluation

History

- Determining the reason for failure is crucial.
  - Technical
  - Trauma
  - Biological
- Failure within 6 months without an interlude of full functional activity may indicate biological graft issues or technical issues.
- Difficulty achieving motion with rehabilitation may indicate technical tunnel placement issues.
- Failure and giving way with minimal trauma may indicate that the graft failed before the recent trauma.
- A significant period of full functional activity followed by a significant traumatic episode—pure traumatic failure and an approach similar to that used in the primary anterior cruciate ligament reconstruction (ACLR) may be successful.

Physical Examination

- Should focus on knee motion and other ligament or structural laxities that may contribute to graft stretching and ultimate failure.
  - Range of motion—emphasis on knee extension; significant hyperextension usually requires graft fixation with knee in full extension
  - Effusion
  - Posterior drawer to evaluate posterior cruciate ligament
  - Medial and lateral collateral testing
  - Dial test to evaluate posterolateral corner
  - Gait observation to demonstrate subtle valgus thrust issues

Imaging

- Imaging should focus on issues that will require modification of the primary procedure.
- *Radiographs*
  - Long-leg bilateral standing film to demonstrate varus or valgus alignment that may affect symptom outcomes and graft stretching.

   - Standing lateral view can demonstrate any tibial slope issues.
   - Weight-bearing (bent-knee 45-degree posteroanterior) radiographs to evaluate for degenerative changes.
   - Full extension lateral, with bolster under the ankle, shows tibial tunnel position.
- *Other imaging modalities used at surgeon's discretion*
   - CT scans give best information regarding precise tunnel location and size.
      - If tibial or femoral tunnels have enlarged to 15 mm or larger in diameter, some form of single-stage or two-stage bone grafting is indicated.
   - MRI shows meniscal and cartilage damage.

Sterile Instruments/Equipment

- Previous operative note
- C-arm fluoroscopy
- Implant removal set
- Microfracture awls
- Osteochondral autografting sets
- Meniscal repair equipment
- Bone-graft harvesting instruments if indicated
- Allograft for primary or backup use as graft choice

Surgical Procedure

- Surgical approach
   - Previous incisions are used or extended if possible.
   - Skin bridges <7 cm wide should be avoided.
   - Anteromedial.
   - Transtibial.
   - Rear-incision or two-entry—can utilize new femoral bone vs anteromedial or transtibial based on different angle of tunnel (Figs. 44-1 to 44-4).
- Graft choice
   - Autograft three times less likely to rupture per multicenter ACL revision study (MARS data)—soft tissue (hamstrings) equal results to bone-patellar tendon-bone

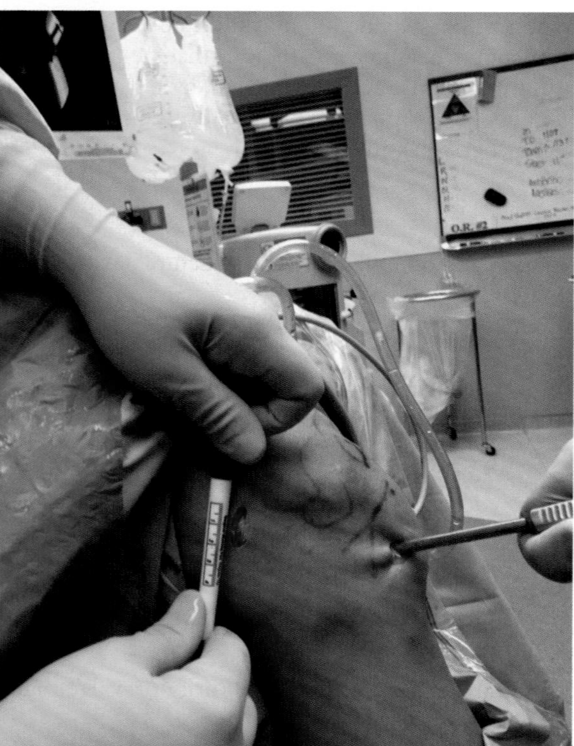

Figure 44-1 | Lateral thigh incision for rear entry approach.

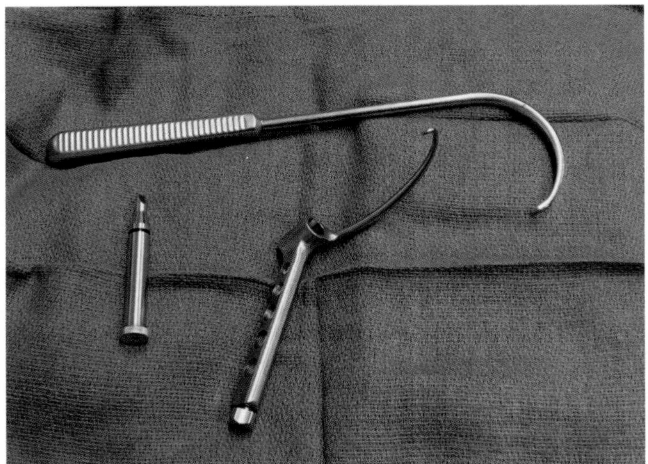

Figure 44-2 | Guides for rear entry femoral approach.

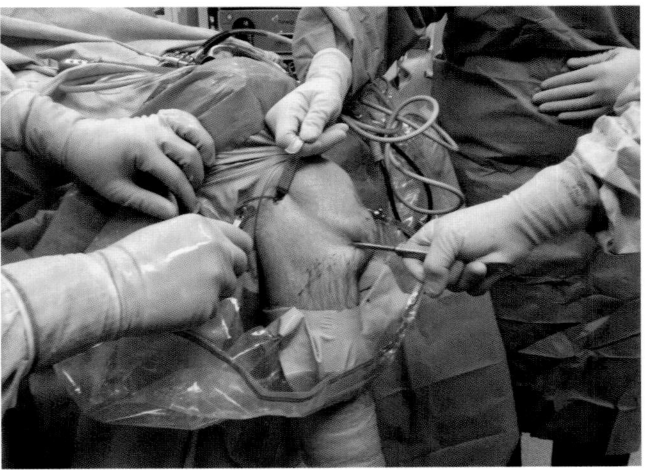

Figure 44-3 | Rear entry guide being pulled into notch with curved hook.

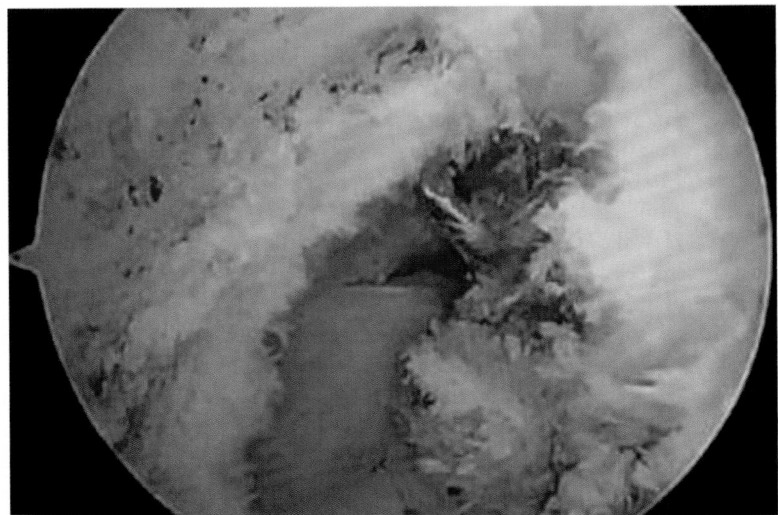

Figure 44-4 | Demonstrates ability to independently determine guidewire/tunnel position. High in the notch as in Figure 44-4 to low in Figure 44-5 or anywhere in between.

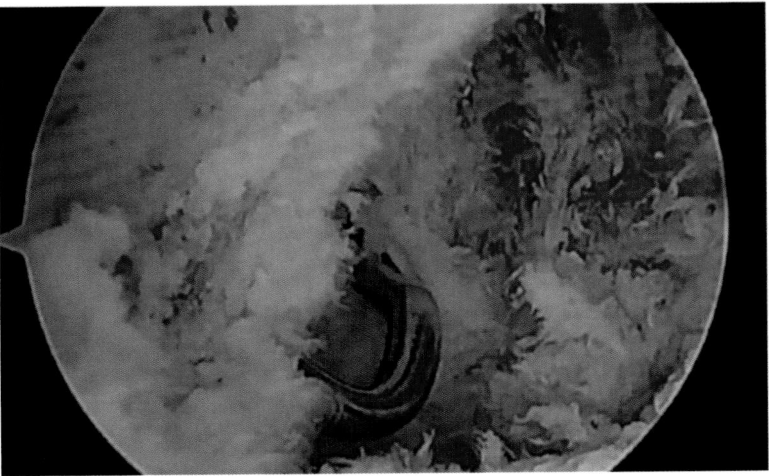

Figure 44-5 | Low wire/tunnel position.

        - Bone-patellar tendon-bone: ipsi- or contralateral, avoid poor results of reharvest.
        - Hamstring—ipsi- or contralateral—semitendinosus and gracilis—may be smaller and previous tunnel—current graft size mismatch must be accommodated.
        - Quadriceps tendon.
    - Allografts: advantages include no donor site morbidity, smaller incision, shorter tourniquet and operative times, and no size limitations; disadvantages include cost, risk of disease transmission, questionable potential for rejection, lower patient-reported outcomes, and higher graft rupture rate per MARS data.
- Implant removal
    - Unnecessary removal creates defects that must be treated.
    - Usually femoral implants are more difficult to remove, especially if the screw is buried.
        - It is important to make sure that the angle and seating of the screwdriver are accurate. If the metal has softened, one turn of an improperly seated screwdriver may strip the screw head.
        - With cannulated screws, a guide pin placed through the screw is helpful.
        - Image intensification can help locate a screw that has been buried by or overgrown in bone.
        - Attempts to remove a bioabsorbable screw may cause fragmentation; best to leave it intact if possible and ream through part or all of it.
        - Femoral or tibial implants from a previous endoscopic technique or two-incision technique can be left intact, depending on their location and choice of a different approach.
- Grafting of bony defects
    - Cylinder-shaped graft can be taken from the tibia with a handheld trephine harvester.
    - Allograft dowels are popular in filling tunnel defects.
    - Two-stage bone grafting typically requires 6 months of incorporation.
    - Defects can be filled with oversized absorbable or metal interference screws, which can be stacked adjacent to one another to fill the defect.
    - A large bone block allograft can be used.
    - Posterior wall deficiency may require conversion to an over-the-top technique, two-incision technique, or use of an Endobutton.
- Tunnel preparation
    - Tunnels with appropriate size and place can be reused; grossly inappropriate tunnels require new tunnels to be drilled; and "almost right" tunnels remain a challenge.
    - Femoral tunnels generally can be developed based on the surgeon's usual approach—blended tunnels are not a predictor for worse outcome per MARS data.
    - Tibial tunnels are more challenging: drill guides do not as reliably hit the predetermined aiming spot; the guidewire can hit sclerotic tunnel walls or previous bone plugs and be diverted as it enters the joint.
        - A smaller drill bit can be used to drill a tunnel through which a free guidewire can be positioned and malleted into the femur to hold the new position after adjustments to improve position in the anteroposterior or mediolateral direction. Then, a larger drill bit is used over the guidewire.
- Graft fixation
    - A variety of alternative or adjunct fixation devices should be available, including buttons, staples, and a screw set with spiked washers.
    - The use of a metal screw for graft fixation has been shown to be an independent predictor of improved patient outcomes per MARS data.
    - Larger screws may be helpful for slightly enlarged tunnels that do not require grafting.

Postoperative Protocol

- Rehabilitation evaluated by MARS group
- Immediate weight bearing no harm
- Immediate passive and active motion no harm
- Rehabilitative postoperative braces no advantage
- Functional derotation braces used at return to sports improved patient-reported outcomes—no difference in graft failure rates

Suggested Readings

Group M. Factors influencing graft choice in revision anterior cruciate ligament reconstruction in the MARS group. *J Knee Surg*. 2016;29(6):458-463.

MARS Group. Effect of graft choice on the outcome of revision anterior cruciate ligament reconstruction in the Multicenter ACL Revision Study (MARS) cohort. *Am J Sports Med*. 2014;42(10):2301-2310.

MARS Group. Meniscal and articular cartilage predictors of clinical outcome after revision anterior cruciate ligament reconstruction. *Am J Sports Med*. 2016;44(7):1671-1679.

Wright RW. Two-incision anterior cruciate ligament reconstruction. *J Knee Surg*. 2014;27(5):343-346.

Wright RW, Gill CS, Chen L, et al. Outcome of revision anterior cruciate ligament reconstruction: a systematic review. *J Bone Joint Surg Am*. 2012;94(6):531-536.

Chapter 45
Anterolateral Ligament Reconstruction

JACOB M. KIRSCH
MOIN KHAN
ASHEESH BEDI

Relative Indications for Anterolateral Ligament (ALL) Reconstruction

- Persistent pivot shift test following anterior cruciate ligament (ACL) reconstruction
- Preoperative grade 3 pivot shift test
- Knee hyperlaxity with ACL injury (Beighton criteria ≥ 6)
- Revision ACL reconstruction with rotary instability

Sterile Instruments/Equipment

- Thigh tourniquet
- Leg holder
- Disposable 2.4-mm guide pins, 2X
- 4.5- and 7.0-mm cannulated drills
- 4.75-mm biocomposite SwiveLock anchor and 7-mm biocomposite tenodesis SwiveLock anchor (Arthrex, Naples, FL)
- Disposable tap (available, although not routinely needed)
- No. 2 FiberLoop sutures, 2X (Arthrex, Naples, FL)
- No. 2 FiberWire suture (Arthrex, Naples, FL)

Positioning

- The patient is positioned supine on the operating table.
- An arthroscopic leg holder is used on the operative extremity.
- A well-leg holder is used to position the nonoperative extremity in a flexed and abducted position to protect the femoral and peroneal nerves.
- A sterile tourniquet is placed high on the operative thigh.
- The foot of the operating table is dropped to allow for maximal knee flexion.

Examination Under Anesthesia

- After induction of anesthesia, the following examination maneuvers are performed and compared to the contralateral extremity:
  - Lachman test
  - Pivot shift
  - Dial test

- Posterolateral drawer, drawer in internal rotation (for posterolateral and anteromedial rotatory instability, respectively)
- Varus/valgus stress
- Internal rotation stress of tibia in >35 degrees flexion

Relevant ALL Anatomy

- Proximal origin of the ALL is variable; however, it is typically 5 mm proximal and posterior to the origin of the lateral collateral ligament.[1]
- Distal insertion is more broad and inserts approximately midway between the center of the fibular head and Gerdy tubercle,[2] ~10-11 mm distal to the lateral tibial plateau.[1,3]
- The ALL is ~4 cm long.[3]

Surgical Approach

- The anatomic landmarks of the knee are identified (Fig. 45-1).

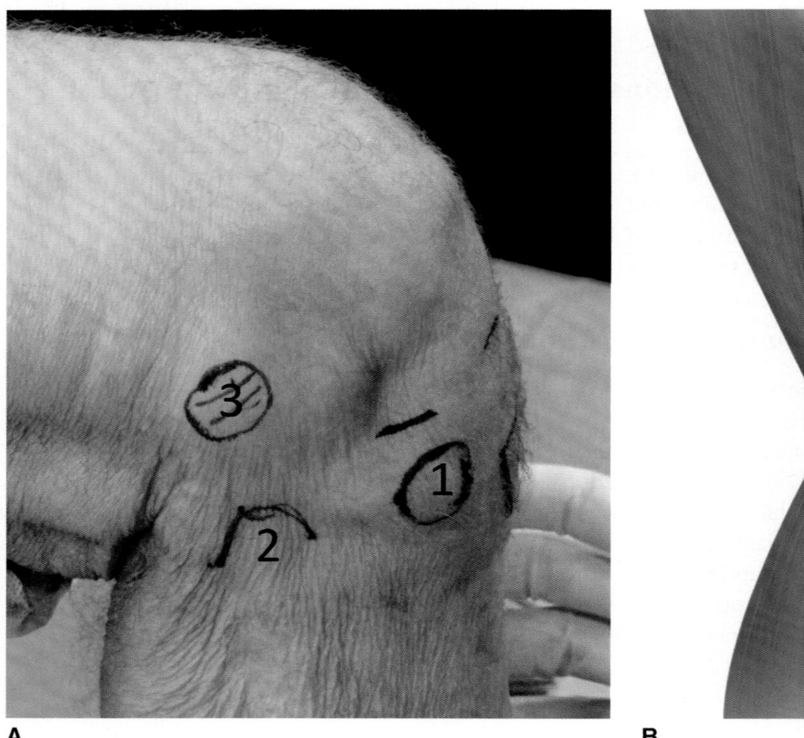

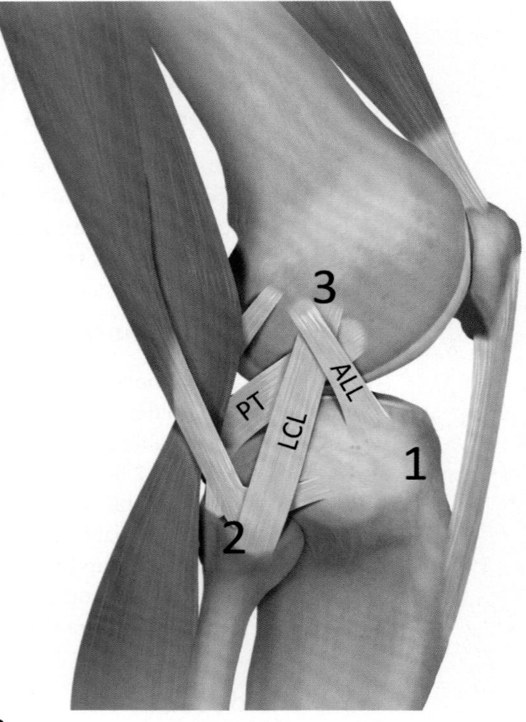

Figure 45-1 | Surface anatomic landmarks of the knee **(A)** and a diagrammatic illustration of the ligamentous anatomy of the lateral knee **(B)**. Important landmarks are Gerdy tubercle (*1*), the fibular head (*2*), and the lateral femoral epicondyle (*3*). ALL, anterolateral ligament; LCL, lateral collateral ligament; PT, popliteal tendon. (Courtesy of Arthrex, Inc.)

- Distal landmarks
  - Inferior pole of the patella and tibial tubercle
  - Lateral joint line
  - Gerdy tubercle
  - Head of the fibula
- Proximal landmark
  - Lateral femoral epicondyle

- The ALL origin proximal and posterior to the lateral femoral epicondyle is identified (Fig. 45-2).

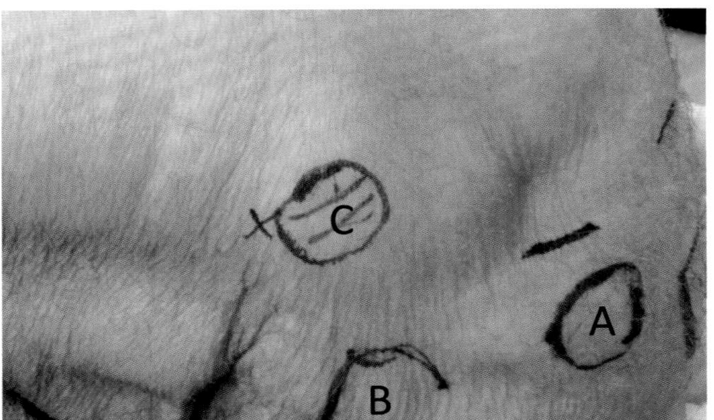

Figure 45-2 | The origin of the anterolateral ligament is just proximal and posterior to the lateral femoral epicondyle. It is marked with an "X". Important landmarks are Gerdy tubercle (*A*), the fibular head (*B*), and the lateral femoral epicondyle (*C*). (Courtesy of Arthrex, Inc.)

- With the knee in flexion, a small incision is made ~8 mm proximal and 4 mm posterior to the lateral femoral epicondyle (Fig. 45-3).
- The incision is carried deep through subcutaneous tissue, and the iliotibial band is split in line with its fibers.

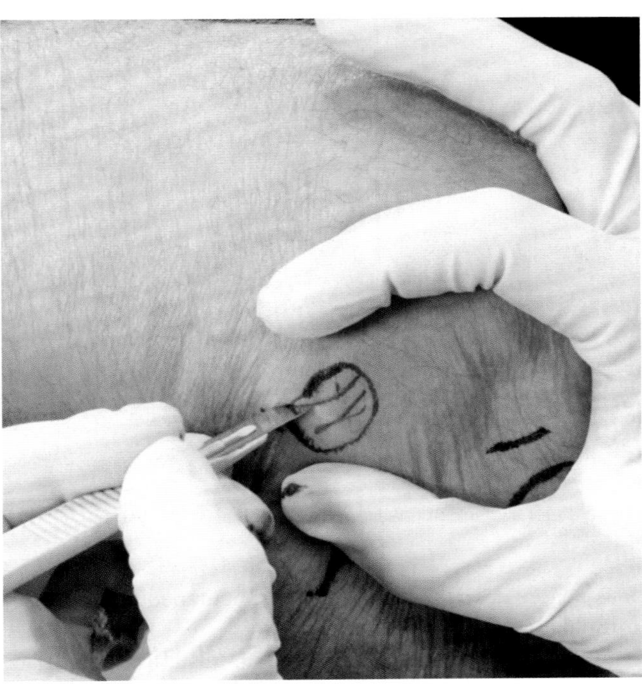

Figure 45-3 | An incision is made centered over the origin of the anterolateral ligament and carried deep through the iliotibial band. (Courtesy of Arthrex, Inc.)

Guide Pin Placement

- Proximal guide pin
  - The proximal origin of the ALL is ~5 mm proximal and posterior to the origin of the lateral collateral ligament.[1]
  - A 2.4-mm guide pin is inserted at the origin of the ALL and advanced in a slightly superior and anterior trajectory to avoid mechanical conflict with the ACL femoral tunnel (Fig. 45-4).
- Distal guide pin
  - The distal insertion of the ALL is ~10-11 mm distal to the distal lateral joint line and ~24 mm posterior to Gerdy tubercle[1] (Fig. 45-5).

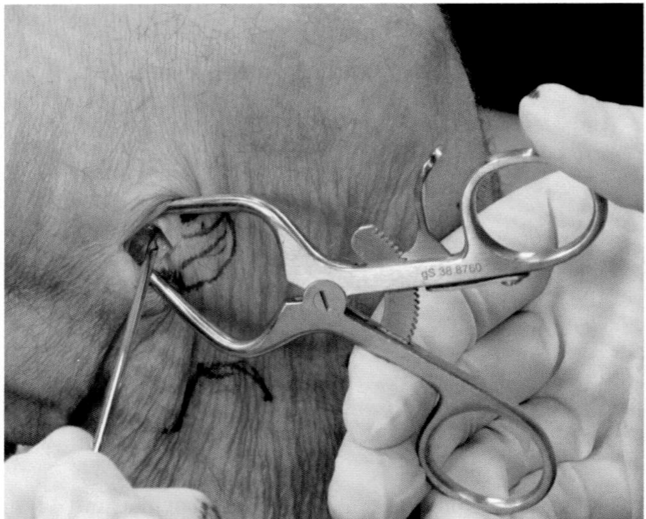

Figure 45-4 | Proximal guide pin position at the origin of the anterolateral ligament. (Courtesy of Arthrex, Inc.)

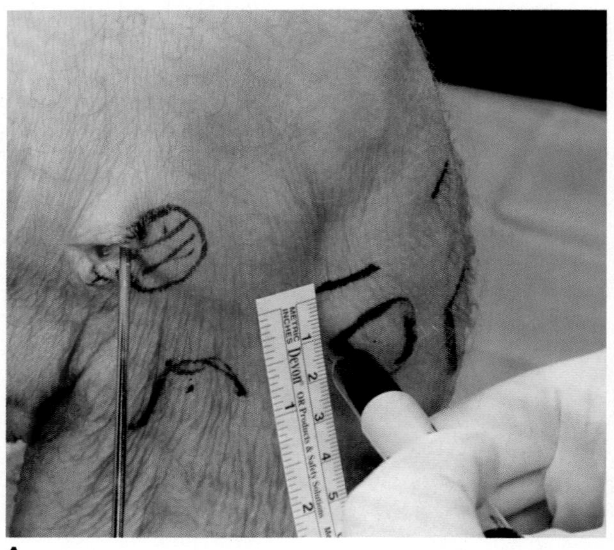

A

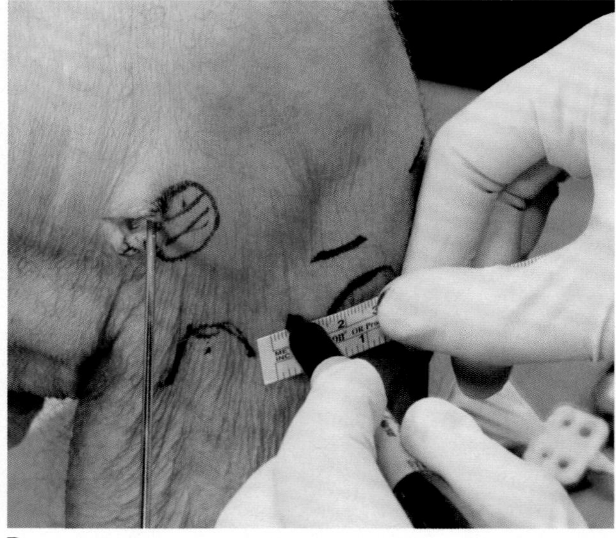

B

Figure 45-5 | The distal insertion of the anterolateral ligament relative to the lateral joint line **(A)** and Gerdy tubercle and the fibular head **(B)**. (Courtesy of Arthrex, Inc.)

- Sharp dissection is carried deep through skin and subcutaneous tissue just proximal to the anterior compartment musculature.
- The second 2.4-mm guide pin is placed with care to stay distal and parallel to the joint line (Fig. 45-6).
- Radiographic verification of landmarks
  - Although not a routine part of our procedure, intraoperative fluoroscopy can be used to evaluate accurate guide pin placement.
  - On an anteroposterior radiograph of the knee, the femoral guide pin should be 22.3 mm proximal to the proximal joint line, whereas the tibial guide pin is ~7.5 mm distal to the distal joint line.[1]
  - On a lateral radiograph of the knee, the femoral guide pin should be roughly 47.5% of the distance from the anterior aspect of the femoral condyle and ~4 mm distal to Blumensaat line. The tibial guide pin is ~53.2% of the distance from the anterior aspect of the lateral tibial plateau.[4]

Test for Isometry

- Graft isometry can be evaluated by wrapping a no. 2 FiberWire suture around the proximal and distal guide pins and ranging the knee in flexion and extension (Fig. 45-7).
- The FiberWire should remain taut throughout range of motion.
- If excessive laxity is encountered, the guide pins should be removed and repositioned.

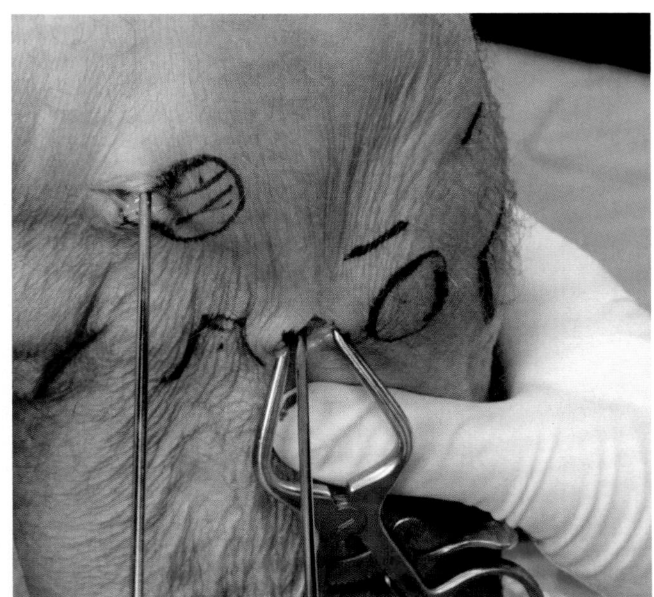

Figure 45-6 | Distal guide pin placement. (Courtesy of Arthrex, Inc.)

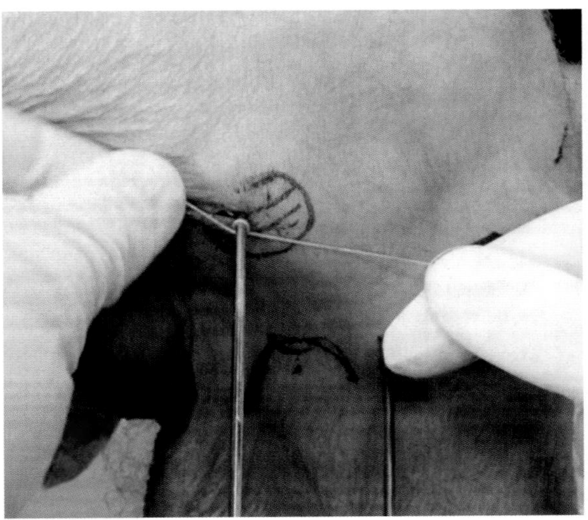

A

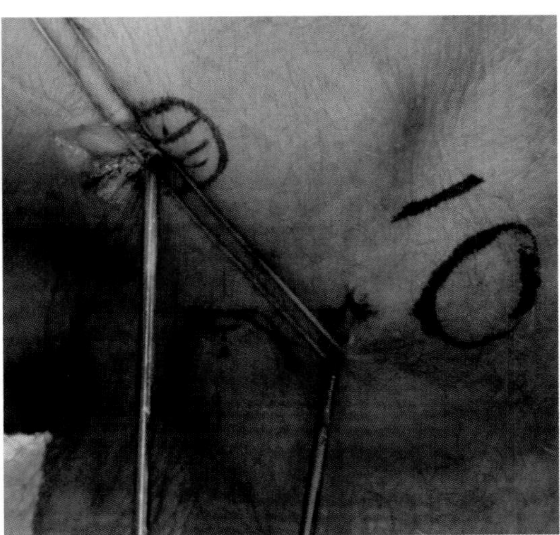

B

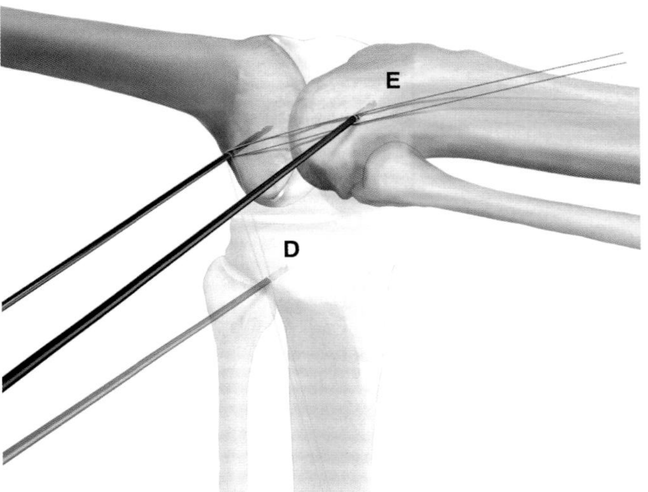

C

Figure 45-7 | Evaluation of graft isometry by tying a suture around the proximal **(A)** and distal **(B)** guide pins. The knee is ranged **(C)** in both flexion **(D)** and extension **(E)** while the suture is observed for laxity. (Courtesy of Arthrex, Inc.)

Socket Preparation

- After graft isometry is verified, the proximal guide pin is overreamed with a 4.5-mm cannulated drill to a depth of ~20 mm (Fig. 45-8).
- Similarly, the distal guide pin is overreamed with a 7-mm cannulated drill to a depth of 20 mm.

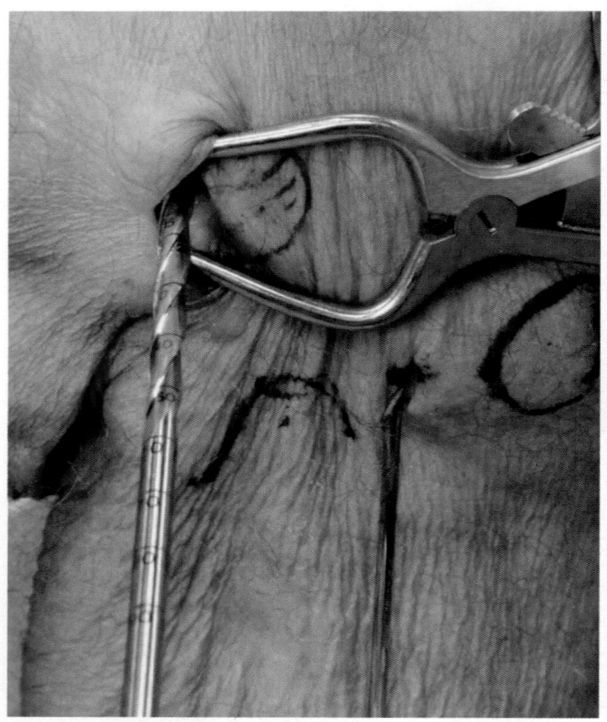
A

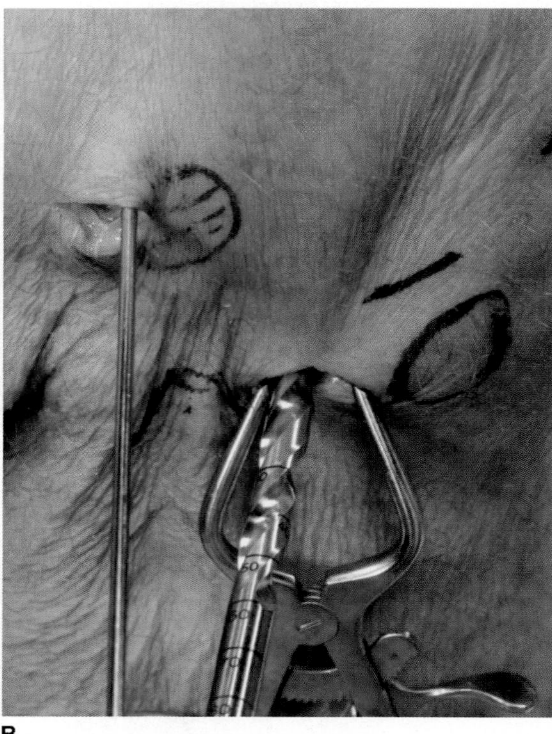
B

Figure 45-8 | Overreaming of the proximal **(A)** and distal **(B)** guide pins to a depth of 20 mm. (Courtesy of Arthrex, Inc.)

Graft Preparation and Proximal Fixation

- We routinely use a gracilis autograft for ALL reconstruction.
- The proximal 20 mm of the graft is whipstitched and tubularized with a no. 2 FiberWire suture.
- The suture is then passed through the eyelet of a 4.75-mm biocomposite SwiveLock anchor, and the anchor is advanced into the blind socket (Fig. 45-9).
- After the graft is gently impacted into the socket, it is advanced in the usual fashion.

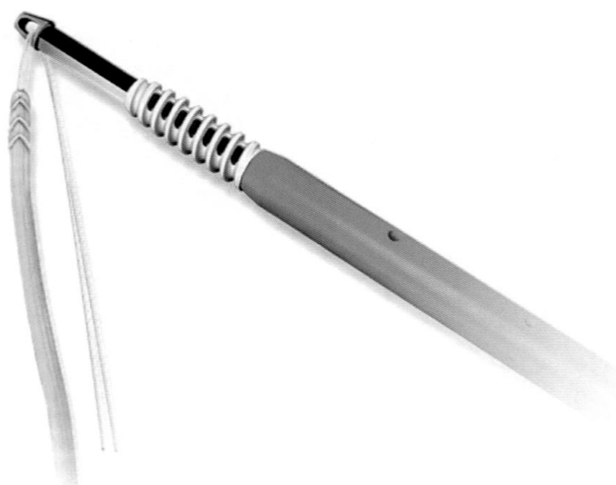
A

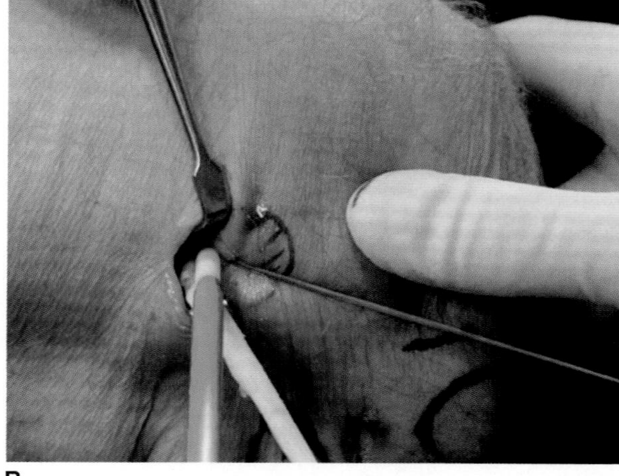
B

Figure 45-9 | The suture is passed through the anchor eyelet **(A)** and advanced into the blind socket **(B, C)**. (Courtesy of Arthrex, Inc.)

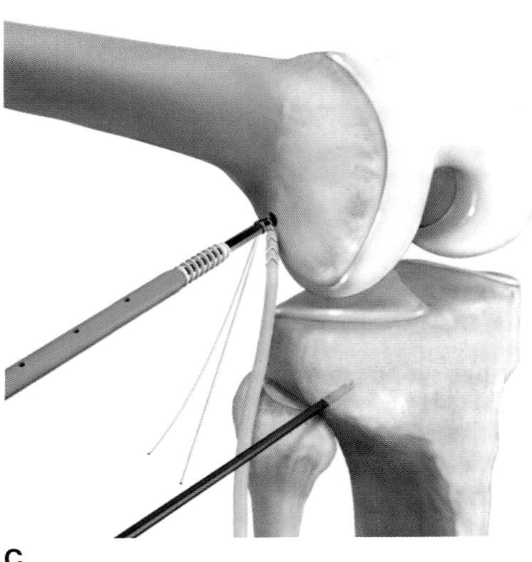

C

Figure 45-9 | *(Continued)*

Graft Tunneling

- A hemostat is used to tunnel the graft between the proximal and distal aspects of the reconstruction.
- It is important to remain deep to the iliotibial band while being superficial to the lateral collateral ligament.
- A loop stitch is used to shuttle the graft distally (Fig. 45-10).

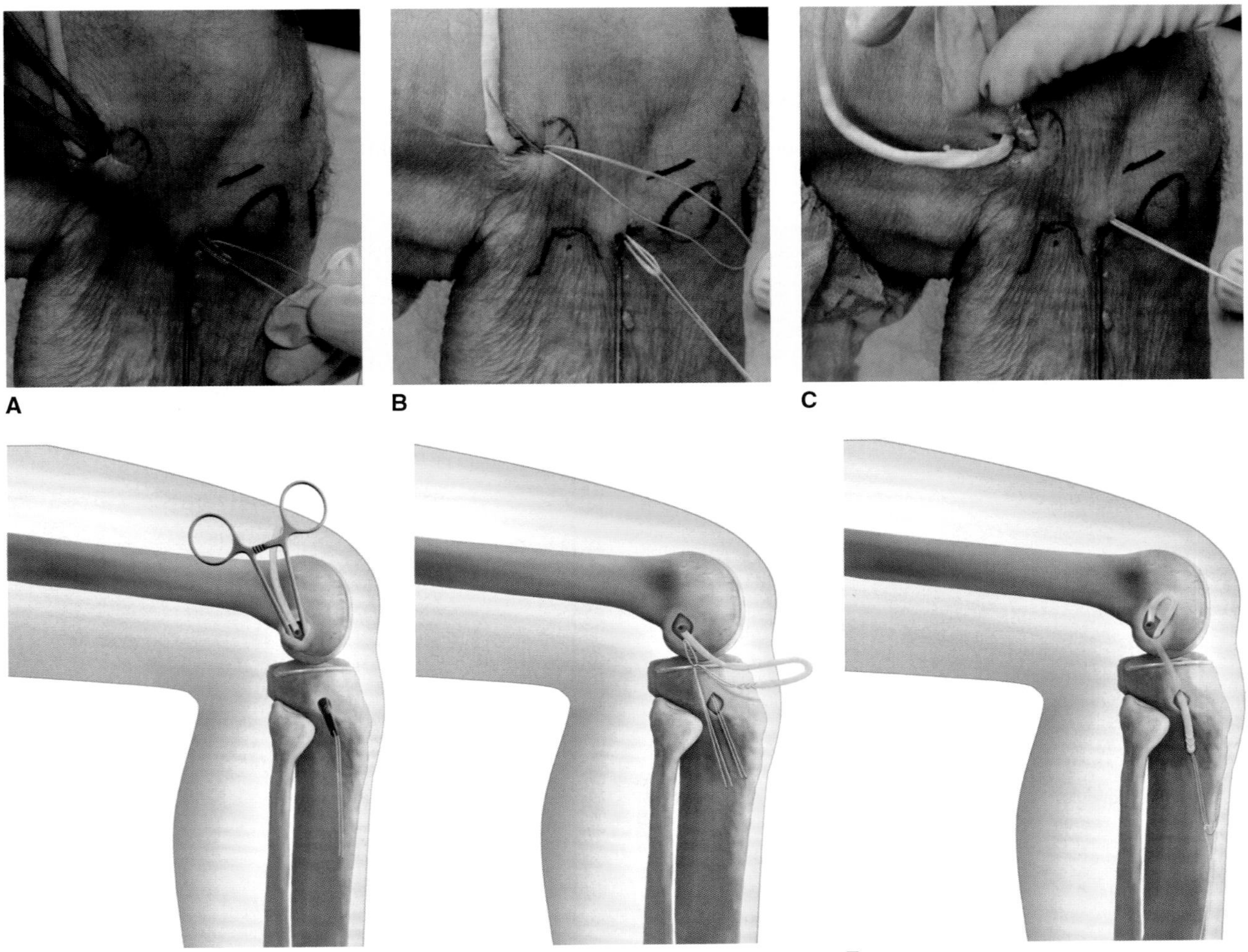

A B C

D E F

Figure 45-10 | Tunneling of the graft distally depicted both intraoperatively **(A-C)** and diagrammatically **(D-F)**. (Courtesy of Arthrex, Inc.)

- The graft is pulled taut once completely tunneled (Fig. 45-11).

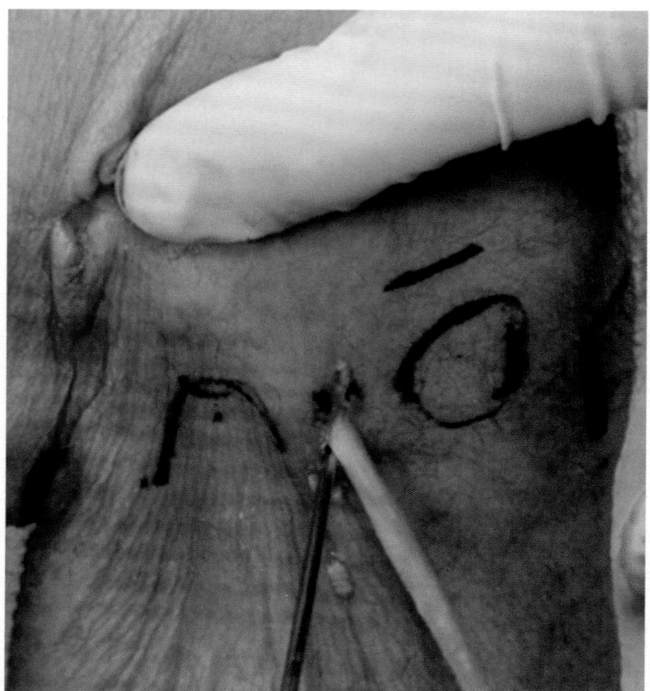

Figure 45-11 | The graft is pulled taut through the distal incision. (Courtesy of Arthrex, Inc.)

Graft Preparation and Distal Fixation

- The graft is marked as it exits the distal incision and at a point ~20 mm distally (Fig. 45-12).

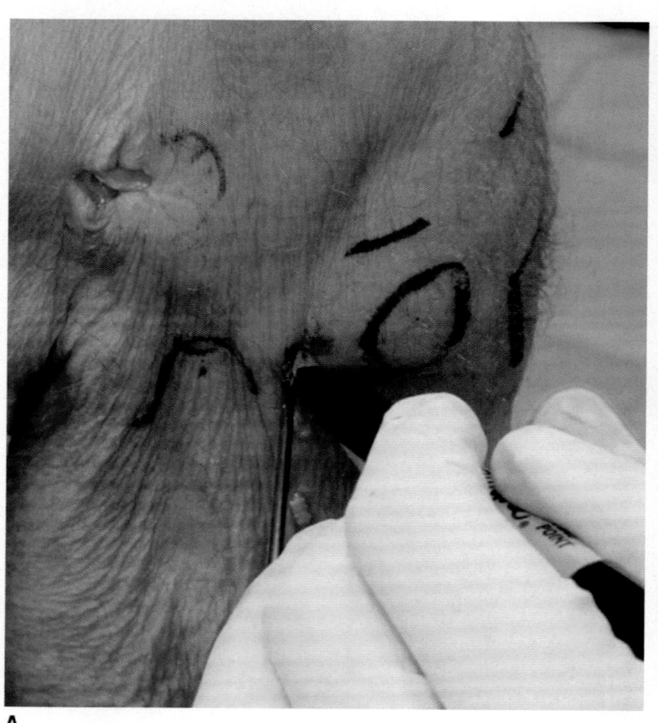

A

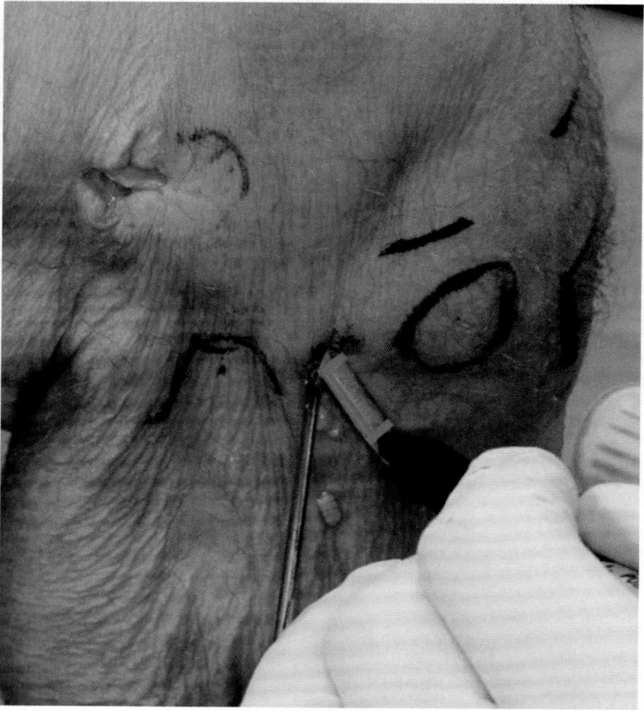

B

Figure 45-12 | The graft is marked as it exits the distal incision **(A)** and at a point 20 mm distal **(B)**. (Courtesy of Arthrex, Inc.)

- The graft between the marks is whipstitched and tubularized with a no. 2 FiberWire suture (Fig. 45-13).

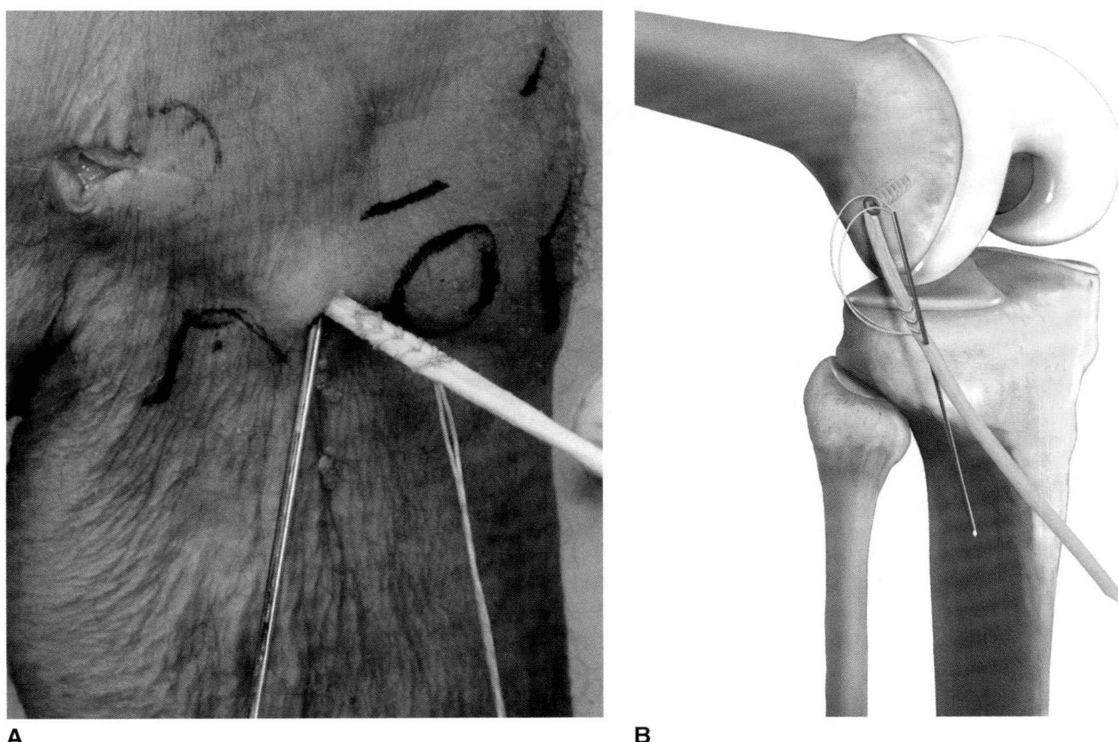

Figure 45-13 | Tubularization of the distal graft **(A, B)** with a whipstitched pattern. (Courtesy of Arthrex, Inc.)

- The knee is brought into extension and neutral rotation.
- A 7.0-mm biocomposite tenodesis SwiveLock anchor is used to dock the graft over the distal blind socket. The graft is subsequently tensioned, and the anchor is advanced (Fig. 45-14).

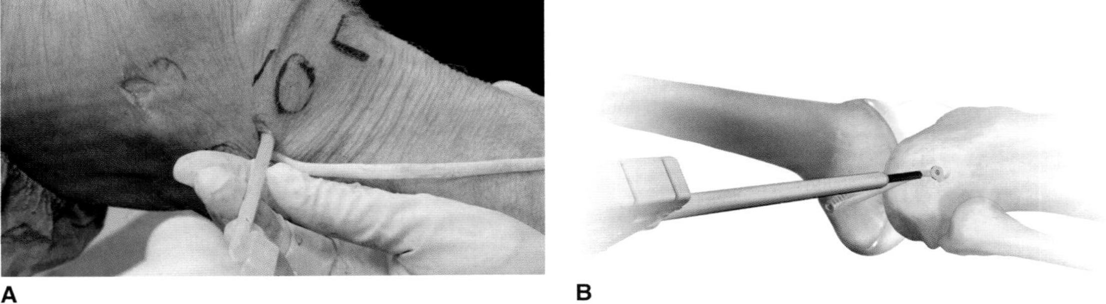

Figure 45-14 | Fixation of the distal aspect of the graft with the knee in extension and neutral rotation **(A, B)**. (Courtesy of Arthrex, Inc.)

- The excess part of the graft can be excised at this point, leaving the final reconstruction (Fig. 45-15).

Final Examination

- After the procedure is complete, the knee is thoroughly examined and compared to the contralateral side.
- The knee is brought through full range of motion, and rotational stability is assessed with the pivot shift examination.

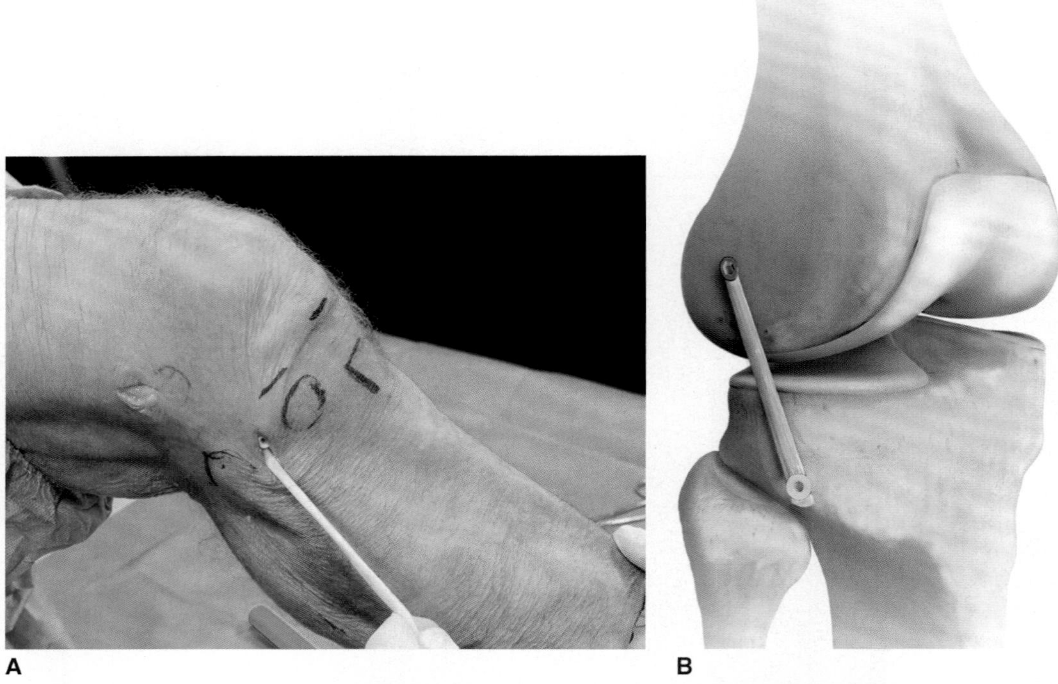

Figure 45-15 | Excess graft is removed **(A)** revealing the final reconstruction **(B)**. (Courtesy of Arthrex, Inc.)

- Resistance to internal rotation of the tibia is assessed in deeper degrees of knee flexion (>35 degrees flexion), as this appears to be an essential function of the ALL.[5]

Closure

- All wounds are irrigated.
- The iliotibial band is closed with absorbable suture.
- The subcutaneous tissue and skin are closed in the usual fashion.

References

1. Kennedy MI, Claes S, Fuso FA, et al. The anterolateral ligament: an anatomic, radiographic, and biomechanical analysis. *Am J Sports Med.* 2015;43:1606-1615.
2. Van der Watt L, Khan M, Rothrauff BB, et al. The structure and function of the anterolateral ligament of the knee: a systematic review. *Arthroscopy.* 2015;31:569-582, e563.
3. Claes S, Vereecke E, Maes M, et al. Anatomy of the anterolateral ligament of the knee. *J Anat.* 2013;223:321-328.
4. Helito CP, Demange MK, Bonadio MB, et al. Radiographic landmarks for locating the femoral origin and tibial insertion of the knee anterolateral ligament. *Am J Sports Med.* 2014;42:2356-2362.
5. Parsons EM, Gee AO, Spiekerman C, et al. The biomechanical function of the anterolateral ligament of the knee: response. *Am J Sports Med.* 2015;43:NP22.

Chapter 46

Endoscopic PCL Reconstruction

RYAN P. COUGHLIN
CLAUDE T. MOORMAN III

Sterile Instruments and Equipment

- Tourniquet
- Fluoroscopy
- 30- and 70-degree arthroscope
- Arthroscopic cannulas
- Achilles allograft
- FiberLoop and no. 2 FiberWire sutures (Arthrex, Naples, FL)
- Gore Smoother graft passer (Arthrex, Naples, FL)
- Milagro biocomposite screws (DePuy Synthes, Raynham, MA)
- 6.5-mm cancellous screw and 12-mm washer

Patient Positioning

- Preoperative regional anesthesia is administered in the anesthetic holding area. The patient is brought to the operating room and placed supine on the operating table.
  - A tourniquet is placed around the upper thigh. A padded lateral post is used to assist with valgus stress to the extremity. In the operating room, general orotracheal anesthesia is induced. The operative extremity is then examined under anesthesia. The affected knee is then prescrubbed with Hibiclens (Mölnlycke Health Care, Norcross, GA) and alcohol, prepared with ChloraPrep (Becton, Dickinson and Co., Franklin Lakes, NJ), and draped with sterile drapes and towels.

Graft Preparation

- An Achilles allograft prepared with Biocleanse (RTI Biologics, Alachua, FL) is removed from the freezer and allowed to thaw on a back table (Fig. 46-1).
  - The bone block is cut with an oscillating saw blade and contoured so that it can be passed smoothly through a 10-mm tunnel.
  - Two no. 2 FiberWire sutures are passed through the bone block for graft passage. The graft is then marked for orientation during passage.
  - The tendinous part of the graft is placed under tension and tubularized with a running 2-0 Vicryl suture. A FiberLoop suture is used to whipstitch the tendinous part of the graft. The graft is then placed on a tension board and covered with a saline-soaked sponge.

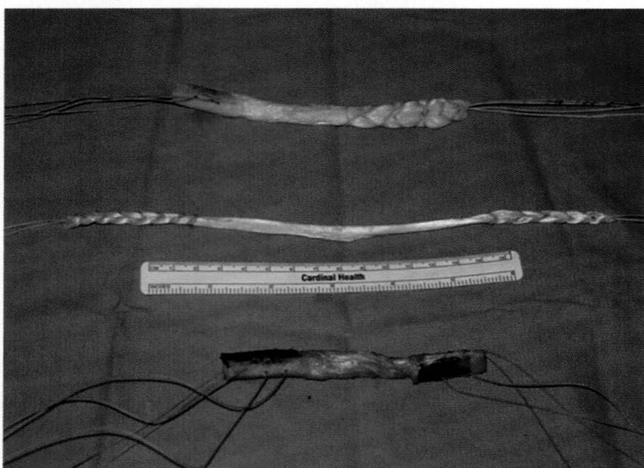

Figure 46-1 | The Achilles allograft is shown on the top of the image. No. 2 FiberWire sutures passed through the bone plug with the cortical side marked with a blue marking pen. The tendinous part is tubularized and whipstitched with FiberLoop suture.

Diagnostic Arthroscopy

- The 30-degree arthroscope is introduced into the knee through a standard anterolateral portal. The anteromedial portal is created under direct vision using a spinal needle for localization.
  - The knee is systematically examined beginning at the suprapatellar pouch area, followed by the medial compartment, the intercondylar notch, and the lateral compartment.

PCL Footprint Preparation

- The torn posterior cruciate ligament (PCL) is debrided with a mechanical shaver leaving some residual fibers attached to the femoral footprint.
  - A low medial wall notchplasty can be performed to improve visualization and graft passage. Viewing of the tibial attachment site can be improved using a 70-degree scope from the anterolateral portal or by placing a 30-degree scope through a posteromedial accessory portal (Table 46-1).
  - A full-radius shaver is used to remove remnant fibers of the PCL tibial attachment. A trough is created between the midline septum and medial meniscal root to allow the neurovascular bundle to retract posteriorly and allow better access to the PCL facet.[1] A curved rasp or curette is inserted through the notch to remove the PCL remnant from the posterior slope of the tibial facet. Adequate debridement is achieved once the mammillary bodies on either side of the PCL facet are seen.

Table 46-1 | Technical tips and pearls to endoscopic PCL reconstruction

PCL footprint preparation	Improved visualization: low medial wall notchplasty, posteromedial portal, 70-degree scope
Tunnel placement	A more vertical tibial tunnel can decrease graft killer turn
	Tibial tunnel: fluoroscopic control and reaming completed by hand to avoid neurovascular breach
Graft passage	Arthrex Gore Smoother used to chamfer tunnel edges for easier graft passage
	Probe used through the posteromedial portal as a fulcrum to redirect the graft into tibial tunnel
	Cancellous bone plug faced posteriorly in femoral tunnel to minimize graft abrasion
Fixation	Anterior drawer applied with 90-degree knee flexion

PCL Tunnel Placement

- The PCL tibial guide marking hook is attached to the adapter drill guide C-ring and inserted through the anteromedial portal (Fig. 46-2).
  - The distal end of the marking hook is placed on the PCL facet ~10 mm distal to the posterior tibial articular cartilage and 7 mm anterior to the posterior cortex as measured along the PCL facet (Fig. 46-3).[2]

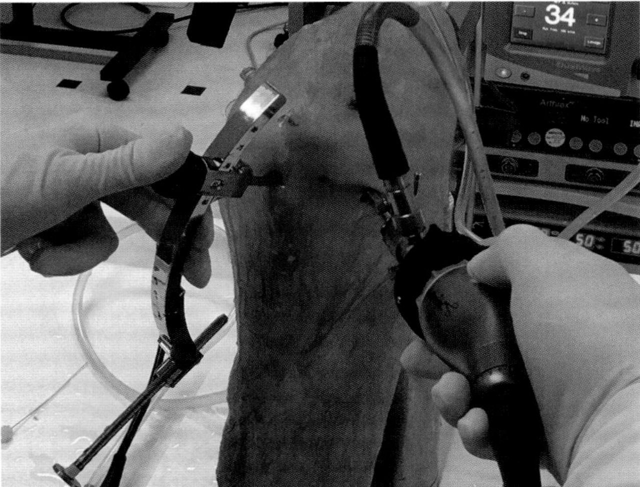

Figure 46-2 | PCL tibial guide is inserted through the anteromedial portal with the drill sleeve directed just medial and inferior to the tibial tuberosity.

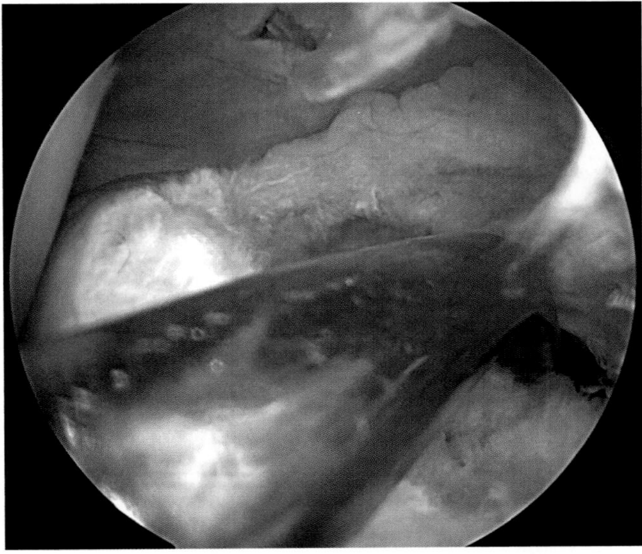

Figure 46-3 | The PCL guide is positioned in the trough on the back of the tibia, resting on the PCL facet as viewed from the anterolateral portal.

- The drill guide is oriented ~60 degrees to the articular surface of the tibia, starting just inferior and medial to the tibial tuberosity (Table 46-1).
- A 2.4-mm guide pin is drilled under fluoroscopy through the posterior cortex (Fig. 46-4).

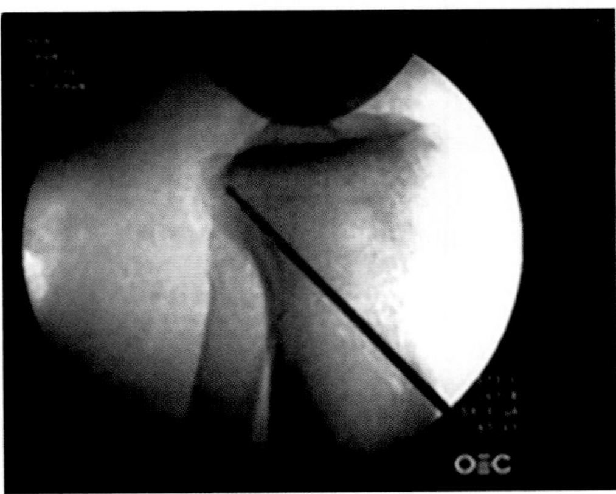

Figure 46-4 | Lateral fluoroscopic image showing advancement of the 2.4-mm guide pin towards the PCL tibial footprint.

- The pin can be tapped the final 1 cm to prevent penetration. While tapping the pin, a curved curette can be placed through the posteromedial portal to protect the neurovascular structures from pin penetration during advancement.
- Fluoroscopic control is used for reaming the tunnel to a diameter of 10 mm (Fig. 46-5). The final portion of the reaming is completed by hand so as not to breach into the neurovascular structures (Table 46-1).

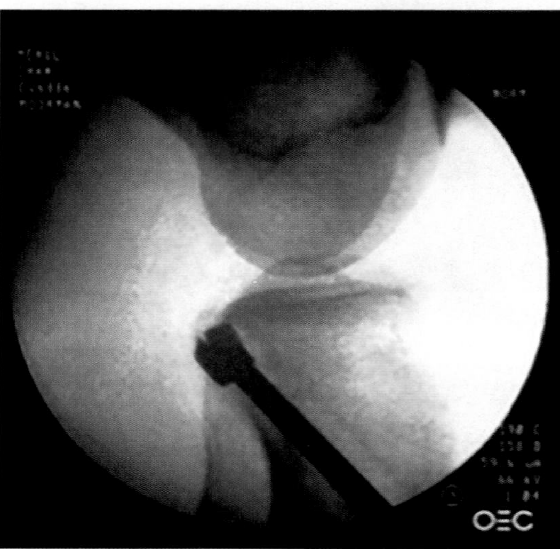

Figure 46-5 | Lateral fluoroscopic image showing advancement of the 10-mm reamer towards the PCL tibial footprint.

- The femoral footprint is identified at the junction of the roof wall 1 cm posterior to the articular surface (Fig. 46-6).[3]

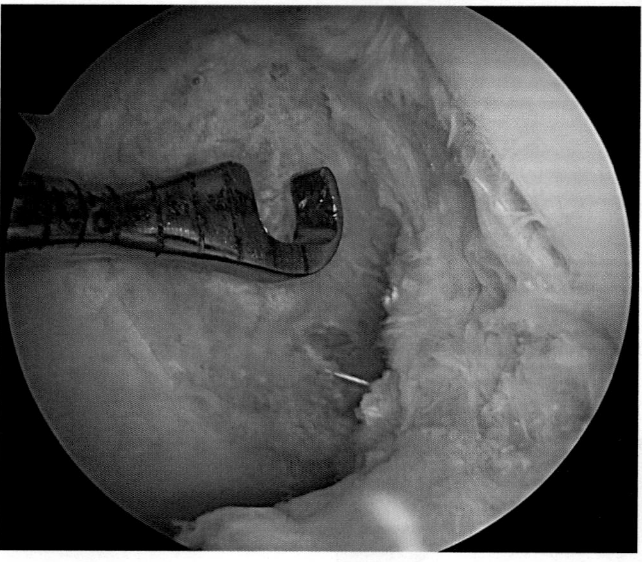

Figure 46-6 | Femoral guide resting on the PCL femoral footprint.

- The PCL guide is placed through the anteromedial portal, and the tip aimer is placed directly on the PCL femoral footprint.
- The drill sleeve is placed on the skin to determine the area in which to make a small longitudinal skin incision (Fig. 46-7). Dissection is carried down to the vastus medialis, which is then incised in line with the skin incision.

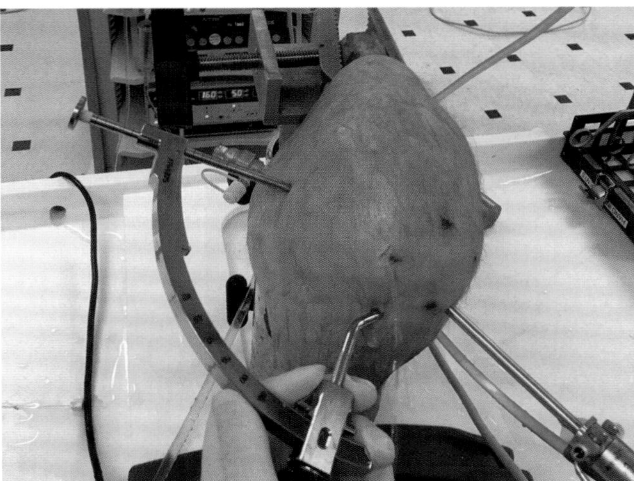

Figure 46-7 | Left cadaveric knee showing the PCL femoral guide. The tip aimer is placed through the anteromedial portal with the drill sleeve resting on the medial femoral cortex.

- The drill sleeve is placed on the medial femoral cortex. The 2.4-mm guide pin is then drilled outside-in to the notch (Fig. 46-8). The guide is removed, and a 10-mm reamer is used to ream the femoral tunnel (Fig. 46-9). All bone debris is removed with suction from the mechanical shaver.

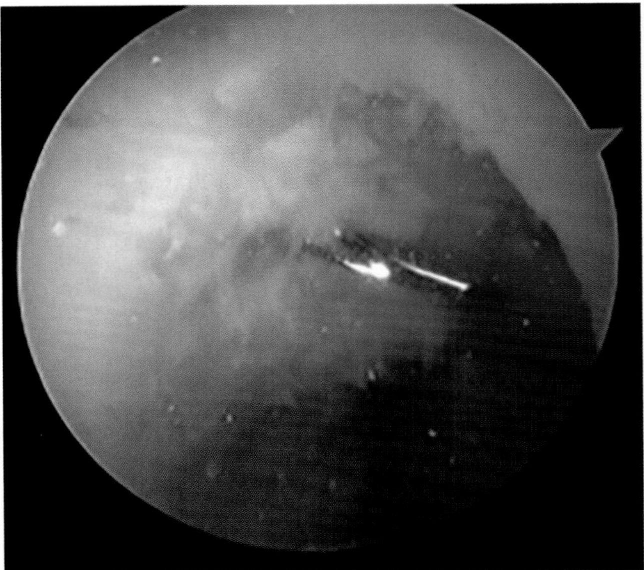

Figure 46-8 | The 2.4-mm pin is drilled outside-in entering the PCL femoral footprint.

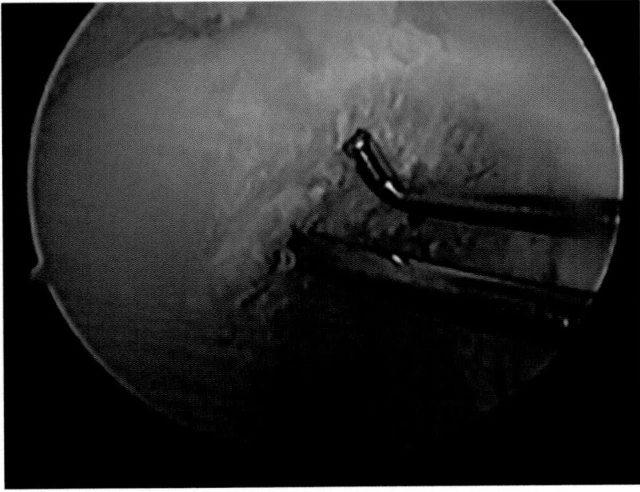

Figure 46-9 | The 10-mm reamer is shown entering the PCL femoral footprint.

Graft Passage

- A Gore Smoother is passed retrograde through the tibial tunnel and out the anteromedial portal (Fig. 46-10). The smoother is cycled until the tibial tunnel edges are smooth, facilitating graft passage (Table 46-1). The suture from the tendinous part of the graft is passed through the smoother loop, and the smoother is pulled distally, shuttling the sutures out the tibial tunnel. Hyperflexion of the knee can help pass the graft through the tibial tunnel (Table 46-1).
- A grasper is inserted through the femoral tunnel into the notch to grab the sutures on the bone block. The bone plug is pulled flush with the femoral tunnel aperture (Table 46-1).

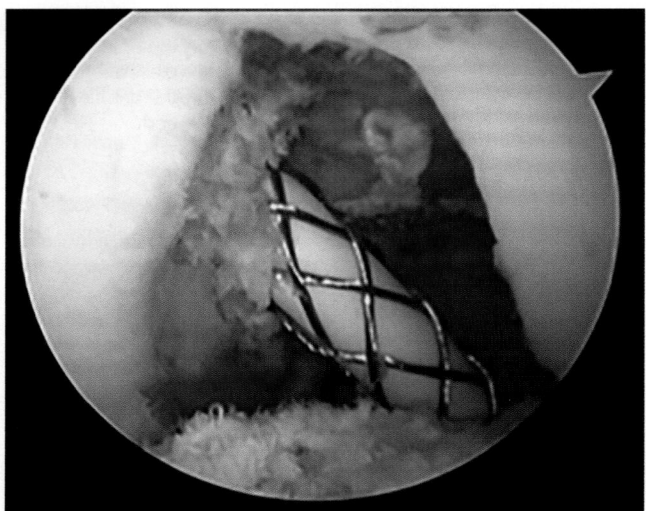

Figure 46-10 | The Gore Smoother is being passed retrograde up the tibial tunnel into the posterior part of the knee.

Graft Fixation

- A guidewire is placed between the bone block and the tunnel wall at the desired location of the screw.
- The tunnel notcher is inserted over the guidewire to notch the femoral tunnel to a depth that matches the desired screw length.
- The full length of the notch and bone block are tapped with a Milagro Screw Tap. A Milagro screw that is 2 mm smaller than the femoral tunnel is inserted over the guidewire.
- The soft tissue portion of the graft is fixed into the tibia with a post and washer (low-profile 12-mm washer and 6.5-mm cancellous screw) just distal to the PCL tibial tunnel and supplemented by a retrograde biocomposite interference screw.
  - PCL fixation is done with the knee in 90 degrees of flexion while an anterior drawer is applied to the tibia (Table 46-1).

Postoperative Care

- The patient is allowed weight bearing as tolerated with crutches in a hinged knee brace locked in extension with passive range of motion restricted to 0-90 degrees for the first 4 weeks.
- Patellar mobilizations, quadriceps sets, and straight leg raises are begun immediately.
- The hinged brace is unlocked for gait training at 4 weeks and is discontinued along with crutches at 8 weeks postoperatively.
- If good quadriceps control is achieved, closed chain strengthening can begin at 6 weeks.
- Hamstring activation is limited for the first 12 weeks.
- Return to sports as tolerated is allowed at 9 months.

References

1. Ahn JH, Wang JH, Lee SH, Yoo JC, Jeon WJ. Increasing the distance between the posterior cruciate ligament and the popliteal neurovascular bundle by a limited posterior capsular release during arthroscopic transtibial posterior cruciate ligament reconstruction: a cadaveric angiographic study. *Am J Sports Med.* 2007;35(5):787-792.
2. Moorman CT III, Murphy Zane MS, Bansai S, et al. Tibial insertion of the posterior cruciate ligament: a sagittal plane analysis using gross, histologic, and radiographic methods. *Arthroscopy.* 2008;24(3):269-275.
3. Wind WM Jr, Bergfeld JA, Parker RD. Evaluation and treatment of posterior cruciate ligament injuries: revisited. *Am J Sports Med.* 2004;32:1765-1775.

Chapter 47
Tibial Inlay Technique for Posterior Cruciate Ligament Reconstruction

VICTOR ANCIANO
MARK D. MILLER

Advantages of Tibial Inlay over Transtibial Approach

- The transtibial approach has been shown to increase graft abrasion, attenuation, and failure of patellar tendon grafts undergoing cyclic loading protocols.
- The transtibial approach has a risk of popliteal artery damage during reaming of the tibial tunnel and exiting from the posterior tibial cortex (Figs. 47-1 and 47-2).
- The tibial inlay technique, as described, does not require intraoperative repositioning.
- Functional outcomes are similar between transtibial and tibial inlay techniques.

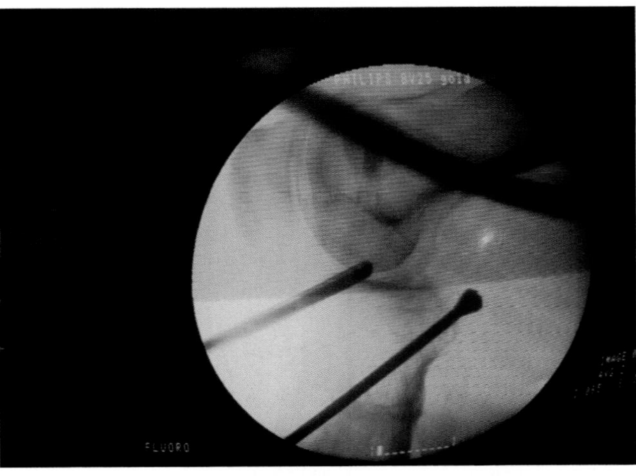

Figure 47-1 | Transtibial approach: drilling of tibial tunnel. Fluoroscopy showing risk of tibial posterior cortex breaching during drilling.

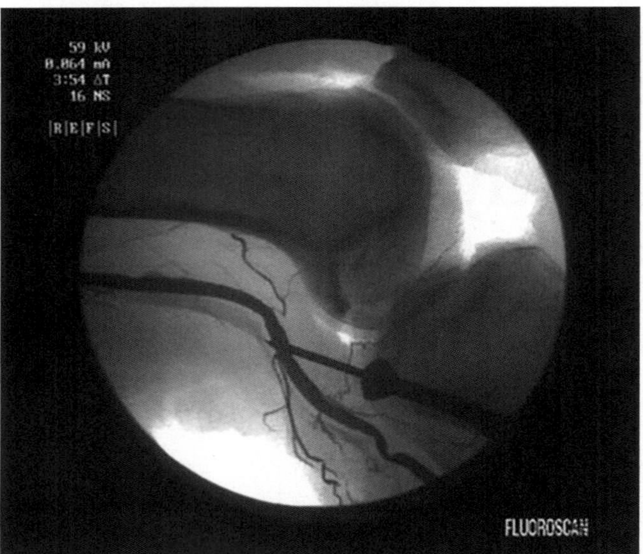

Figure 47-2 | Transtibial tunnel approach with angiogram showing proximity of popliteal artery to transtibial tunnel and risk of injury with guidewire placement.

Sterile Instruments/Equipment

- Beanbag
- Ankle-foot orthosis–type leg holder
- Positioning foam
- Arthroscopic equipment
- Looped 18-gauge guidewire

Positioning

- The patient is positioned in the lateral decubitus position with the use of an ankle-foot orthosis–type leg holder on the operative side. The lateral decubitus position is achieved with a beanbag positioner with the "bed roll" technique (Fig. 47-3).
  - The bed roll technique involves using positioning foam to wrap the nonoperative leg and securing it with elastic bandaging (Fig. 47-3).

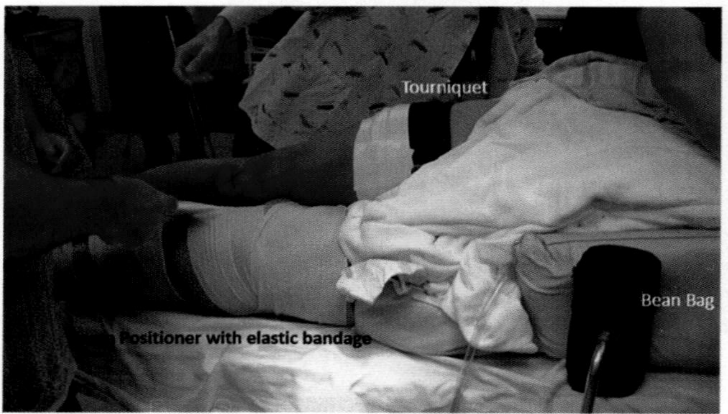

Figure 47-3 | Lateral decubitus position with use of beanbag positioner and bed roll technique of nonoperative extremity.

- The positioning should allow for comfortable transition between an abducted hip with a flexed knee for arthroscopy to a position of neutral abduction, with a partially flexed hip and knee to allow posterior access to the popliteal fossa (Fig. 47-4).
- If a bed roll technique is not used, close attention should be paid to padding the contralateral, nonoperative leg. Padding should be applied to the fibular head and lateral malleolus to protect against common peroneal nerve palsy and pressure ulcers, respectively. The use of an axillary roll prevents brachial plexus injury. Positioning the patient's ipsilateral arm over the body with padding protects the ulnar nerve.

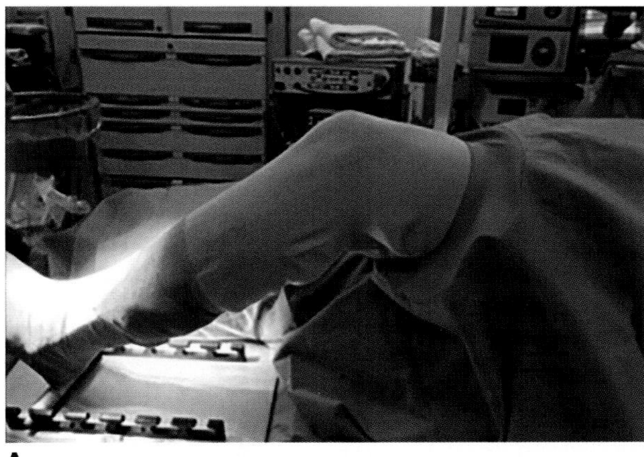

A

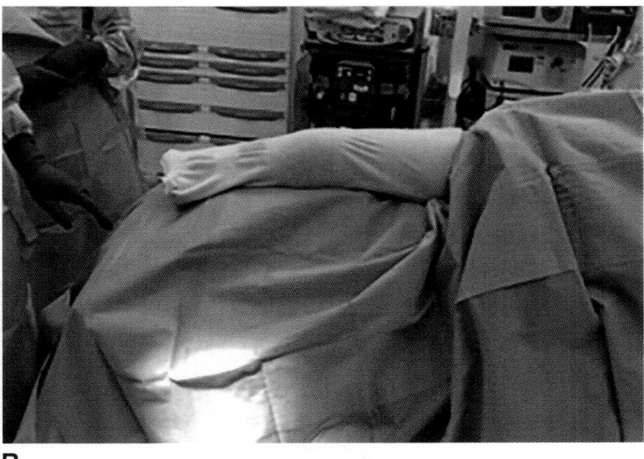

B

Figure 47-4 | A. Positioning of the operative extremity with foot-ankle orthosis–type leg holder for arthroscopy. **B.** Positioning of the leg in the lateral decubitus position for posterior approach.

Graft Selection

- There are numerous graft options, both autografts and allografts. The most common autologous grafts are bone-patellar tendon-bone (BPTB), hamstrings, and quadriceps. Allografts are usually BPTB, Achilles tendon, or soft tissue grafts.
  - There is no current evidence favoring a specific graft choice with respect to outcomes and functional scores. However, if autografts have lower failure rates in anterior cruciate ligament (ACL) reconstruction, it could be inferred that autografts would perform better in posterior cruciate ligament (PCL) reconstruction as well.
  - BPTB offers an ideal graft length for the tibial inlay technique.
  - When harvesting BPTB grafts, we recommend a 11- to 12-mm-diameter graft.
  - Double-bundle reconstruction has shown superior stability in biomechanical studies, with decreased posterior tibial translation, but no advantages have been shown with respect to functional outcomes.

Surgical Technique

- The procedure begins with a diagnostic arthroscopy using inferolateral and inferomedial portals. The inferolateral portal is the primary viewing portal, and the inferomedial portal is the primary instrumentation portal. They can be used interchangeably as needed to improve visualization and access.
  - During arthroscopy, residual fibers of the injured PCL are debrided. The posteromedial bundle may be preserved as well as meniscofemoral ligaments if they are not injured.
  - Note: Preserving the PCL remnant as augmentation of the graft may enhance healing through supplementation of soft tissue for vascular ingrowth and enhanced proprioception.
  - If an autologous graft is being used, graft harvesting should be done after diagnostic arthroscopy.
  - Next, the femoral tunnel is drilled. An 11- to 12-mm tunnel is recommended.
  - Note: If using a BPTB graft, we recommend using a fluted drill bit and a sizer to save bone graft. This may be used later to graft the defects created in the patella.
  - A one- or two-tunnel technique can be used with the tibial inlay technique. For one-tunnel, the anterolateral bundle footprint is used: 1 o'clock position (for a right knee) between 6 and 8 mm posterior to the articular margin of the medial arch point and 7-8 mm inferior to the trochlear point.
  - If a two-tunnel technique is used, placement of the anterolateral tunnel is the same as for the one-tunnel technique. The posteromedial tunnel is placed posterior and inferior to the anterolateral tunnel: 3:30 position (right knee) 11 mm posterior and inferior to the articular margin of the medial arch point and 10-11 mm superior to the posterior point of the articular cartilage margin.
  - We recommend outside-in femoral tunnel placement. There is less angle divergence using this technique. Vastus medialis obliquus (VMO) fibers can be split or a subvastus approach can be used. Femoral tunnel placement PCL guides can be used.

- Once the femoral tunnel(s) is completed, the posterior approach is made by placing the leg on a Mayo stand in the standard lateral decubitus position allowing posterior access (Fig. 47-5).
- The tibial inlay is approached through a transverse incision in the popliteal crease with careful subcutaneous dissection. A transverse horizontal incision is preferred over a curvilinear incision for better cosmetic results and fewer wound complications (Fig. 47-5).
- The fascia over the gastrocnemius is incised, and a hockey stick incision is made in the gastrocnemius fascia extending distally on the medial aspect.

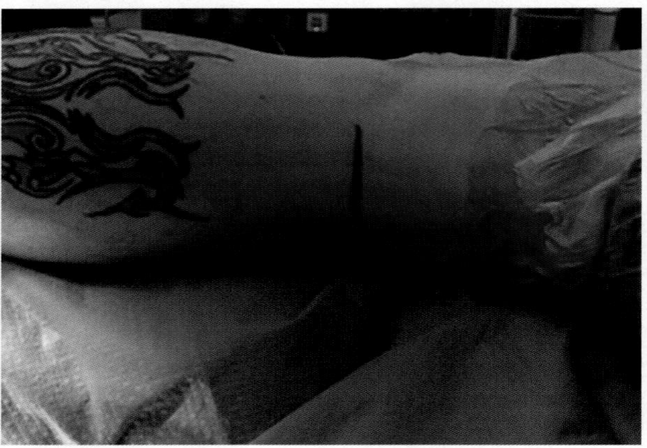
A

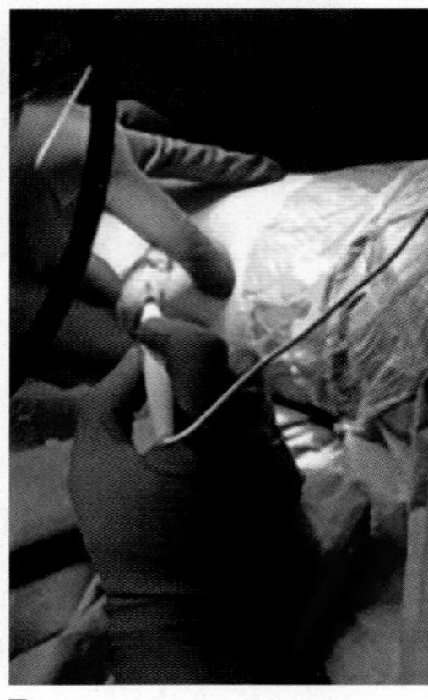
B

Figure 47-5 | A. Horizontal posterior transverse incision at popliteal crease. **B.** Dissection of subcutaneous tissue superficial to gastrocnemius fascia.

- The medial head of the gastrocnemius is mobilized to gain access to the back of the knee. Unlike the lateral head, the medial head of the gastrocnemius is quite mobile. Using Steinmann pins during lateral retraction of the gastrocnemius allows hands-free retraction. Bending the Steinmann pin away from the incision improves exposure (Fig. 47-6).
- Electrocautery and a burr are used to create a trough in the posterior tibial sulcus. To position the inlay, the medial and lateral posterior tibial eminences are palpated. The medial eminence is the more prominent. The inlay is placed directly in between these landmarks (Fig. 47-6).

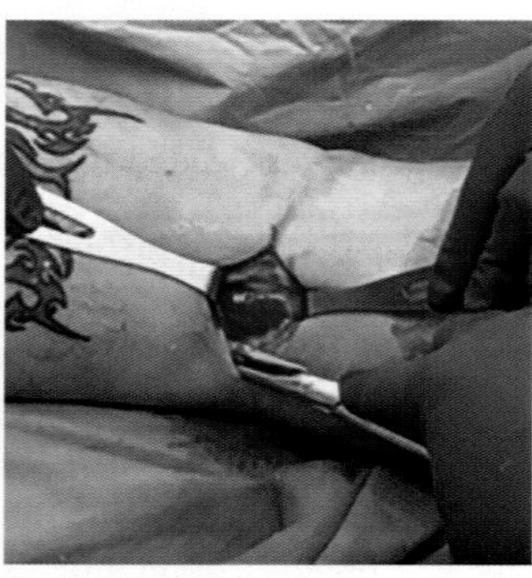
A

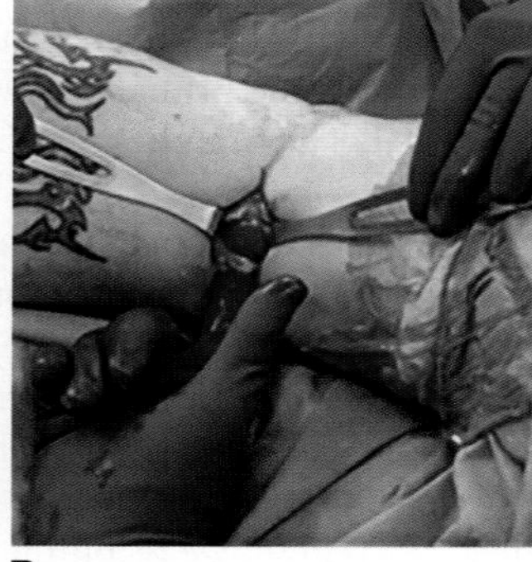
B

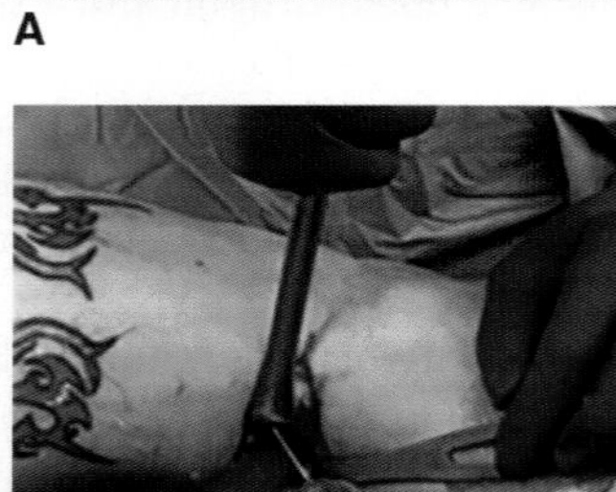
C

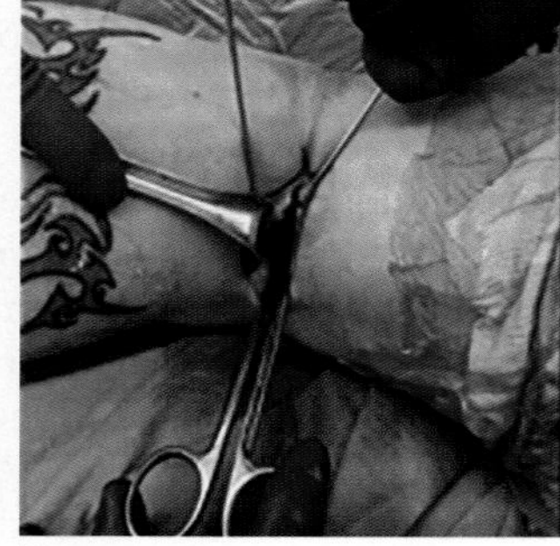
D

Figure 47-6 | A. Visualization of medial gastrocnemius. **B.** Palpation of posterior tibial eminences with finger retraction of medial gastrocnemius muscle. **C.** Placement of Steinmann pin for hands-free retraction of medial gastrocnemius. **D.** Two Steinmann pins bent away from surgical field to improve exposure of posterior tibia.

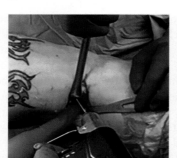

- Beginning at the top of the trough and extending proximally, a posterior arthrotomy is made in the posterior aspect of the knee.
- Note: Passing a finger easily through the arthrotomy will facilitate the graft's passage through the arthrotomy.
- The looped 18-gauge guidewire is passed through the arthrotomy and retrieved anteriorly using the arthroscope (Fig. 47-7).

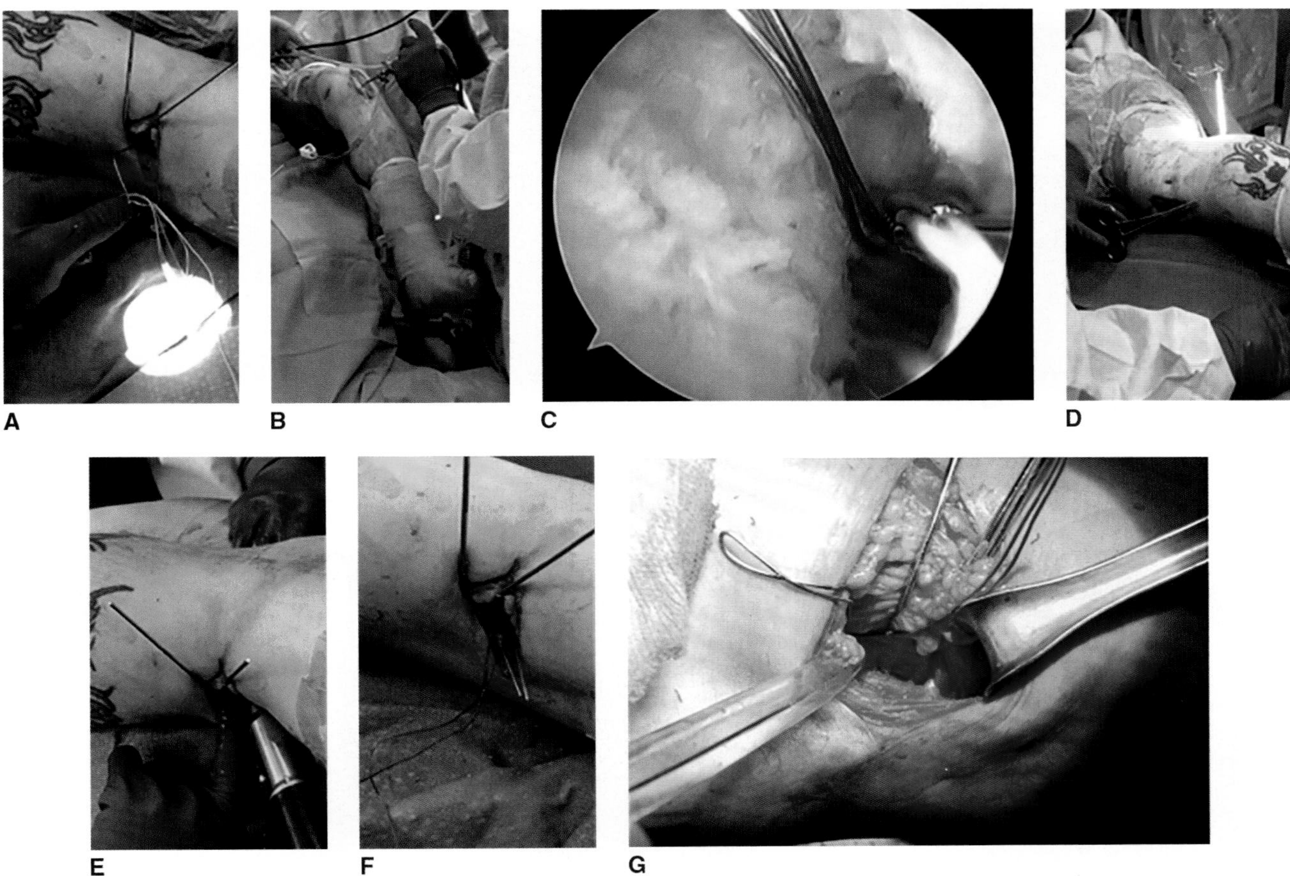

Figure 47-7 | Stepwise sequence of passage of the graft from posterior to anterior. **A.** Graft's tibial block sutures through looped guidewire. **B.** Arthroscopic-assisted securing of guidewire from posterior arthrotomy. **C.** Arthroscopic picture of looped guidewire through posterior arthrotomy being retrieved with grasper. **D.** Securing of looped guidewire anteriorly with hemostat clamp. **E.** Drilling of graft's tibial bone block guidewires into tibial inlay. **F.** Demonstrations of temporary fixation of the graft's tibial bone block with two guidewires. **G.** Visualization of tibial inlay is made possible by excellent exposure with phrenic retractor and Steinmann pins.

- Before graft passage, two guidewires are drilled into the tibial bone block of the graft. This will permit the bone graft to be fixed with posteroanterior bicortical 4.5-mm cannulated screws with washers and achieve temporary fixation before screw fixation (Fig. 47-8). It is often helpful to obtain intraoperative fluoroscopy AP and lateral views to ensure that the graft is in an ideal position before final screw fixation (Fig. 47-9).

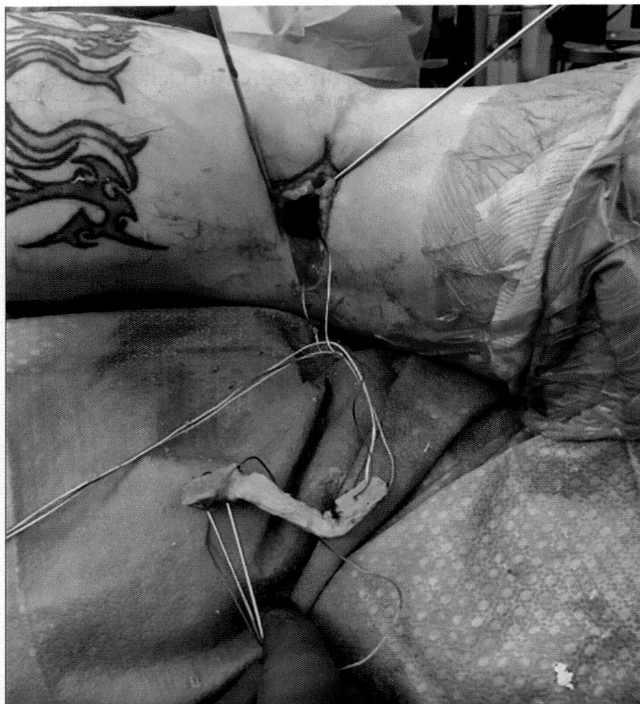

Figure 47-8 | Looped guidewire through posterior arthrotomy with graft sutures in loop. The graft's tibial bone block shows the two guidewires drilled for improved handling and temporary fixation.

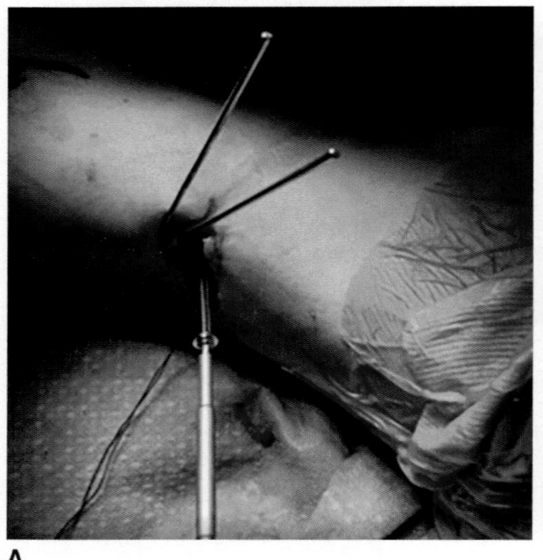

A

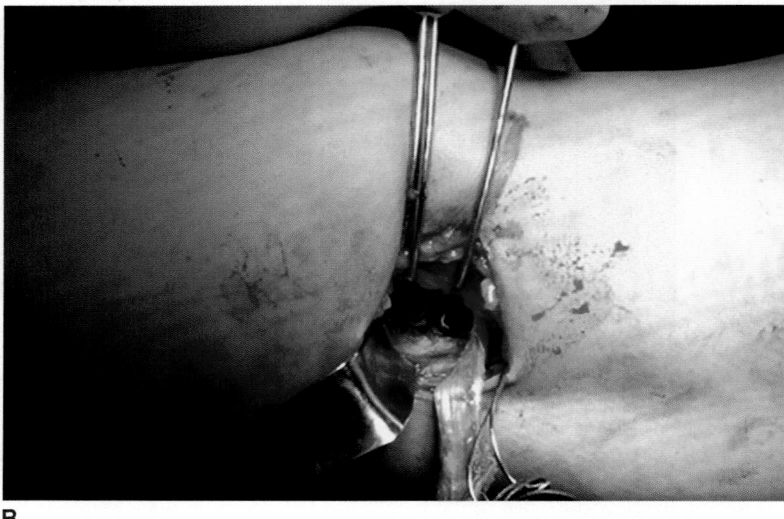

B

Figure 47-9 | **A.** Definite fixation of graft's tibial bone block to tibial inlay with screw fixation and soft tissue washer. **B.** Fixation of graft's tibial bone block to tibial inlay with two cannulated screws.

- With the guidewire, the sutures are passed from the patellar bone block into the knee. Graft sutures are placed in a perpendicular fashion.
- Note: If when passing the graft into the knee, it "hangs up," pulling the graft forward and redirecting with an arthroscopic probe into the femoral tunnel can facilitate passage. The use of a right angle to pull the bone plug anterior before passing it into the tunnel can also be helpful.
- With a femoral tunnel suture passer, the femoral bone block is passed into the femoral tunnel. If using a double-bundle technique, the posteromedial bundle is passed first.
- The knee should be cycled several times before fixation to eliminate residual laxity.
- An interference screw, button, or staple can be used as secondary fixation on the femoral side. We recommend backup fixation for all cases.
- Note: When fixing the graft in the femoral tunnel, an anterior drawer maneuver can be used to reduce the knee. In patients with grossly unstable knees, it may be helpful to evaluate the reduction with fluoroscopy before final fixation (Fig. 47-10).

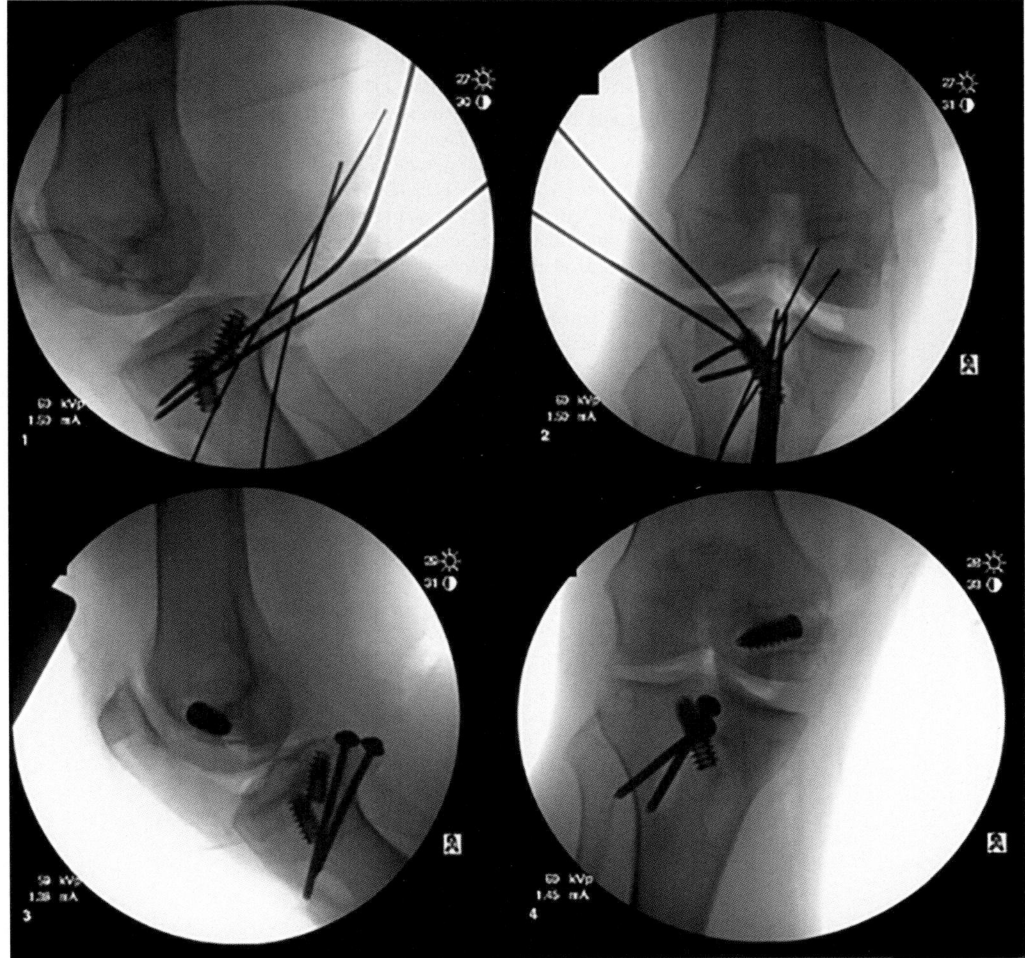

Figure 47-10 | AP and lateral fluoroscopic intraoperative images of PCL inlay revision case. *Top Row*: Temporary fixation of graft's tibial bone block with guidewires to tibial inlay. *Bottom Row*: Tibial fixation of graft with two cannulated bicortical screws with soft tissue washers.

Pediatric Considerations

- PCL tibial inlay reconstruction is possible in skeletally immature patients using the same approach and technique for the tibial portion. However, a hamstring graft is used and is looped over a screw and soft tissue washer, and the free ends are passed through an all-epiphyseal femoral tunnel.

Postoperative Rehabilitation

- Patients are placed in an extension brace and are allowed protected weight bearing.
- Physical therapy can start 2-3 days after surgery.
- During physical therapy, range of motion exercises in the prone position should be started early.
- Quadriceps exercises are recommended, but hamstring exercises are discouraged.
- Protective weight bearing can be advanced by 6 weeks.
- The brace can be discontinued at 6 weeks, and flexion can progress as tolerated.
- Return to sports is expected between 9 and 12 months postoperatively.

Suggested Readings

Anderson CJ, Ziegler CG, Wijdicks CA, Engebretsen L, LaPrade RF. Arthroscopically pertinent anatomy of the anterolateral and posteromedial bundles of the posterior cruciate ligament. *J Bone Joint Surg Am.* 2012;94(21):1936-1945. doi:10.2106/JBJS.K.01710.

Chahla J, Nitri M, Civitarese D, Dean CS, Moulton SG, LaPrade RF. Anatomic double-bundle posterior cruciate ligament reconstruction. *Arthrosc Tech.* 2016;5(1):e149-e156. doi:10.1016/j.eats.2015.10.014.

Dempsey I, Gwathmey FW, Miller MD. Section III, Procedure 22. Posterior cruciate ligament repair and reconstruction. In: Miller M, Cole B, Cosgarea A, Owens B, Browne J, eds. *Operative Techniques: Knee Surgery*. Elsevier Health Sciences; 2017.

Harner CD, Janaushek MA, Kanamori A, Yagi M, Vogrin TM, Woo SL. Biomechanical analysis of a double-bundle posterior cruciate ligament reconstruction. *Am J Sports Med.* 2000;28(2):144-151. doi:10.1177/03635465000280020201.

Johannsen AM, Anderson CJ, Wijdicks CA, Engebretsen L, LaPrade RF. Radiographic landmarks for tunnel positioning in posterior cruciate ligament reconstructions. *Am J Sports Med.* 2013;41(1):35-42. doi:10.1177/0363546512465072.

LaPrade CM, Civitarese DM, Rasmussen MT, LaPrade RF. Emerging updates on the posterior cruciate ligament: a review of the current literature. *Am J Sports Med.* 2015;43(12):3077-3092. doi:10.1177/0363546515572770.

Miller MD, Kline AJ, Gonzales J, Beach WR. Vascular risk associated with a posterior approach for posterior cruciate ligament reconstruction using the tibial inlay technique. *J Knee Surg.* 2002;15(3):137-140.

Nuelle CW, Milles JL, Pfeiffer FM, et al. Biomechanical comparison of five posterior cruciate ligament reconstruction techniques. *J Knee Surg.* 2017;30(6):523-531.

Osti M, Hierzer D, Seibert FJ, Benedetto KP. The arthroscopic all-inside tibial-inlay reconstruction of the posterior cruciate ligament: medium-term functional results and complication rate *J Knee Surg.* 2017;30(30):233-243.

Song EK, Park HW, Ahn YS, Seon JK. Transtibial versus tibial inlay techniques for posterior cruciate ligament reconstruction: long-term follow-up study. *Am J Sports Med.* 2014;42(12):2964-2971. doi:10.1177/0363546514550982.

Tompkins M, Keller TC, Milewski MD, et al. Transtibial tunnel placement in posterior cruciate ligament reconstruction: how it relates to the anatomic footprint. *Orthop J Sports Med.* 2014;2(2). doi:10.1177/2325967114523384.

Chapter 48
Double-Bundle Anterior Cruciate Ligament Reconstruction

THIERRY PAUYO
MARCIO BOTTENE VILLA ALBERS
FREDDIE H. FU

Preoperative Considerations

- Anterior cruciate ligament (ACL) reconstruction should focus on the restoration of the ACL to its native dimensions, collagen orientation, and insertion sites, according to individual anatomy. This concept can be applied to single-bundle (SB) and double-bundle (DB) ACL reconstruction.[1]
- Ultimately, the graft choice is based on graft characteristics and particularly on the estimated graft size. Based on the preoperative measurements of the tibial ACL footprint on sagittal and coronal cuts of the MRI, the native tibial footprint area is estimated (Fig. 48-1).[2]
- The target graft size is from 50% to 70% of the estimated native tibial insertion area.[3] If the ACL footprint is more than 14 mm, a double-bundle ACL reconstruction is safe (Fig. 48-2).

Sterile Instrument/Equipment

- Tourniquet
- 30-degree arthroscopic camera
- Arthroscopic shaver
- ACL tibial guide
- Cannulated arthroscopic standard and flexible reamers
- Arthroscopic tunnel dilators
- Arthroscopic ruler
- Suspensory fixation for the femur
- Polyether ether ketone (PEEK) interference screw fixation for the tibia

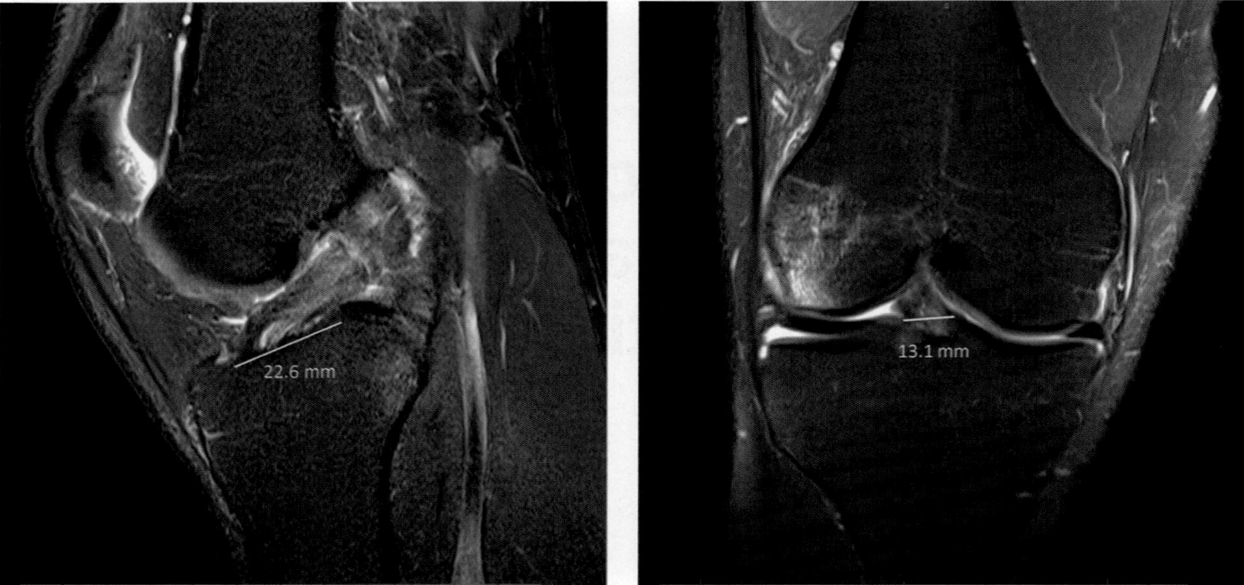

Figure 48-1 | Sagittal **(left)** and coronal **(right)** MRI T2 of the injured ACL. The ACL footprint measures 22.6 mm, which is large enough to have a double-bundle ACL reconstruction.

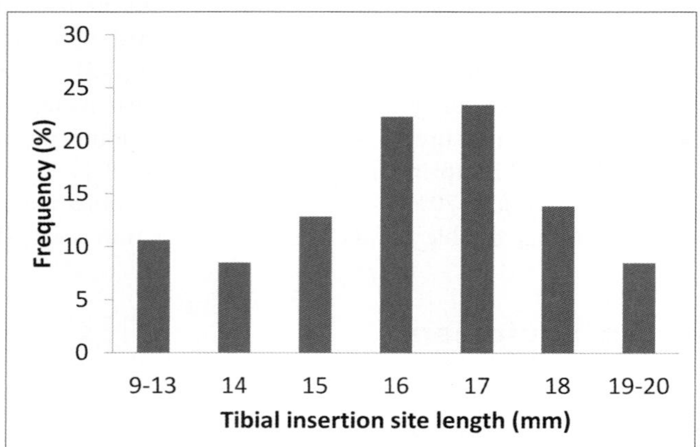

Figure 48-2 | Reference table to decide between single- and double-bundle ACL reconstruction. The target graft size should be from 50% to 70% of the estimated native tibial insertion area. If the ACL footprint is more than 14 mm on the sagittal MRI, double-bundle ACL reconstruction is safe.

Positioning

- The patient is positioned supine, and the affected leg is placed in a circumferential leg holder (Fig. 48-3).
- Care is taken to pad all bony prominences, including the greater trochanter, the fibular head (peroneal nerve), and the elbow (radial nerve).
- A pneumatic tourniquet is placed on the upper thigh of the affected extremity.
- With the foot of the table dropped, the knee can be moved from full extension to 120 degrees of flexion.
- The affected leg is elevated for 3 minutes, and the tourniquet is inflated.

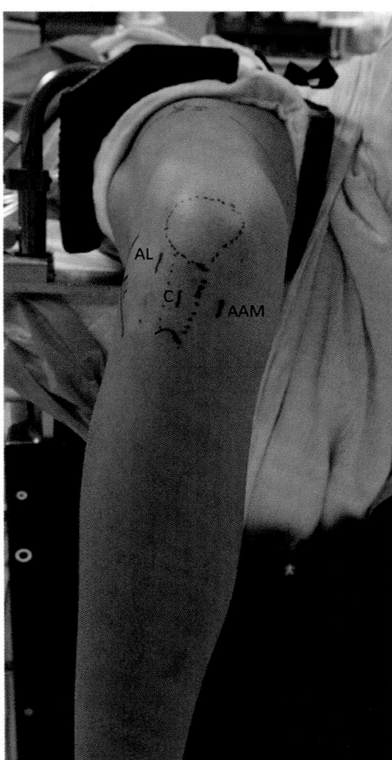

Figure 48-3 | The affected leg is placed in a circumferential leg holder.

Portals

- A three-portal technique is used to view the ACL footprint and perform the reconstruction.
  - Anterolateral (AL), central (C), and accessory anteromedial (AAM) are used (Fig. 48-4).
- The AL portal is made first.
  - It is just lateral to the patellar tendon and superior to the inferior pole of the patella.

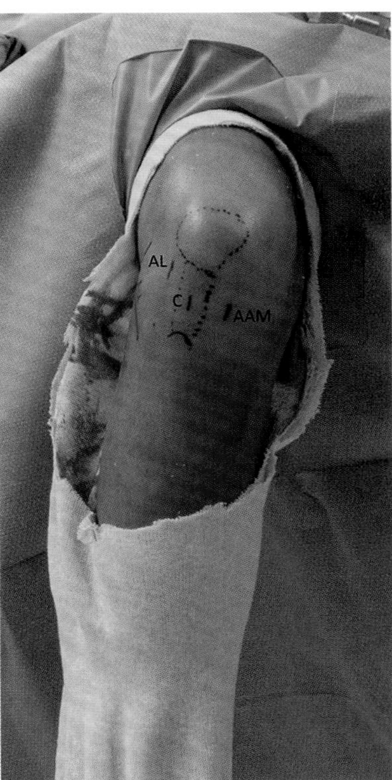

Figure 48-4 | Portal placement of the three-portal technique for individualized anatomic double-bundle ACL reconstruction. Portals: AL, Anterolateral; AAM, accessory anteromedial; C, central.

- The C and AAM portals are placed under direct visualization with an 18-gauge needle.
- The C portal is placed along the medial border of the inferior patellar tendon.
  - The 18-gauge needle should be in line with the native ACL.
  - If this cannot be achieved, the C portal can be placed with a transtendinous technique.
    - Care should be taken not to injure the intermeniscal ligament.
- The AAM portal is placed at the level of the joint line.
  - This is ~1.5 cm medial to the C portal.
  - Debridement of the fat pad can improve viewing during placement of this portal.
  - During portal placement, the spinal needle should:
    - Pass safely above the medial meniscus
    - Reach the center of the femoral ACL footprint
    - Allow safe passage of instruments to prevent damage to the medial femoral condyle

Procedure

- A diagnostic arthroscopy is done, with evaluation of all compartments for injuries that may have been missed on MRI.
- The ACL tear is examined by placing the arthroscopic camera in each portal (Fig. 48-5).
  - The tear pattern and location are noted.
  - The anteromedial (AM) and posterolateral (PL) bundles of the ACL are identified.

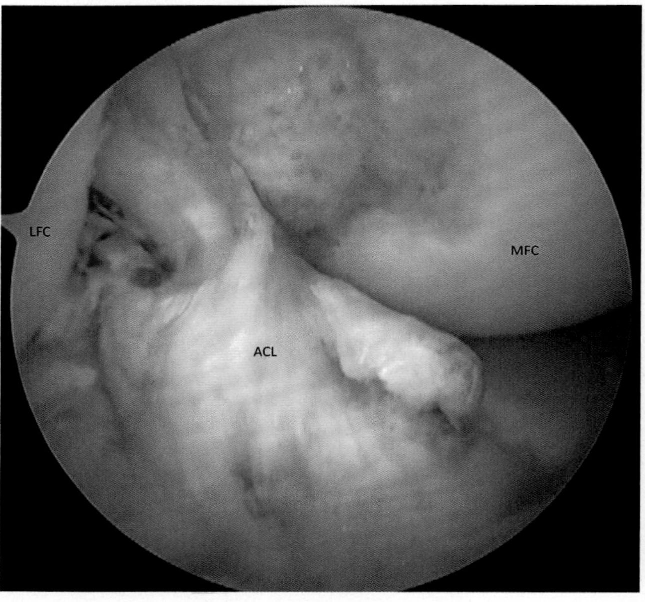

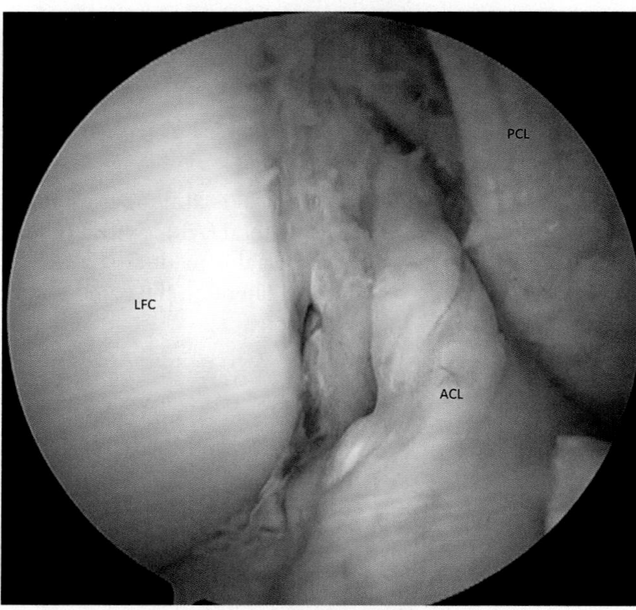

Figure 48-5 | Native injured anterior cruciate ligament (ACL). LFC, lateral femoral condyle; MFC, medial femoral condyle.

- The ACL footprint is uncovered by cutting the ACL stump with a no. 11 blade scalpel (Fig. 48-6).
  - This will ensure the preservation of the native site of the ACL footprint.
- The width and length of the AM and PL bundle insertions on the tibia are measured with an arthroscopic ruler placed in the C portal (Fig. 48-7).
- The smaller size measured for the AM and PL bundles determines the ACL graft size.
  - The diameter of the AM bundle typically measures 7-9 mm, and the diameter of the PL typically measures 5-7 mm.
    - The insertion site must be >14 mm to proceed with a double-bundle reconstruction (See Preoperative Considerations).
- The height and width of the femoral notch are measured to ensure that the size of the notch is adequate.

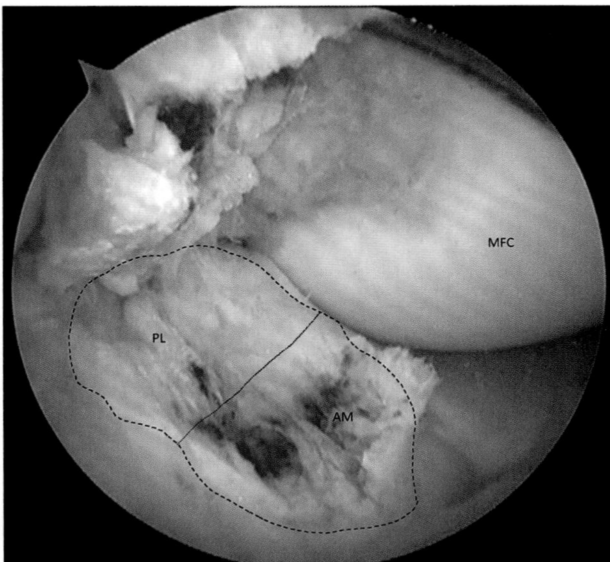

Figure 48-6 | ACL tibial footprint exposed. The posterolateral (PL) and anteromedial (AM) bundles are demarcated by the *dotted line*. MFC, medial femoral condyle.

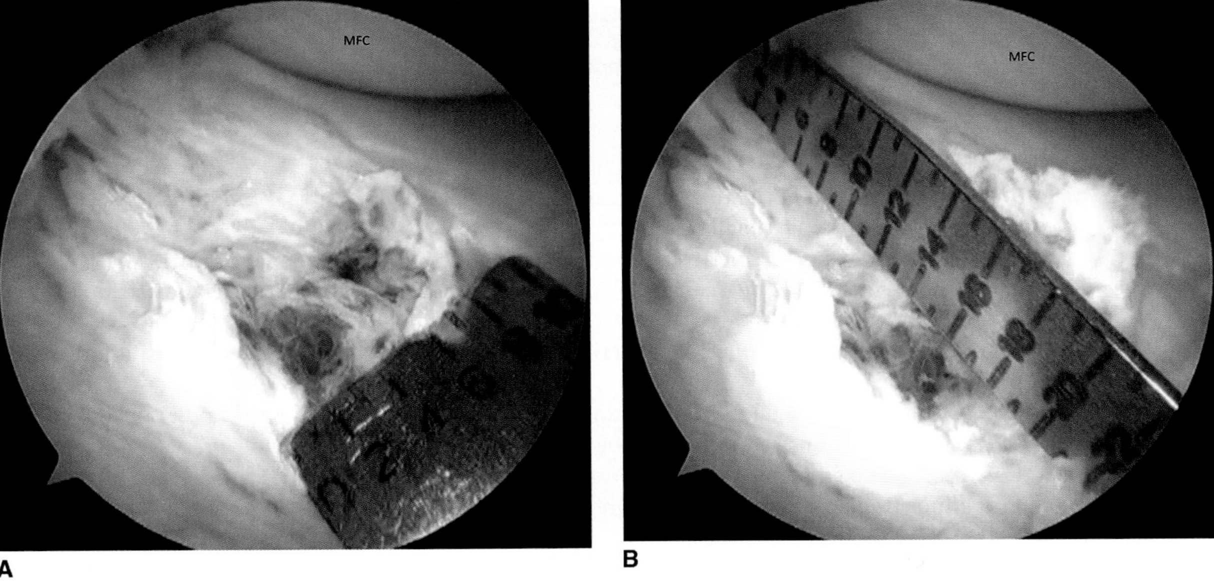

Figure 48-7 | A, B. Measurements of the tibial ACL footprint with the arthroscopic ruler. MFC, medial femoral condyle.

Tunnel Placement

Femoral Tunnels

- The PL femoral tunnel is placed through the AAM portal.
  - The starting point is marked with an awl at the center of the PL femoral insertion.
  - Correct placement of the PL tunnel starting point is confirmed by evaluation through all three portals.
  - A flexible guidewire is placed through the AAM portal to the marked center of the PL femoral insertion (Fig. 48-8).
  - The guidewire is advanced through the lateral femoral cortex and then the skin while the knee in hyperflexion.
  - The length of the tunnel is measured.
    - An ideal length is 30-40 mm to ensure 20 mm of graft is in the tunnel while enough length is maintained for the suspensory fixation.
  - A cannulated flexible reamer is placed over the guidewire while being careful not to damage the medial femoral condyle.
    - This tunnel is 1-2 mm smaller than the graft diameter.
- The AM femoral tunnel is made in the same fashion (Fig. 48-9).

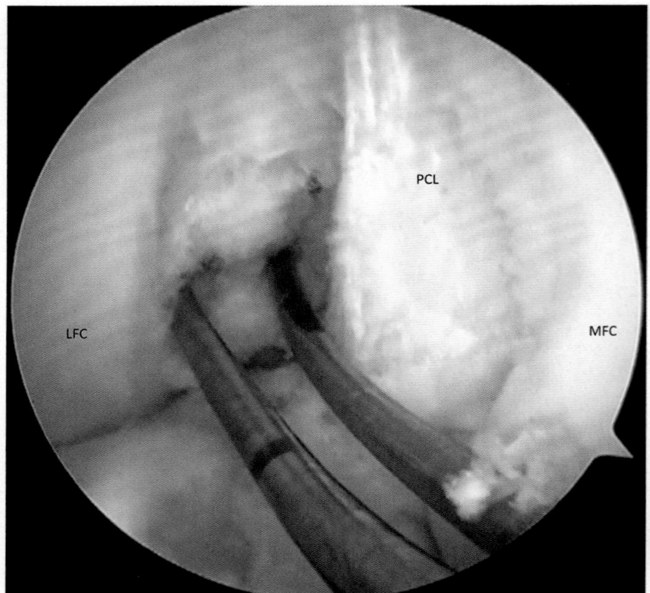

Figure 48-8 | Placement of the guidewires during positioning of the femoral tunnels in the AM and PL ACL footprint. PCL, posterior cruciate ligament; LFC, lateral femoral condyle; MFC, medial femoral condyle.

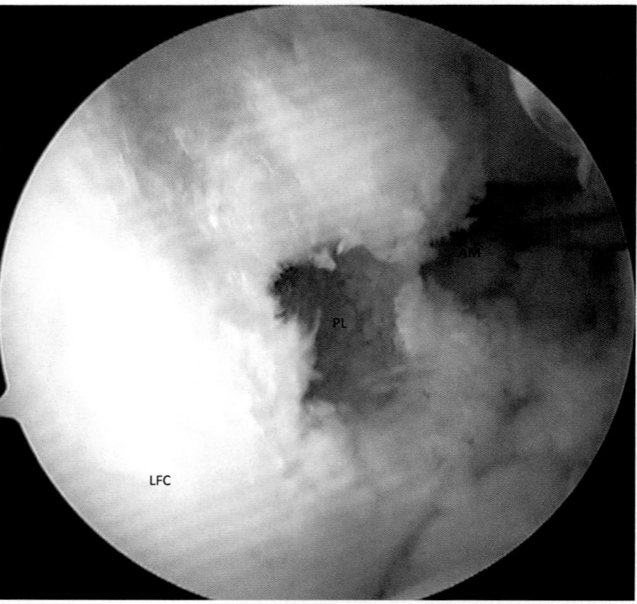

Figure 48-9 | The posterolateral (PL) and anteromedial (AM) tunnels on the femoral ACL footprint. The two tunnels are distinct and separated by a 1- to 2-mm wall. LFC, lateral femoral condyle.

Tibial Tunnels

- A 5-cm vertical incision is made over the anterior medial proximal tibia, 2 cm distal to the joint line and 1-2 cm medial to the tibial tubercle.
- If hamstring tendons are harvested, the same incision can be used for tibial drilling.
- The ACL guide is set to 45 degrees and placed at the center of the PL bundle tibial insertion through either the C or AAM portal.
- The guidewire is advanced until it is seen intra-articularly (Fig. 48-10); proper positioning of the guidewire is confirmed.
- The ACL guide is then set at 55 degrees and placed at the center of the AM bundle tibial insertion.
  - The starting point on the tibia should be 1-1.5 cm away from the PL guidewire.
  - Care must be taken to ensure that the tunnels do not merge.
  - Proper positioning of the AM guidewire is confirmed.

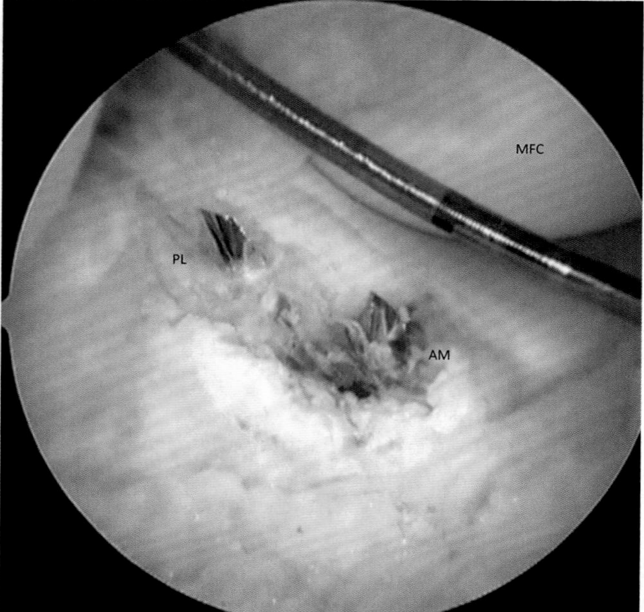

Figure 48-10 | Placement of the guidewires during positioning of the tibial tunnels in the anteromedial (AM) and posterolateral (PL) ACL footprint. MFC, medial femoral condyle.

- The knee is moved through a range of motion (ROM) to ensure that no graft impingement is present in extension.
- Cannulated reamers are placed over each guidewire, and the tunnels are reamed to a size 1-2 mm smaller than the measured graft.
- Each tunnel is dilated by hand to the final graft diameter (Fig. 48-11).

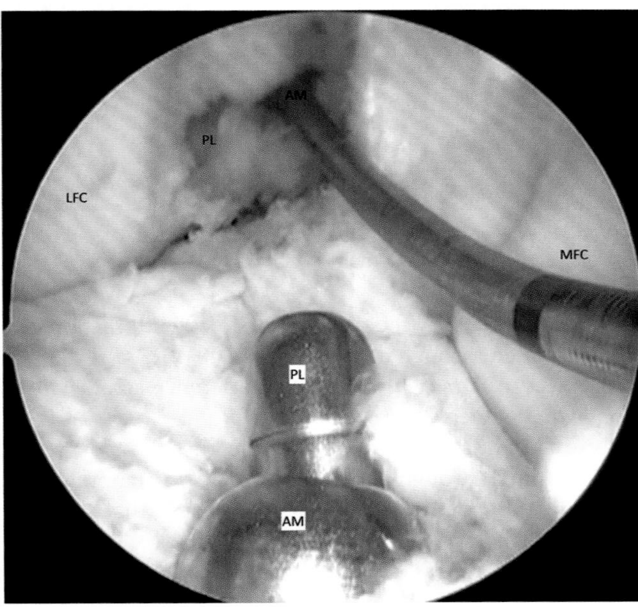

Figure 48-11 | View through the central portal of the anteromedial (AM) and posterolateral (PL) femoral tunnels with the dilators in the tibial tunnels. LFC, lateral femoral condyle; MFC, medial femoral condyle.

ACL Graft Passage and Fixation

- A Beath pin, with a loop suture attached to it, is placed through the AAM portal into the femoral PL tunnel and brought out through the anterolateral thigh.
- A suture-grasping device is placed through the PL tibial tunnel, and the suture is retrieved through it.
- A second Beath pin is placed for the AM femoral tunnel, and the suture is retrieved in a similar fashion.
- The PL bundle is passed first, from the tibia to the femur, with arthroscopic guidance, and the suspensory device on the lateral femoral cortex is "flipped" (Fig. 48-12).
- The AM bundle is passed in a similar fashion.

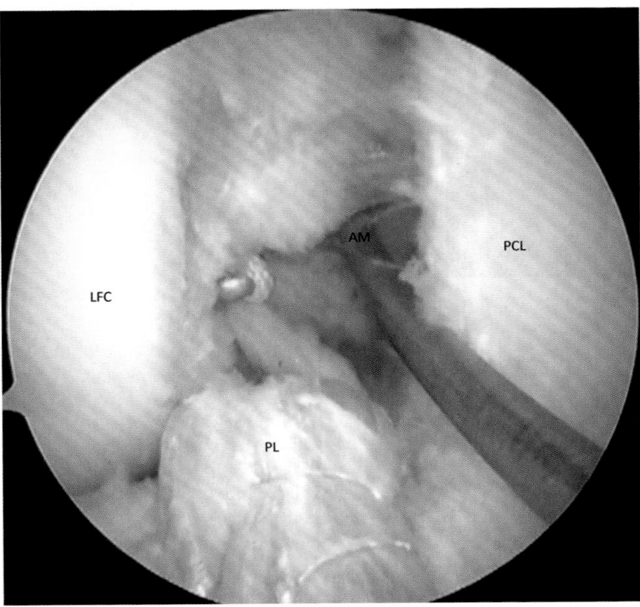

Figure 48-12 | Passage of the posterolateral (PL) bundle graft with the suspensory fixation. AM, anteromedial; LFC, lateral femoral condyle; PCL, posterior cruciate ligament.

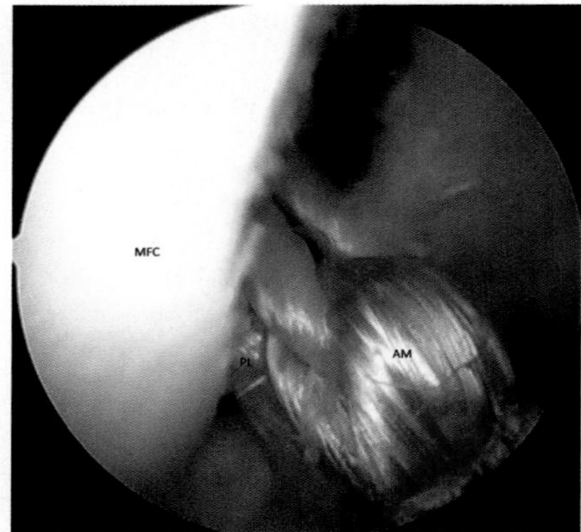

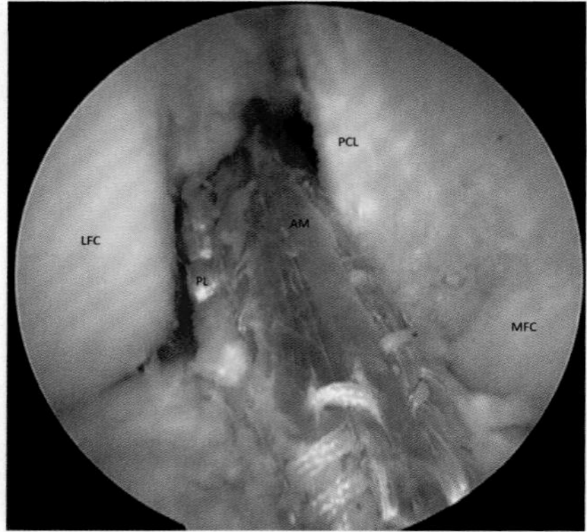

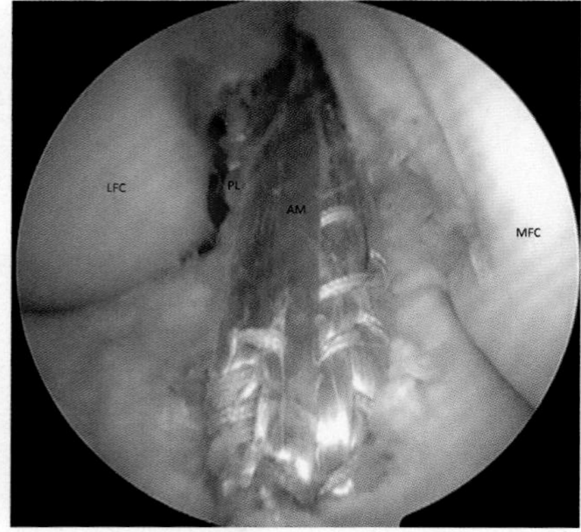

Figure 48-13 | Final ACL graft viewed through the anterolateral, central, and accessory medial portals. AM, anteromedial; LFC, lateral femoral condyle; PCL, posterior cruciate ligament; PL, posterolateral; MFC, medial femoral condyle.

- Correct placement for the suspensory fixation is confirmed with the image intensifier.
- The two bundles are examined through all portals (Fig. 48-13).
- The PL bundle graft is secured first with a PEEK interference screw with the knee in 0 degrees of flexion while tension is maintained on the sutures.
- The AM bundle is secured in a similar fashion with the knee in 30 degrees of flexion.
- The two bundles are examined through all portals to confirm anatomic position.
- The knee is moved from full extension to flexion to ensure that there is no graft impingement (Fig. 48-14).
- Anatomic tunnel placement is best assessed by postoperative computed tomography (CT) scan of the knee (Fig. 48-15).

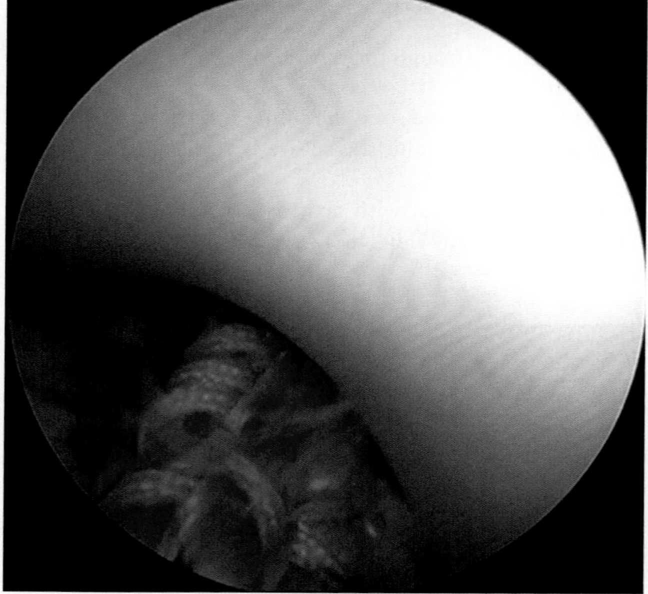

Figure 48-14 | View of the ACL graft with the knee in full extension demonstrates no impingement.

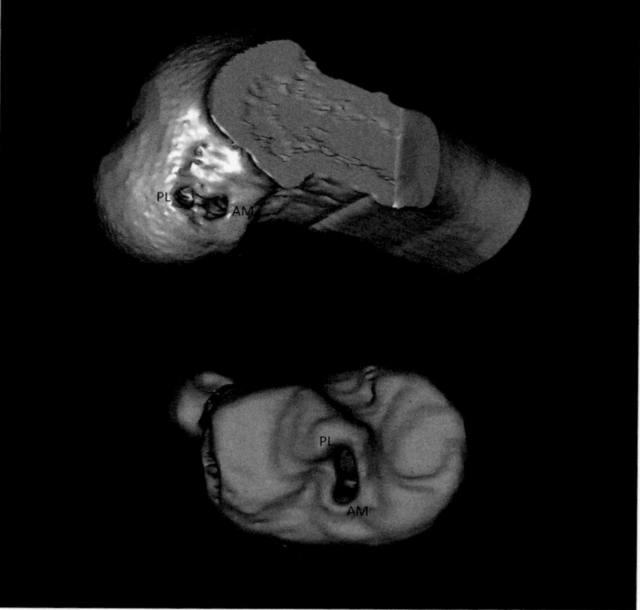

Figure 48-15 | CT scan of the tibial and femoral tunnels demonstrates anatomic position of the double-bundle ACL reconstruction. AM, anteromedial; PL, posterolateral.

References

1. Hofbauer M, Muller B, Murawski CD, van Eck CF, Fu FH. The concept of individualized anatomic anterior cruciate ligament (ACL) reconstruction. *Knee Surg Sports Traumatol Arthrosc.* 2014;22(5):979-986.
2. Guenther D, Irarrazaval S, Albers M, et al. Area of the tibial insertion site of the anterior cruciate ligament as a predictor for graft size. *Knee Surgery Sports Traumatol Arthrosc.* 2017;25(5):1576-1582.
3. Fujimaki Y, Thorhauer E, Sasaki Y, Smolinski P, Tashman S, Fu FH. Quantitative in situ analysis of the anterior cruciate ligament: length, midsubstance cross-sectional area, and insertion site areas. *Am J Sports Med.* 2016;44(1):118-125.

Chapter 49

Knee Dislocation: PCL-ACL-Medial Reconstruction

GREGORY C. FANELLI
MATTHEW G. FANELLI

Sterile Instruments/Equipment

- Fanelli posterior cruciate ligament (PCL)/anterior cruciate ligament (ACL) Guide and instrumentation system (Biomet Sports Medicine, Warsaw, Indiana) (Figs. 49-1 and 49-2).
- Fanelli Magellan suture retriever (Biomet Sports Medicine, Warsaw, Indiana)

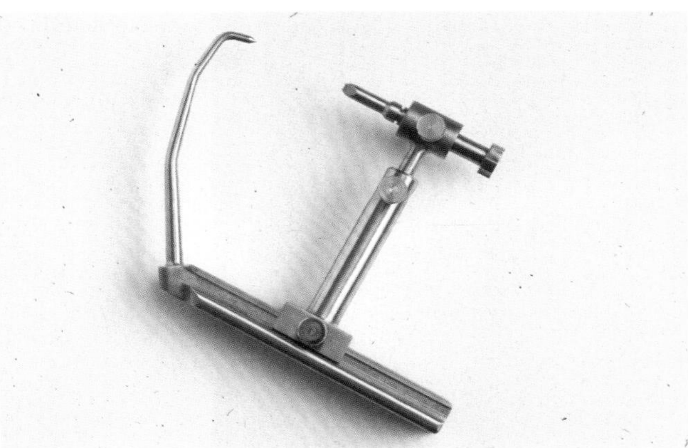

Figure 49-1 | Fanelli PCL ACL Guide and instrumentation system.

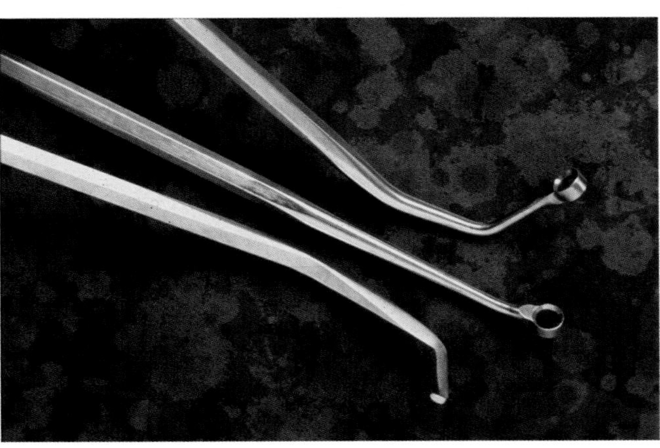

Figure 49-2 | Fanelli PCL ACL Guide and instrumentation system.

- Graft-tensioning boot (Biomet Sports Medicine, Warsaw, Indiana) (Fig. 49-3).
- Double-bundle aimers (Biomet Sports Medicine, Warsaw, Indiana)
- Gentle Thread Interference Screws (Biomet Sports Medicine, Warsaw, Indiana)
- Poly Suture Buttons 15 and 19 mm (Biomet Sports Medicine, Warsaw, Indiana)

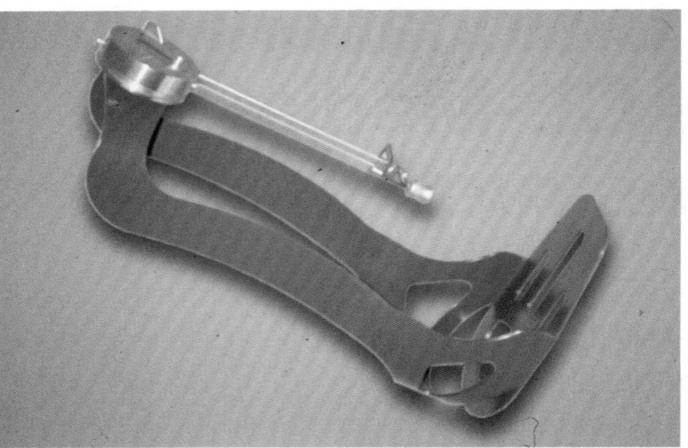

Figure 49-3 | Graft-Tensioning Boot.

Graft Selection

- PCL reconstruction
  - Achilles tendon allograft, anterolateral bundle (Fig. 49-4)
  - Anterior tibial tendon allograft, posteromedial bundle

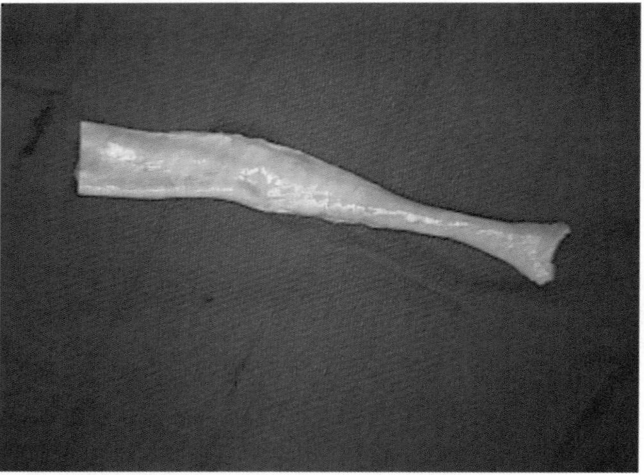

Figure 49-4 | Achilles tendon allograft, anterolateral bundle.

- ACL reconstruction
  - Achilles tendon allograft
- Medial posteromedial reconstruction
  - Primary repair
  - Posteromedial capsular shift
  - Semitendinosus allograft
- Allograft tissue is prepared before the patient is brought into the operating room to minimize anesthesia time for the patient and to facilitate the flow of the surgical procedure.

Positioning

- The patient is placed supine on the fully extended operating room.
- A tourniquet is applied to the upper thigh of the operative extremity, and that extremity is prepared and draped in a sterile fashion. Tourniquet use is minimized during the procedure.

Instability Confirmation

- PCL instability
  - Positive posterior drawer and diminished or negative tibial step-off.
- ACL instability
  - Positive Lachman and pivot shift tests.
- Medial and posteromedial instability
  - There are three different types of posteromedial instability patterns.
    - Type A (axial rotation instability only).
    - Type B (axial rotation instability combined with valgus laxity with a soft endpoint).
    - Type C (axial rotation instability combined with valgus laxity with no endpoint).
    - The axial rotation posteromedial instability (Type A) is most frequently overlooked and is often the cause of failed bicruciate ligament reconstruction since this allows continued axial rotation instability with chronic repetitive microtrauma damaging the PCL and ACL reconstruction.
    - Positive posteromedial and anteromedial drawer tests and valgus laxity tests.

Arthroscopic Approach

- The arthroscopic instruments are inserted with:
  - Inflow through the superolateral patellar portal
  - Instrumentation and visualization through the inferomedial and inferolateral patellar portals (Fig. 49-5)
  - Additional portals are established as necessary.

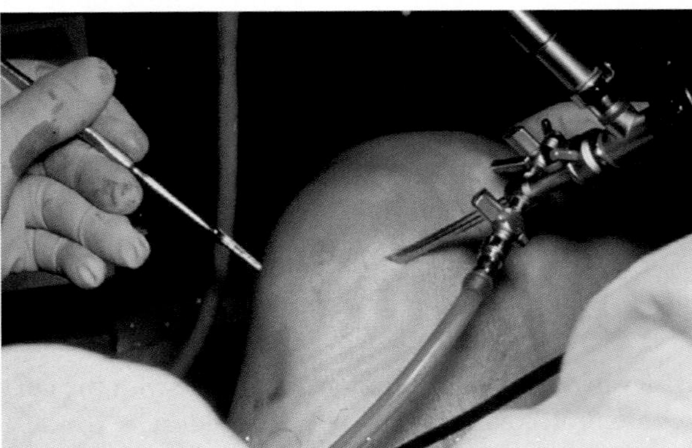

Figure 49-5 | Instrumentation and visualization through the inferomedial and inferolateral patellar portals.

- Exploration of the joint consists of evaluation of the patellofemoral joint, the medial and lateral compartments, the medial and lateral menisci, and the intercondylar notch (Figs. 49-6 and 49-7).

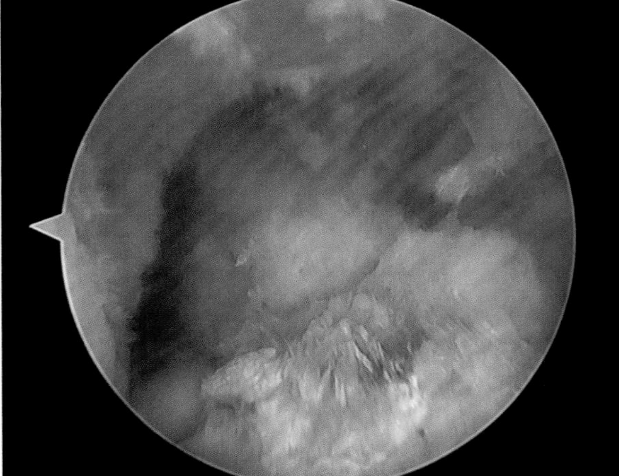

Figure 49-6 | Exploration of the joint consists of evaluation of the patellofemoral joint, the medial and lateral compartments, medial and lateral menisci, and the intercondylar notch.

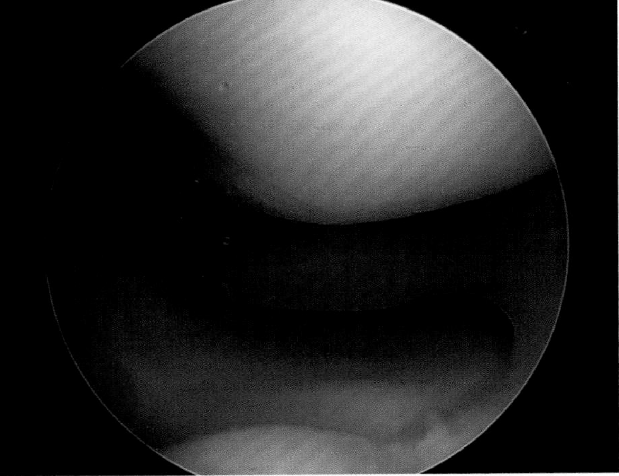

Figure 49-7 | Exploration of the joint consists of evaluation of the patellofemoral joint, the medial and lateral compartments, medial and lateral menisci, and the intercondylar notch.

Posterior Cruciate Ligament Reconstruction

- The PCL reconstruction is performed with the knee flexed between 90 and 110 degrees.

Posteromedial Safety Incision

- An extracapsular extra-articular posteromedial safety incision is made by creating an incision ~1.5-2 cm long starting at the posteromedial border of the tibia ~1-2 in below the level of the joint line and extending distally, with dissection carried to the level of the crural fascia, which is incised longitudinally.
- An interval is developed between the medial head of the gastrocnemius muscle posterior and the capsule of the knee joint anterior.
- The surgeon's index finger is inserted in the posteromedial safety incision to protect the neurovascular structures and to confirm the position of the PCL tibial tunnel in proximal-distal and mediolateral placement (Figs. 49-8 and 49-9).

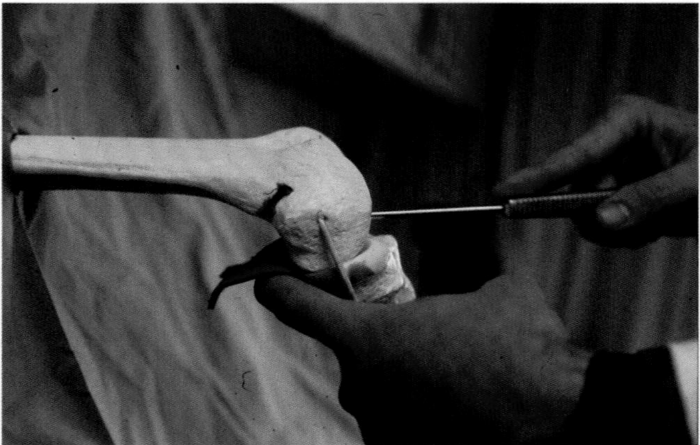

Figure 49-8 | The surgeon's index finger is inserted in the posteromedial safety incision to protect the neurovascular structures and to confirm the position of the PCL tibial tunnel in proximal distal and mediolateral placement.

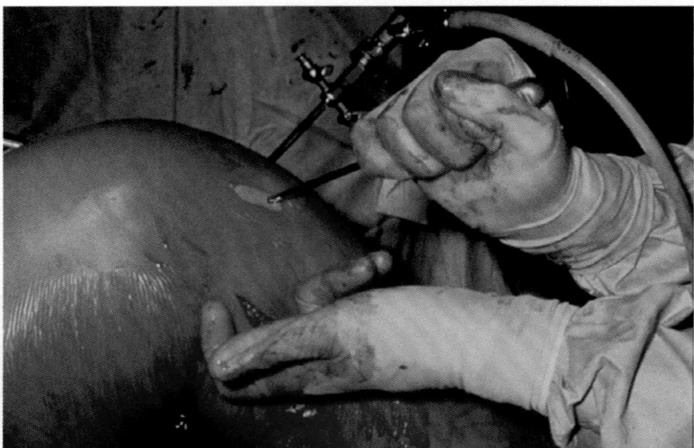

Figure 49-9 | The surgeon's index finger is inserted in the posteromedial safety incision to protect the neurovascular structures and to confirm the position of the PCL tibial tunnel in proximal distal and mediolateral placement.

- The posterior capsule is elevated from the posterior tibial ridge with the curved PCL instruments.
- Neurovascular structures are protected throughout the procedure.

PCL Tibial Tunnel

- The arm of the PCL/ACL guide is inserted through the inferomedial patellar portal.
- The tip of the guide is positioned at the inferolateral aspect of the PCL anatomic insertion site.
- The bullet portion of the guide contacts the anteromedial surface of the proximal tibia at a point midway between the posteromedial border of the tibia and the tibial crest anterior, ~1 cm below the tibial tubercle (Fig. 49-10).

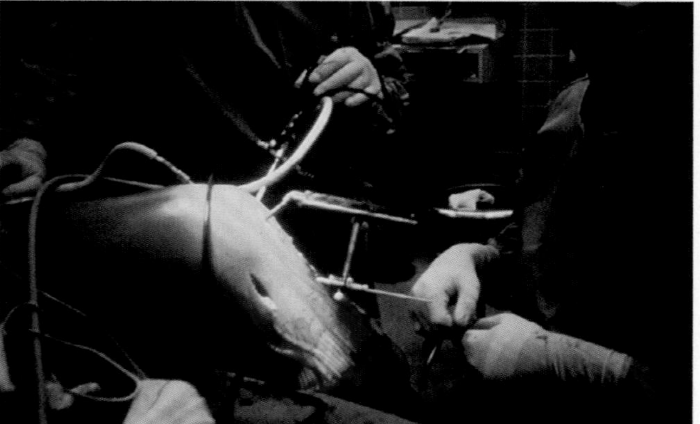

Figure 49-10 | The bullet portion of the guide contacts the anteromedial surface of the proximal tibia at a point midway between the posteromedial border of the tibia and the tibial crest anterior, ~1 cm below the tibial tubercle.

- This will provide an angle of graft orientation such that the graft will turn two very smooth 45-degree angles on the posterior aspect of the tibia.
- The tip of the guide in the posterior aspect of the tibia is confirmed with the surgeon's index finger through the extracapsular extra-articular posteromedial safety incision (see Fig. 49-9).
- When the PCL/ACL guide is positioned in the desired area, a blunt spade-tipped guidewire is drilled from anterior to posterior.
- The surgeon's index finger confirms the position of the guidewire through the posteromedial safety incision.
- The appropriately sized standard cannulated reamer is used to create the tibial tunnel.
- The curved PCL closed curette is positioned to cup the tip of the guidewire.
- The surgeon's finger through the posteromedial safety incision monitors the position of the guidewire.
- When the drill is engaged in bone, the guidewire is reversed, blunt end pointing posterior for additional patient safety.
- The drill is advanced until it reaches the posterior cortex of the tibia (Fig. 49-11).
- The chuck is disengaged from the drill, and the tibial tunnel is completed by hand.

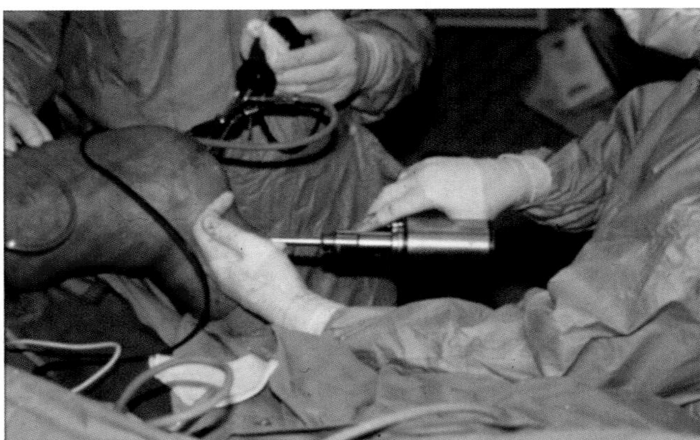

Figure 49-11 | The drill is advanced until it reaches the posterior cortex of the tibia.

PCL Femoral Tunnel

- The PCL single-bundle or double-bundle femoral tunnels are made from inside out using the double-bundle aimers.
- The double-bundle aimer is inserted through a low anterolateral patellar arthroscopic portal and is positioned directly on the footprint of the femoral anterolateral bundle PCL insertion site.
- The appropriately sized guidewire is drilled through the aimer, through the bone, and out a small skin incision.
- Care is taken to insure that there is no compromise of the articular surface.
- The double-bundle aimer is removed, and an acorn reamer is used to endoscopically drill from inside out the anterolateral PCL femoral tunnel (Fig. 49-12).
- For a double-bundle double-femoral tunnel PCL reconstruction, the same process is repeated for the posteromedial bundle of the PCL.
- An adequate bone bridge (~5 mm) between the two femoral tunnels before drilling is essential.

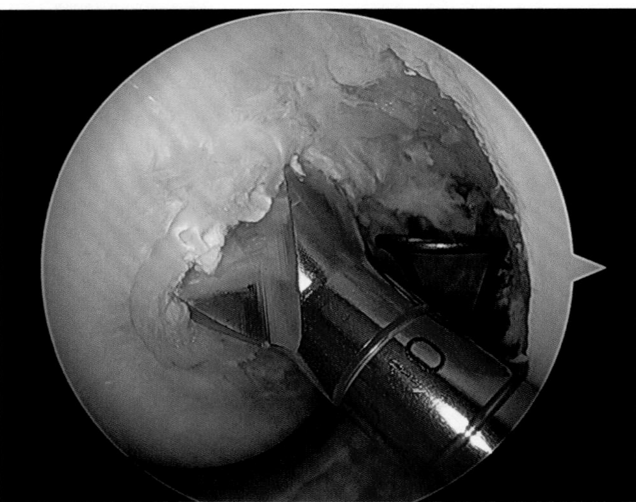

Figure 49-12 | The double-bundle aimer is removed, and an acorn reamer is used to endoscopically drill from inside out the anterolateral PCL femoral tunnel.

PCL Graft Passage, Tensioning, and Fixation

- A Fanelli Magellan suture retriever is introduced through the tibial tunnel into the joint and retrieved through the femoral tunnel (Fig. 49-13).
- The traction sutures of the graft material are attached to the loop of the Magellan suture retriever, and the graft is pulled into position (Fig. 49-14).

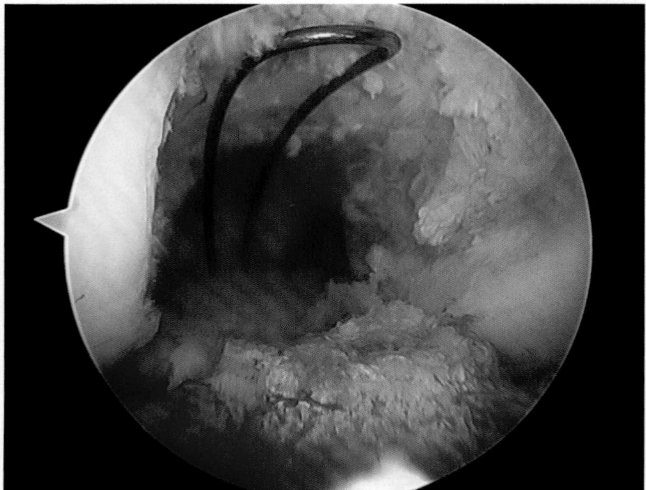

Figure 49-13 | A Fanelli Magellan suture retriever is introduced through the tibial tunnel into the joint and retrieved through the femoral tunnel.

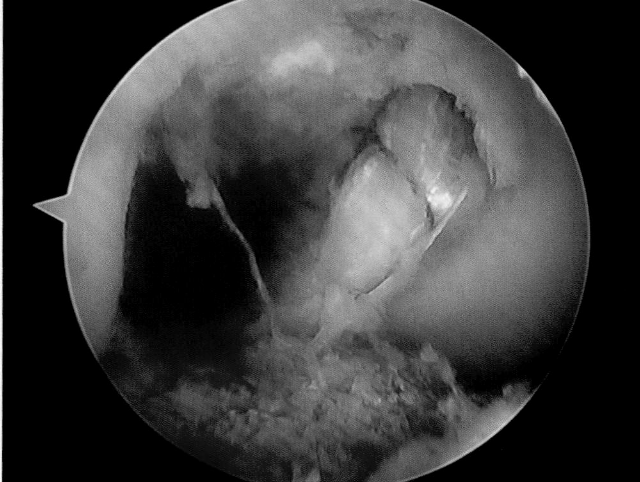

Figure 49-14 | The traction sutures of the graft material are attached to the loop of the Magellan suture retriever, and the graft is pulled into position.

- The graft material is secured on the femoral side with a resorbable interference screw for primary aperture opening fixation and a polyethylene ligament fixation button for cortical suspensory backup fixation.
- Tension is placed on the PCL graft distally using the Biomet graft-tensioning boot to restore the anatomic tibial step-off (Fig. 49-15).
- The knee is cycled through a full range of motion multiple times to allow pretensioning and settling of the graft.
- The process is repeated until there is no change in the torque setting on the graft tensioner.
- The knee is placed in 70-90 degrees of flexion, and fixation is achieved on the tibial side of the PCL graft with a resorbable interference screw and cortical suspensory backup fixation with a bicortical screw and spiked ligament washer.

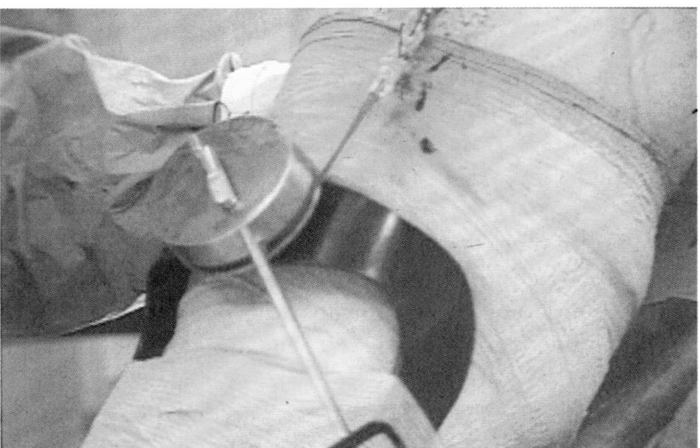

Figure 49-15 | Tension is placed on the PCL graft distally using the Biomet graft-tensioning boot to restore the anatomic tibial step-off.

Anterior Cruciate Ligament Reconstruction

- The ACL reconstruction is performed with the knee in ~90-115 degrees of flexion using a transtibial femoral tunnel surgical technique.

ACL Tibial Tunnel

- The arm of the drill guide enters the knee joint through the inferomedial patellar portal.
- The bullet of the drill guide contacts the anteromedial proximal tibia externally ~1 cm proximal to the tibial tubercle midway between the posteromedial border of the tibia and the tibial crest anteriorly.
- The guidewire is drilled through the guide to emerge through the center of the stump of the ACL tibial footprint.
- A standard cannulated reamer is used to create the tibial tunnel.

ACL Femoral Tunnel

- With the knee in ~90-110 degrees of flexion, an over-the-top femoral aimer is introduced through the tibial tunnel and used to position a guidewire on the medial wall of the lateral femoral condyle approximating the anatomic insertion site of the ACL (Fig. 49-16).
- ACL graft fixation is achieved on the femoral side with a resorbable interference screw and backup fixation with a polyethylene ligament fixation button.

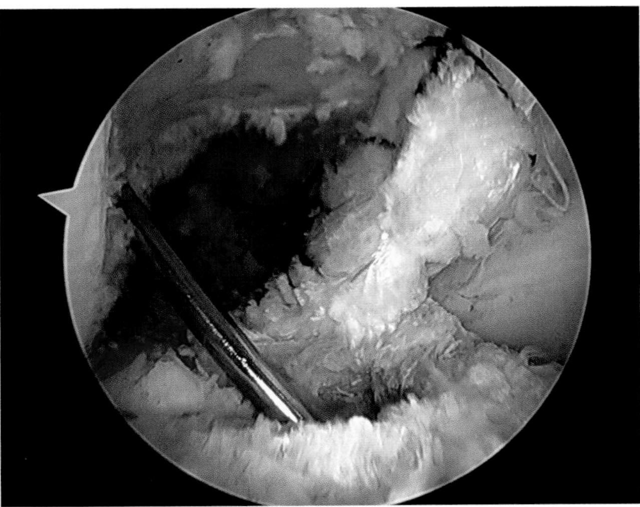

Figure 49-16 | With the knee in ~90-110 degrees of flexion, an over-the-top femoral aimer is introduced through the tibial tunnel and used to position a guidewire on the medial wall of the lateral femoral condyle approximating the anatomic insertion site of the ACL.

ACL Graft Tensioning and Tibial Fixation

- The ACL graft is tensioned on the tibial side using the Biomet graft-tensioning boot.
- Tension is gradually applied to the ACL graft sutures until the Lachman and pivot shift tests are normal.
- The knee is cycled through a full range of motion multiple times to allow pretensioning and settling of the graft.
- The process is repeated until there is no change in the torque setting on the graft tensioner.
- The knee is placed in 30 degrees of flexion, and fixation is achieved on the tibial side of the ACL graft with a resorbable interference screw for aperture opening interference fixation and cortical suspensory backup fixation with a polyethylene ligament fixation button (Fig. 49-17).

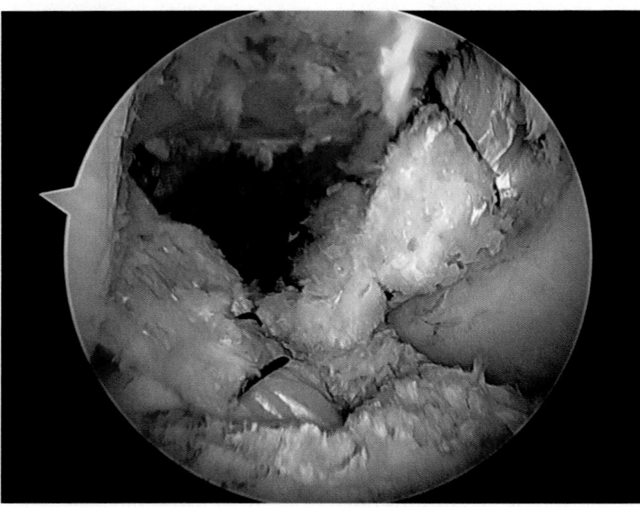

Figure 49-17 | The knee is placed in 30 degrees of flexion, and fixation is achieved on the tibial side of the ACL graft with a resorbable interference screw for aperture opening interference fixation and cortical suspensory backup fixation with a polyethylene ligament fixation button.

Medial and Posteromedial Reconstruction

- The surgical leg is positioned on the fully extended operating room table in a supported flexed-knee position.
- Posteromedial and medial reconstructions are performed through a medial curved incision.
- Primary repair of all acute medial-side injured structures is done with suture anchors, screws and washers, and permanent sutures through drill holes as indicated.
- The primary repair is then augmented with an allograft tissue reconstruction.

Posteromedial Capsular Shift

- Posteromedial capsular shift is performed in chronic cases.
- The sartorius fascia is incised and retracted, exposing the superficial medial collateral ligament (sMCL) and the posteromedial capsule.
- Nerves and blood vessels are protected throughout the procedure.
- A longitudinal incision is made just posterior to the posterior border of the sMCL.
- Care is taken not to damage the medial meniscus during the capsular incision.
- Avulsed capsular structures are primarily repaired with suture anchors and permanent no. 2 sutures.
- The interval between the posteromedial capsule and medial meniscus is developed.
- The posteromedial capsule is shifted in an anterior and superior direction.
- The medial meniscus is repaired to the new capsular position.
- The shifted capsule is sewn into the deep and sMCL with three no. 2 permanent braided Ethibond sutures (Ethicon, Somerville, NJ) in horizontal mattress fashion.
- That suture line is reinforced with a running no. 2 ethibond suture (Fig. 49-18).

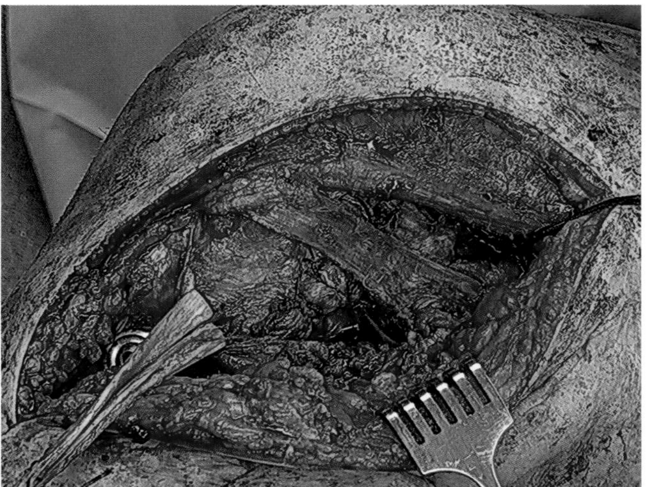

Figure 49-18 | Suture line is reinforced with a running no. 2 ethibond suture.

Superficial Medial Collateral Ligament Reconstruction

- Superficial medial collateral ligament (sMCL) reconstruction is performed using allograft tissue after completion of the primary capsular repair and posteromedial capsular shift procedures.
- The semitendinosus allograft is attached at the anatomic insertion sites of the sMCL on the tibia with a screw and spiked ligament washer or suture anchors (Fig. 49-19).
- Final graft tensioning and graft fixation position is ~40-45 degrees of knee flexion.
- The tibial insertion site is secured first.
- Final tensioning and fixation of the allograft tissue is performed on the femoral side.
- Femoral side fixation is accomplished with a screw and spiked ligament washer or by looping the allograft tissue around the adductor magnus tendon and sewing the graft back on itself with permanent braided no. 2 Ethibond suture (Fig. 49-20).

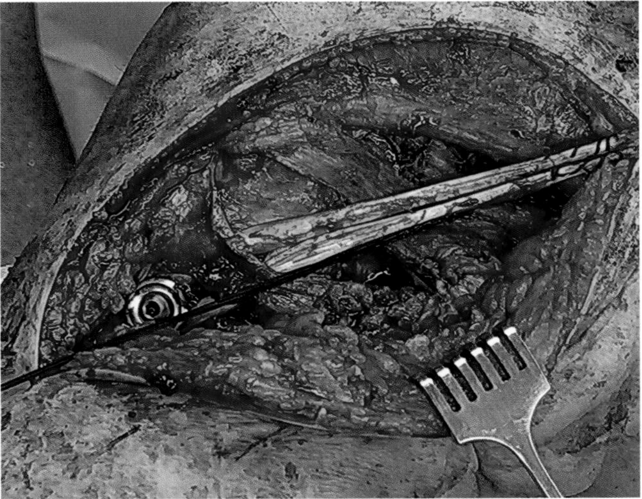

Figure 49-19 | The semitendinosus allograft is attached at the anatomic insertion sites of the superficial medial collateral ligament on the tibia with a screw and spiked ligament washer or suture anchors.

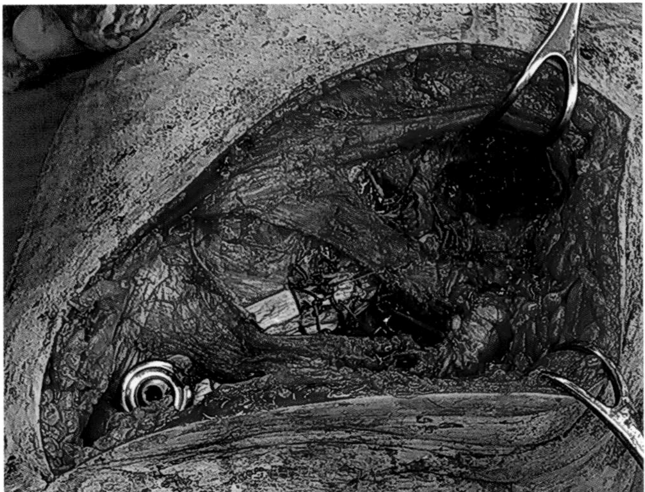

Figure 49-20 | Femoral side fixation is accomplished with a screw and spiked ligament washer or by looping the allograft tissue around the adductor magnus tendon and sewing the graft back on itself with permanent braided no. 2 Ethibond suture.

- No. 2 ethibond suture is used to sew the tails of the graft together proximal to the washer to prevent slipping and also to sew the allograft to the deep capsular layers for additional reinforcement (Fig. 49-21).

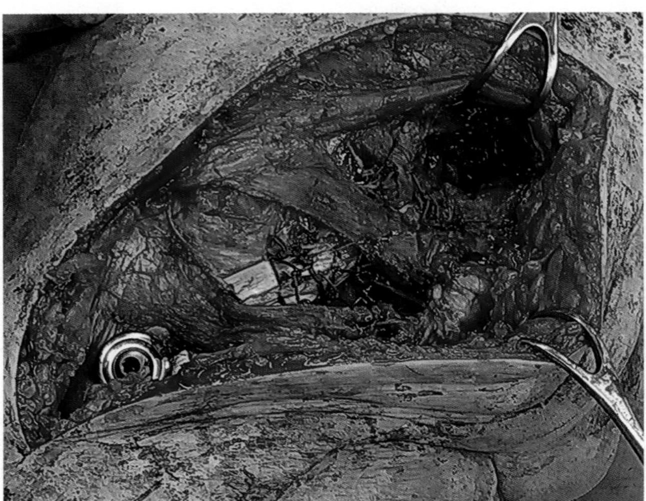

Figure 49-21 | No. 2 Ethibond suture is used to sew the tails of the graft together proximal to the washer to prevent slipping and also to sew the allograft to the deep capsular layers for additional reinforcement.

Postoperative Rehabilitation

- The knee is maintained in full extension for 3-5 weeks non–weight bearing.
- Progressive range of motion occurs during postoperative week 3-5 through 10.
- Progressive weight bearing occurs at the beginning of postoperative weeks 3 through 5.
- Progressive closed kinetic chain strength training, proprioceptive training, and continued motion exercises are initiated very slowly beginning at postoperative week 12.
- The long leg range of motion brace is discontinued after the 8th to 10th week.
- Return to sports and heavy labor occurs after the 9th to 12th postoperative month when sufficient strength, range of motion, and proprioceptive skills have returned.
- It is very important to carefully observe these complex knee ligament injury patients and get a feel for the "personality of the knee."
- The surgeon may need to make adjustments and individualize the postoperative rehabilitation program as necessary.
- Careful and gentle range of motion under general anesthesia is a very useful tool in the treatment of these complex cases and is used as necessary.

Suggested Readings

Fanelli GC. *Rationale and Surgical Technique for PCL and Multiple Knee Ligament Reconstruction*. 3rd ed. Warsaw, Indiana: Biomet Sports Medicine; 2012.

Fanelli GC, ed. *The Multiple Ligament Injured Knee. A Practical Guide to Management*. New York: Springer-Verlag; 2013.

Fanelli GC, ed. *Posterior Cruciate Ligament Injuries: A Practical Guide to Management*. 2nd ed. New York: Springer; 2015.

Fanelli GC, Stannard JP, Stuart MJ, et al. Management of complex knee ligament injuries. *J Bone Joint Surg Am*. 2010;92:2235-2246.

Chapter 50
Knee Dislocation—ACL/PCL/PLC

JARRET M. WOODMASS
BRUCE A. LEVY
MICHAEL J. STUART

Chronic ACL/PCL/PLC Injuries

- A thorough physical examination is performed to assess knee range of motion, ligament laxity, limb alignment, gait, and neurovascular status.[1–3]
- Anteroposterior, lateral, patellar, and full-length standing (hip-knee-ankle) radiographs along with magnetic resonance imaging are essential to confirm the clinical examination findings and rule out concomitant pathology (eg, malalignment, meniscus, articular cartilage, subchondral bone injuries).
- Multiple reconstruction techniques exist for posterolateral corner injuries (PLC).[4]
- Author's approach:[5]
  - All-inside anterior cruciate ligament (ACL) and posterior cruciate ligament (PCL) allograft reconstructions with suspensory fixation.
  - PLC reconstruction using an anatomic single graft technique.[6]
    - Note: Stress radiographs showing asymmetric varus instability of 10 mm (at 30 degrees of knee flexion) represent disruption of the lateral collateral ligament (LCL), popliteofibular ligament, popliteus tendon, and lateral capsular avulsion.[7] In this circumstance, a dual graft reconstruction is performed as described by Laprade (not shown here).[8]

Sterile Instruments/Equipment

- Standard arthroscopy setup
- Spider limb positioner (Tenat Medical, Smith & Nephew, Calgary, AB)
- Allograft tissue: 3 or 4 tendons
- RetroConstruction Drill Guide Set (Arthrex, Naples, FL)
- FiberTape (Arthrex, Naples, FL)
- TightRope (Arthrex, Naples, FL)
- TightRope Attachable Button System (ABS) (Arthrex, Naples, FL)
- BioComposite screws (Arthrex, Naples, FL)
- Passport cannula (Arthrex, Naples, FL)
- Vessel loop

Patient Preparation/Positioning

- The patient is positioned supine with a tourniquet applied to the upper thigh.
- Both knees are examined under anesthesia to confirm the instability pattern.
- Fluoroscopic imaging is used to measure the amount of medial and lateral joint space opening (grade of instability) compared to the contralateral knee.
- The operative leg is stabilized in a Spider knee positioner.
  - This allows stable knee positioning at various flexion angles and decreases reliance on assistants.

Graft Selection/Preparation

- All-inside ACL—quadrupled semitendinosus allograft (Fig. 50-1)
  - Length: >260 mm total (65-70 mm quadrupled graft); width: 8-10 mm
  - FiberTape passed through femoral button and incorporated into (but not sutured to) the graft (internal brace)
  - Femoral fixation—TightRope; tibial fixation—TightRope ABS; 5.5-mm SwiveLock anchors (1—GraftLink supplementary fixation; 2—internal brace)

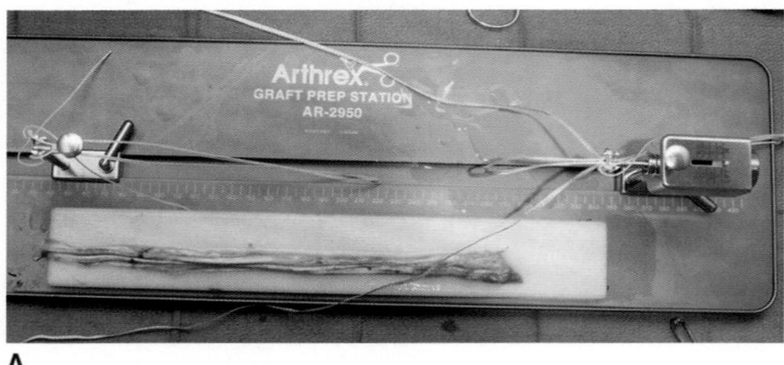

A

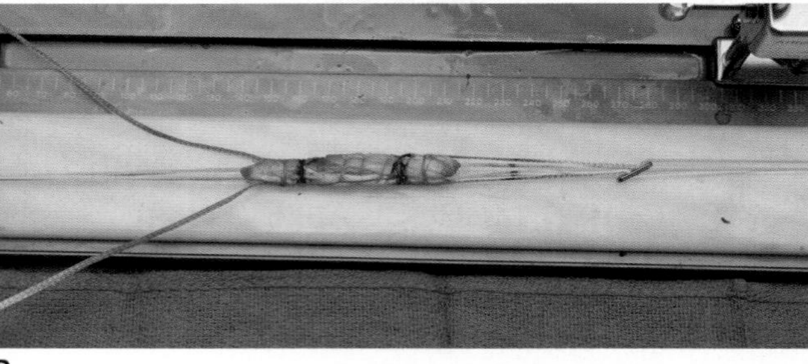

B

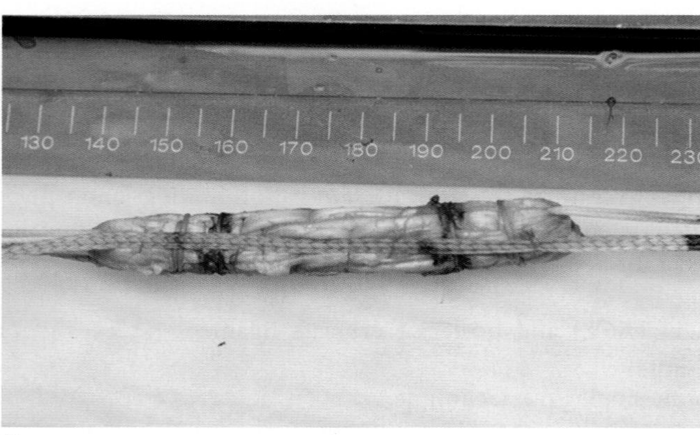

C

Figure 50-1 | All-inside ACL graft preparation using semitendinosus allograft and an internal brace. **A.** Semitendinosus allograft tendon. **B.** Quadrupled semitendinosus allograft with TightRope ABS tibial fixation and TightRope femoral fixation. **C.** Final construct demonstrating the internal brace (FiberTape) being loosely apposed to the allograft with Monocryl suture allowing independent tensioning.

- All-inside PCL—quadrupled anterior tibial tendon allograft
  - Length: >320 mm total (80-90 mm quadrupled graft); width: 10-12 mm
  - FiberTape passed through femoral button and incorporated into (but not sutured to) the graft (internal brace)
  - Femoral fixation—TightRope; tibial fixation—TightRope ABS, 5.5-mm SwiveLock anchors (1—GraftLink supplementary fixation; 2—internal brace)
- PLC reconstruction: anatomic single-graft transfibular reconstruction
  - Achilles tendon allograft (minimum of 20 cm length) with bone block
    - Bone block is contoured to press fit into a 9- × 25-mm femoral socket

All-inside ACL Reconstruction Socket Preparation

- A superomedial outflow portal, both standard and low inferomedial portals, and an inferolateral working portal are established.
- Femoral tunnel creation
  - The knee is flexed 100-120 degrees to prevent injury to the peroneal nerve.
  - A spade-tipped pin is advanced through femoral footprint.
  - The transosseous distance is measured.
  - A low-profile reamer (equal to graft diameter) is advanced 20 mm (Fig. 50-2A).
  - The spade tip is pulled through, leaving a passing suture.
- Tibial tunnel creation
  - A transtibial drill guide directs a 3.5-mm drill into the center of the ACL footprint (Fig. 50-2B).
  - The drill is replaced by a FlipCutter (Arthrex, Naples, FL) reamer (equal to graft diameter).
    - A tibial socket is retroreamed to a depth of 30 mm.

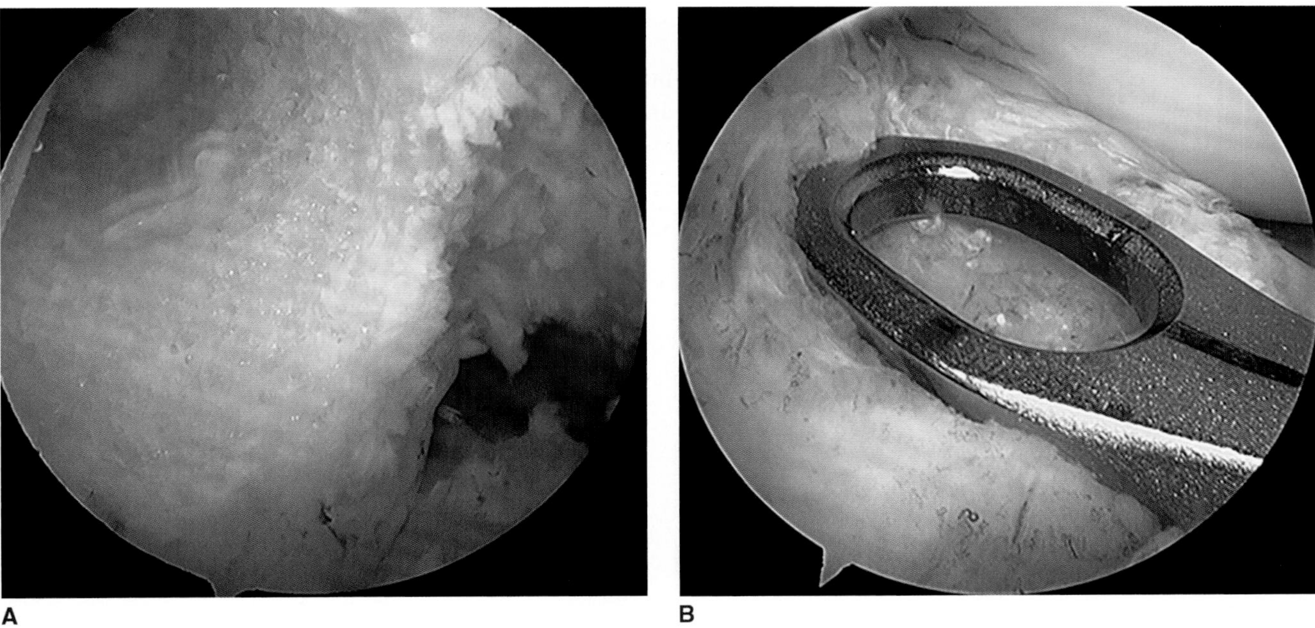

Figure 50-2 | ACL tunnel preparation. **A.** ACL femoral socket post reaming. **B.** The transtibial guide resting over the anatomic tibial footprint.

All-inside PCL Reconstruction Socket Preparation[9,10]

- A posteromedial portal is established under arthroscopic vision (Fig. 50-3).
- The PCL footprint, mammillary bodies, and the posterior horns of the menisci are identified.
  - The shaver and radiofrequency probe inserted through the posteromedial portal are used to expose the PCL facet while viewing with a 70-degree scope through the inferomedial portal.
  - Soft tissue is released until both the medial and lateral mammillary bodies and the popliteus muscle belly are exposed (Fig. 50-4A).
- Tibial tunnel creation[10]

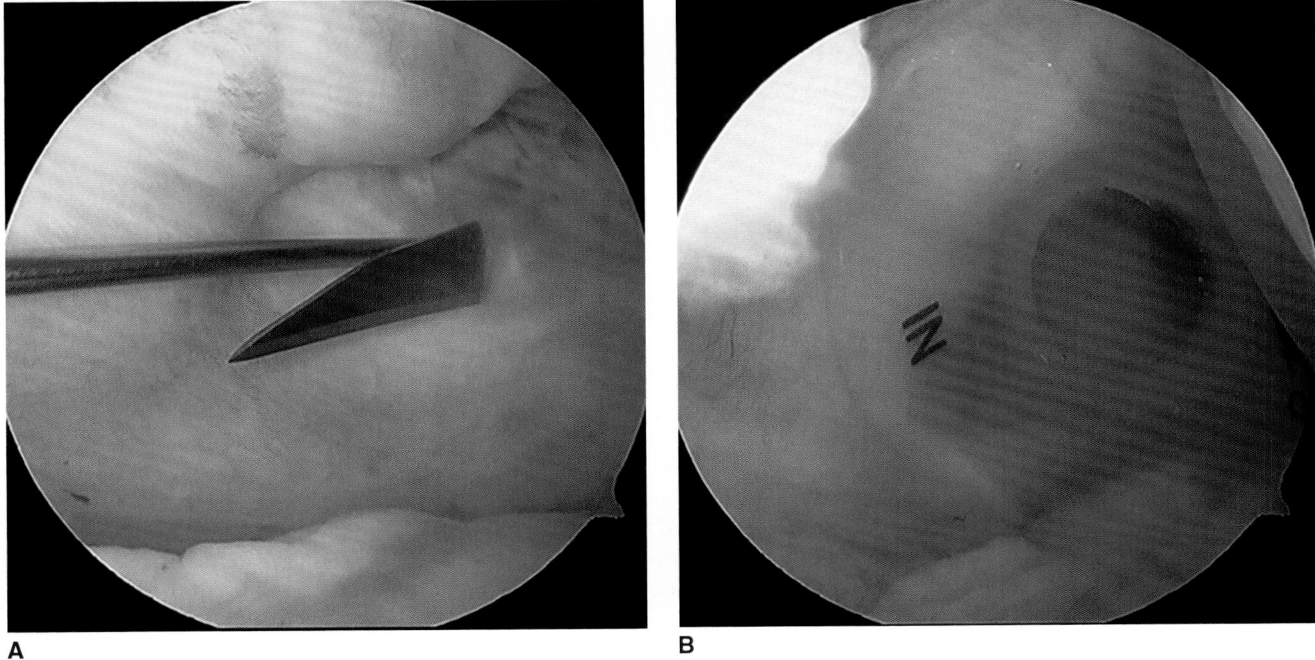

Figure 50-3 | Establishing a posteromedial portal. **A.** While viewing from the anterolateral portal, a "needle-and-knife" technique is used to incise the capsule. **B.** A flexible cannula has been inserted to allow easy passage of instruments during tibial preparation.

- A precontoured transtibial guide is inserted through the inferomedial portal while viewing from the posteromedial portal.
- A FlipCutter reamer is advanced into the joint (Fig. 50-4B). Anatomic positioning is confirmed with AP and lateral fluoroscopy,[11] and a 40-mm socket is created (Fig. 50-4C).
- A FiberStick (Arthrex, Naples, FL) is used to insert a passing suture.

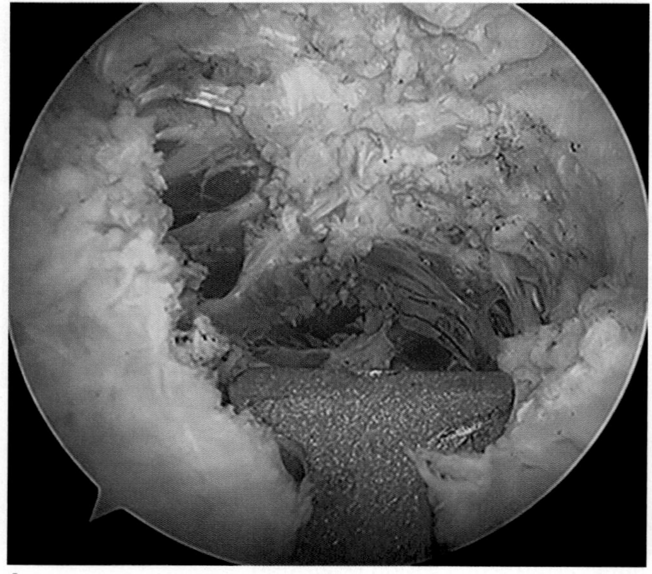

A

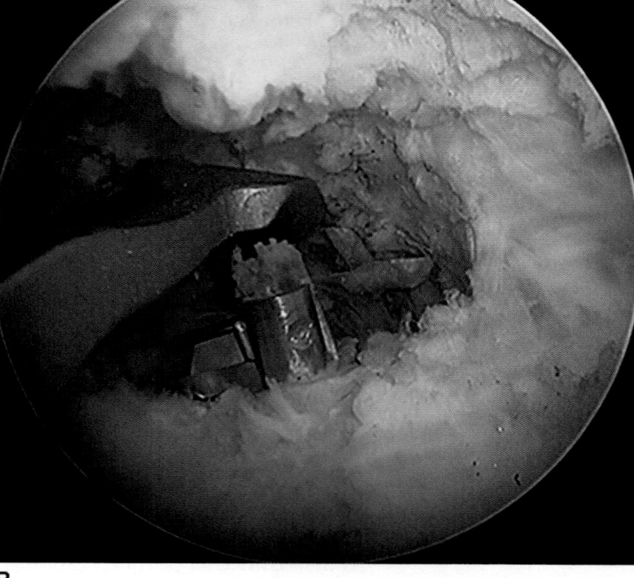

B

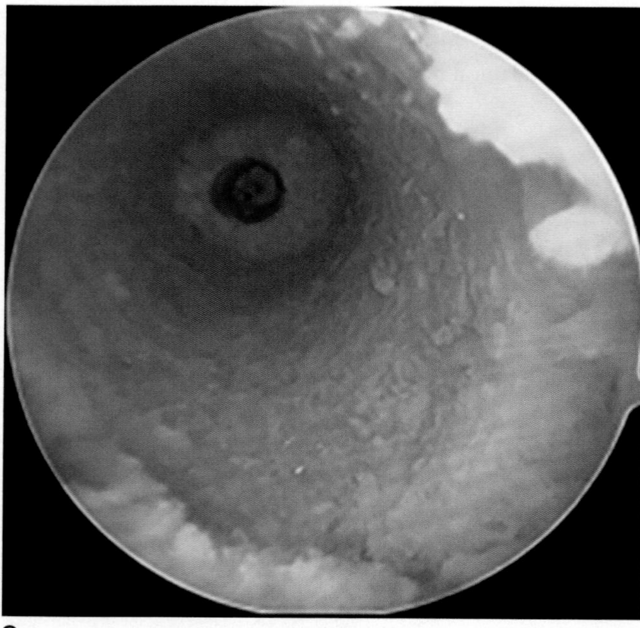

C

Figure 50-4 | Tibial tunnel creation. **A.** Transtibial guide resting over the anatomic PCL footprint showing posterior dissection to the popliteus muscle belly. **B.** FlipCutter reamer deployed in the knee prior to retroreaming the socket to a 40 mm depth. **C.** View of the PCL tibial socket from the posteromedial portal using a 70-degree arthroscope.

- Femoral tunnel creation
  - A low, accessory inferolateral portal is established.
  - A spade-tipped pin is advanced through the center of the PCL anterolateral bundle footprint (Fig. 50-5) adjacent to the articular cartilage of the medial femoral condyle, and the transosseous length is measured. Positioning is confirmed with fluoroscopy.[11]
  - A low-profile reamer is drilled to a depth of 25 mm (equal to graft diameter).
  - The spade-tipped pin is removed, and a passing suture is left in place.

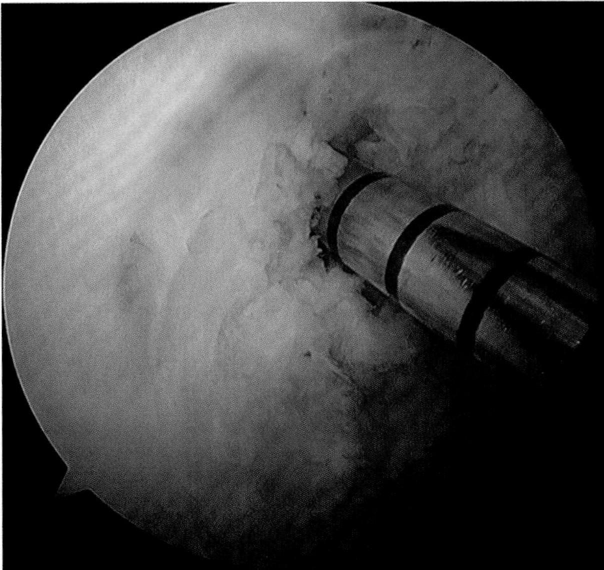

Figure 50-5 | View from the anteromedial portal showing guide pin placement into the center of the anterolateral bundle fibers. (Reprinted from King AH, Prince MR, Reardon PJ, Levy BA, Stuart MJ. All-Inside Posterior Cruciate Ligament Reconstruction. *Oper Tech Sports Med*. 2015;23:302-306, Copyright 2015, with permission from Elsevier.)

ACL/PCL Graft Passage and Tensioning

- The PCL is passed intra-articular (but not tensioned).
  - The tibial side is passed first and pulled to the base of the socket to facilitate easier femoral passage.
  - The FiberTape and a suture grasper are used to create back tension as the femoral TightRope is passed and the button is flipped on the femoral cortex.
  - The TightRope is used to advance the graft into the femoral tunnel.
  - An ABS button is applied on the tibial end.
- The ACL is then passed intra-articular (but not tensioned).
  - The femoral TightRope is passed, and the button is flipped on the femoral cortex.
  - The tibial end is then pulled into the tibial socket, and an ABS button is applied.
- The knee is cycled several times.
  - The PCL is provisionally tensioned with the knee in full extension and then at 90 degrees of flexion to create the normal tibial step-off; backup fixation with a 5.5-mm SwiveLock anchor can be used. A 5.5-mm SwiveLock is used to secure the FiberTape once the PCL tensioning is complete.
  - The ACL is tensioned with the knee in full extension. Backup fixation with a 5.5-mm SwiveLock anchor can be used. A 5.5-mm SwiveLock is used to secure the FiberTape once the ACL tensioning is complete.
  - Final reconstruction is viewed through the anteromedial portal (Fig. 50-6).

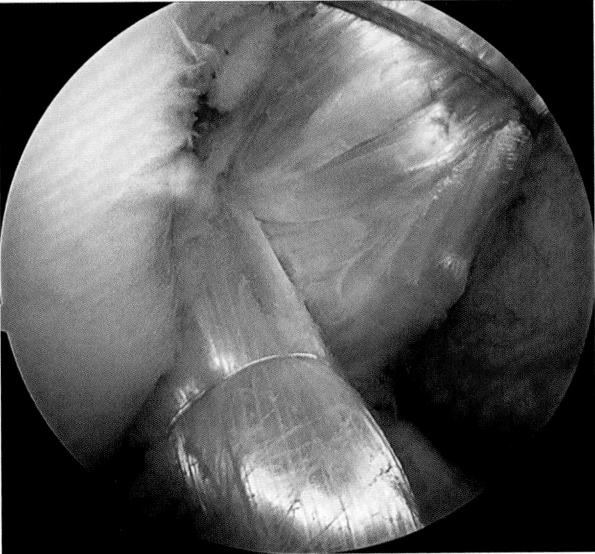

Figure 50-6 | View from the anteromedial portal of the final all-inside ACL and PCL reconstruction.

Posterolateral Corner Reconstruction

- Exposure
  - The thigh tourniquet is inflated.
  - A curvilinear lateral incision is centered over the lateral epicondyle and the anterior border of the fibula.
    - Full-thickness skin flaps are created to expose the biceps femoris and iliotibial band.
  - The common peroneal nerve is carefully identified and protected for the remainder of the procedure.
  - The fibular head is exposed anteriorly and posteriorly.
    - Posterior dissection should allow palpation of the posteromedial tubercle (exit point for the transfibular tunnel) and posterolateral tibia.
    - Anterior dissection exposes the insertion of the LCL on the anterolateral fibula (28.4 mm from the fibular styloid).
  - The iliotibial band is split longitudinally to the level of Gerdy tubercle.
  - A capsulotomy is performed proximal to the joint line.
    - Care is taken not to damage the meniscus or its capsular attachments.

Posterolateral Corner Reconstruction (Fig. 50-7)[6]

- Step 1: Popliteus tendon socket creation and graft fixation
  - The anatomic insertion is identified at the anterior one-fifth of the popliteal sulcus.
  - A guide pin is advanced in a slightly anterior and proximal direction avoiding the femoral notch and ACL socket.

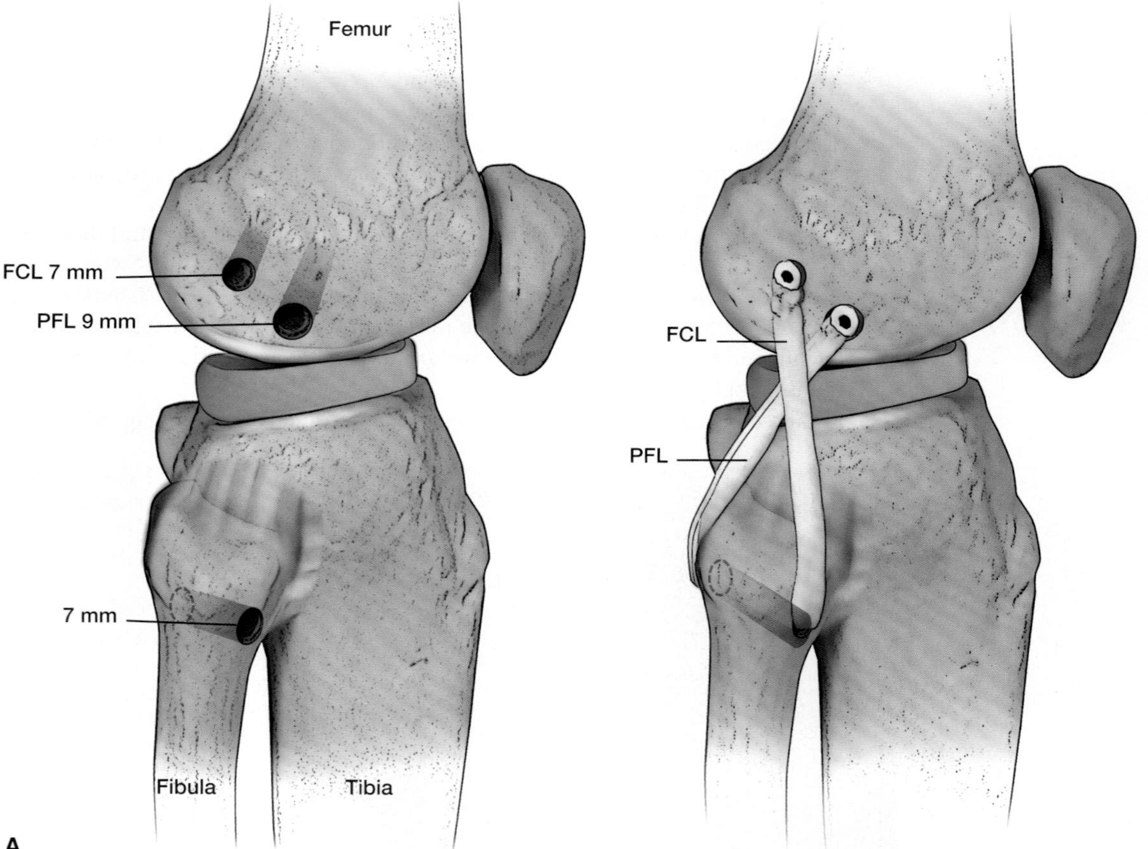

Figure 50-7 | Posterolateral corner reconstruction is performed using a single Achilles tendon allograft. Tunnels are made at the popliteal sulcus, the LCL anatomic origin and through the fibula **(A)**. The Achilles bone block is fixed in the popliteal sulcus with an interference screw. The graft is then tensioned through the fibular head tunnel and secured with a bioabsorbable interference screw. Finally, the graft is tensioned and fixed in the femoral socket at the LCL anatomic origin with both a cortical suspensory fixation device and a bioabsorbable interference screw **(B)**. FCL, fibular collateral ligament; PFL, popliteofibular ligament.

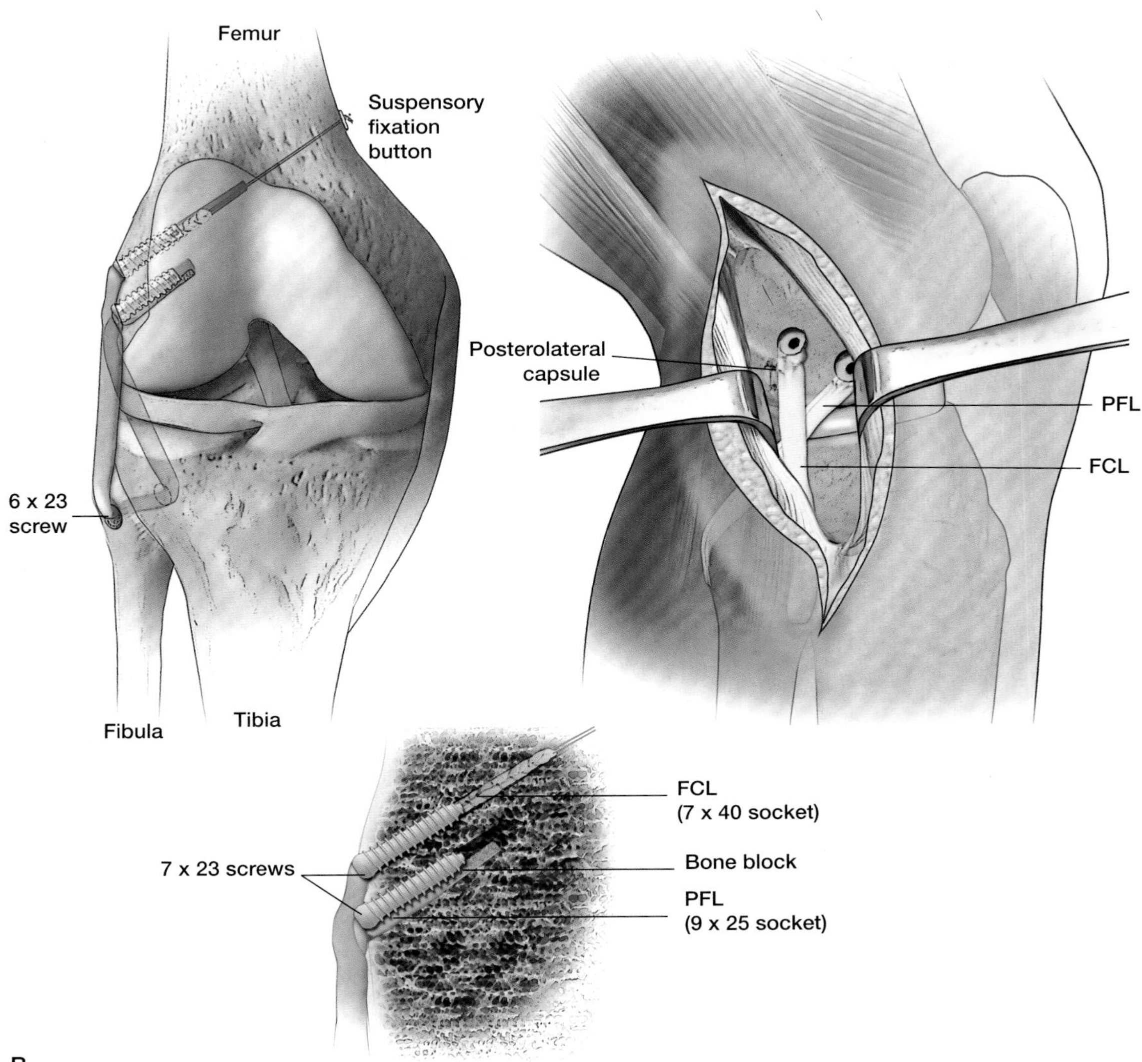

Figure 50-7 | (*Continued*)

- A 9-mm cannulated reamer is used to create a 25-mm deep socket.
- The Achilles allograft bone block is inserted into the socket and secured with a 7- × 23-mm bioabsorbable screw.

- Step 2: Fibular tunnel creation and graft passage
  - A guide pin is passed from the insertion site of the LCL (palpable tubercle on the proximal anterolateral fibula) in a proximal and medial direction, exiting at the posteromedial tubercle.
  - Accurate position is confirmed with fluoroscopic imaging (anterior wire insertion should be 28.4 mm distal to the styloid immediately before the "champagne glass" drop-off).
  - The graft is passed from posterior to anterior through the fibular tunnel.
- Step 3: LCL femoral socket creation
  - A guide pin is placed parallel to the popliteus tunnel at the anatomic origin of the LCL (3.1 mm posterior and 1.4 mm proximal to the lateral epicondyle; 18.5 mm from the center of the popliteus insertion).[12]
  - The Achilles allograft is wrapped around the pin, marked with a pen with the knee in full extension, and the knee is moved through a range of motion to confirm isometry (Fig. 50-8).
  - After isometry has been confirmed, a 7-mm reamer is used to create a 40-mm-deep socket.

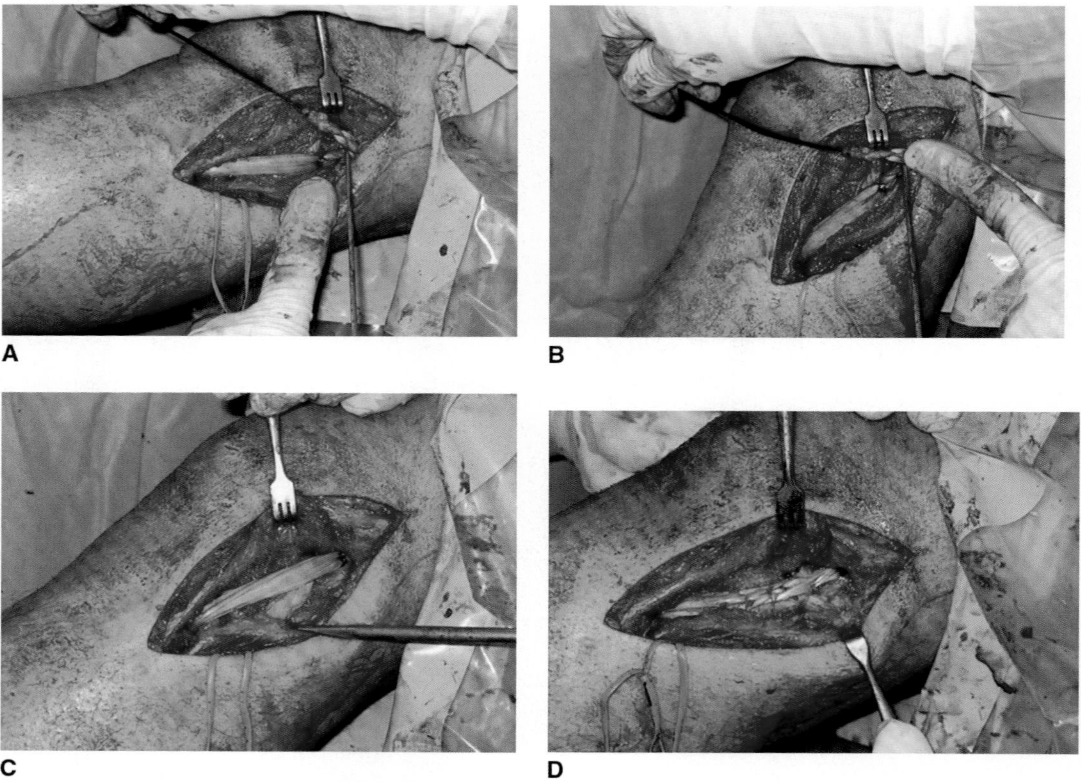

Figure 50-8 | **A.** Graft isometry evaluated in extension. **B.** Graft isometry evaluated in flexion. **C.** Graft construct. **D.** Imbrication of posterolateral capsule to graft construct. (Reprinted from Levy B, Stuart M, Whelan D. Posterolateral Instability of the Knee: Evaluation, Treatment, Results. *Sports Med Arthrosc Rev.* 2010;18:254-262, with permission.)

- Step 4: Final fixation
  - The soft tissue end of the Achilles allograft is trimmed to allow 25-30 mm of graft within the socket. A TightRope is secured to the end of the graft with a looped, locking whipstitch suture.
  - The guide pin is replaced by a spade-tip pin to allow measurement of the transosseous distance.
  - The graft is tensioned at 45-60 degrees of knee flexion with neutral rotation and fixed in the fibular tunnel with a 6- × 23-mm BioComposite screw.
  - The TightRope is passed through the femur, and the button is flipped on the medial femoral cortex. The graft is pulled into the femoral socket and tensioned at 30 degrees of knee flexion with valgus load and neutral rotation.
  - A 7- × 23-mm bioabsorbable screw is inserted into the LCL femoral socket to secure the graft.
- Step 5: Soft tissue repair and capsular plication (Fig. 50-9)

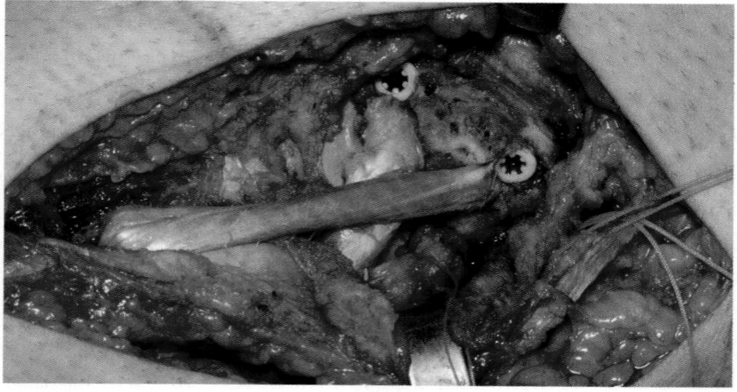

Figure 50-9 | Soft-tissue repair and capsular plication.

  - The native popliteus is tensioned and sutured to the allograft reconstruction (no. 1 ethibond).
  - Three FASTak suture anchors (Arthrex, Naples, FL) are placed on the articular margin of the femur.
  - The anchor sutures are passed through the capsule and tied with the knee in full extension.

References

1. Levy BA, Boyd JL, Stuart MJ. Surgical treatment of acute and chronic anterior and posterior cruciate ligament and lateral side injuries of the knee. *Sports Med Arthrosc Rev.* 2011;19(2):110-119.
2. Levy BA, Stuart MJ, Whelan DB. Posterolateral instability of the knee: evaluation, treatment, results. *Sports Med Arthrosc Rev.* 2010;18(4):254-262.
3. Levy BA, Fanelli GC, Whelan DB, et al. Controversies in the treatment of knee dislocations and multiligament reconstruction. *J Am Acad Orthop Surg.* 2009;17(4):197-206.
4. Geeslin AG, Moulton SG, LaPrade RF. A systematic review of the outcomes of posterolateral corner knee injuries, part 1: surgical treatment of acute injuries. *Am J Sports Med.* 2016;44(5):1336-1342.
5. Levy BA, Stuart MJ. Treatment of PCL, ACL, and lateral-side knee injuries: acute and chronic. *J Knee Surg.* 2012;25(4): 295-305.
6. Schechinger SJ, Levy BA, Dajani KA, Shah JP, Herrera DA, Marx RG. Achilles tendon allograft reconstruction of the fibular collateral ligament and posterolateral corner. *Arthroscopy.* 2009;25(3):232-242.
7. Fanelli GC, Orcutt DR, Edson CJ. The multiple-ligament injured knee: evaluation, treatment, and results. *Arthroscopy.* 2005;21(4):471-486.
8. LaPrade RF, Johansen S, Wentorf FA, Engebretsen L, Esterberg JL, Tso A. An analysis of an anatomical posterolateral knee reconstruction: an in vitro biomechanical study and development of a surgical technique. *Am J Sports Med.* 2004;32(6):1405-1414.
9. Prince MR, Stuart MJ, King AH, Sousa PL, Levy BA. All-inside posterior cruciate ligament reconstruction: graftLink technique. *Arthrosc Tech.* 2015;4(5):e619-e624.
10. Levy BA. Pearls: how i create the tibial socket for PCL reconstruction. *Clin Orthop Relat Res.* 2016;474(5):1113-1121.
11. Johannsen AM, Anderson CJ, Wijdicks CA, Engebretsen L, LaPrade RF. Radiographic landmarks for tunnel positioning in posterior cruciate ligament reconstructions. *Am J Sports Med.* 2013;41(1):35-42.
12. LaPrade RF, Ly TV, Wentorf FA, Engebretsen L. The posterolateral attachments of the knee: a qualitative and quantitative morphologic analysis of the fibular collateral ligament, popliteus tendon, popliteofibular ligament, and lateral gastrocnemius tendon. *Am J Sports Med.* 2003;31(6):854-860.

Chapter 51
Acute Repair of Ruptured Patellar Tendon

JUSTIN H. BARTLEY
KRISTINA L. WELTON
ERIC C. McCARTY

Sterile Instruments/Equipment (Fig. 51-1)

- Tourniquet (optional—rarely used by authors)
- Skin retractors
- Scalpel (no. 10 or no. 15 blade)
- Dissection scissors
- Pickups
- Needle driver
- ACL tibial guide (optional)
- 2.5-mm drill
- Hewson suture passer
- Two no. 5 nonabsorbable, braided, high–tensile strength, polyfilament suture
- One to two no. 2 nonabsorbable, braided, polyfilament suture
- One no. 2 absorbable, monofilament suture

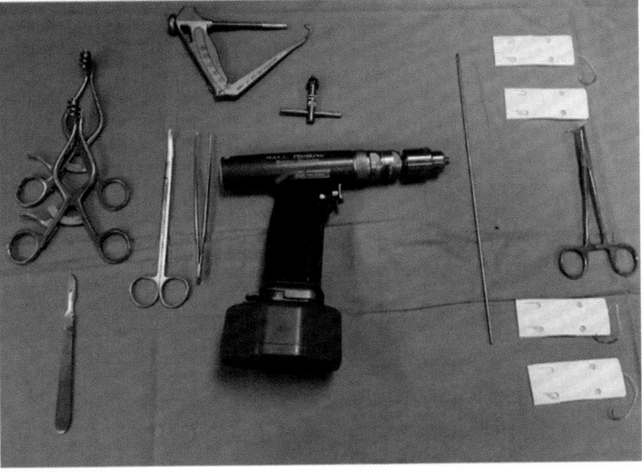

Figure 51-1 | Sterile instruments and equipment.

Positioning (Fig. 51-2)

- The patient is positioned supine on a regular operative bed, small bump beneath the hip such that the knee is point straight upwards, tourniquet in place on operative extremity—but not inflated unless deemed necessary, large sterile bump beneath the operative knee to allow ~30 degrees of flexion during the surgery.

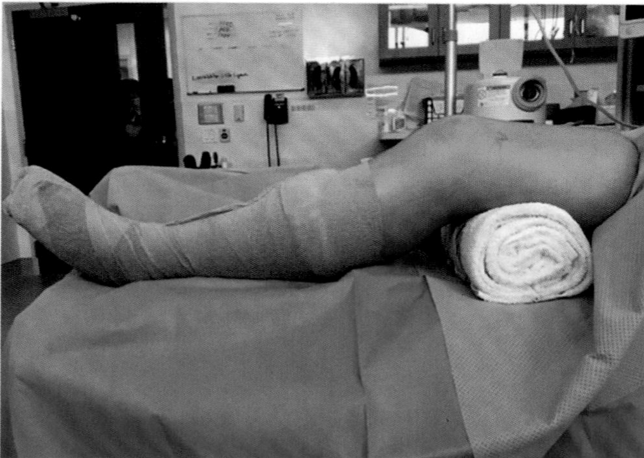

Figure 51-2 | Supine positioning of patient with extremity draping and sterile bump beneath knee.

Surgical Approach (Fig. 51-3)

- Midline incision is made from two fingerbreadths proximal to the patella, inferiorly to the mid-aspect of the tibial tubercle through subcutaneous fat to fascia.
- Medial and lateral flaps are developed to expose the entire patellar and ruptured patellar tendon and retinaculum.

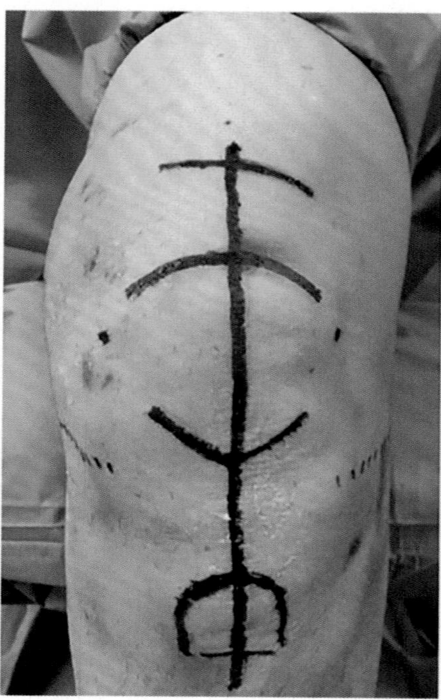

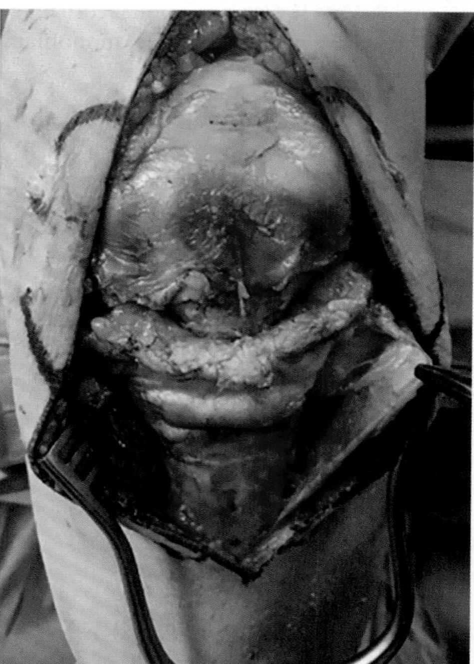

Figure 51-3 | Midline surgical approach demonstrating disrupted patellar tendon, paratenon, and retinaculum.

- Typically the paratenon, medial and lateral patellar retinaculum, and the patellar tendon are completely disrupted.
  - However, if the paratenon can be developed in a separate plane, then this should be performed so that closure can be done in layers at the end of the case.
- Any friable and nonviable tissue is debrided from the edges of the retinaculum and patellar tendon sharply with a fresh blade and/or small rongeur.

Suture Technique

- Two no. 5 nonabsorbable, braided, high–tensile strength, polyfilament sutures are used to perform Krackow locking sutures, running inferiorly down the outsides of tendon, followed by running the suture superiorly up the middle of the tendon, resulting in four sutures exiting the most proximal aspect of the ruptured patellar tendon (Fig. 51-4).

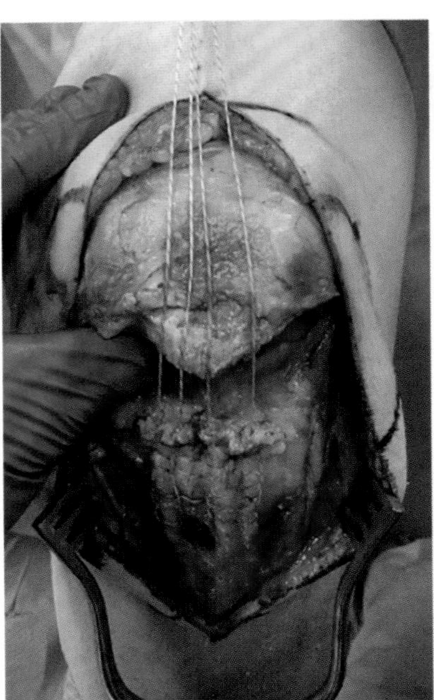
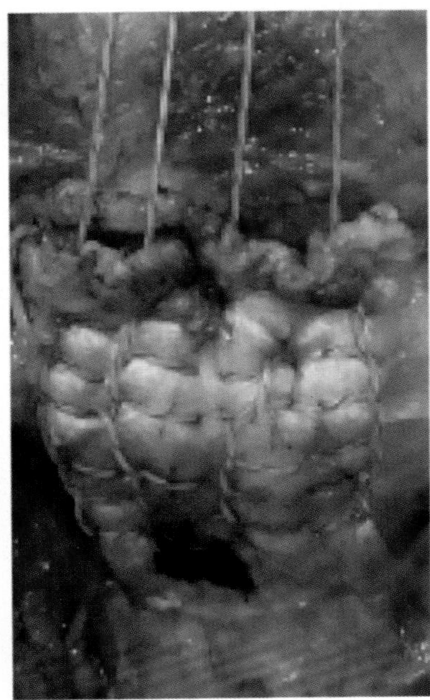
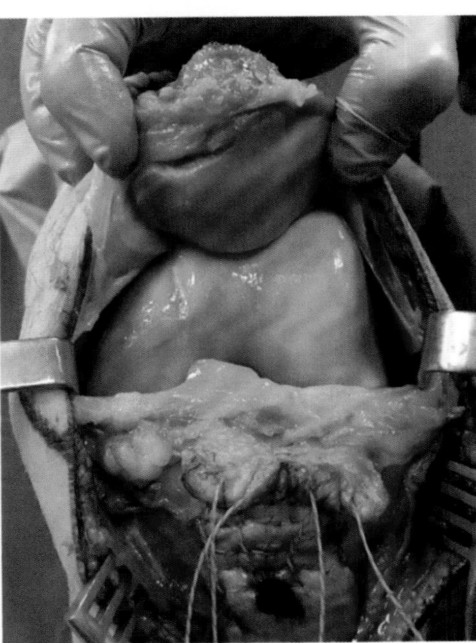

Figure 51-4 | Krackow suture technique in patellar tendon and exposure of articular cartilage.

  - The starting point must be within the proximal substance of the patellar tendon and not within the remaining paratenon and prepatellar bursal tissue as this can result in a consequential lengthening of the patellar tendon.
- The patella is reflected superiorly, utilizing the traumatic interval to allow exposure of articular cartilage to assess for injury and treat appropriately.

Fixation Technique

- The distal patella is prepared by using a rongeur and/or small curette to develop a healthy bed of bleeding subchondral bone, taking care to not disrupt the articular cartilage surface of the patella.
- With or without the aid of the tibial ACL guide, three 2.5-mm longitudinal tunnels are drilled at the medial third, middle, and lateral third of the patella from inferior to superior at the mid-axial thickness of the patella, avoiding the patellar cartilage.
- Once the drill has penetrated the first cortex, the surgeon's hand is dropped to expose the proximal pole of the patella and an Army-Navy or other retractor is used to place the quadriceps muscle under tension, allowing the drill to exit superiorly.
- A small incision with a no. 15 blade in the quadriceps tendon can be made to help expose the drill tip after it has penetrated the second cortex for each of the three passes (Fig. 51-5).

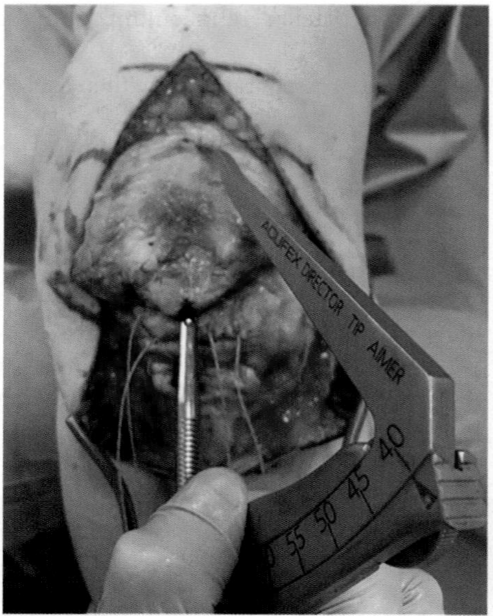

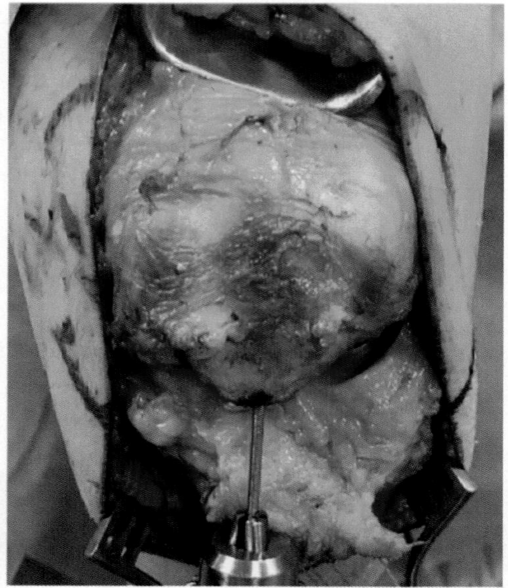

Figure 51-5 | Drilling 3 longitudinal tunnels from inferior pole to superior pole with or without aid of an ACL guide.

- As the drill is withdrawn, it is followed from proximal to distal with the Hewson suture passer to allow shuttling of the suture from distal to proximal.
- The two middle limbs of suture will be shuttled through the middle, longitudinal drill hole, and the lateral and medial limbs of suture will be shuttled out the lateral and medial drill holes, respectively, using an identical technique (Fig. 51-6)

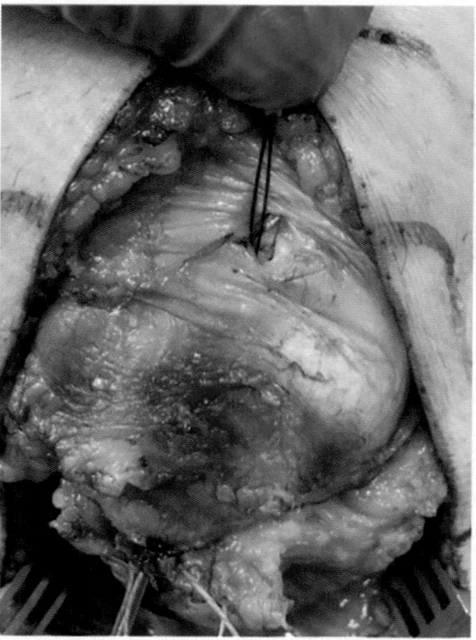

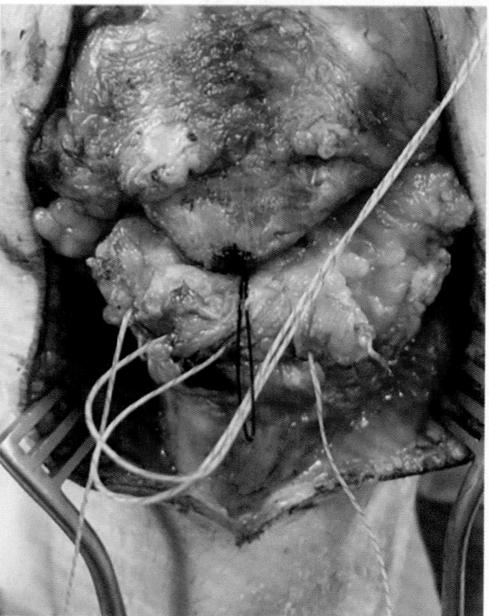

Figure 51-6 | Using Hewson suture passer to shuttle limbs of suture through longitudinal patellar tunnels.

- Once all four limbs of the suture have been shuttled to the superior pole of the patella, we recommend that the middle two limbs of the suture are moved to join the lateral and medial limbs, beneath the quad tendon, using a curved hemostat (Fig. 51-7).

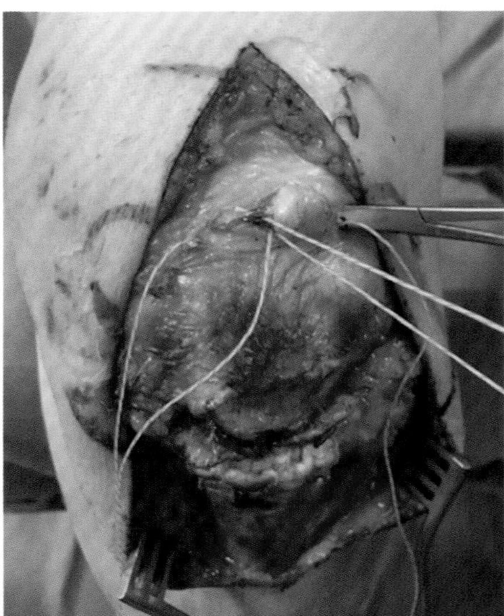
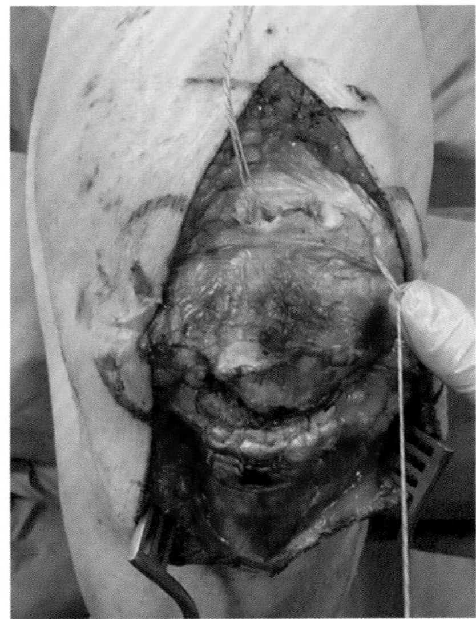
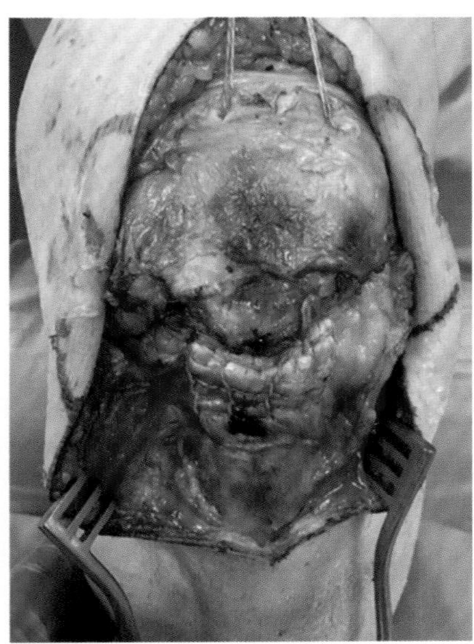

Figure 51-7 | Moving suture limbs beneath quad tendon, tying suture at superior pole, and completed patellar tendon repair.

- The suture can now be tensioned appropriately with the leg in full extension, tied over the patellar bone bridge, without placing tension on the quad insertion at the superior pole of the patella.
- After tying, passively flex the knee to at least 90 degrees to ensure that this does not disrupt the repair and that the patellar tracks appropriately.
- We do not routinely check patellar height after repair, but this can be performed intraoperatively by taking a lateral radiograph with the knee in 30 degrees of flexion and comparing it to the contralateral knee.

Soft Tissue Repair (Fig. 51-8)

- Next, the medial and lateral retinacula are repaired with a no. 2 nonabsorbable, braided, polyfilament suture in an interrupted fashion.
- Routinely, to help protect the repair during healing, a no. 5 nonabsorbable, braided, high-tensile strength, polyfilament suture is used as a cerclage suture; it is placed circumferentially around the proximal pole of the patella and through a transverse 2.5-mm tunnel in the tibial tubercle with the knee in 30 degrees.
- The wound is irrigated and the soft tissues and skin are closed in layers.

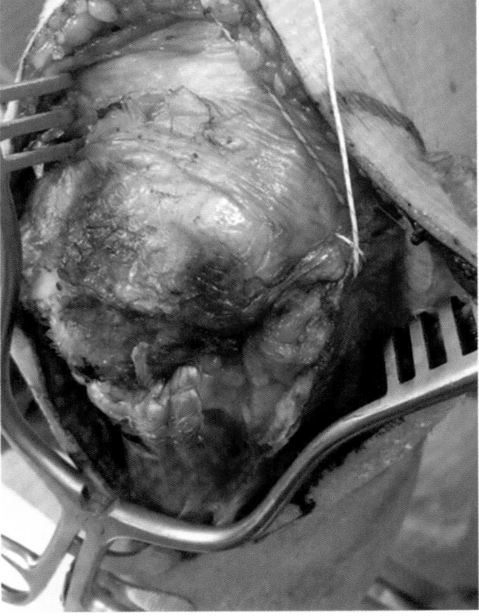
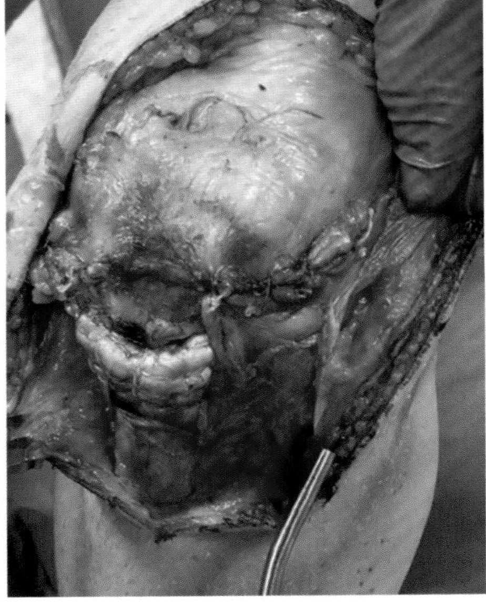

Figure 51-8 | Soft tissue repair.

Postoperative Protocol

- Week 1-2: Partial weight bearing in a hinged knee brace locked in extension for first 2 weeks, initiate quad sets.
- Week 2-3: Initiate straight leg raises.
- Week 3-5: Start range of motion (0-30 degrees) at postoperative week 3 and increase motion by 30 degrees per week; progress to weight bearing as tolerated with knee locked in extension.
- Week 6: Goal of 90 degrees of flexion and walking in hinged knee brace (0-60 degrees) by postoperative week 6.
- Week 6-8: Slowly progress with active range of motion, quad/hamstring/calf strengthening; progress to walking in hinged knee brace with 0-90 degrees of allowable motion by week 8.
- Week 8-14: Progress strengthening as appropriate; discontinue use of hinged knee brace at 10 weeks postoperatively.
- Week 16: Progress to jogging.
- Week 20: Progress to running and agility exercises.
- Month 7-9: Return to sports.

Chapter 52
Quadriceps Tendon Repair

NATALIE L. LEONG
GINA M. MOSICH
DAVID R. McALLISTER

Sterile Instruments/Equipment

- Beath pin
- No. 5 braided polyester suture
- Power wire driver/drill
- Allis clamps ×2
- Senn retractors ×2
- Army-Navy retractors ×2
- Periosteal elevator
- Metzenbaum scissors
- Rongeur

Positioning

- The patient is positioned supine on the operating room table.
- A sterile bump is used to put slight tension on the extensor mechanism. This is especially helpful during the surgical approach.
- A tourniquet is placed on the thigh but not inflated unless necessary.

Surgical Approach

- A direct midline approach to the quadriceps tendon and patella is used, centered over the rupture site, which usually is at its attachment to the proximal pole of the patella.
- The knee is slightly flexed over a sterile bump.
- The skin incision over the quadriceps tendon and patella is 10 cm long.
- The skin and subcutaneous fat are incised sharply down to the level of the extensor mechanism.
- Medial and lateral skin flaps are elevated to expose the quadriceps tendon and the medial and lateral retinacula. Metzenbaum scissors and a periosteal elevator covered with a sponge also are used to mobilize the quadriceps tendon.
- Two Allis clamps are placed on the distal quadriceps tendon and pulled to the level of the superior pole of the patella as the knee is extended.
- A small rongeur is used to debride and roughen the attachment of the quadriceps tendon on the superior patella down to bleeding bone (Fig. 52-1). The distal end of the ruptured quadriceps tendon is sharply debrided of degenerative tendon.

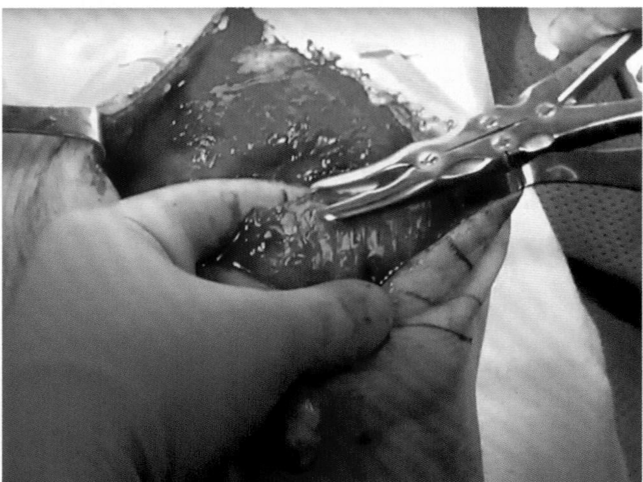

Figure 52-1 | A small rongeur is used to remove soft tissue from the proximal edge of the patella.

Repair of Quadriceps Tendon

- A 4-strand repair using running locked suture technique similar to that described by Krackow et al.[1] is performed with no. 5 braided polyester suture, tensioning the suture with each passage (Fig. 52-2).

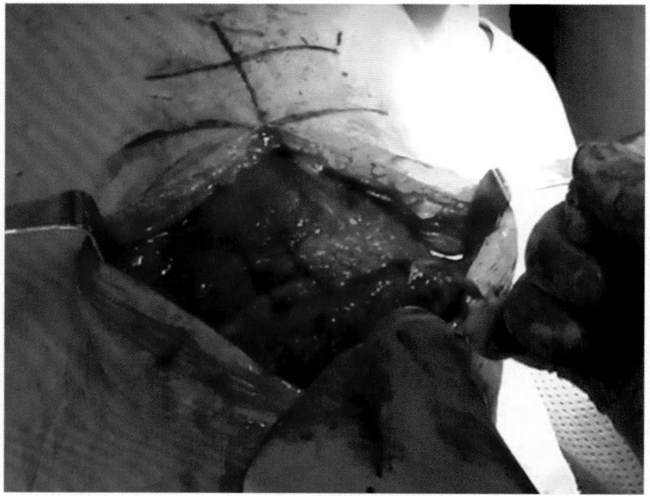

Figure 52-2 | Suture is placed in the quadriceps tendon in a Krackow-like fashion.

- Three parallel osseous tunnels are drilled longitudinally through the patella with a Beath pin; this is a smooth flexible pin with an eyelet (Fig. 52.3) as previously described by Azar and Pickering.[2] The 4 suture strands are passed through these tunnels (1 suture through lateral tunnel, 2 sutures through middle tunnel, and 1 suture through medial tunnel). The sutures enter the superior pole and exit the inferior pole of the patella. It is easiest to pass the pin from proximal to distal with the knee in full extension. A Senn retractor can be used to identify the pin just as it exits the distal patella. The suture(s) are passed through the eyelet, and the pin is manually pulled through the tunnels (Fig. 52-4). The sutures are tied over the inferior pole of the patella with the knee in full extension.
- The knee is gently flexed to 30 degrees to verify that there is no gapping at the repair site.

- Each limb of the graft is placed into the previously drilled tunnels using a SwiveLock interference screw (Arthrex, Naples, FL) (Fig. 53-7).
  - Before the second limb is secured to the patella, the ToggleLoc construct is placed through the graft.

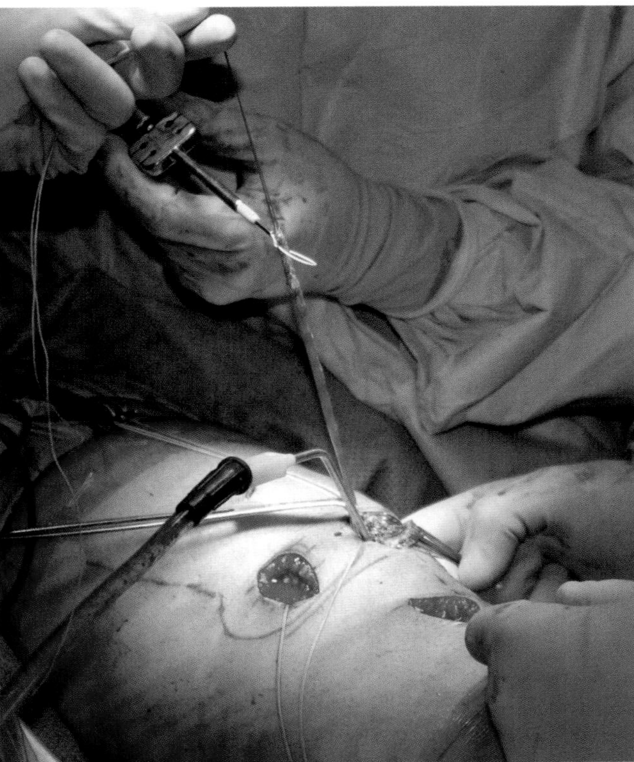

Figure 53-7 | Each limb of the graft is placed into the previously drilled tunnels using a SwiveLock interference screw. (Arthrex, Naples, FL.)

- Each limb is now in its respective tunnel and ready for passage to the femoral insertion site (Fig. 53-8).

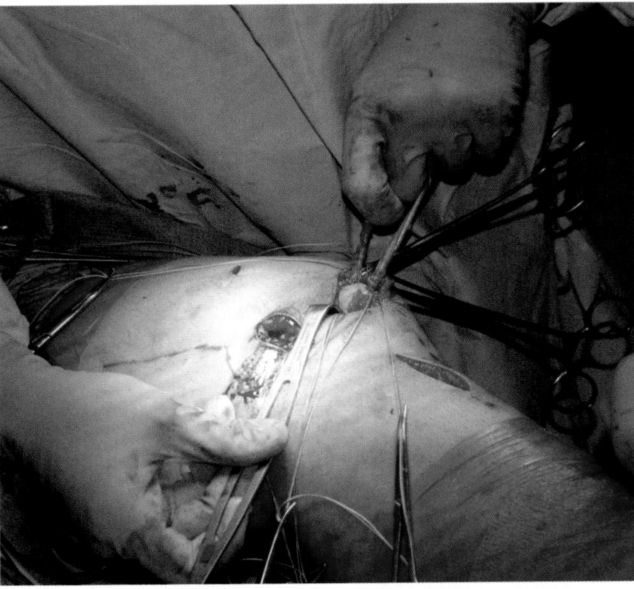

Figure 53-8 | Each limb is now in its respective tunnel and ready for passage to the femoral insertion site.

Femoral Site Preparation

- A 2- to 3-cm longitudinal incision is made over the medial femoral epicondyle.
- A curved hemostat is passed through the appropriate layers of the medial aspect of the knee.
- Once the fascial planes are developed, a passing suture is placed adjacent to the patella and medial femoral condyle in preparation for graft passage (Fig. 53-9).

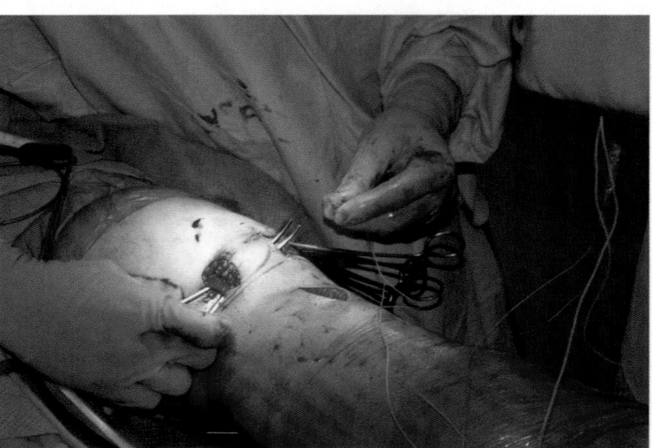

Figure 53-9 | A passing suture is placed in the appropriate layers of the knee in preparation for graft passage.

- The graft is then passed adjacent to the femur while the femoral fixation is prepared.
- An interference screw or button cortical fixation can be used to secure the femoral site.
- For button fixation, the MPFL insertion site on the femur is identified with a guide pin under fluoroscopy.
- The guide pin is drilled from medial to lateral, directed slightly anterior and superior, through the lateral cortex.
- A reamer sized to the doubled graft is drilled over the guide pin to a depth of 30 to 40 mm.
- A 4.5-mm cannulated drill bit is then drilled through the lateral cortex.

Final Graft Fixation

- The graft is passed with the aid of the previously placed passing suture (Fig. 53-10).

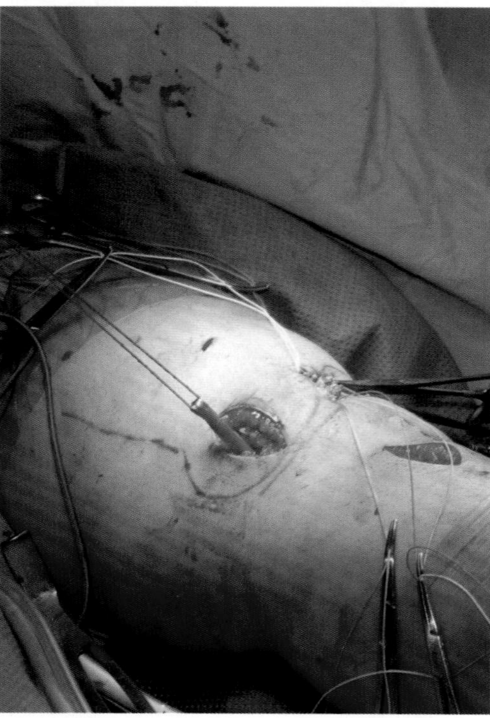

Figure 53-10 | The graft is passed with aid of the previously placed passing suture.

- A Beath pin is placed through the femoral tunnel, and the button is passed through and secured on the lateral cortex (Fig. 53-11).

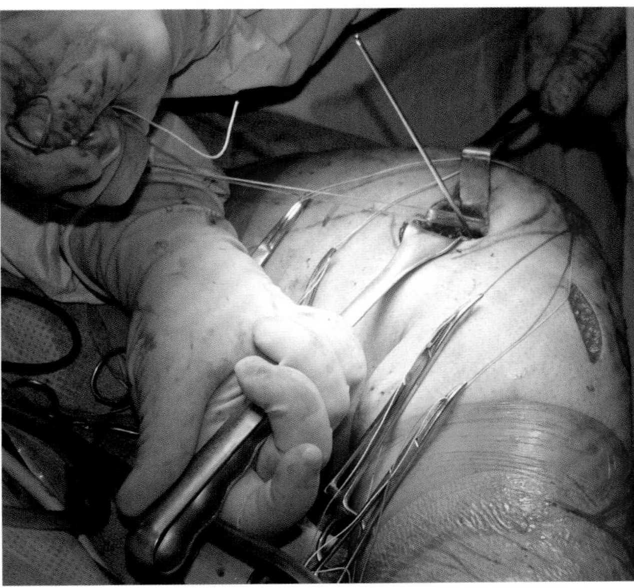

Figure 53-11 | With the aid of fluoroscopy, the MPFL insertion site is located, and a guide pin is drilled through the lateral cortex. A reamer sized to the doubled graft is then drilled from 30 to 40 mm.

- The graft is tensioned into the tunnel initially at 30 degrees.
- The knee is then flexed to 120 degrees, and the graft is fully tensioned into the tunnel.
- The knee is brought back to 30 degrees, patellar stability is assessed, and final fixation is applied (Fig. 53-12).

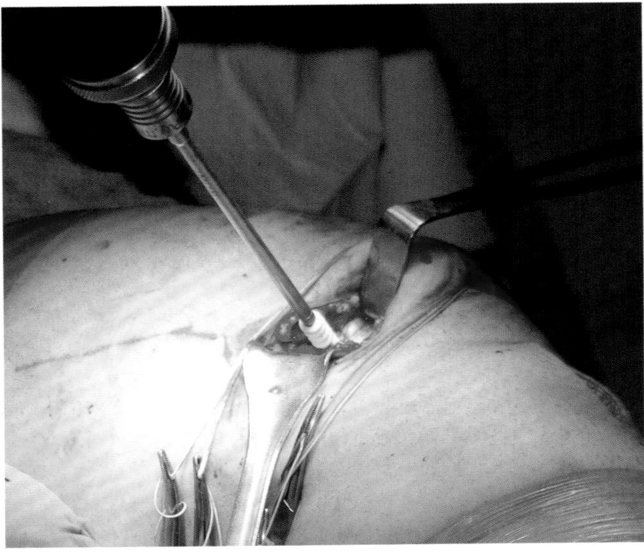

Figure 53-12 | A button or interference screw can be used to secure the graft to the femoral side with the knee initially at 30 degrees of flexion.

- Tension can be increased as needed.
- The wounds are closed in a standard fashion.
- Postoperative radiographs can be obtained at the first postoperative visit (Fig. 53-13).

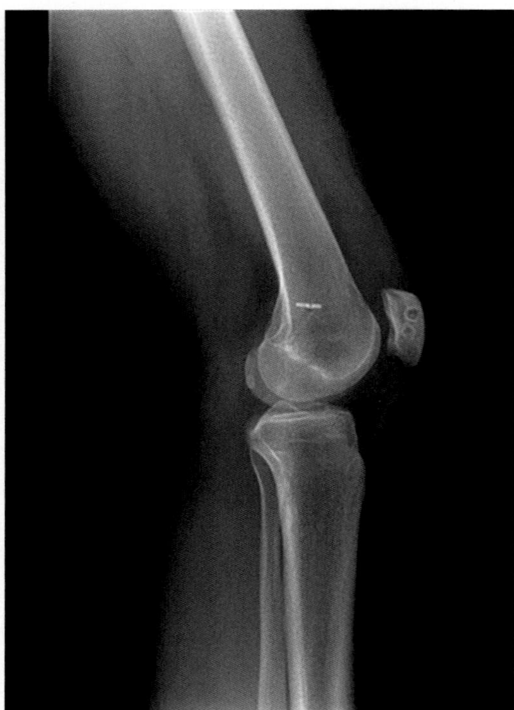

Figure 53-13 | Postoperative lateral view radiograph demonstrating patellar and femoral tunnels.

Postoperative Care

- The patient is placed in a knee brace locked in extension immediately following the procedure.
  - Bracing usually is continued for ~6 to 8 weeks as the patient regains lower limb strength and control.
- Protected (50%) weight bearing is allowed immediately after surgery.
- Knee flexion to 90 degrees is allowed as tolerated.
- Postoperative pain usually is managed with oral narcotics.
- At 4 weeks, full weight bearing is allowed, and the brace is unlocked.
- The crutches are discontinued at 6 weeks; the brace is discontinued at 8 weeks.
- The core components of postoperative rehabilitation are restoration of range of motion, quadriceps strengthening, and enhancement of proximal lower limb control.
- Return to unrestricted activities/sports should be individualized; currently, there are no validated criteria for determining safe return to play.
- If a patient does not achieve at least 90 degrees of flexion by 6 weeks, the intensity of the physical therapy regimen should be increased.

Complications

- According to a systematic review, the overall complication rate for MPFL reconstruction is 26.1%.[6]
- Complications following MPFL reconstruction include
  - Arthrofibrosis
  - Wound complications (eg, infection)
  - Patellar fracture
  - Symptomatic implants
  - Residual or recurrent patellar instability
  - Patellofemoral arthritis

Acknowledgments

We would like to thank Bradford Tucker, MD for contributing to the images included in this chapter.

References

1. van Duijvenbode D, Stavenuiter M, Burger B, et al. The reliability of four widely used patellar height ratios. *Int Orthop.* 2016;40(3):493-497.
2. Dejour H, Walch G, Nove-Josserand L, et al. Factors of patellar instability: an anatomic radiographic study. *Knee Surg Sports Traumatol Arthrosc.* 1994;2(1):19-26.
3. Seitlinger G, Scheurecker G, Högler R, et al. Tibial tubercle-posterior cruciate ligament distance: a new measurement to define the position of the tibial tubercle in patients with patellar dislocation. *Am J Sports Med.* 2012;40(5):1119-1125.
4. Weinberger JM, Fabricant PD, Taylor SA, et al. Influence of graft source and configuration on revision rate and patient-reported outcomes after MPFL reconstruction: a systematic review and meta-analysis. *Knee Surg Sports Traumatol Arthrosc.* 2017;25(8):2511-1519.
5. Burrus MT, Werner BC, Conte EJ, et al. Troubleshooting the femoral attachment during medial patellofemoral ligament reconstruction: location, location, location. *Orthop J Sports Med.* 2015;3(1):2325967115569198.
6. Shah JN, Howard JS, Flanigan DC, et al. A systematic review of complications and failures associated with medial patellofemoral ligament reconstruction for recurrent patellar dislocation. *Am J Sports Med.* 2012;40(8):1916-1923.

Chapter 54
Tibial Tubercle Transfer

JAMES D. WYLIE
JOHN P. FULKERSON

Patient Evaluation/Indications

- Patient history
  - Patellofemoral complaints can be due to instability or pain or both.
  - Patients with patellofemoral pain commonly complain of pain with walking up/down stairs and inclines or sitting for long periods of time.
  - Onset of pain is often insidious, related to patellofemoral lateral malalignment/arthrosis or associated with patella instability with lateral tracking.[1]
- Physical examination
  - Gait evaluation may show valgus coronal plane alignment or excessive femoral anteversion/internal rotation and compensatory external tibial torsion.[2]
  - An overloaded lateral patellar facet related to malalignment is commonly tender to compression or palpation, often with crepitus.[1]
  - The J-sign is common in patients with lateral patellar maltracking.
  - Patients with instability commonly complain of apprehension with lateral patellar translation.
  - Apprehension with increasing degrees of flexion can be a sign of trochlear dysplasia.[3]
  - Resisted knee extension at varying degrees of flexion can be suggestive of a cartilage lesion in the patellofemoral articulation.[1]
  - Pain on stepping down with the contralateral leg suggests an articular lesion.[2]
- Imaging
  - Standard radiographs (anteroposterior, 3-degree knee flexion weight-bearing posteroanterior, true lateral, and 30-degree knee flexion Merchant views)[1,4]
    - Patellofemoral arthrosis is most commonly seen on the lateral and Merchant views.
    - Patellar tilt seen on Merchant view suggests lateral facet overload.[4]
  - Magnetic resonance imaging (MRI)
    - This can be valuable in evaluating patellofemoral articular cartilage integrity.
    - Axial imaging can investigate the integrity of the medial retinacular structures in patients with traumatic dislocation.[4]
    - MRI allows measurement of the tibial tubercle-trochlear groove (TT-TG) distance, with >20 mm being abnormal.[4]
    - Can be used to measure the tibial tubercle-posterior cruciate ligament (TT-PCL) distance, with more than 24 mm being abnormal.[5]
  - Computed tomography (CT)
    - In lieu of MRI, CT can measure the TT-TG distance with >15-20 mm being abnormal.
    - Mid-patella axial images at 15-, 30-, and 45-degree knee flexion can evaluate patellar tracking.[1]

- Indications for anteromedial tibial tubercle transfer osteotomy
  - Failed conservative measures for lateral patellofemoral arthrosis including physical therapy focused on the patellofemoral joint with emphasis on core strengthening and lower extremity mechanics/gait.
  - Recurrent patellar instability or patellofemoral pain with radiographic and clinical lateral tracking. This can be performed in combination with medial patellofemoral reconstruction in recurrent patella instability patients.
  - Intact medial facet and medial trochlear articular cartilage are needed to accept the transferred load for optimal outcomes.[6]

Sterile Instruments/Equipment

- Tourniquet (nonsterile)
- Arthroscope
- Arthroscopic cautery
- Two Army-Navy (Parker-Langenbeck) retractors
- Tonsil (Schnidt) clamp
- Electrocautery (Bovie)
- Cobb elevator
- Handheld sagittal saw (Smith & Nephew, Stryker Total Performance System [TPS] or equivalent) with a minimum ½-inch-wide, 2-inch-long straight blade
- Osteotome set, preferably Lambotte osteotomes
- Large-fragment set with 4.5-mm screws, including drill and countersink

Positioning and Diagnostic Arthroscopy

- The patient is positioned supine on a regular operating table with a nonsterile tourniquet.
- A bump can be placed under the ipsilateral hip if the patient exhibits excessive external rotation of the leg on the operating table.
- The leg is exsanguinated, and a thigh tourniquet is inflated.
- Diagnostic arthroscopy is performed with standard anterolateral and anteromedial portals.
  - Starting with an anteromedial viewing portal can allow optimal anterolateral portal placement to complete the lateral release as needed.
  - Diagnostic arthroscopy focuses on the patellofemoral joint, specifically detailing the state of the articular cartilage.
  - An anteromedializing tubercle osteotomy most efficiently unloads the lateral facet and the distal pole of the patella.
  - If the lateral retinacular tissues are too tight to allow medialization of the patella, an arthroscopic lateral release is performed at this time. Open lateral lengthening is also an option.

Approach and Exposure

- A 7- to 8-cm incision is made just lateral to the tibial tubercle starting just above the distal aspect of the patellar tendon.
- Full-thickness skin flaps are raised proximally 1-2 cm above the insertion of the patellar tendon and distally along the level of the proposed osteotomy. This is usually 6-10 cm distal to the patellar tendon insertion.
- The medial and lateral aspects of the patellar tendon insertion are dissected so that a tonsil retractor can be placed between the tendon and the bone (Fig. 54-1).
- The anterior compartment is then incised and elevated off the anterior and lateral tibia to allow complete exposure of the proposed osteotomy cut.
  - This allows protection of the neurovascular structures in the posterior aspect of the anterior compartment (the anterior tibial artery and deep peroneal nerve run just behind the lateral tibia at this level) (Fig. 54-2).

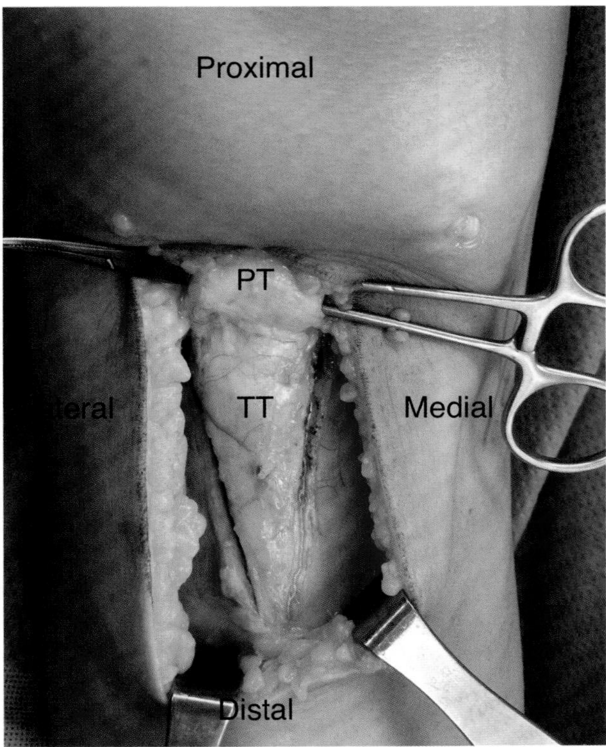

Figure 54-1 | Dissection taken down to the tibial tubercle (TT) with medial and lateral skin flaps and isolation of medial and lateral aspects of the patellar tendon (PT).

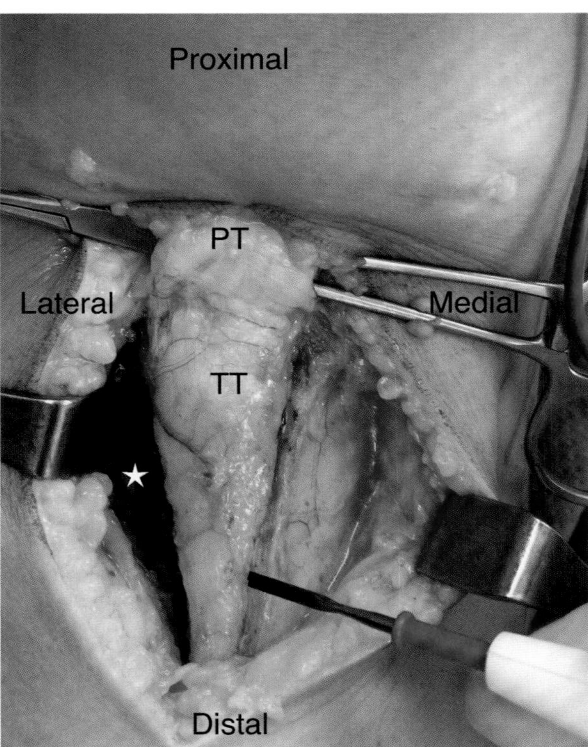

Figure 54-2 | The anterior compartment of the lower leg is dissected off of the lateral aspect of the anterior tibia (*star*) with the electrocautery to allow visualization of the lateral cortex of the tibia where the osteotomy will exit. TT, tibial tubercle; PT, patellar tendon.

Osteotomy

- The osteotomy is made from medial to lateral.
- Electrocautery is used to mark just medial to the patellar tendon insertion in a linear fashion, exiting about 6-8 cm distally on the anterior cortex.
- A handheld Total Performance System (TPS) (Stryker, Kalamazoo, MI) or Dyonics Power (Smith & Nephew, Andover, MA) saw is used to score the cortex and confirm a straight osteotomy.
- The osteotomy is then made through the medial cortex with care to make a straight osteotomy that tapers out the anterior cortex, avoiding a notch in the tibia.
  - A cortical hinge can be left anteriorly to increase the stability of the osteotomy.
  - The obliquity of the cut can be altered based on the degree of desired anterior displacement.
  - Patients with more degenerative change, especially at the distal pole, will benefit from more anterior displacement.[6]
    - Patients with a primary complaint of instability typically benefit more from medialization.
- The osteotomy cut is then completed through the lateral cortex starting distally and progressing proximally. This entire cut must be perfectly flat to allow stable transfer of the osteotomy and secure early bone healing of the transferred osteotomy.
  - The anterior compartment musculature is retracted so that the tip of the saw blade can be seen at all times (Figs. 54-3 and 54-4).
- As this progresses more proximally to the flare of the tibia, a wide osteotome is used to continue the osteotomy more proximally from lateral to medial. This connects the proximal posterolateral cut to the region just lateral to the patellar tendon insertion. Great care should be taken at all times to avoid exiting the posterior tibia in steeper osteotomies (Fig. 54-5).

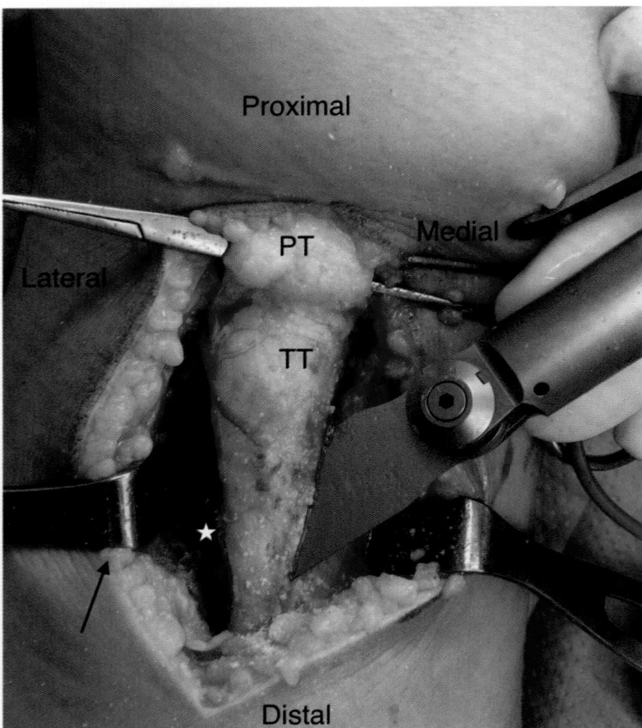

Figure 54-3 | The osteotomy is started from anteromedial to posterolateral. An Army-Navy retractor or equivalent (*arrow*) is used to retract the anterior compartment to allow complete visualization of the saw blade (*star*) during osteotomy. TT, tibial tubercle; PT, patellar tendon.

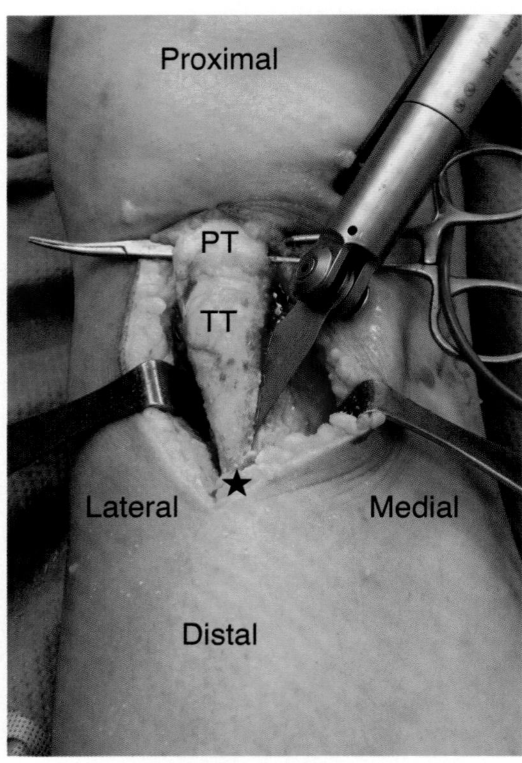

Figure 54-4 | The osteotomy is completed in an anteromedial to posterolateral direction. An anterior cortical hinge can be left distally to improve stability of the fragment (*star*). TT, tibial tubercle; PT, patellar tendon.

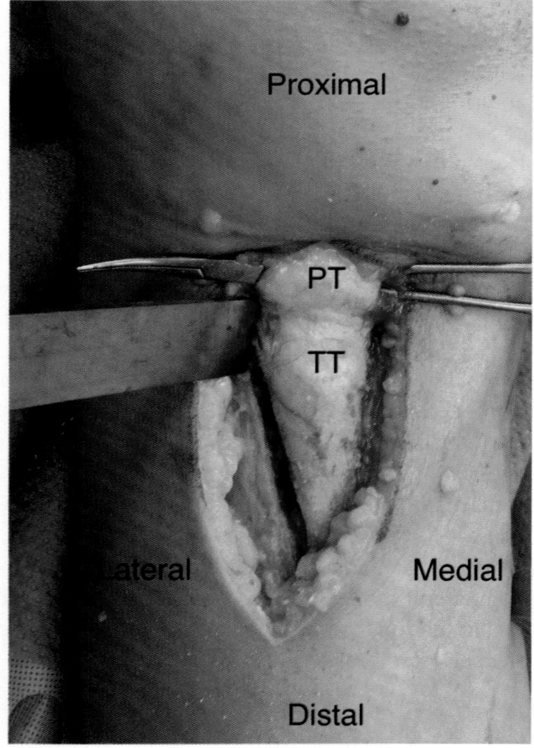

Figure 54-5 | A 1-inch osteotome is used to make the osteotomy from the proximal aspect of the saw cut to the posterior aspect of the patellar tendon in a lateral to medial direction at about a 45-degree angle. TT, tibial tubercle; PT, patellar tendon.

- A ½-inch osteotome is used from medial to lateral and lateral to medial behind and above the patellar tendon to complete the osteotomy through the superior cortex of the tibia. This cut should be made such that the tubercle can be moved freely.
  - This prevents fracture propagation into the tibial plateau with attempted manipulation of the tubercle fragment (Figs. 54-6 and 54-7).

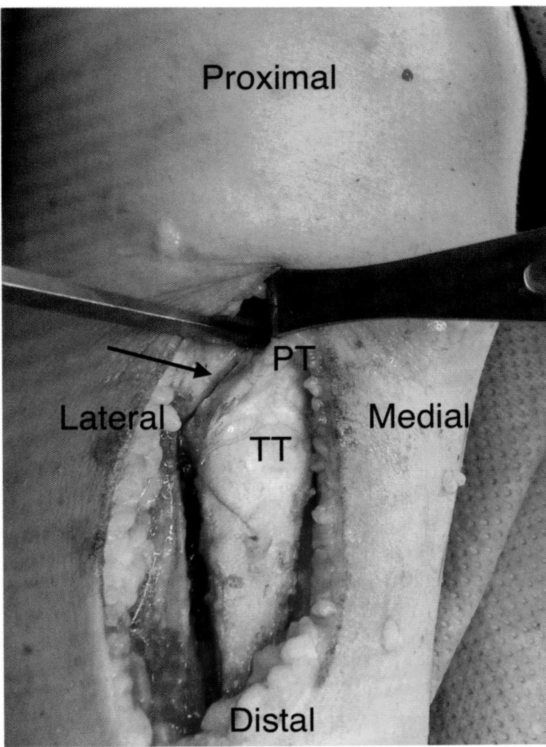

Figure 54-6 | A ½-in osteotome is used to make the osteotomy behind the patellar tendon in a medial to lateral and lateral to medial direction. The osteotomy shown in Figure 54-5 is just distal and lateral to the osteotome (*arrow*). TT, tibial tubercle; PT, patellar tendon.

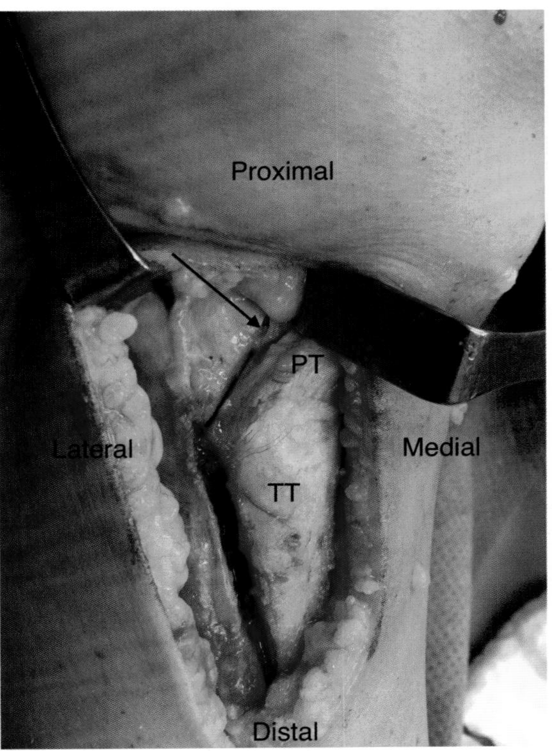

Figure 54-7 | The entire proximal lateral cortex is visualized to confirm that the osteotomy is completed through all cortical bone (*arrow*). TT, tibial tubercle; PT, patellar tendon.

- Electrocautery is used to release any remaining soft tissue tethers to the tubercle fragment and also to assure release of any infrapatellar scar or contracture,
  - If a lateral release was done arthroscopically, this can be confirmed to be complete through the superior aspect of the incision by palpation of the lateral retinacular structures (Fig. 54-8).
- When the fragment is free, it should slide anteromedially along the osteotomy.
  - Normally, 1 cm of displacement along the osteotomy provides appropriate anteromedialization (Figs. 54-9 and 54-10).
  - Arthroscopic observation of patellar tracking is the best way to judge appropriate displacement.
    - This can be done using provisional fixation with Kirschner wires or, with more experience, can be done after placing the first fixation screw when the surgeon thinks appropriate displacement has been achieved.

Fixation and Closure

- The proximal screw, ~1 cm distal to the tendon insertion, is placed in lag fashion.
  - The tubercle fragment is drilled as perpendicular to the osteotomy as possible with a 4.5-mm drill and the tibia with a 3.2-mm drill (Fig. 54-11).
  - A 4.5-mm cortical screw of the measured length is then countersunk in the osteotomy fragment, compressing it against the tibia.
  - Countersinking the screws is important given the frequent need for implant removal because of the prominence of the tibial tubercle.

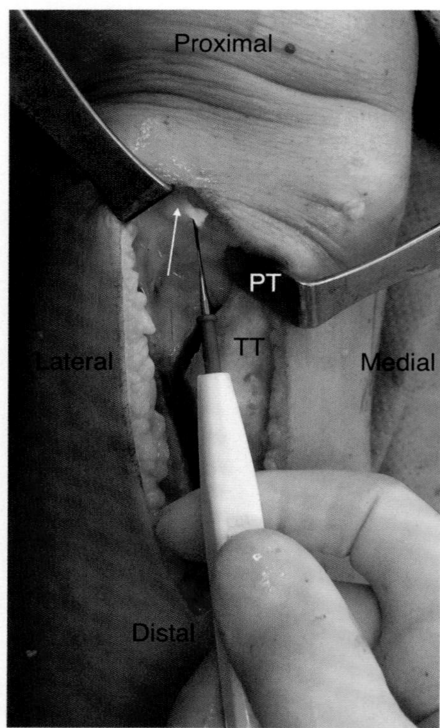

Figure 54-8 | The electrocautery is used to release the soft tissue tether from the lateral retinacular structures (*arrow*) that would prevent anteromedialization of the tubercle. TT, tibial tubercle; PT, patellar tendon.

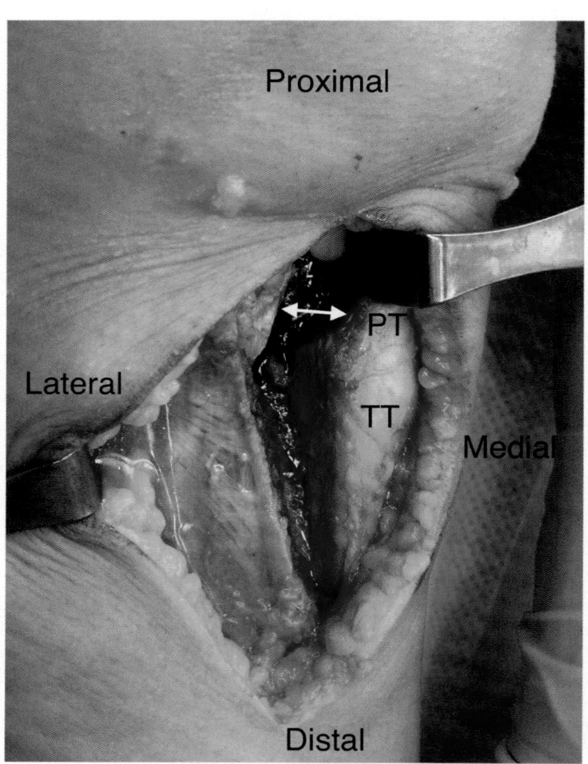

Figure 54-9 | Visualized from anterolaterally, the tubercle is medialized after osteotomy is completed with displacement visualized (*arrow*). TT, tibial tubercle; PT, patellar tendon.

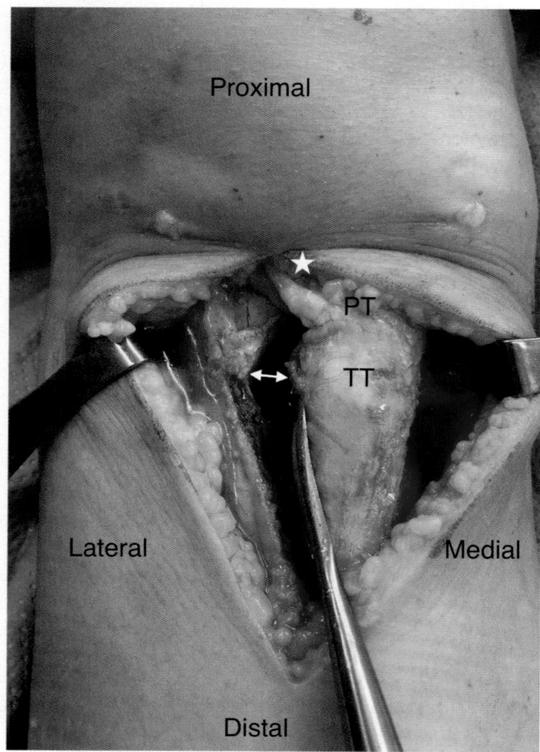

Figure 54-10 | Visualized from anteriorly, the Cobb elevator is used to hinge the tubercle anteromedially (*arrow*). If any further soft tissue tethers are identified (*star*), these can be further released if they do not allow medialization of the patella. TT, tibial tubercle; PT, patellar tendon.

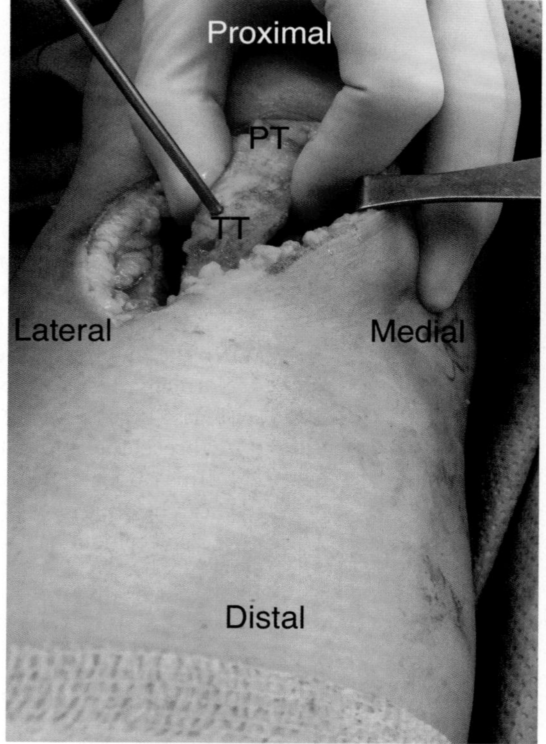

Figure 54-11 | The drill is used in lag fashion in a slightly anterolateral to posteromedial direction to allow compression of the osteotomy surface while the tubercle is held in the desired amount of correction. TT, tibial tubercle; PT, patellar tendon.

- If alignment was not checked before placement of the first screw, arthroscopic observation of patellar tracking can be done at this time to confirm appropriate anteromedialization and unloading of the distal and/or lateral articular lesion(s).
  - The distal pole of the patella should be slightly tipped up off the trochlear cartilage, and the medial patellar facet should be articulating with the medial trochlea. The lateral patellar facet should be decompressed compared to the preoperative examination.
  - Care should be made not to overmedialize the patella, which can lead to medial overload and possible medial instability.
- The second screw is placed 1-2 cm distal in the same lag fashion as above (Figs. 54-12 and 54-13).

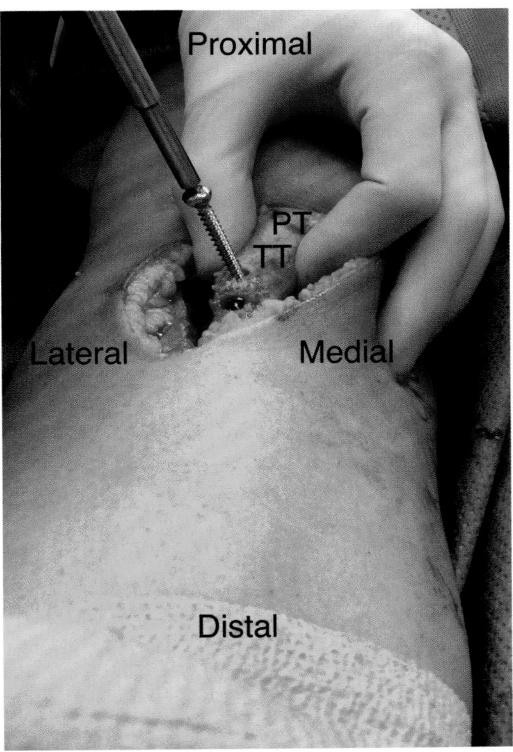

Figure 54-12 | Two 4.5-mm large fragment cortical screws are countersunk in the tubercle fragment with bicortical fixation in an anterolateral to posteromedial direction. TT, tibial tubercle; PT, patellar tendon.

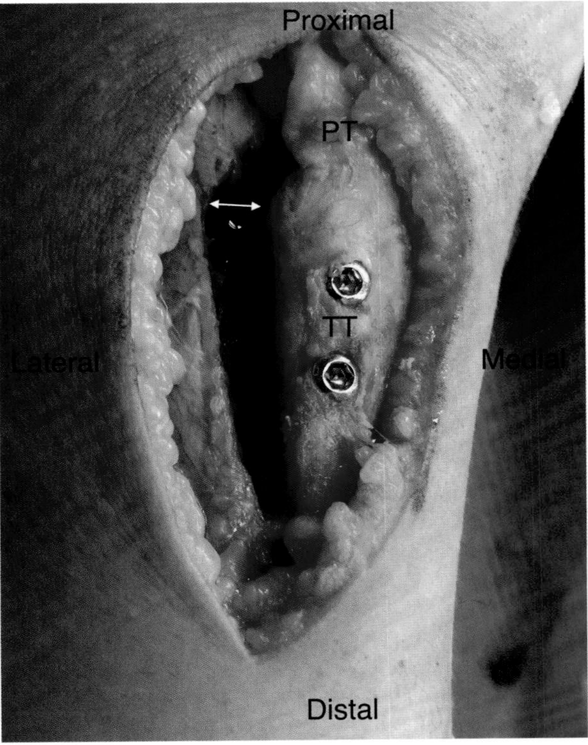

Figure 54-13 | Final fixation of the osteotomy illustrating the medial displacement (*arrow*) of the proximal aspect of the tibial tubercle (TT). PT, patellar tendon.

- Fluoroscopy can be used intraoperatively to confirm appropriate implant placement and length but is not required.
- The tourniquet is then released, hemostasis is obtained using the electrocautery, and the wound is closed in layered fashion with dermal and skin sutures. We normally close the skin with Zipline (Zipline Medical, Campbell, CA) or staples.
- A sterile dressing, continuous cooling pad, and knee immobilizer are placed.

Postoperative Recovery and Rehabilitation

- Anticoagulation with aspirin 325 mg daily or Lovenox is continued for 2 to 4 weeks depending on risk stratification.
- Rest, ice, and elevation and ankle pumps are continued for the first 1 to 2 weeks.
- A knee immobilizer is used for 4 to 5 weeks.
  - Starting on postoperative day 3, patients begin knee range-of-motion exercises once daily. A single bend daily is sufficient. The goal is 90 degrees of flexion by 3 weeks and 120 degrees of flexion by 6 weeks.

- The patient is restricted to toe-touch weight bearing for 6 weeks with crutches.
- The patient can then progress to weight bearing as tolerated at 6 weeks.
- With guidance of a physical therapist, progressive range-of-motion and strengthening exercises continue after 6 weeks.
- Patients generally return to straight line running at 6 months and contact sports at 1 year.

References

1. Fulkerson JP. Anteromedialization of the tibial tuberosity for patellofemoral malalignment. *Clin Orthop Relat Res.* 1983;(177):176.
2. Manske RC, Davies GJ. Examination of the patellofemoral joint. *Int J Sports Phys Ther.* 2016;11:831-853.
3. Bollier M, Fulkerson JP. The role of trochlear dysplasia in patellofemoral instability. *J Am Acad Orthop Surg.* 2011;19:8-16.
4. Thomas S, Rupiper D, Stacy GS. Imaging of the patellofemoral joint. *Clin Sports Med.* 2014;33(3):413-436.
5. Seitlinger G, Scheurecker G, Hogler R, et al. Tibial tubercle-posterior cruciate ligament distance: a new measurement to define the position of the tibial tubercle in patients with patellar dislocation. *Am J Sports Med.* 2012;40:1119-1125.
6. Pidoriano AJ, Weinstein RN, Buuck DA, et al. Correlation of patellar articular lesions with results from anteromedial tibial tubercle transfer. *Am J Sports Med.* 1997;25:533-537.

Chapter 55
Arthroscopic Internal Fixation of Osteochondritis Dissecans

CHRISTIAN N. ANDERSON
ALLEN F. ANDERSON

Background

- Osteochondritis dissecans (OCD) is an idiopathic lesion of the subchondral bone that can compromise the articular cartilage if healing fails to occur.[1,2]
- While the etiology remains controversial, clinical[3] and basic science[4] studies in the older literature support trauma as a pathogenesis of OCD.
- More recently, evidence from animal studies indicates that OCD in the classic location of the medial femoral condyle is caused by occlusion of the epiphyseal vascular arcade.[5–7]
- OCD lesions can be reliably classified into six arthroscopic categories—three immobile types and three mobile types, based on the Research in Osteochondritis of the Knee (ROCK) study group classification system (Fig. 55-1).[1]
- Treatment for OCD is dictated by skeletal maturity of the patient and stage of the lesion at the time of presentation.
- The goal of treatment is to preserve the articular cartilage through healing of the OCD fragment.

Preoperative Planning

Radiographic Evaluation

- Plain radiographs: anteroposterior (AP), 45-degree posteroanterior (PA) flexed, lateral, and sunrise weight-bearing views.
- Long-leg radiograph to determine the mechanical axis of the extremity.
- Magnetic resonance imaging (MRI) can determine the integrity of the articular cartilage and lesion stability. The MRI criteria for OCD instability include high T2 signal behind the fragment, surrounding cysts, a cartilage fracture line, and a fluid-filled defect.

Treatment Algorithm

- Skeletally immature patients with immobile lesions and healthy articular cartilage
  - Non–weight bearing for 6 weeks, followed by activity restriction until radiographic healing is achieved
  - If noncompliant, immobilization for 6 weeks
  - If patient is within 6 months of skeletal maturity or OCD lesion has failed to heal despite 6 months of conservative treatment, antegrade or retrograde drilling is indicated.
- Patients with unstable or loose fragments are candidates for operative fixation with or without bone grafting.
- Patients who have OCD lesions that have failed to heal despite operative fixation or who have irreparable lesions are candidates for a resurfacing procedure.

	Type	Description	Diagrams
Immobile Lesions	Cue Ball	No abnormality detectable arthroscopically.	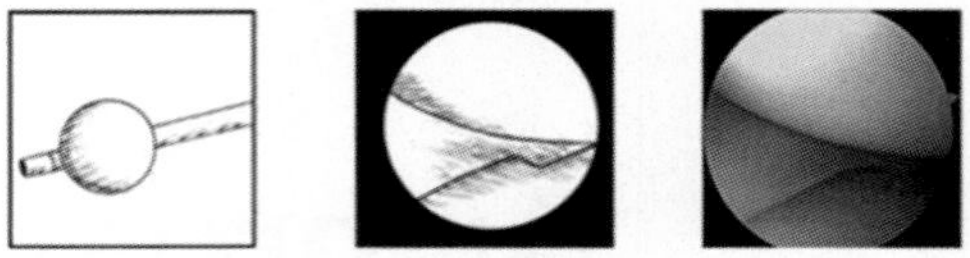
	Shadow	Cartilage is intact and subtly demarcated (possibly under low light).	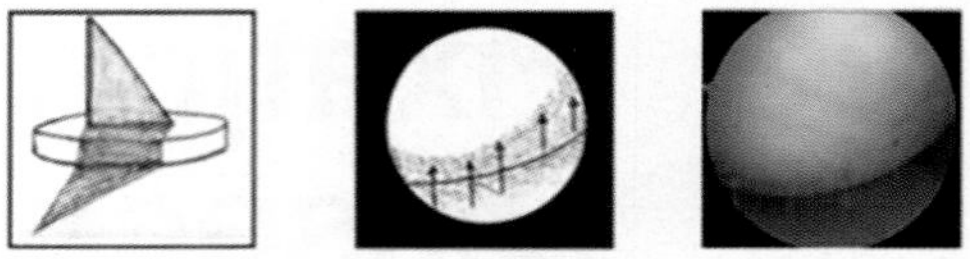
	Wrinkle in the Rug	Cartilage is demarcated with a fissure, buckle, and/or wrinkle.	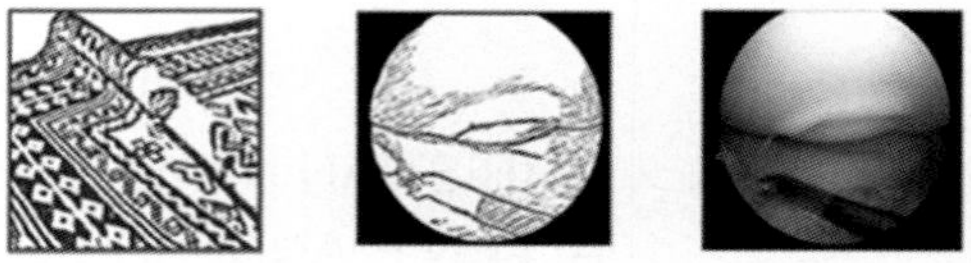
Mobile Lesions	Locked Door	Cartilage fissuring at periphery, *unable* to hinge open.	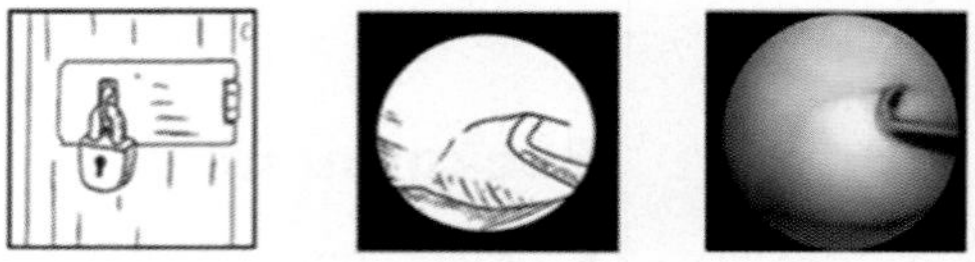
	Trap Door	Cartilage fissuring at periphery, *able* to hinge open.	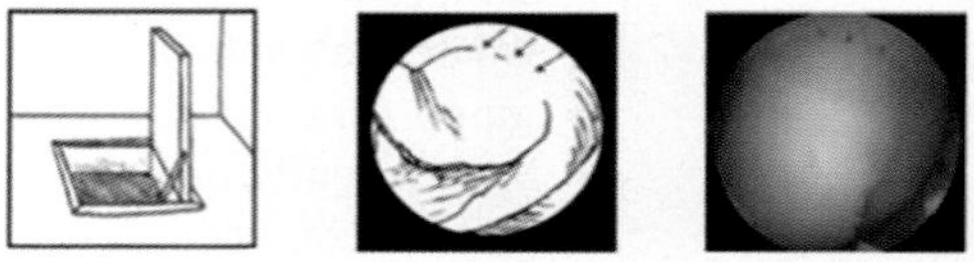
	Crater	Exposed subchondral bone defect.	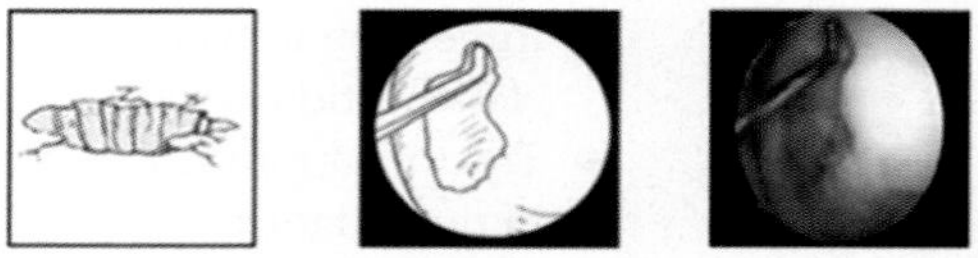

Figure 55-1 | The ROCK study group classification for OCD lesions.[4]

Surgical Technique: Antegrade Drilling

Setup (Fig. 55-2)

- The patient is positioned supine on the operating table.
- The operative leg is placed in an arthroscopic leg holder one handbreadth above the patella.
- The leg holder is raised to elevate the operative knee above the contralateral extremity for viewing in the lateral plane while using fluoroscopy.

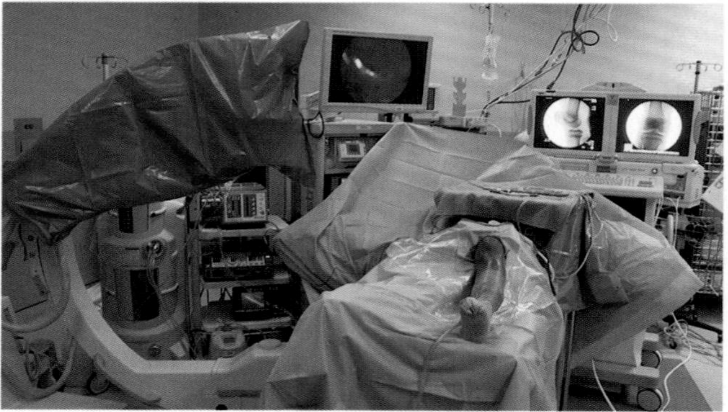

Figure 55-2 | Operating room setup. The C-arm and video monitor are placed on the contralateral side of the injured knee, while the C-arm monitor is placed on the ipsilateral side.

- The leg holder should be set up to allow the surgeon to remove the leg if needed so that the lesion can be accessed through an arthrotomy with the knee in flexion.
- The C-arm is placed on the opposite side of the injured extremity, and the monitor is placed on the same side as the operative extremity (Fig. 55-2).
- Before preparing and draping the extremity, fluoroscopic images of the knee in the AP and lateral planes are obtained, and the location of the lesion is identified, if possible (Fig. 55-3A).

Drilling

- Standard arthroscopic portals are established, and a diagnostic arthroscopy is completed.
- In stable lesions (cue ball), the articular surface may have good subchondral support and may look and feel completely normal. The articular cartilage over the lesion also may be softer than the surrounding cartilage.
- When the lesion cannot be identified arthroscopically (Fig. 55-3B), a 0.045-in smooth Kirschner wire (K-wire) is inserted into the suspected location of the lesion (Fig. 55-3C). Fluoroscopic imaging in the AP and lateral planes is then used to confirm that the K-wire is in the lesion (Fig. 55-3D).
- Once the lesion is identified, a 0.062-in or 0.045-in smooth K-wire is placed in a Jacob drill chuck so that it is 1.5 cm longer than a standard 5-mm arthroscopic cannula.
- The 0.045-in K-wire damages less of the articular cartilage and is just as efficacious as the 0.062-in K-wire (Fig. 55-3E and F).
- The cannula is inserted into the knee adjacent to the lesion and is used to prevent iatrogenic articular cartilage damage and overpenetration of the K-wire into the physis.
- Multiple holes are drilled through the articular cartilage and subchondral bone to uniformly cover the lesion (Fig. 55-3E and F). Bleeding should occur after the tourniquet is deflated (Fig. 55-3G).

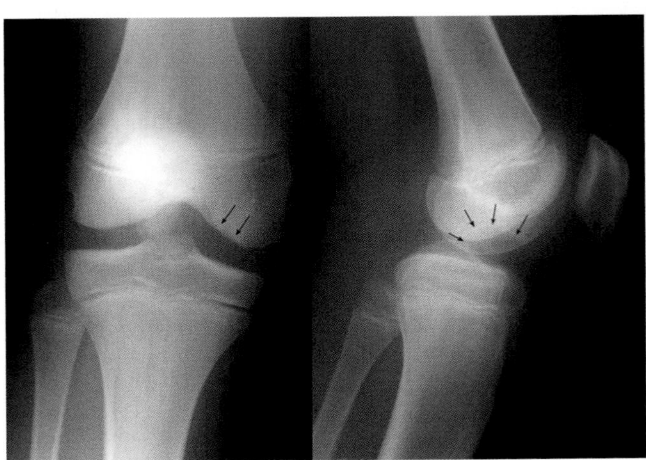

A

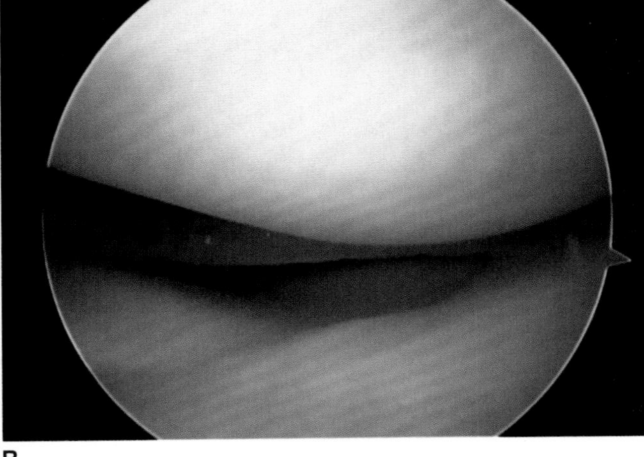

B

C

Figure 55-3 | A. AP and lateral fluoroscopic images demonstrating the lesion location on the medial femoral condyle (*black arrows*). **B.** In lesions that cannot be located arthroscopically, a 0.45 K-wire is inserted in the suspected location of the lesion and it is confirmed with fluoroscopy **(C).**

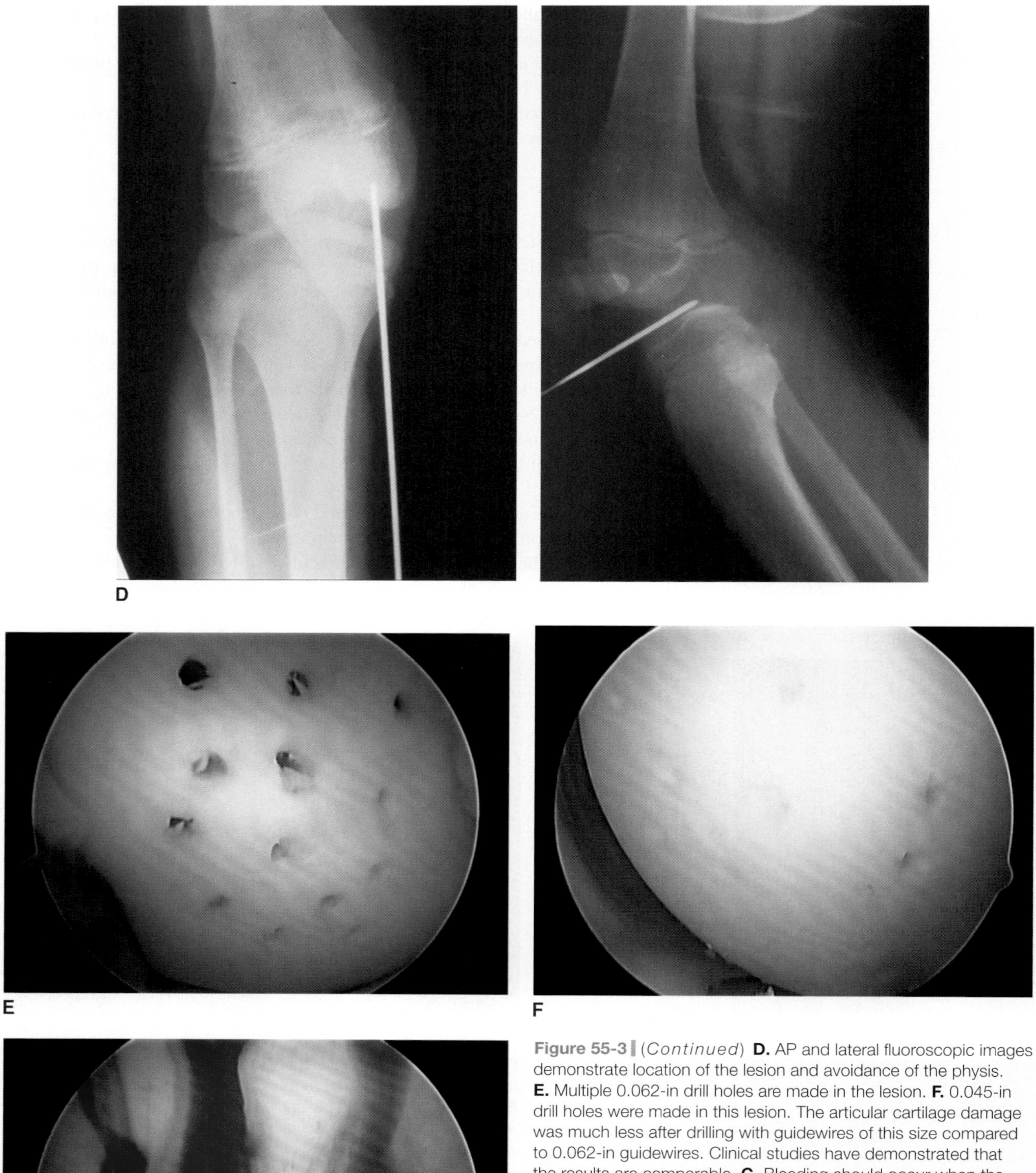

D

E

F

G

Figure 55-3 | (*Continued*) **D.** AP and lateral fluoroscopic images demonstrate location of the lesion and avoidance of the physis. **E.** Multiple 0.062-in drill holes are made in the lesion. **F.** 0.045-in drill holes were made in this lesion. The articular cartilage damage was much less after drilling with guidewires of this size compared to 0.062-in guidewires. Clinical studies have demonstrated that the results are comparable. **G.** Bleeding should occur when the tourniquet is deflated.

- The knee flexion angle can be changed to create multiple drill holes that are perpendicular to the joint surface.
- Lesions on the medial femoral condyle can be drilled through the anteromedial or anterolateral portal.
- Lesions of the lateral femoral condyle typically are more posterior and are generally more accessible when drilled through the anterolateral portal with the knee in flexion.

Operative Fixation

- The decision to perform arthroscopic or open fixation of an unstable OCD lesion depends on several lesion-specific variables.
  - Arthroscopic fixation generally is indicated for accessible lesions that are mobile (locked door, trap door) and do not require bone grafting to restore congruency.
  - Open fixation usually is indicated for large lesions, lesions that are difficult to access, loose bodies, and fragments with bone deficiency requiring bone grafting (trap door, crater).
- **Arthroscopic fixation with bioabsorbable nails (Fig. 55-4A-D):**
  - *Advantages*
    - Good compression

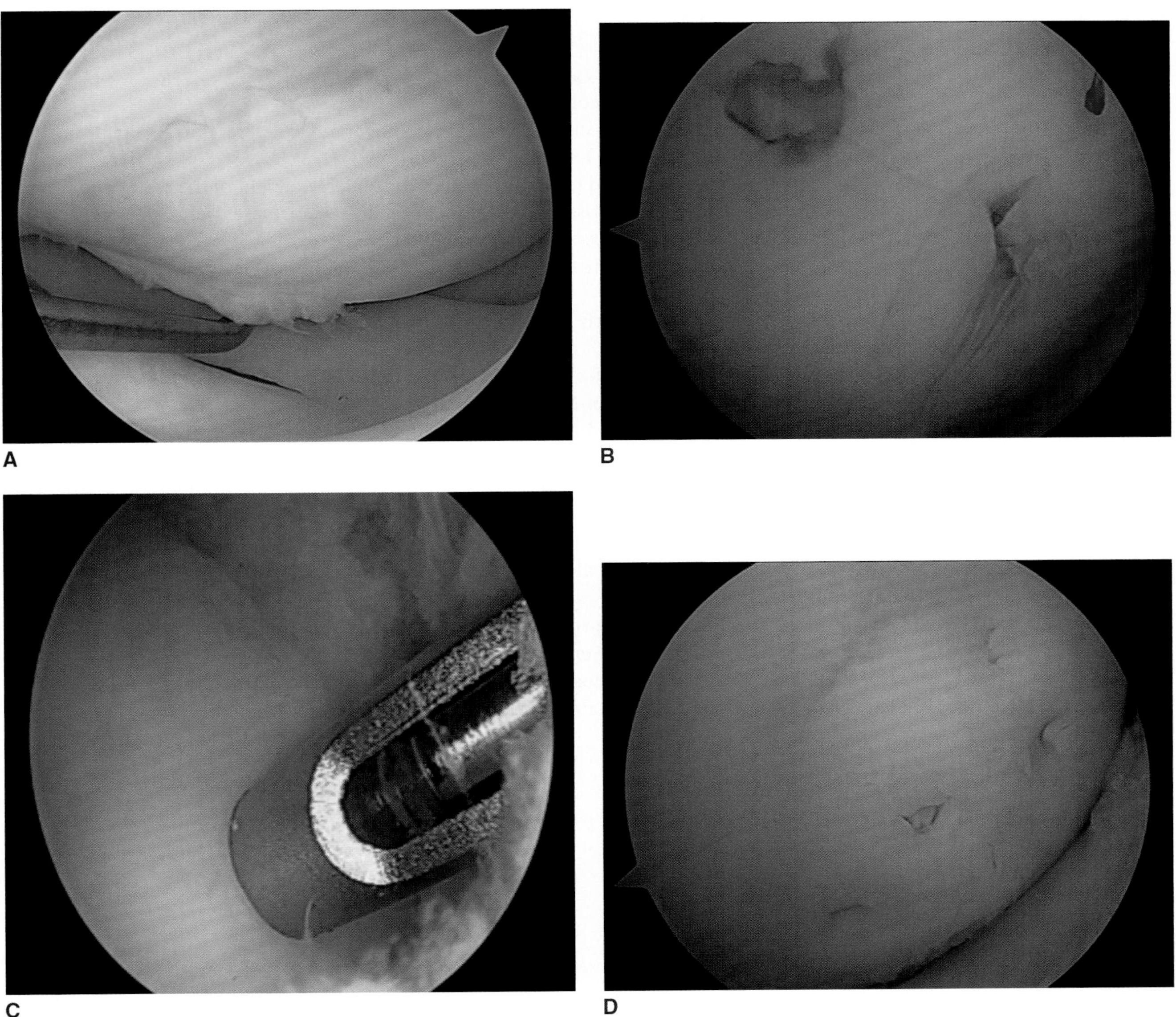

Figure 55-4 | **A.** Unstable "locked door" lesion as classified by the ROCK group[4]. **B.** After lesion preparation and provisional fixation, the lesion is drilled with a K-wire to improve vascularity, as visualized by blood outflow from the cartilage perforations. **C.** Placement of a ConMed SmartNail. Final fixation construct **(D)** and second look 1 year after surgery **(E)**.

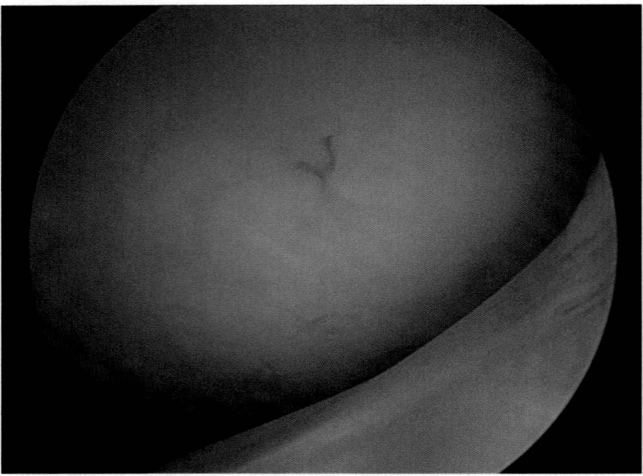

E

Figure 55-4 | (*Continued*)

- MRI compatible
- No need for secondary surgery for removal
- *Disadvantages*
  - Possible implant breakage and cartilage damage
  - Foreign body reaction and osteolysis
- The arthroscope can be placed in either the anteromedial or anterolateral portal depending on the trajectory needed to stabilize the lesion.
- A standard 4.5-mm shaver is used to perform a superficial debridement of the crater and fragment to remove all interposed fibrous tissue. A 3.5-mm curved shaver can be useful for debriding areas of the lesion that are hard to access with the straight shaver.
- Curettes (curved and straight) are used to clean any residual fibrous tissue from within the base of the lesion.
- Multiple holes are drilled with a 0.045-in K-wire to improve vascularity to the lesion (Fig. 55-4B).
- The lesion is reduced with a probe and provisionally fixed with a 0.045-in K-wire in the location where it can be replaced with ConMed SmartNail system (Linvatec, Ithaca, NY). The K-wire can be placed percutaneously to avoid instrument crowding during internal fixation.
- The 1.5-mm drill guide for the SmartNail system is introduced into the knee through either the anteromedial or anterolateral portal to achieve an angle orthogonal to the lesion (Fig. 55-4C).
- The guide is left in place to maintain the trajectory of the drill hole, and a 1.5- × 16-mm SmartNail is inserted using the tamp that allows the implant to be countersunk 2 mm when fully seated (Fig. 55-4C).
- Implants are placed at even intervals to stabilize the lesion. The implants are angled at different trajectories to increase pullout strength and lesion stability (Fig. 55-4D).
- The lesion is probed to ensure stability and to check for implant prominence.
- SmartNails also can be used to stabilize displaced lesions (Fig. 55-5A-C).

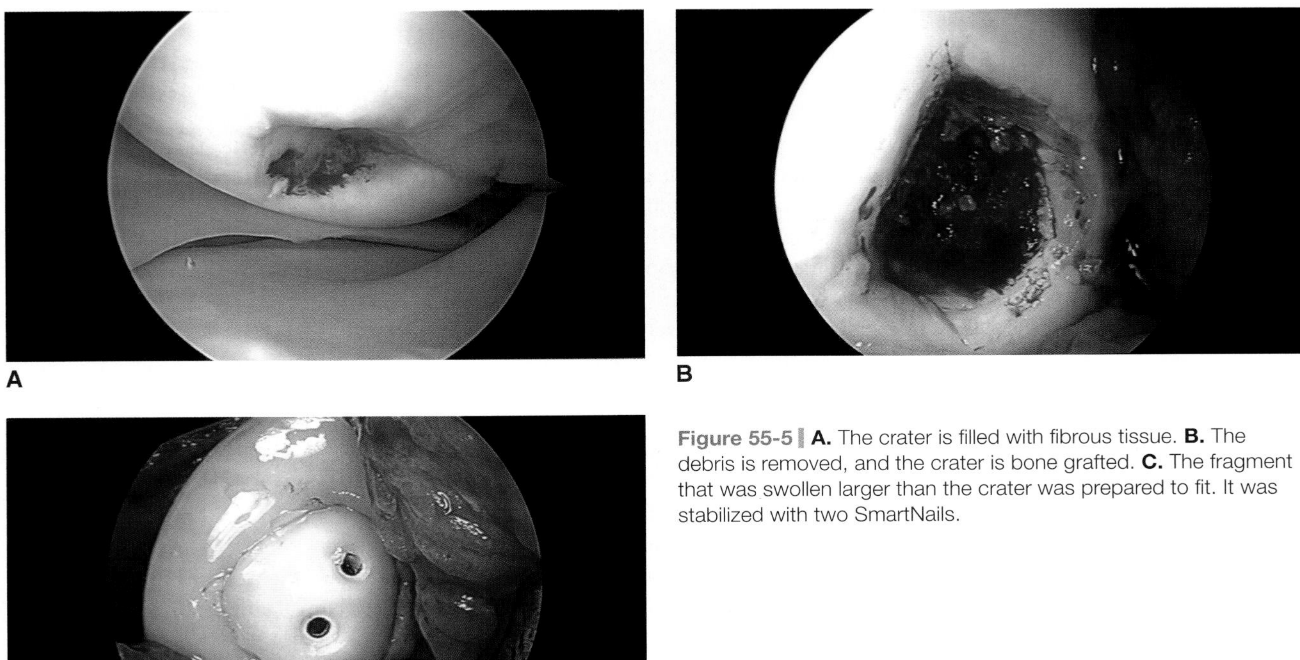

Figure 55-5 | **A.** The crater is filled with fibrous tissue. **B.** The debris is removed, and the crater is bone grafted. **C.** The fragment that was swollen larger than the crater was prepared to fit. It was stabilized with two SmartNails.

- **Operative fixation with metal screws (Fig. 55-6A-C):**
  - *Advantages*
    - Provides most rigid fixation and compression of all techniques
    - High healing rate

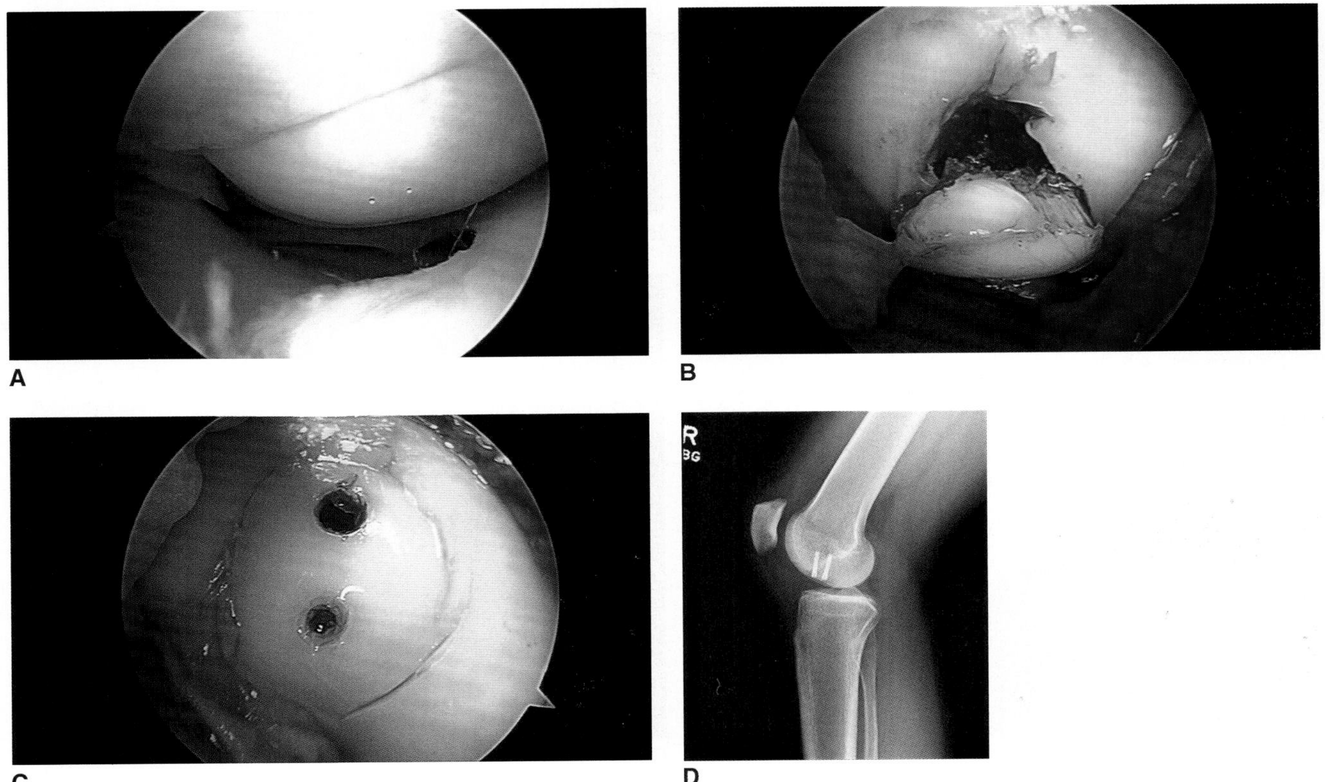

Figure 55-6 | A "trap door" lesion **(A** and **B)** as classified by the ROCK group.[4] **C.** Two titanium variable pitch headless compression screws are used to fix the fragment. **D.** Postoperative lateral radiograph demonstrates that the screw heads are positioned flush with the subchondral bone.

- *Disadvantages*
  - Subsequent surgery needed for removal
- Metal screws can be used during either open or arthroscopic fixation depending on the lesion-specific variables previously mentioned.
- The lesion and crater are prepared as previously described, and autologous bone graft can be obtained from the femoral metaphysis if bone grafting is necessary to restore congruency (Fig. 55-6A and B).
- Cannulated titanium variable pitch headless compression screws are used: 2.5-mm-diameter screws for small fragments and 3.5-mm screws for large fragments.
  - These are low profile and offer good compression but need bone in the fragment for compression to occur.
- Partially threaded mini-fragment screws
  - These offer good compression but need to be countersunk to avoid articular cartilage damage.
- Technique
  - Once preparation, bone grafting, and reduction of the fragment are complete, a guidewire is introduced into the lesion, and a second guidewire is placed in a similar fashion to prevent rotation of the fragment.
  - The first guidewire is overdrilled, and the screw is seated until the head is flush with the subchondral bone of the OCD fragment.
  - Subsequent screws can be placed as needed to complete fixation of the lesion (Fig. 55-6C).
  - Fluoroscopy should be used to ensure that the screw heads are beneath the subchondral bone and avoid the physis (Fig. 55-6D).

- **Open reduction and internal fixation with osteochondral autograft plugs (Fig. 55-7A-D):**

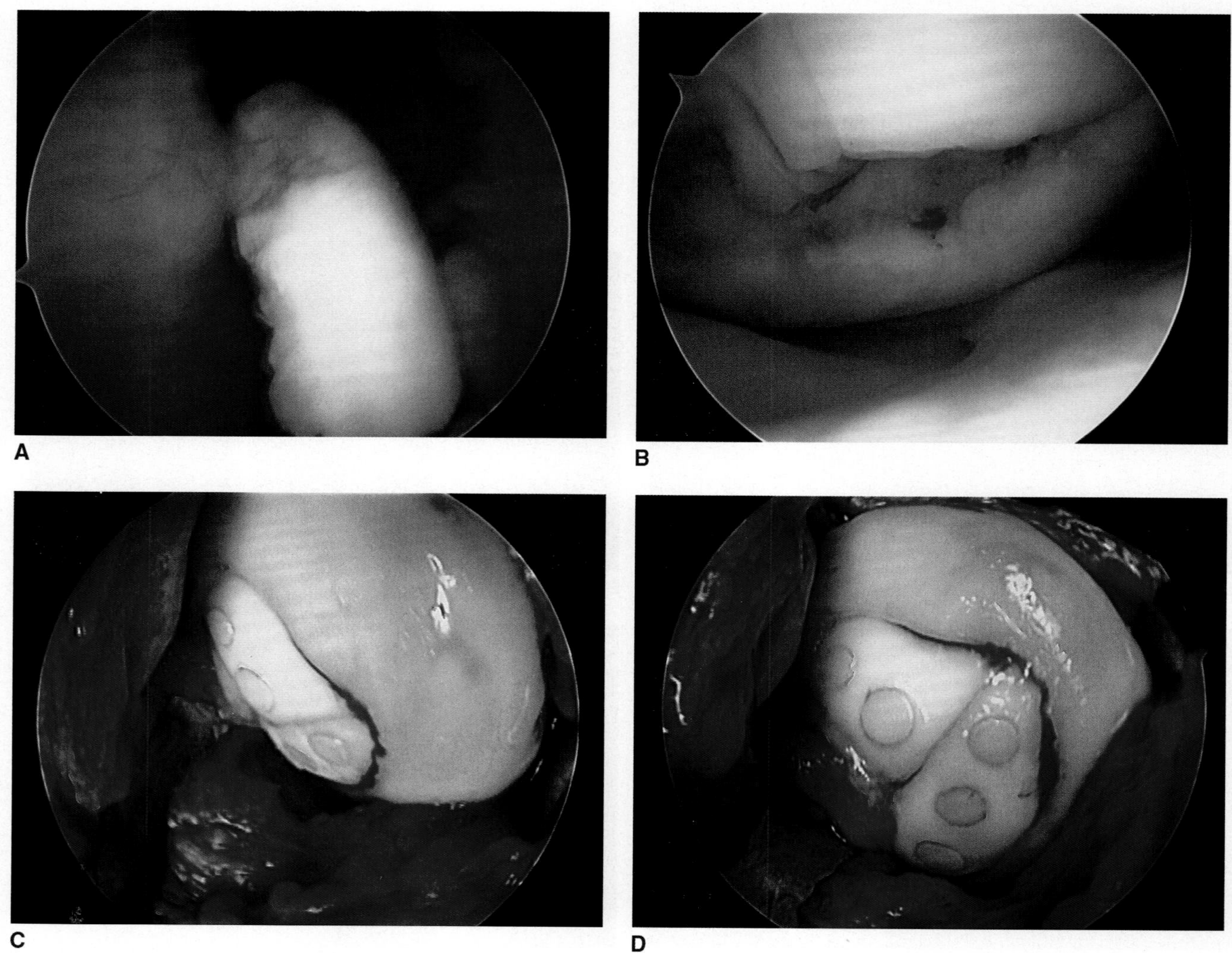

Figure 55-7 | A loose body **(A)** from a "crater" lesion **(B)** as classified by the ROCK group.[4] **C.** The crater is prepared by curetting and removing the fibrous tissue and drilling the base of the crater. Bone graft is added to restore congruency with the surrounding articular cartilage. **D.** The lesions are secured using multiple osteochondral plugs for fixation.

- *Advantages*
  - Provides stability and bone graft
  - No risk of implant causing tibial articular cartilage damage
  - No need for secondary surgery for removal
- *Disadvantages*
  - Less compression than metal screws or bioabsorbable nails
  - Donor site morbidity
- A medial or lateral arthrotomy is made over the location of the lesion with enough length to allow harvesting of the osteochondral plug from the superior trochlea on the same side.
- If the fragment is displaced, it frequently swells larger than the crater (Fig. 55-7A). The crater is cleaned of fibrous tissue and the edges are freshened (Fig. 55-7B). A small threaded K-wire is placed in the fragment at the site where subsequent fixation will enter the fragment. This K-wire is used to hold the fragment as it is being carefully pared down to fit the crater.
- The lesion is then reduced and checked for congruency.
- If there is a step-off between the normal articular surface and the OCD fragment after reduction, bone grafting from the femoral metaphysis is necessary to restore congruency.
  - The osteochondral plugs should be 5 or 6 mm in diameter. The initial literature suggested using 3.5- or 4-mm mosaicplasty plugs. Harvesting plugs of this diameter in pediatric patients often results in crushing of the bone. A plug that is 15 mm long may be crushed to only 5 mm long, and that is not long enough to stabilize the lesion. In our experience, this complication has not occurred with plugs that are 5 or 6 mm in diameter.
  - The donor harvester is inserted to a depth of 15 mm.
  - The lesion is provisionally fixed at the site where one of the OATS plugs will be inserted to increase stability during the insertion of the initial OATS plug.
- Osteochondral autograft bone plugs are then placed into the lesion using the osteochondral autograft transfer system (OATS) system (Arthrex, Naples, FL).
- Osteochondral plugs are placed at even intervals to achieve adequate fixation of the lesion (Fig. 55-7C and D).
- If additional compression is desired, a headless compression screw or countersunk mini-fragment screw can be used to supplement the OATS fixation.

Pearls

- For lesions that are mobile (locked door, trap door), a no. 15 blade knife can be used to take down part of the lesion so that it can be hinged open for improved access during arthroscopy.
- Care should be taken not to remove normal bone on the lesion or within the crater during debridement.
- Intact articular cartilage that acts as a hinge for the fragment should be preserved to assist in reduction and improve stability of the fragment.
- If an anatomic reduction is not possible during arthroscopy, open reduction should be performed.
- Loose bodies often are hypertrophied, and the subchondral bone can undergo metaplasia,[8] resulting in a purely chondral fragment. If the cartilage is not deteriorated, the fragment can be reshaped with a no. 15 blade knife and fixed with bioabsorbable nails, OATS plugs, or metal screws.[9]
- During drilling, provisional fixation, and final fixation, fluoroscopy should be used to avoid damaging the femoral physis.

References

1. Carey JL, Wall EJ, Grimm NL, et al. Novel arthroscopic classification of osteochondritis dissecans of the knee. *Am J Sports Med.* 2016;44(7):1694-1698.
2. Twyman RS, Desai K, Aichroth PM. Osteochondritis dissecans of the knee. A long-term study. *J Bone Joint Surg (Br).* 1991;73(3):461-464.
3. Anderson AF, Lipscomb AB, Coulam C. Antegrade curettement, bone grafting and pinning of osteochondritis dissecans in the skeletally mature knee. *Am J Sports Med.* 1990;18(3):254-261.
4. Aichroth P. Osteochondral fractures and their relationship to osteochondritis dissecans of the knee. An experimental study in animals. *J Bone Joint Surg (Br).* 1971;53(3):448-454.
5. Oldstad K, Hendrickson EH, Ekman S, et al. Local morphological response of the distal femoral articular-epiphyseal cartilage complex of young foals to surgical stab incision and potential relevance to cartilage injury and repair in children. *Cartilage.* 2013;4(3):239-248.

6. Toth F, David FH, LaFonde E, et al. In vivo visualization using MRI T_2 mapping of induced osteochondritis and osteochondritis dissecans lesions in goats undergoing controlled exercise. *J Orthop Res.* 2017;35(4):868-875.
7. Ytrehus B, Grindflek E, Teige J, et al. Experimental ischemia of porcine growth cartilage produces lesions of osteochondrosis. *J Orthop Res.* 2004;22(6):1201-1209.
8. Uozumi H, Sugita T, Aizawa T, et al. Histologic findings and possible causes of osteochondritis dissecans of the knee. *Am J Sports Med.* 2009;37(10):2003-2008.
9. Anderson CN, Magnussen RA, Block JJ, et al. Operative fixation of chondral loose bodies in osteochondritis dissecans in the knee: a report of 5 cases. *Orthop J Sports Med.* 2013;1(2):232596713496546.

Chapter 56
Arthroscopic Microfracture of Osteochondritis Dissecans Lesions of the Knee

THOMAS R. CARTER
MATTHEW BROWN

Sterile Instruments/Equipment

- Arthroscopic instrumentation
- Probe
- Wireless driver/drill
- 0.062-in Kirschner wire
- Biocompression screw/chondral dart

Preoperative Preparation

- Radiograph suggesting OCD lesion (Fig. 56-1).

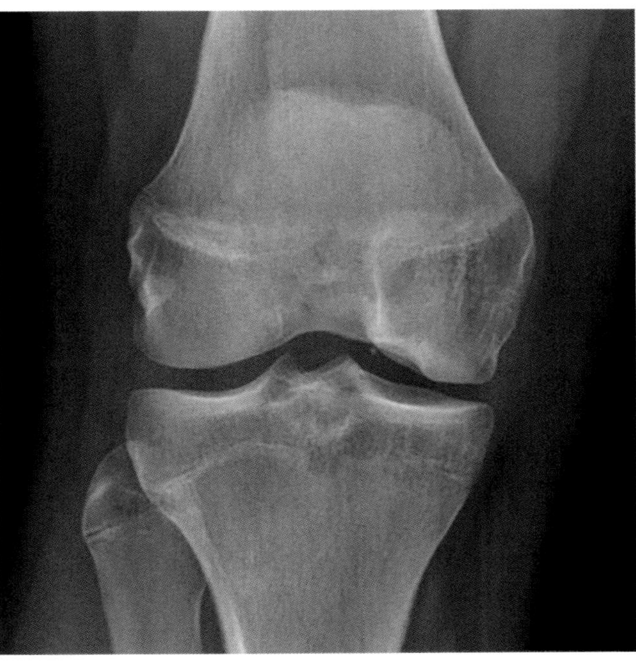

Figure 56-1 | Radiograph demonstrating medial femoral condylar OCD lesion of the right knee.

- MRI demonstrating OCD lesion (Fig. 56-2).
- Treatment plans for OCD lesions may change based on intraoperative findings (Fig. 56-3).

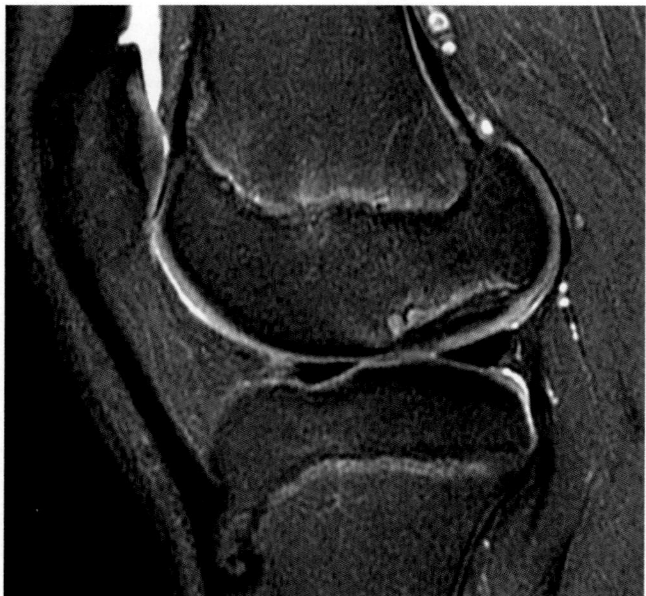

Figure 56-2 | MRI demonstrating lateral femoral condylar OCD lesion.

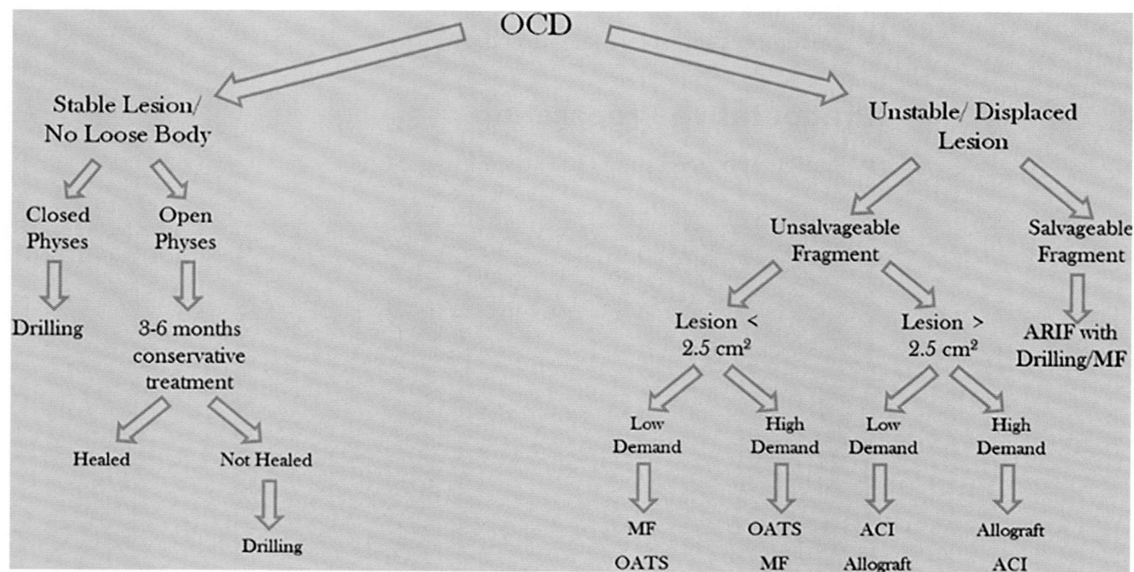

Figure 56-3 | Flow sheet demonstrating options for OCD lesions. (From Erickson BJ, Chalmers PN, Yanke AB, et al. Surgical management of osteochondritis dissecans of the knee. *Curr Rev Musculoskelet Med.* 2013;6:102-114.)

Positioning

- The patient is placed supine on a table with the foot of the table dropped.
- A tourniquet is placed on the operative leg but is used only if needed.
- If transarticular (antegrade) drilling is to be done, the leg holder is positioned similar to the position used for anteromedial anterior cruciate ligament (ACL) portal drilling to enable flexion and to reach posterior lesions (Fig. 56-4).

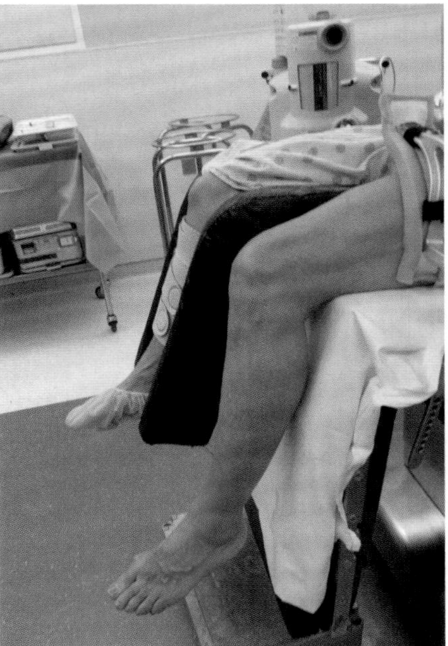

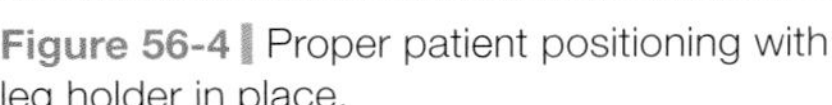

Figure 56-4 | Proper patient positioning with leg holder in place.

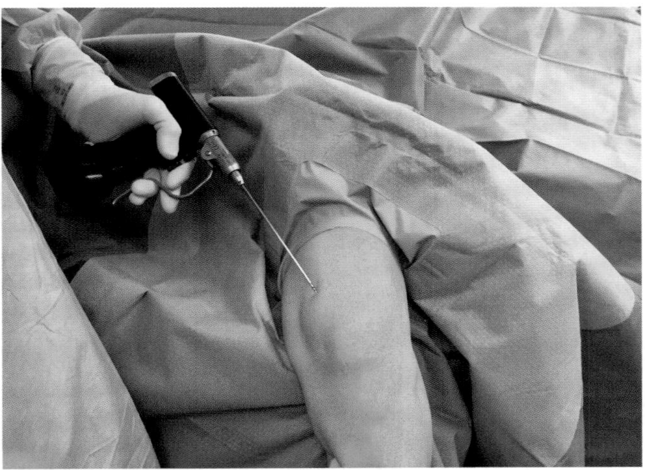

Figure 56-5 | Ensure sufficient room for retrograde drilling.

- If retrograde drilling is being considered, the nonoperative leg is placed in a position similar to that used for posterior cruciate ligament (PCL) repair.
- This provides adequate room to reach the lesion and enables C-arm use for localizing the lesion (Fig. 56-5).

Surgical Approach

- The initial portal should be opposite the lesion to be treated.
- A working portal is made second, with spinal needle localization to aid in perpendicular portal placement relative to the lesion (Fig. 56-6).
- The entire knee is inspected for other pathology before treating the OCD lesion.

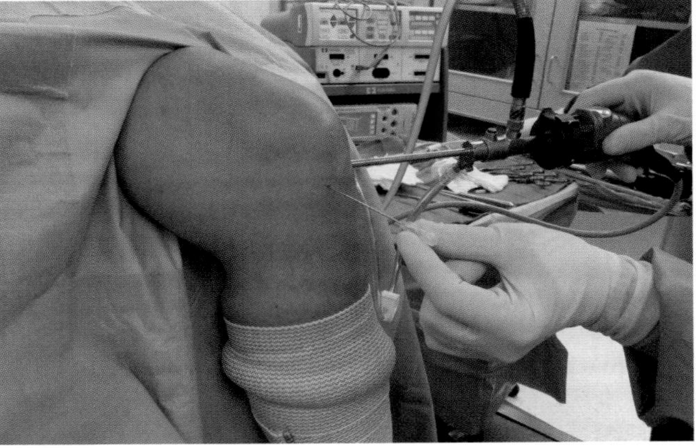

Figure 56-6 | Initial portal opposite the lesion to be treated, with needle localization of second portal.

Fixation Techniques

- The lesion is inspected and probed to evaluate chondral integrity (Fig. 56-7).

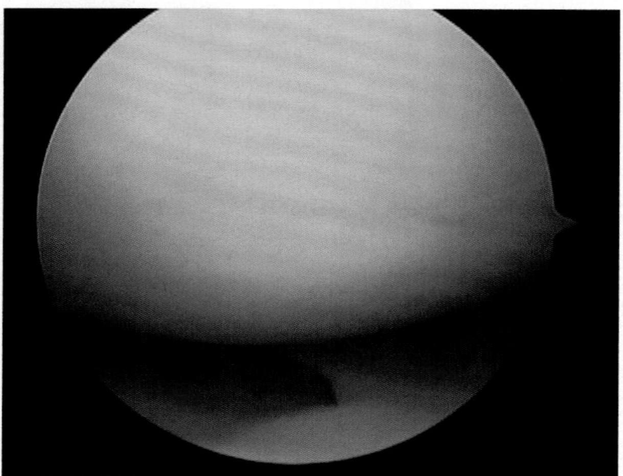

Figure 56-7 | Arthroscopic lesion inspection.

- If the lesion is stable, a 0.062-in Kirchner wire is drilled into the lesion to promote bleeding.
- The avascular bone is perforated, with spacing ~3 to 4 mm apart (6 to 10 holes depending on lesion size).
- If articular cartilage is intact but there is a concern about stability, a biocompression screw or chondral dart can be used for support (Fig. 56-8).
- If the lesion is unstable, the base needs to be debrided of the fibrous layer, the bone drilled, and the osteochondral fragment replaced and secured.

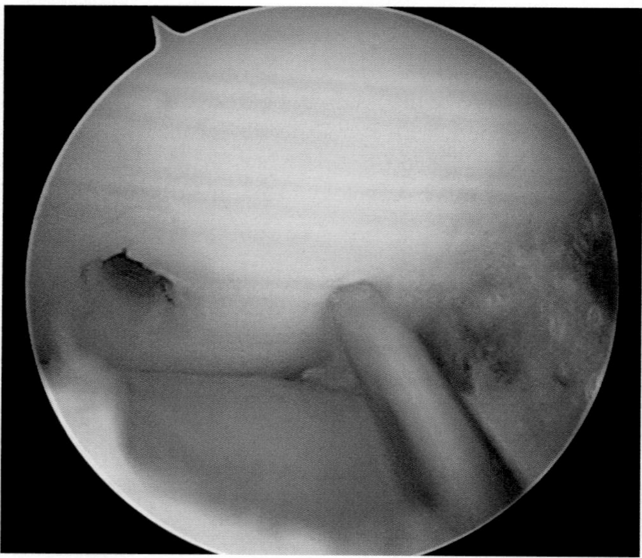

Figure 56-8 | Lesion secured and drilled transarticularly.

Suggested Readings

Erickson BJ, Chalmers PN, Yanke AB, et al. Surgical management of osteochondritis dissecans of the knee. *Curr Rev Musculoskelet Med.* 2013;6:102-114.

Kocher MS, Micheli LJ, Yaniv M, et al. Functional and radiographic outcome of juvenile osteochondritis dissecans of the knee treated with transarticular arthroscopic drilling. *Am J Sports Med.* 2001;29:562-566.

Shea KG, Carey JL, Brown GA, et al. Management of osteochondritis dissecans of the femoral condyle. *J Am Acad Orthop Surg.* 2016;24:e102-e104.

Chapter 57

Open Osteochondral Autograft Transfer System (OATS)/Mosaicplasty for Osteochondral Lesions of the Knee

THOMAS J. GILL

Indications

- Symptomatic grade III-IV femoral condyle defect 1-4 cm^2
- MRI demonstrates focal osteochondral defect of the weight-bearing femoral condyle, with mild associated subchondral femoral condylar edema as seen on sagittal image (Fig. 57-1).
- Cartilage fragment displaced toward intercondylar notch.
- First- or second-line treatment
- High physical demand patient

Equipment

- Standard operating room table
- Lateral post at level of distal femoral metaphysis
- Tourniquet (usually 34″ cuff)
- U-drape 1015
- Bovie
- Disposable OATS kit (plugs come in 6, 8, and 10 mm)
- Z retractors
- Rongeur
- Curette
- Microfracture pick set
- Open knee retractor kit

Prep/Drape

1. Well-padded thigh tourniquet as high as possible, 1015 U-drape (Fig. 57-2A).
2. Supine with lateral leg post (Fig. 57-2B).
3. Horizontal post or "bump" at the level of the mid-tibial diaphysis to hold the knee in hyperflexion (more than 90 degrees) when the knee is flexed after draping and the foot placed just proximal to the post (Fig. 57-2C).
4. Prepare thigh, knee, and ankle.
5. Draping: half sheet down, half sheet up, and blue U-drape. Foot in blue impervious stockinette. Leg wrapped with Coban (3M, St. Paul, MN). Lower extremity drape.

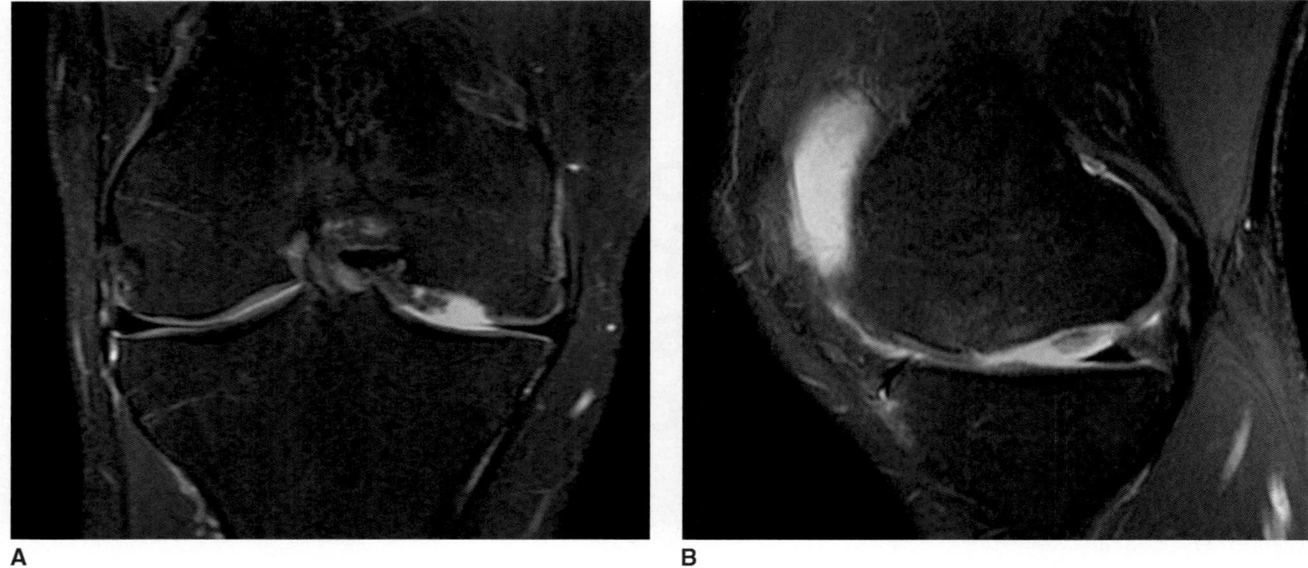

Figure 57-1 | A. Coronal T_2-weighted fat-suppressed. B. Sagittal T_2-weighted fat-suppressed.

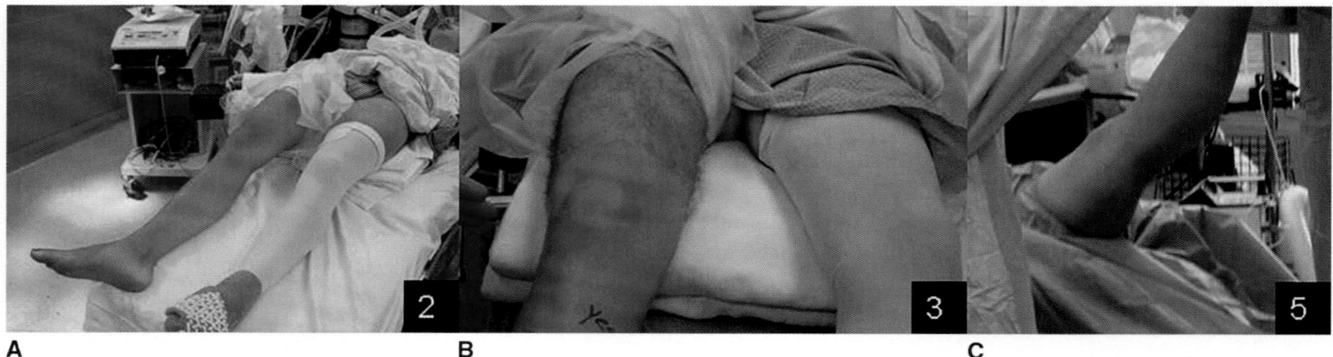

Figure 57-2 | A. Well-padded thigh tourniquet as high as possible, 1015 U-drape. B. Supine with lateral leg post. C. Horizontal post or "bump" at the level of the mid-tibial diaphysis to hold the knee in hyperflexion (more than 90 degrees) when the knee is flexed after draping and the foot placed just proximal to the post.

Technique

Surgical Approach

- Knee arthroscopy is performed first to evaluate the chondral lesion, confirm planned method of treatment, and treat associated pathology such as a meniscus tear or removal of a loose body (Fig. 57-3).
- Decision is made whether to perform the OATS procedure arthroscopically vs open technique.
- My preference for any lesion over 8 mm is to perform an open approach. The surgical outcome is highly dependent on a near-perfect reconstruction of the convex surface of the femoral condyle and articular surface, and I believe this is best accomplished with an open approach.
- After arthroscopy is complete, the limb is exsanguinated, and the thigh tourniquet is inflated to 280 mm Hg.
- Knee is placed in 90-100 degrees of flexion.
- A 3- to 4-cm incision is made for a medial parapatellar approach (medial inferior pole of the patella coursing distally) with a no. 15 blade. Care is taken to maintain well-vascularized skin flaps.

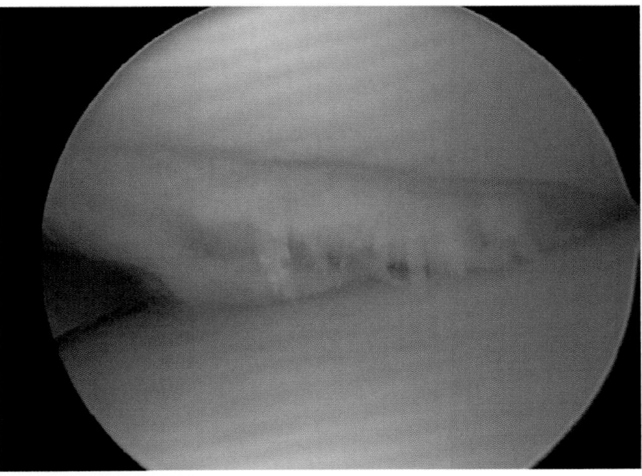

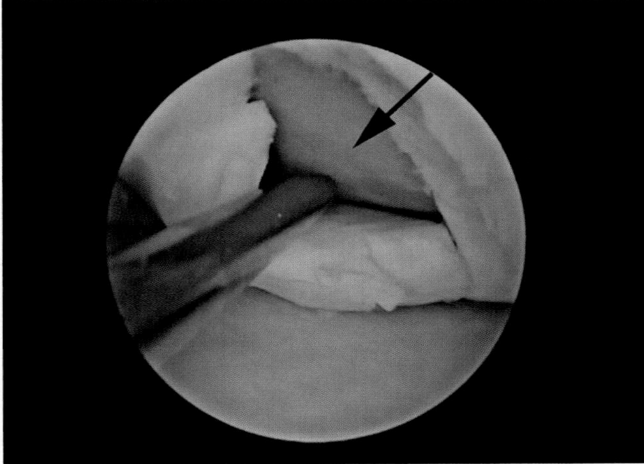

Figure 57-3 ‖ Knee arthroscopy is performed first to evaluate the chondral lesion, confirm planned method of treatment, and treat associated pathology such as a meniscus tear or removal of a loose body.

- Z retractors are used in the intercondylar notch and deep to the medial collateral ligament (MCL) (Fig. 57-4).
- The fat pad is excised anteriorly if necessary to expose the femoral condyle.

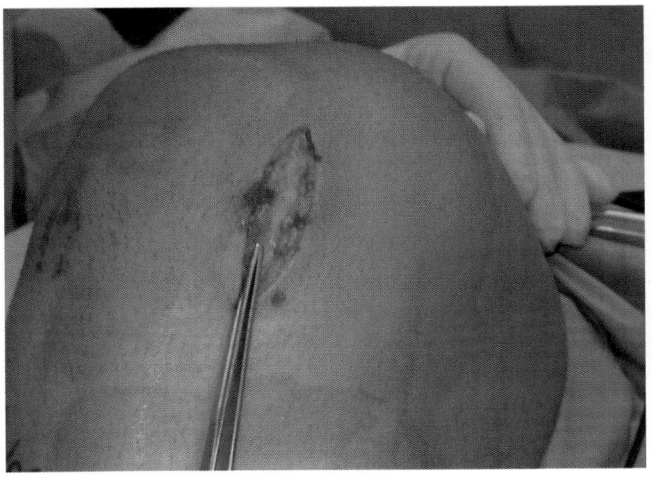

A

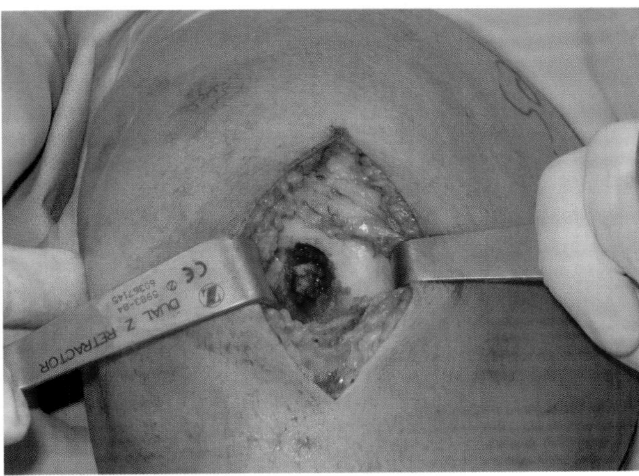

B

Figure 57-4 ‖ A. Medial-based incision. **B.** Right knee medial femoral condyle.

Evaluation and Preparation of the Lesion

- The knee is maintained in 60-90 degrees of flexion.
- A curette and knife are used to produce a sharp border to the defect.
- The enclosed tamp in the OATS kit is used to plan how many donor plugs will be needed to reconstruct the defect.
- Disposable OATS kit (Arthrex, Naples, FL) (Fig. 57-5).
- First, a plug is removed from the chondral defect with the white recipient harvester (6, 8, or 10 mm).
  - Must be absolutely perpendicular
  - The plug is tapped into the medial femoral epicondyle:
    - 15 mm for chondral defect
    - 20 mm for osteochondral defects

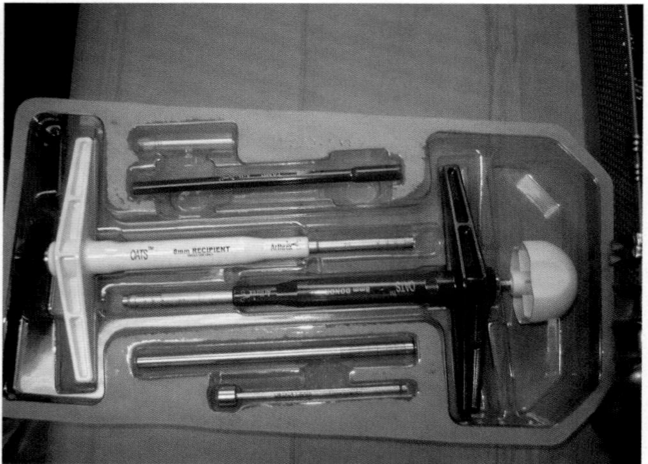

Figure 57-5 | Disposable OATS kit. (Arthrex, Naples, FL.)

- Quick rotational turns are used to disconnect the plug for complete removal (Fig. 57-6A).
- The plug is removed and placed in the cup for later use as backfill for donor site (Fig. 57-6B).

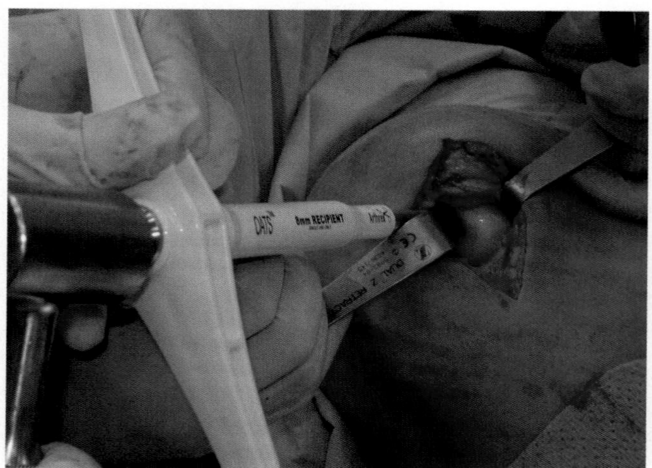

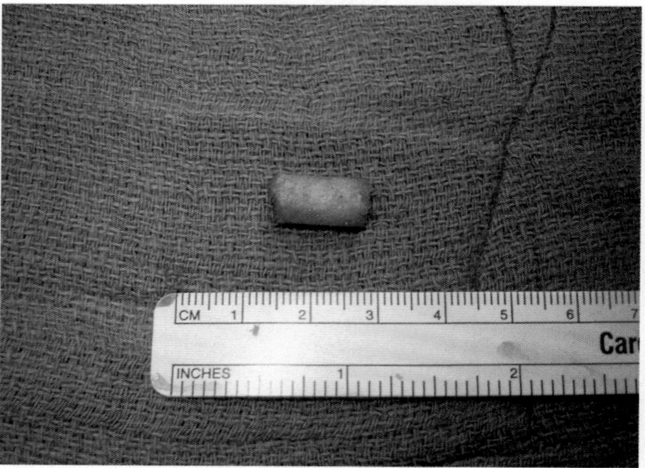

A B

Figure 57-6 | A and **B**. Recipient plug (to be used as backfill for donor site).

- Removal of donor graft:
  - The knee is placed in extension.
  - Recommended order of donor plugs based on articular contact pressure
    - Medial trochlear ridge from distal to proximal
    - Lateral trochlear ridge from distal to proximal
    - Roof of intercondylar notch
    - Sulcus terminalis
  - Donor plug is tapped into place (same distance as recipient).
    - If multiple plugs are taken, removal should start distally and subsequent plugs are taken distal to proximal.
  - Quick turns are used to remove the plug completely in one piece (Fig. 57-7A).
  - The alignment rod is inserted into the recipient site and tamped to the 15-mm depth (Fig. 57-7B).

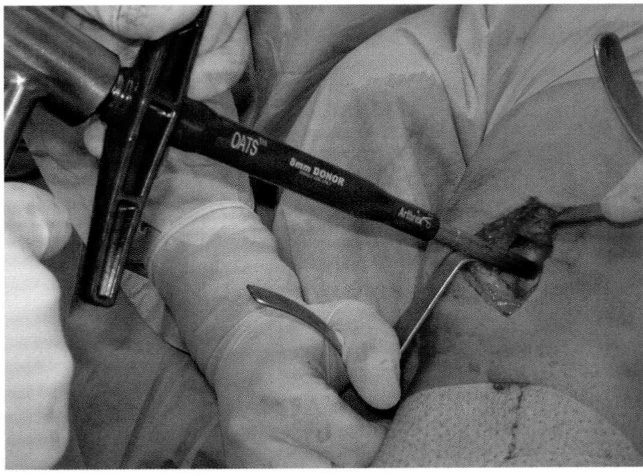

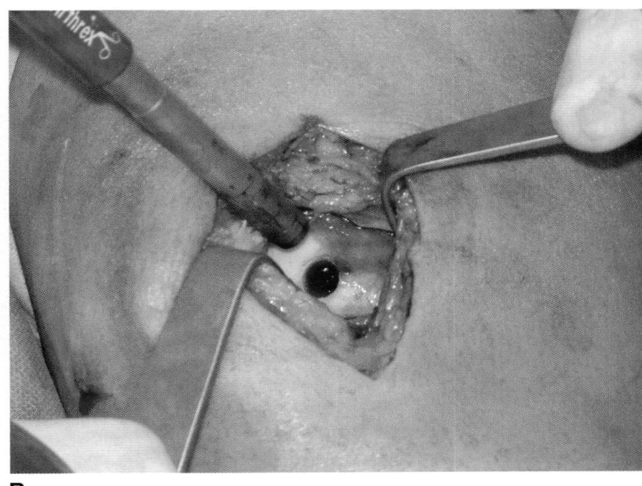

A B

Figure 57-7 | **A.** Quick turns are used to remove the plug completely in one piece. **B.** The alignment rod is inserted into the recipient site and tamped to the 15-mm depth recipient plug (to be used as backfill for donor site).

- Placement of donor plug into the defect:
  - The clear delivery tube is placed on the end of the donor harvester containing the donor plug.
  - The white screw wheel is placed on the donor harvester.
  - The delivery tube is placed into the recipient hole in the defect (making sure to stay perpendicular), and the white knob is turned to advance the plug through the tube (Fig. 57-8).

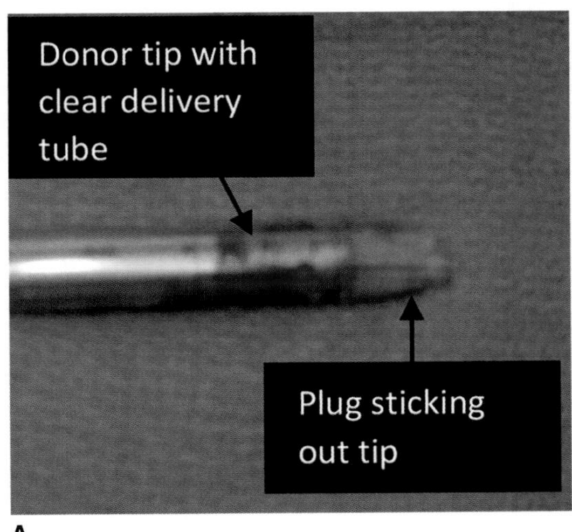

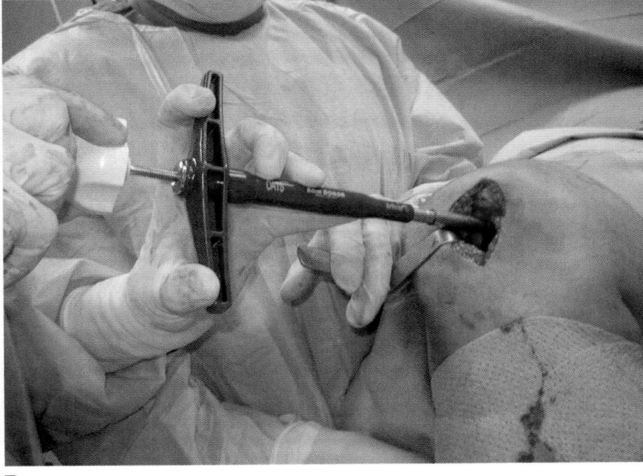

A B

Figure 57-8 | The delivery tube **(A)** is placed into the recipient hole in the defect (making sure to stay perpendicular), and the white knob is turned to advance the plug through the tube **(B)**.

- The insertion device is removed.
- The plug is gently tapped fully in with the blue tamp (must be lined up perpendicular to defect). The blue tamp is placed halfway onto the plug and halfway onto the surrounding native articular surface to prevent over- or underadvancement of the plug.
  - Initially, it is better to err on the side of being too proud, but when finalizing later after all plugs have gone in, it is better to err on side of being too countersunk, or the plugs will experience too much pressure and be more likely to fail (Fig. 57-9).

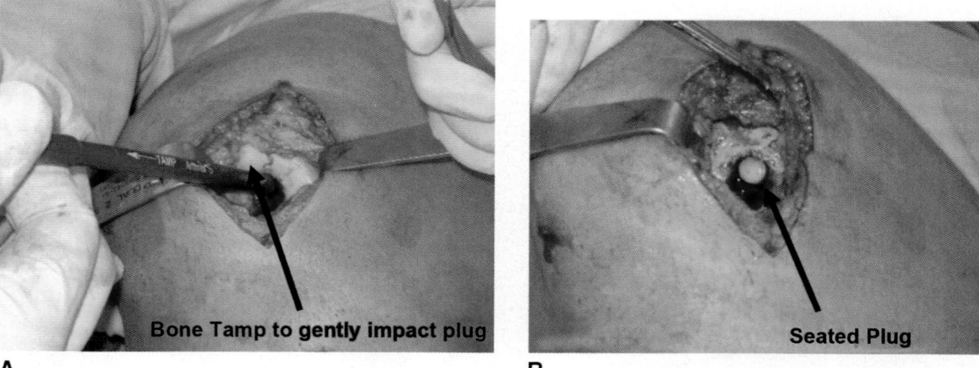

Figure 57-9 | **A.** Bone tamp to gently impact plug. **B.** Seated plug.

- These steps are repeated as needed, going distal to proximal taking new donor plugs.
  - The alignment rod is used if needed to tap holes for plugs.
- A small 1-mm wall of bone is left between plugs to improve donor plug stability in a multiplug, mosaicplasty construct (Fig. 57-10).

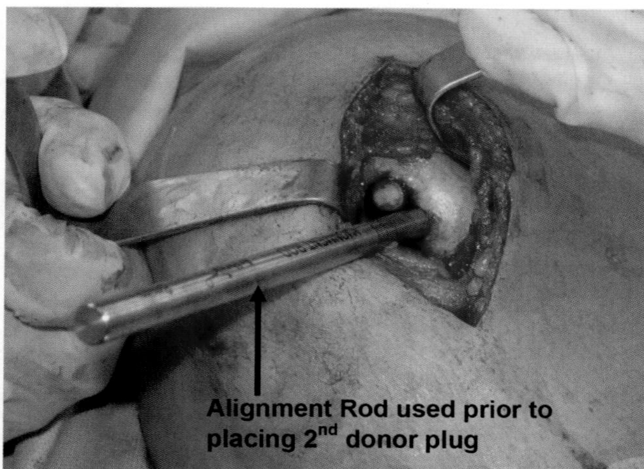

Figure 57-10 | Alignment rod used prior to placing second donor plug.

- The plugs harvested by the recipient harvester are placed into the donor holes as backfill to decrease chance of a postoperative hemarthrosis (Fig. 57-11).
  - Once the perpendicular position of the plug is verified, it is tamped down.

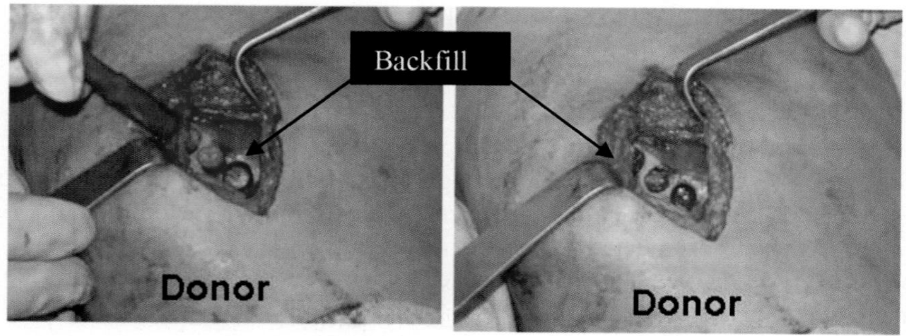

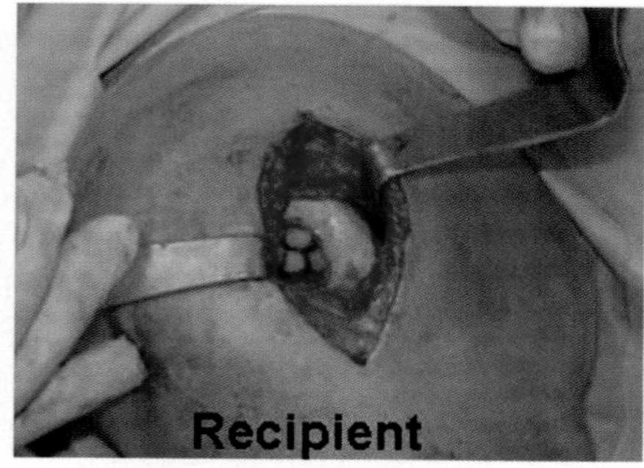

Figure 57-11 | The plugs harvested by the recipient harvester are placed into the donor holes as backfill to decrease chance of a postoperative hemarthrosis.

- The leg is placed in slight hyperextension to reduce the plugs, tamping them down more if needed.
- Running a finger over the defect can confirm plug reduction and recreation of convex articular surface (Fig. 57-12).
  - It is better to err on the side of being too countersunk.

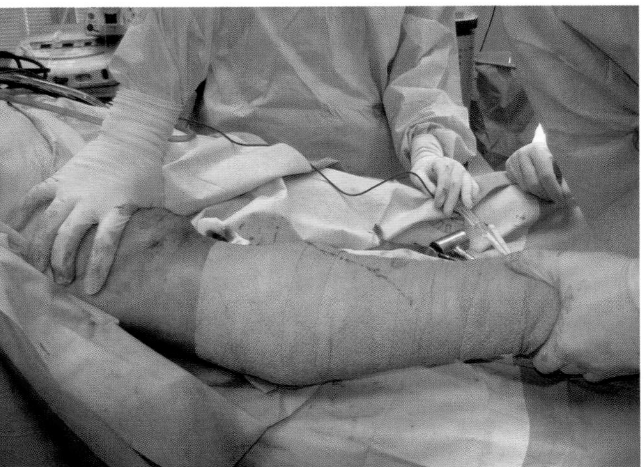

Figure 57-12 | Running a finger over the defect can confirm plug reduction and recreation of convex articular surface.

Closure:

- The joint capsule is closed with no. 1 Vicryl suture.
- 2-0 Vicryl is used for subcutaneous tissue.
- 3-0 Prolene is used for skin.

Post-op

- Cryocuff
- Continuous passive motion is used for 2 weeks (at least 8 hours/day).
- For patellar and trochlear groove lesions, a 0-30 degree brace is used for 6 weeks, with crutches as needed (WBAT).
- For femoral condyle defects, no brace is used, but crutches for 6 weeks of partial weight bearing.
- Limited quadriceps range-of-motion exercises (quad sets, heel prop, heel slide, ankle pumps) are begun at 0-2 weeks.
- A strengthening program is begun at 2-6 weeks.
- At 8 weeks, the brace is discontinued and further strengthening is implemented.
- Return to full activity as tolerated is allowed at 12 weeks.

Chapter 58
Osteochondral Allograft Transplant for Osteochondritis Dissecans Lesions of the Knee

ERIC J. COTTER
DREW A. LANSDOWN
RACHEL M. FRANK
BRIAN J. COLE

Background

- Osteochondritis dissecans (OCD) is a disorder primarily affecting subchondral bone, leading to osseous collapse and destabilization of overlying articular cartilage (Fig. 58-1).[1,2]
- OCD may be present in many joints but most commonly affects the medial femoral condyle of the knee (70% of cases).[3,4]
- While OCD may affect both pediatric and adult populations, the incidence of disease is higher in children and adolescents (9.5 per 100,000 persons age 6 to 19 per year).[5]
- Osteochondral allograft (OCA) transplantation has been shown to be an effective knee joint preservation procedure for OCD of the knee,[6] with high patient satisfaction and low rates of graft failure.[7]

Clinical Indications

- Isolated, unipolar symptomatic chondral or osteochondral lesions of the femoral condyle, trochlea, or patella
- Bipolar lesions of the patellofemoral compartment also can be treated with OCA, though outcomes are less predictable.
- Young (chronologically <50 years of age), high physical demand patients
- Lesion area is typically >10 mm^2.
- Body mass index (BMI) < 35, neutral alignment, and meniscal status are modifiable risk factors that should be considered when deciding if OCA is appropriate.
  - OCA can be successfully performed concomitantly with osteotomy, meniscal procedure, or ligament repair/reconstruction.[6]
- Many patients with symptomatic lesions can be successfully treated with nonoperative measures including injections, physical therapy, and activity modification.
  - OCA can be used as a primary option for patients who remain or become symptomatic and in whom conservative measures have failed. In addition, OCA is a viable option for patients who have failed prior surgical intervention such as arthroscopic debridement, OCA fixation, or fragment excision.[8,9]

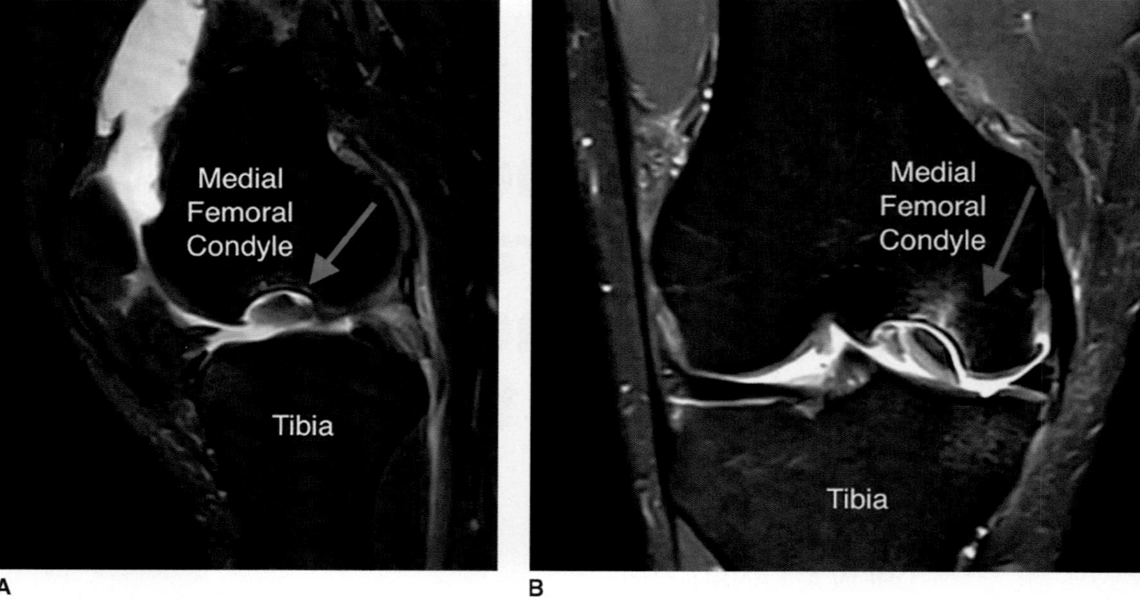

Figure 58-1 | Magnetic resonance images demonstrating an OCD lesion of the medial femoral condyle as denoted by the red arrows in a 31-year-old male. **A.** A sagittal plane, fat-suppressed T2-weighted image; **(B)** coronal plane, fat-suppressed T2-weighted MRI image.

Sterile Instruments/Equipment

- Well-padded tourniquet
- A press-fit technique is commonly used for most contained defects of the femoral condyles by the senior author using commercially available systems (Allograft OATS, Arthrex, Naples, FL) (Fig. 58-2).

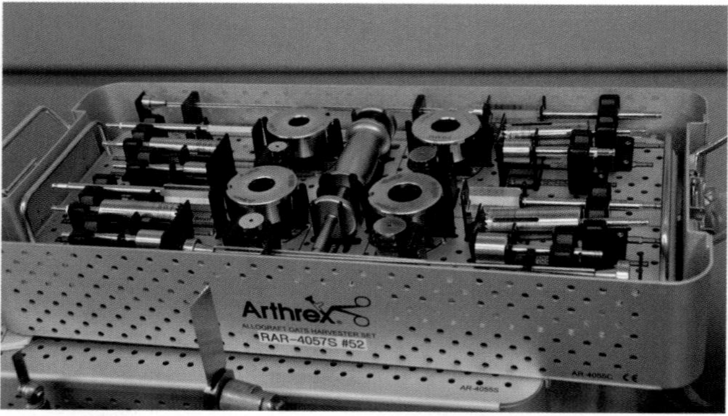

Figure 58-2 | Allograft OATS Harvest Set. (Arthrex Inc., Naples, FL.)

- Instrument and implant considerations (many of the following may not be required and decision-making is based on surgeon experience and defect-specific variables)
  - Cannulated cylindrical sizing guides (15, 18, 20, 25, 30, and 35 mm)
  - Cannulated cutting bore
  - Allograft workstation
  - Donor harvester
- Arthroscopy tower and arthroscope
  - Arthroscopic shaver may be necessary.
- Z retractors (2), large rakes (2), and/or Hohmann retractors (2)
- No. 15 blade scalpel
- Small ruler
- Sterile marking pen
- Hemostat
- Room temperature saline
- Guidewire

- Pulsatile lavage of combination saline and CO_2 (CarboJet, Kinamed, Camarillo, CA)
- Oscillating saw
- Rongeur
- Hand tamp and mallet
- Metallic headless screws (Acutrak 2 mini screws, Acumed, Hillsboro, OR), Bio-Compression screws (Arthrex, Naples, FL), Orthosorb pins (Depuy, Inc., Warsaw, IN)

Positioning

- The patient can be positioned supine, or the limb can be placed in a standard anterior cruciate ligament (ACL) leg holder (Fig. 58-3).

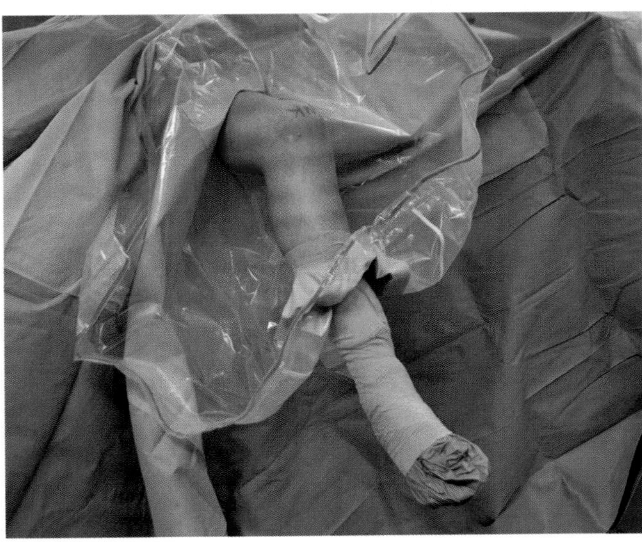

Figure 58-3 | Right knee is flexed to ~80 degrees in an arthroscopic knee holder.

  - For simple OCA transplantation, the patient is supine with the leg placed straight on the bed.
  - For complex OCA transplantation with concomitant procedures, we may use the ACL leg positioner such that the knee is draped free at 90 degrees of flexion allowing circumferential access.
- A well-padded thigh tourniquet is used for the duration of the case and deflated at the end of the case before closure to ensure hemostasis.
- The operative extremity is prepared and draped for a standard anterior approach to the knee.

Portals/Exposure

- This procedure typically is performed through a small parapatellar arthrotomy using a central incision.
  - In general, the arthrotomy is made on the ipsilateral side to the pathology, though this may vary based on the optimal angle to allow a perpendicular approach to the osteochondral lesion.
  - On the medial side, a vastus-sparing approach is preferred.
  - On the lateral side, we prefer to release the lateral retinaculum for exposure, which can largely be left open at the conclusion of the case.
  - The arthrotomy can be extended proximally or distally to improve exposure depending on lesion size and location.
  - The arthrotomy can be extended distally to accommodate a high tibial osteotomy (HTO) when indicated for a medial femoral condyle OCA.
- Z retractors or Hohmann retractors are used to (a) retract soft tissue and (b) retract the patella by placing a retractor in the notch (Fig. 58-4).
- The knee can then be flexed to optimally expose the lesion.
- A lateral approach is preferred for patellofemoral lesions with eversion of the patella to ~90 degrees or more when needed. When concomitant tibial tubercle osteotomy is performed, we do this first to improve visualization but do not elevate the entire shingle of bone or disrupt the fat pad in an effort to minimize morbidity.
- For the remainder of the procedure, the flexion angle is kept the same by the leg positioner.

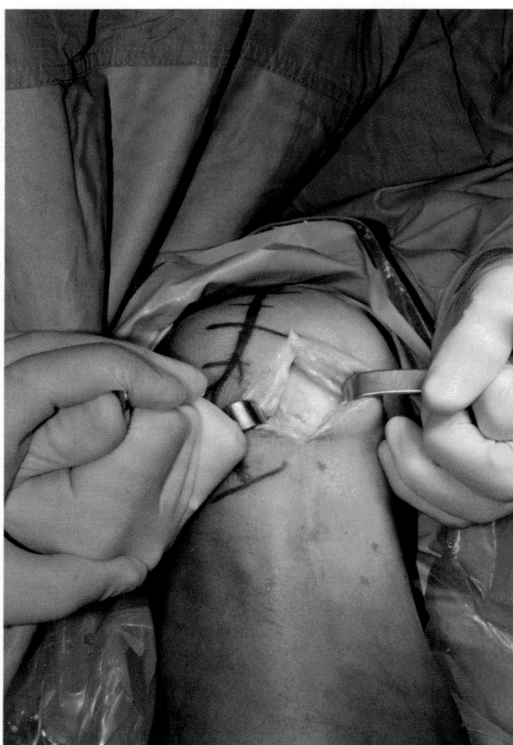

Figure 58-4 | Soft tissue retraction with two Z retractors to allow visualization of a medial femoral condylar defect.

Procedure

Step 1: Exposure

- Before induction of anesthesia, an appropriate-sized OCA is confirmed to be physically on site.
- Before the arthrotomy is made, we prefer to conduct a diagnostic arthroscopy to assess for concomitant pathology and to confirm that the chondral defect is suitable for allograft implantation.
  - If a prior staging arthroscopy was performed recently, the diagnostic arthroscopy can be eliminated at the time of osteochondral allografting.
  - If concomitant pathologies are present, such as ligamentous injury requiring reconstruction, meniscal deficiency requiring meniscus debridement, repair or transplantation, and/or malalignment necessitating osteotomy, these procedures are performed before OCA transplantation.
- Following arthroscopy, a mini-arthrotomy as described previously is made in the standard fashion, exposing the defect along the medial or lateral femoral condyle (Fig. 58-5).

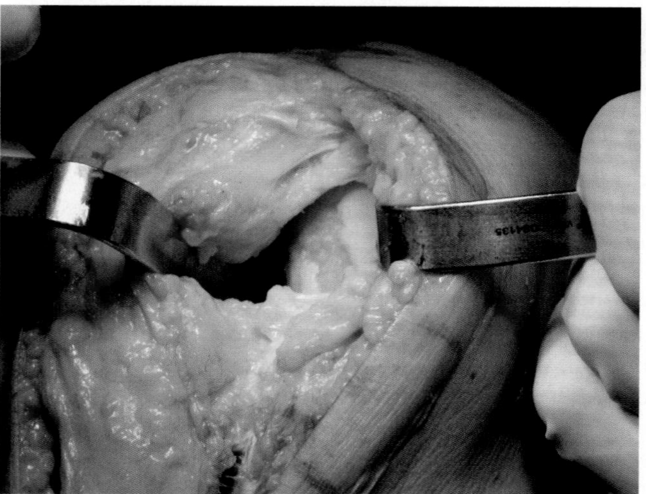

Figure 58-5 | Knee flexion to ~70 to 110 degrees, exposing the osteochondral lesion.

- The allograft is opened (Fig. 58-6) and soaked in room temperature sterile saline on the back table. Sudden changes in temperature may be chondrotoxic and should be avoided.

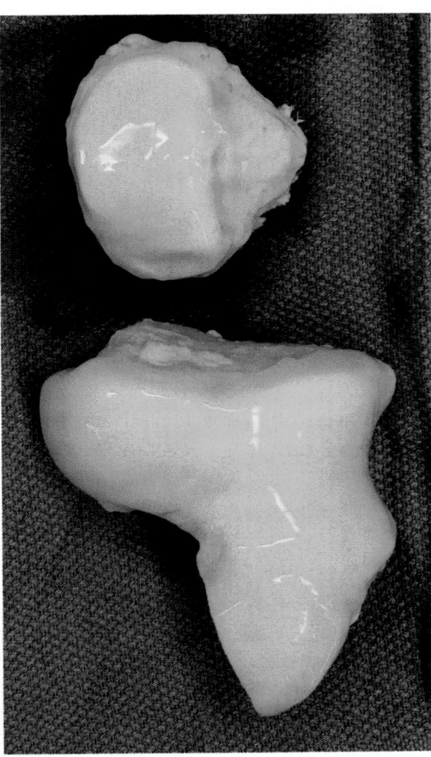

Figure 58-6 | A donor osteochondral allograft hemicondyle and patella.

Step 2: Preparation of the Cartilage Lesion

- The lesion is inspected to define the margins, with any adjacent damaged cartilage debrided to allow accurate sizing of the lesion.
  - The shape of the lesion will determine if a single cylindrical plug or multiple plugs are necessary for larger, oblique lesions. Alternatively, newer instrumentation (Bio-Uni, Arthrex, Naples, FL) can be used for long oblique lesions of the medial femoral condyle.
  - We prefer a press-fit technique rather than a customized hand-cut shell graft.
- Any number of allograft preparation and implantation trays can be used. The following steps describe preparation of the OCD bed and allograft with one of these available systems.
  - The allograft OATS set (Arthrex, Naples, FL) allows allograft implants of 15, 18, 20, 25, 30, and 35 mm.
- Different cannulated, cylindrical sizing guides are placed over the lesion to estimate the appropriate size of the allograft.
  - It is essential to place the sizing guide perpendicular to and flush with the surrounding articular cartilage to ensure congruity.
  - It is better to slightly oversize the lesion than leave marginal quality tissue on its perimeter.
- Once the appropriate size is determined, a cannulated sizer is placed in the center of the lesion so that the sizer completely covers the lesion.
- The same cylindrical sizer is placed perpendicular on the donor condyle to ensure that a plug with similar topographical anatomy can be harvested.
  - A marking pen is used to mark its location along with the 12 o'clock position.
- Once the donor knee is found to be of acceptable size, the cannulated sizer is placed back over the recipient lesion, and a 2.4-mm guide pin is inserted perpendicular through it to a depth of at least 3 cm (Fig. 58-7).
- The sizer is removed leaving the guide pin, and a cannulated cutting bore of the same size is placed on the guide pin. The cutting bore is used to score the peripheral cartilage and a portion of the subchondral bone.

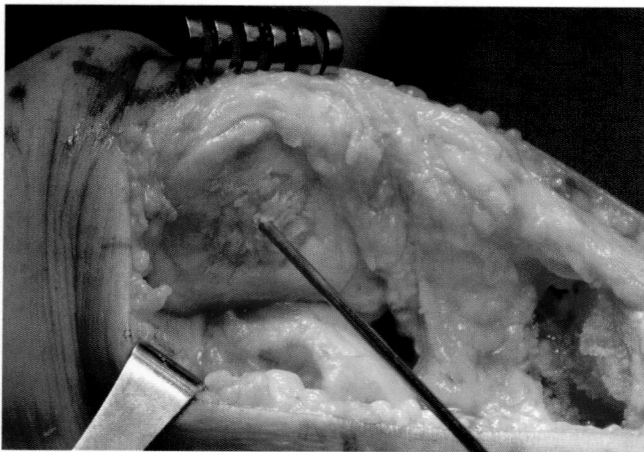

Figure 58-7 | A 2.4-mm guide pin placed into the center of the patellar osteochondral defect.

- A cannulated reamer of the same size is placed on the guide pin and used to create a cylindrical defect in the recipient bone of a depth of 6 to 8 mm (Figs. 58-8 to 58-10).

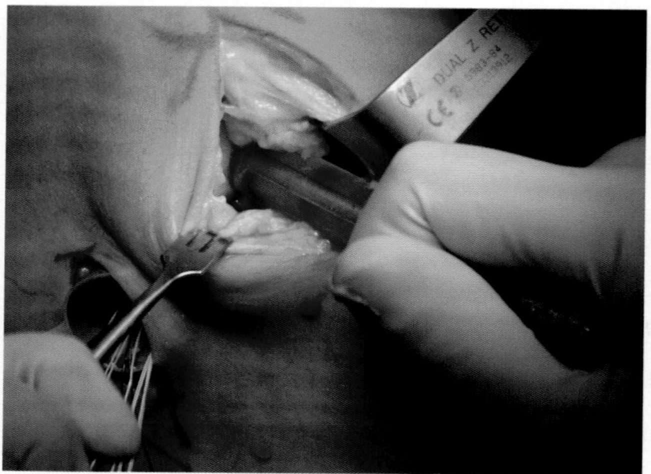

Figure 58-8 | A cylindrical sizing guide placed over the 2.4-mm guide pin to appropriate size of a lateral femoral condyle defect.

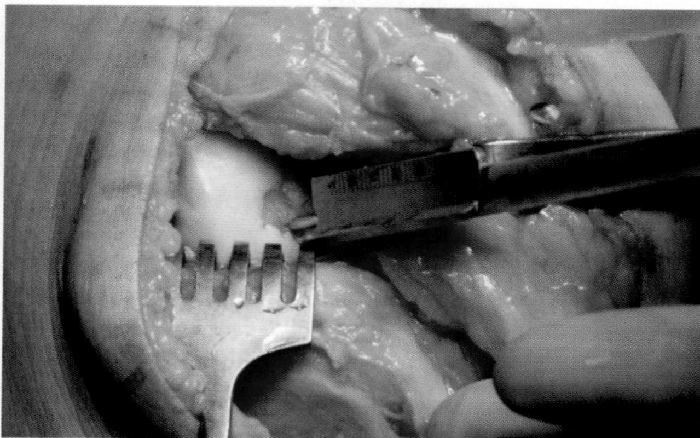

Figure 58-9 | A cannulated reamer used to ream a lateral femoral condylar lesion.

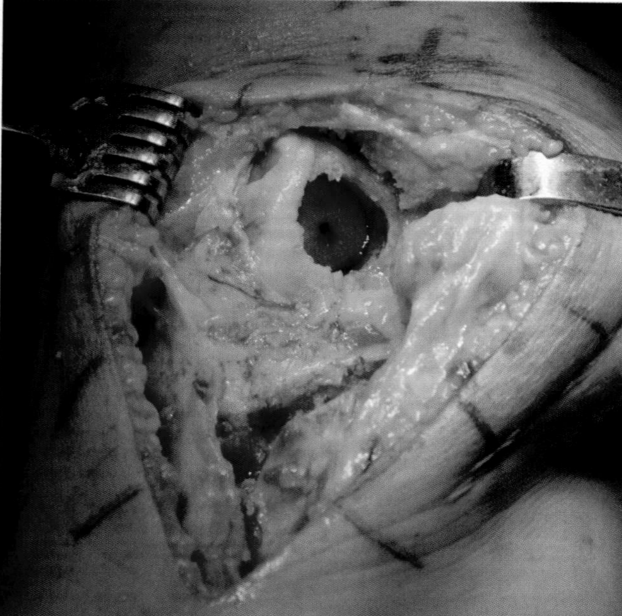

Figure 58-10 | A lateral trochlear defect reamed to a depth of ~6 to 8 mm.

- Cold saline irrigation is used during reaming to decrease the risk of thermal necrosis to the surrounding cartilage.
- The reamer and guidewires are both removed.
- Precise depth measurements are taken of the four quadrants on the recipient lesion (12, 3, 6, and 9 o'clock) using a small paper ruler held with a hemostat (Fig. 58-11).

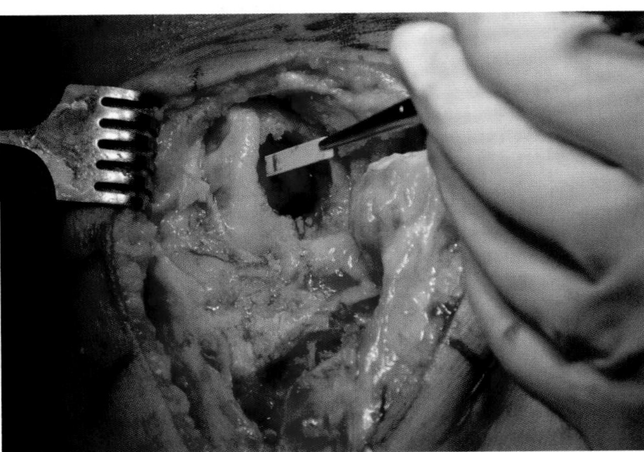

Figure 58-11 | A small ruler attached to a hemostat used to measure depth at 3, 6, 9, and 12 o'clock.

- A fresh no. 15 blade is used to remove any loose or frayed cartilage on the perimeter of the lesion.
- A small Kirschner wire (K-wire) can be used to drill multiple nonconfluent holes in the bed of the socket to induce further bleeding for osseous healing.
- Autologous bone graft can be used from the reamings to graft any cystic change exposed during the reaming.

Step 2 Pearls

- In some OCD lesions, the graft may not be completely contained within the defect and may need additional fixation such as a biocompression screw.
- Maintaining a perfectly perpendicular approach provides the optimal restored surface. If the cannulated guide is not able to reach this position, the flexion angle and varus/valgus position of the knee can be adjusted to improve access.
- Accurate measurements will also lead to a graft that fits well within the created defect. Care should be taken to ensure that the ruler does not bend against the bone, which will alter the measurement.

Step 3: Allograft Preparation

- If a full hemicondyle is received, it may need to be trimmed with a saw to fit on the back table workstation (Fig. 58-12).
- The donor condyle is secured in the workstation using the four screws.
  - Alternatively, if an extra assistant is available, the donor condyle can be held on the table by the assistant while the graft is fashioned.
- The bushing of appropriate size is placed over the graft at the exact position that matches the previously marked 12 o'clock position.

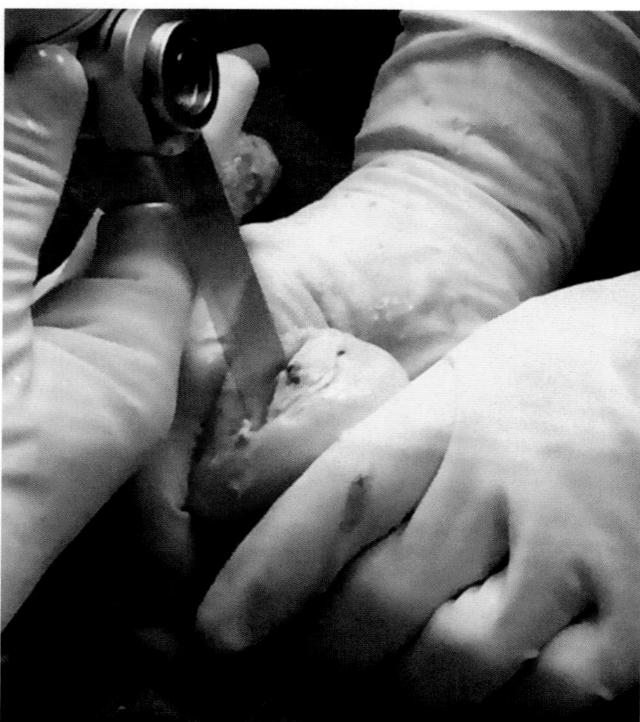

Figure 58-12 | An oscillating saw being used to trim down the donor distal femur.

- The bushing is adjusted three dimensionally so that a sizer placed through the bushing fits directly over the marked spot on the graft. The bushing is secured (Fig. 58-13).

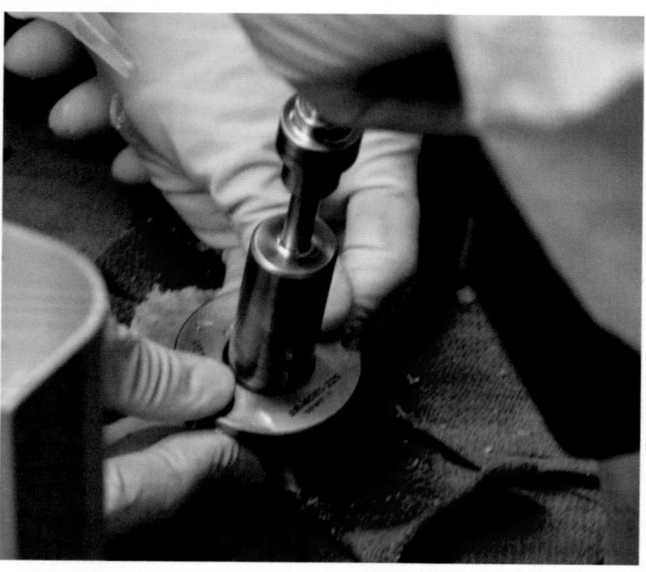

Figure 58-13 | A graft harvester of the appropriate size placed over the bushing and cored through the extent of the donor tissue.

- A donor harvester is used to drill through the entire donor condyle. The graft is then gently extracted (Fig. 58-14).
  - An assistant secures the plug with forceps, taking care to avoid damaging the articular surface.

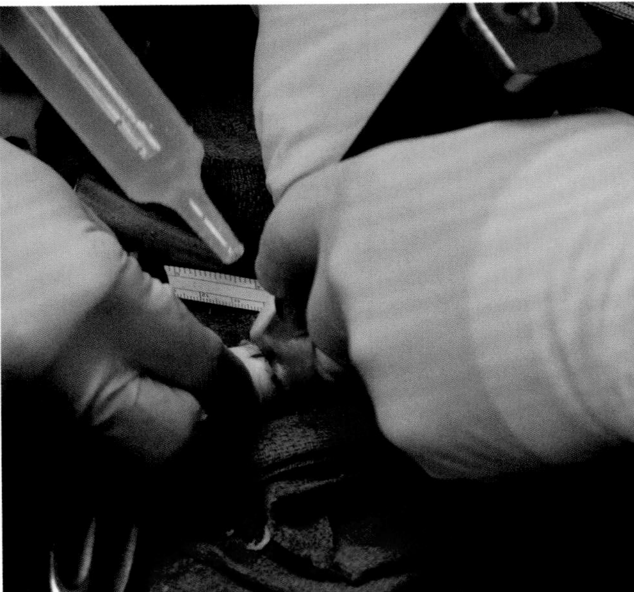

Figure 58-14 | The donor plug being trimmed to ~6 to 8 mm depending on the deepest measurement in the recipient defect.

- The depth measurements previously made in the recipient socket are marked at the four corners of the donor plug taking careful note of 12 o'clock (Fig. 58-15).

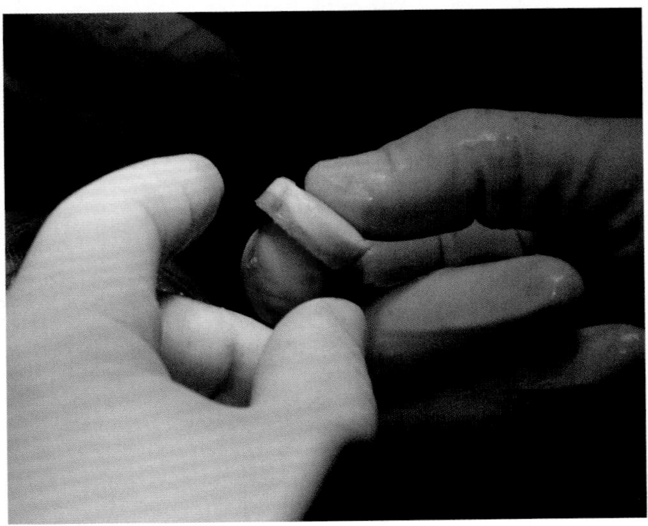

Figure 58-15 | The donor plug being marked at the 12 o'clock position to line up at the 12 o'clock position on the recipient defect.

- The allograft is secured to the holding clamp at the marked positions and trimmed with an oscillating saw.
  - If the four quadrants are of different depths, the saw is used to gently trim subchondral bone to the appropriate depth.

Step 3 Pearls

- Ensuring that the bushing and all instrumentation are perfectly perpendicular is the key point to producing a graft that matches the recipient condyle.
- When marking the depth for trimming the graft, the depths at each quadrant are marked first. Next, a line connecting these can be drawn to plan for the appropriate angle of the cut to reach the appropriate depth at each part of the graft.
- For patellar grafts, the contour of the defect can be especially challenging to match if it involves the vertical ridge. Replicating the appropriate contour will depend on the anatomy of the donor graft and lesion location. The donor patella should be carefully inspected with this in mind to find the optimal location for a graft (or multiple grafts) that will match the topography of the recipient patella.
- Inappropriate trimming of the depth of the donor plug at 3, 6, 9, and 12 o'clock leads to incongruity, with the graft being recessed or sitting too proud relative to the surrounding host.
- Excessive force or a high number of impactions may diminish chondrocyte viability.[10,11]

Step 4: Graft Implantation

- A combination of saline and CO_2 pulsatile lavage is used to remove remaining marrow elements from the donor allograft plug and is applied to the recipient site to remove residual bony debris (Fig. 58-16).[12]
- The graft is gently press fit into the socket, lining up the two 12 o'clock positions on the donor and recipient sides (Fig. 58-17).
- If the graft cannot be fit flush to the surrounding cartilage by hand, a tamp can be used to gently tap the graft in place.

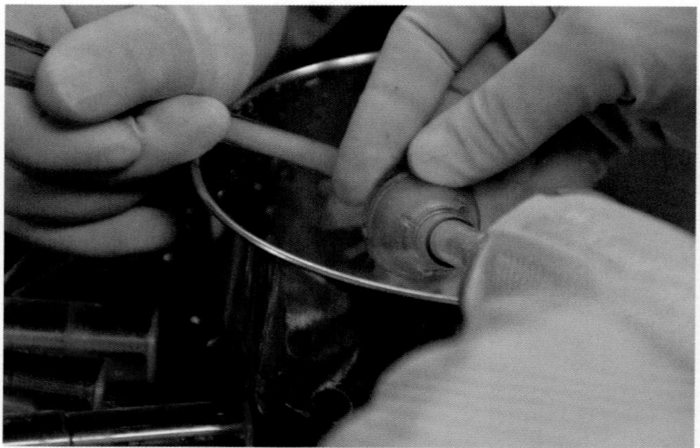

Figure 58-16 | Pulsatile saline lavage of an osteochondral allograft plug.

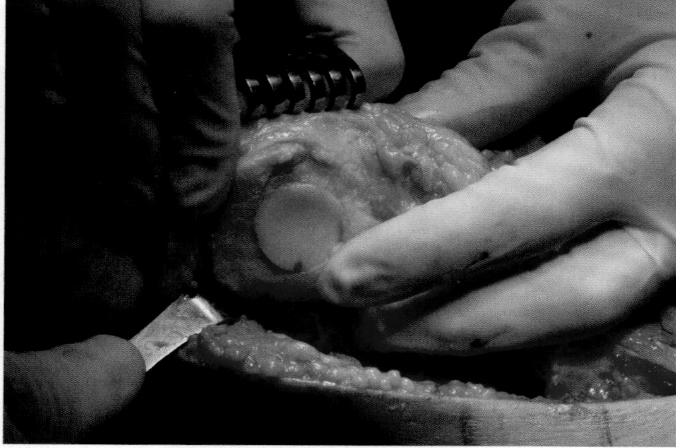

Figure 58-17 | A patellar osteochondral allograft plug being gently press fit into the donor socket.

Step 4 Pearls

- If the graft is too tight, a same-sized dilator can be used to dilate the socket.
- If the graft is too loose, bone grafting can be done on the periphery of the plug. Adjunct fixation also may be necessary through the center of the graft.
- Positioning the graft in the deepest location first and then levering the remainder into the recipient site often is a successful way to place the graft.

Step 5: Graft Fixation

- If a tight press fit cannot be achieved, additional fixation may be necessary. Options for graft fixation:
  - Metallic headless screws (Acutrak 2 mini screws, Acumed, Hillsboro, OR)
    - Useful for large and uncontained plugs

- Bioabsorbable screws (Bio-Compression screws, Arthrex, Naples, FL)
  - Preferred by the authors for large and uncontained plugs
- Orthosorb pins (Depuy, Inc., Warsaw, IN)
  - Made of polydioxanone suture (PDS) (absorbable)
  - Available in 1.3- and 2.0-mm diameters
  - Useful for small plugs (under 20 mm in diameter)
  - Technique
    - The appropriate K-wire from the kit is placed through the center of the plug into the bone.
    - The K-wire is removed and the Orthosorb pin is advanced over a cannulated inserter into the bone.
    - The pin is trimmed to be flush with the bone.
    - If more than one pin is used, they should be placed in a divergent fashion.

Step 5 Pearls

- If the graft does not fit flush against the recipient condyle, the graft size and recipient site should both be checked and rereamed/recut as necessary.
- If the graft needs to be removed, a Freer elevator can be used to work the graft out of its position or a reverse threaded extractor can be used by screwing it into the graft and gently tamping the graft out of position by grasping the extractor post.

Step 6: Closure

- The thigh tourniquet is deflated, and hemostasis is obtained.
- The knee is irrigated with saline, and the arthrotomy is closed in layers.
- Our preference is to place small absorbable sutures (2-0 Vicryl [Ethicon, LLC, San Lorenzo, Puerto Rico]) in the fat pad to limit bleeding from the fat pad.
- The medial retinaculum is closed with interrupted, strong absorbable sutures (no. 1 Vicryl [Ethicon, LLC]).
- If a lateral release was performed, it can be left open.
- A hinged knee brace locked in full extension is applied and is taken off only for physical therapy and continuous passive motion (CPM).

Postoperative Rehabilitation

- Phase I (0 to 6 weeks)
  - Heel-touch weight bearing
  - The hinged knee brace locked in full extension is used for the first 2 weeks, with removal allowed for CPM machine use. The brace is discontinued at 2 weeks.
  - CPM is used ~6 hours per day beginning at 0 to 40 degrees and advancing 5 to 10 degrees daily as tolerated from weeks 0 to 6.
  - Exercises for weeks 0 to 2 include quadriceps sets, calf pumps, passive leg hangs to 90 degrees, and seated leg raises.
  - Passive and assisted active range-of-motion is advanced at 2 weeks. Side-lying hip and core, hamstring, and gluteus medius exercises are initiated.
- Phase II (6 to 8 weeks)
  - Weight bearing is advanced 25% weekly until full.
  - Full range of motion should be achieved.
  - Phase I exercises are advanced.
- Phase III (8 to 12 weeks)
  - Full weight bearing is achieved.
  - Gait training, closed chain activities, wall sits, shuttle movements, mini-squats, and toe raise exercises are initiated.
  - Unilateral stance activities and balance training are advanced.
- Phase IV (12 weeks to 6 months)
  - Phase III exercises are intensified including core, gluteal, pelvic stability, and eccentric hamstring movements.

  - Patients may advance to use of elliptical, stationary bicycle, and pool as tolerated.
- Phase V (6 to 12 months)
  - Functional activity is advanced.
  - Return to sport-specific activity and impact can begin at ~8 months.
- Rehabilitation pearls
  - Rehabilitation protocols may be altered depending on treatment of concomitant pathology such as osteotomy, meniscal allograft transplantation, or ligament reconstruction.

References

1. Crawford DC, Safran MR. Osteochondritis dissecans of the knee. *J Am Acad Orthop Surg.* 2006;14(2):90-100.
2. Kon E, Vannini F, Buda R, et al. How to treat osteochondritis dissecans of the knee: surgical techniques and new trends: AAOS exhibit selection. *J Bone Joint Surg Am.* 2012;94(1):e1.1-e1.8. doi:10.2106/JBJS.K.00748.
3. Cahill BR, Phillips MR, Navarro R. The results of conservative management of juvenile osteochondritis dissecans using joint scintigraphy. A prospective study. *Am J Sports Med.* 1989;17(5):601-605; discussion 605-606. doi:10.1177/036354658901700502.
4. Linden B. The incidence of osteochondritis dissecans in the condyles of the femur. *Acta Orthop Scand.* 1976;47(6):664-667.
5. Kessler JI, Nikizad H, Shea KG, et al. The demographics and epidemiology of osteochondritis dissecans of the knee in children and adolescents. *Am J Sports Med.* 2014;42(2):320-326. doi:10.1177/0363546513510390.
6. Frank RM, Lee S, Levy D, et al. Osteochondral allograft transplantation of the knee: analysis of failures at 5 years. *Am J Sports Med.* 2017;45(4):864-874. doi:10.1177/0363546516676072.
7. Sadr KN, Pulido PA, McCauley JC, et al. Osteochondral allograft transplantation in patients with osteochondritis dissecans of the knee. *Am J Sports Med.* 2016;44(11):2870-2875. doi:10.1177/0363546516657526.
8. Briggs DT, Sadr KN, Pulido PA, et al. The use of osteochondral allograft transplantation for primary treatment of cartilage lesions in the knee. *Cartilage.* 2015;6(4):203-207. doi: 10.1177/1947603515595072.
9. Chahal J, Gross AE, Gross C, et al. Outcomes of osteochondral allograft transplantation in the knee. *Arthroscopy.* 2013;29(3):575-588. doi:10.1016/j.arthro.2012.12.002.
10. Kang RW, Friel NA, Williams JM, et al. Effect of impaction sequence on osteochondral graft damage: the role of repeated and varying loads. *Am J Sports Med.* 2010;38(1):105-113. doi:10.1177/0363546509349038.
11. Pylawka TK, Wimmer M, Cole BJ, et al. Impaction affects cell viability in osteochondral tissues during transplantation. *J Knee Surg.* 2007;20(2):105-110.
12. Hunt HE, Sadr K, Deyoung AJ, et al. The role of immunologic response in fresh osteochondral allografting of the knee. *Am J Sports Med.* 2014;42(4):886-891. doi:10.1177/0363546513518733.

Chapter 59

Fresh Osteochondral Allograft Transplant for Osteochondritis Dissecans of the Femoral Condyle

TIM WANG
DAVID M. DARE
DEAN WANG
RILEY J. WILLIAMS III

Background

- Osteochondral allograft is our preferred method of treatment for medium- to large-sized articular cartilage defects (>15 mm diameter) in the femur.
  - Microfracture
    - Limited durability
  - Osteochondral autograft transplantation
    - Risk of donor-site morbidity[1]
  - Autologous chondrocyte implantation[2,3]
    - Limits to graft size
    - Need for secondary surgery
    - Prolonged recovery
- Allograft tissue is harvested within 24 hours of donor death.
- Chondrocyte viability and extracellular matrix integrity directly affect postoperative outcomes, and their preservation is critical.
  - The recommended maximal storage time is 28 days, which, when appropriately preserved, correlates with 70% chondrocyte viability.[4]
  - Storage in serum-free culture medium improves chondrocyte viability and metabolism compared to lactated Ringer solution.[5]
- More recently, we augment osteochondral allografts with bone marrow aspirate concentrate (BMAC) harvested from the iliac crest at the time of surgery.
- Concomitant opening wedge high tibial osteotomy and opening wedge distal femoral osteotomy are done for associated varus and valgus deformity, respectively.
- Defect sizing can be done with preoperative MRI scans or staged diagnostic arthroscopy to obtain the appropriately sized allograft tissue (Figs. 59-1 and 59-2).

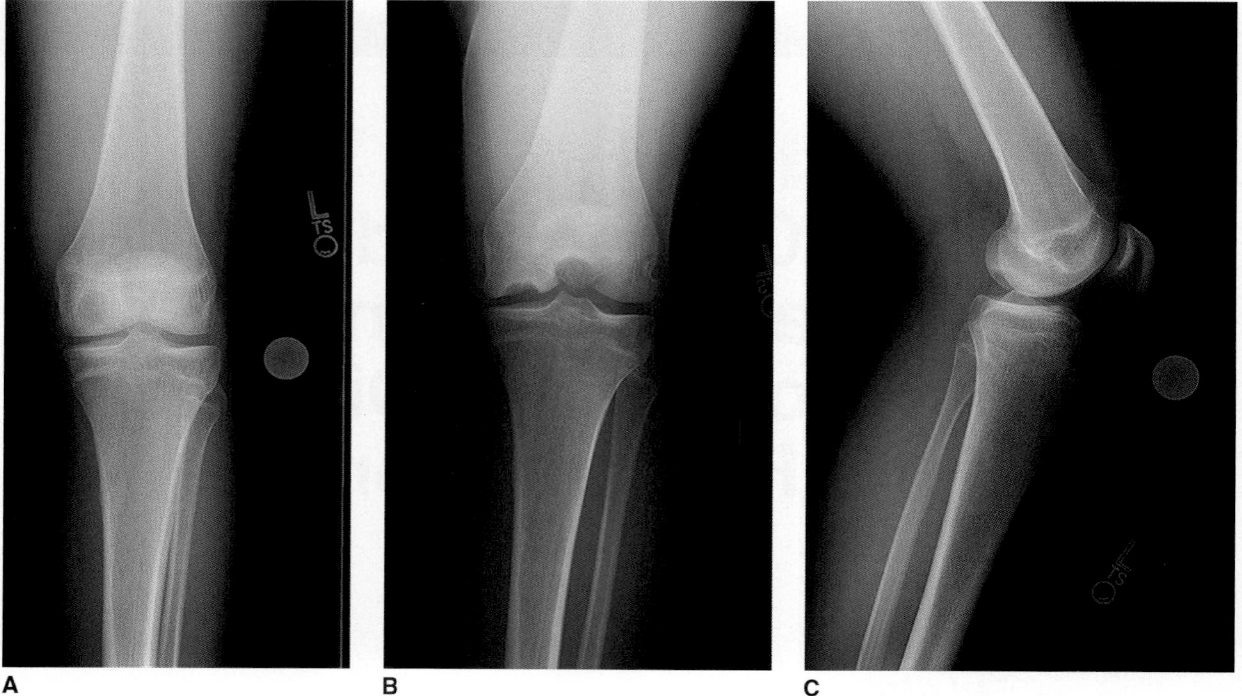

Figure 59-1 | Anteroposterior **(A)** and posteroanterior **(B)** flexed knee and lateral **(C)** radiographs of a 29-year-old patient with osteochondritis dissecans lesion of the left medial femoral condyle.

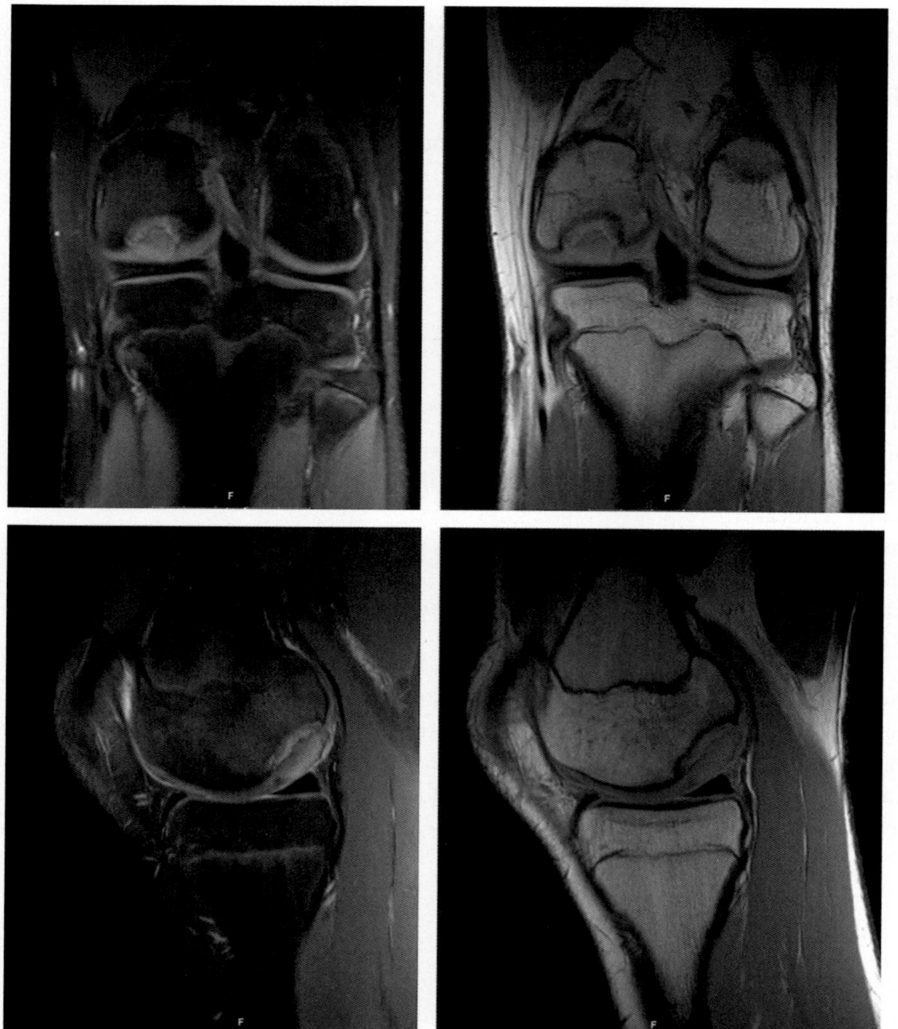

Figure 59-2 | Coronal and sagittal MRI sections of osteochondritis lesion of the left medial femoral condyle.

Positioning

- The patient is positioned supine on a standard operating table.
- A tourniquet is placed on the proximal thigh.
- A lateral post is positioned along the proximal thigh, at the level of the tourniquet, and confirmed to allow application of a valgus-directed force for arthroscopy of the medial compartment.
- After the patient is sedated, BMAC is harvested from the ipsilateral iliac crest.

Arthroscopy

- Standard diagnostic arthroscopy is performed to inspect and size the lesion to confirm optimal treatment strategy (Fig. 59-3). Any concurrent meniscal pathology is treated.
- Typically, a fresh femoral hemicondyle is used for femoral condylar lesions, while a distal femoral specimen is preferred for trochlear lesions. The graft is opened and soaked in antibiotic saline.

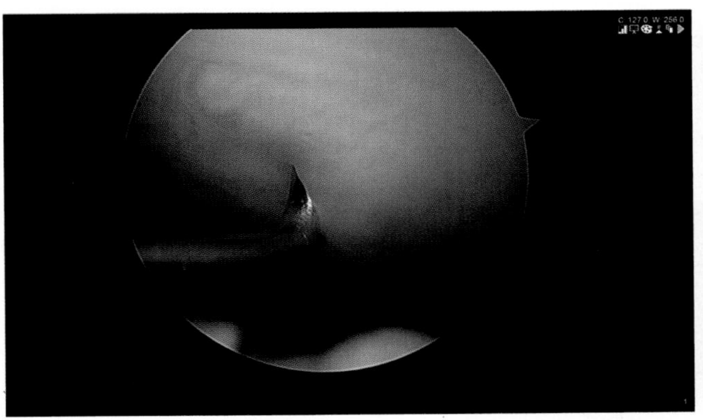

A

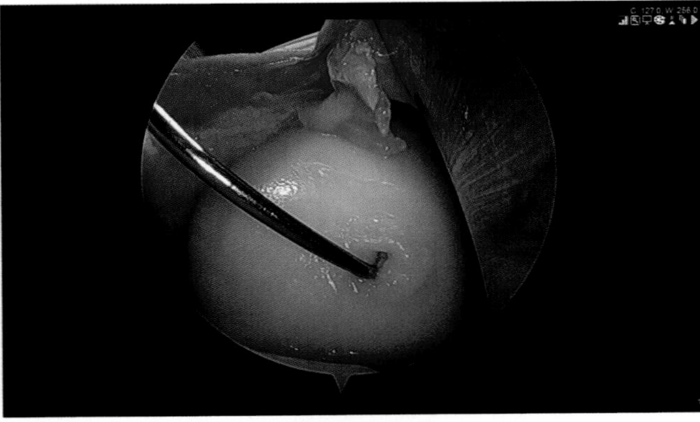

B

Figure 59-3 | Arthroscopic examination of lesion in medial femoral condyle. **A.** Coring reaming guide secured in position on target lesion location. **B.** Coring reamer being used through the guide.

Approach

- A medial or lateral parapatellar arthrotomy is chosen based on the lesion's location. Medial femoral condylar lesions are best approached through a medial parapatellar arthrotomy, whereas lateral femoral condylar lesions are better accessed through a lateral parapatellar arthrotomy (Fig. 59-4).
- After inflation of a thigh tourniquet, dissection is carried sharply through the skin along the medial border of the patella and the patellar tendon until the extensor retinaculum is seen.

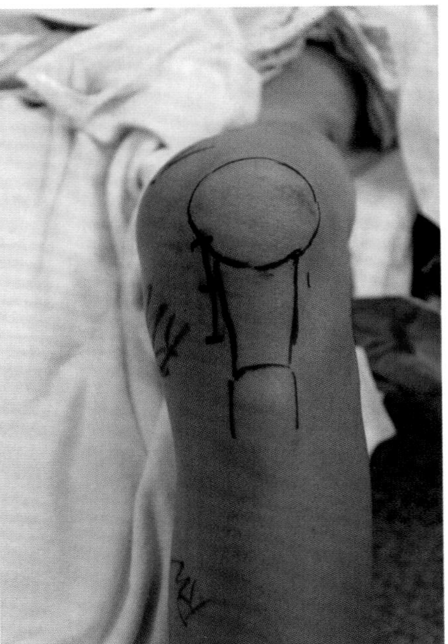

Figure 59-4 | Planned incision and approach for open arthrotomy.

- A parapatellar arthrotomy is made from the mid-patella to just distal to the tibial plateau. A 5-mm cuff of soft tissue is preserved immediately adjacent to the patellar tendon to facilitate arthrotomy closure.
- The infrapatellar fat pad is routinely excised to improve exposure and decrease the risk of infrapatellar scar.
- Exposure is maximized with a Paulson retractor placed along the outside edge of the condyle and a 90-degree sharp Hohmann retractor in the intercondylar notch.
- The knee is flexed to optimize viewing of the lesion through the "window."

Lesion/Recipient Site Preparation

- Using a manufacturer's sizing cylinder, the appropriately sized cannulated cylinder is selected to match the diameter of the lesion.
  - If the graft is oblong or too large for a single circular graft, we prefer to place two stacked grafts in a "snowman" arrangement.
- The tube should be aligned perpendicular to the articular surface, and the lesion should be well shouldered on at least ¾ of its borders. A Kirschner wire is inserted through the guide's central slot.
- A cannulated reamer of the same size as the sizing cylinder is used to drill the lesion to a depth of ~8 to 9 mm (Fig. 59-5).
  - The depth of the recipient site is measured at 12 o'clock, 4 o'clock, and 8 o'clock with a ruler.

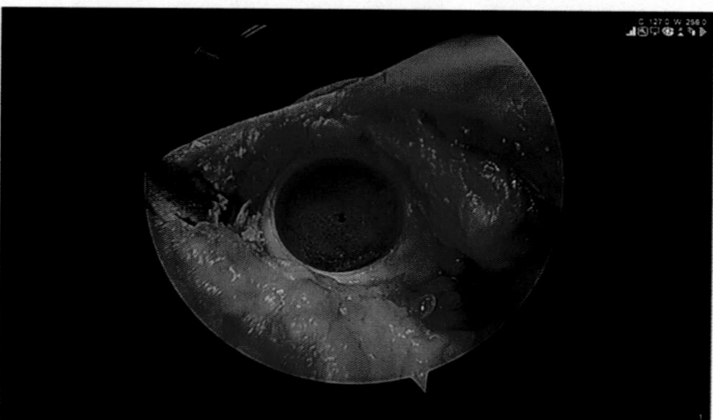

Figure 59-5 | After reaming of the lesion has been completed. At this junction, the depth of the lesion is measured on the clock face to determine the ideal size of the graft.

Donor Site Preparation

- The ideal donor site best matches the overall radius of curvature and contour of the recipient site. The fresh osteochondral allograft (hemicondyle or distal femoral condyle) is oriented to allow the most ergonomically friendly harvest.
- The graft is stabilized with a coring reamer guide (Fig. 59-6).

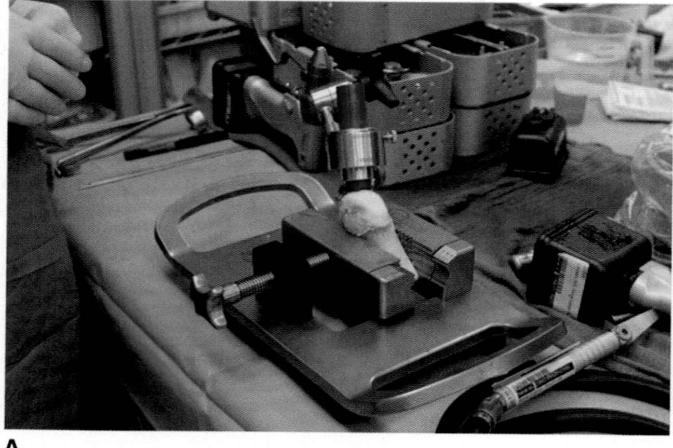

A

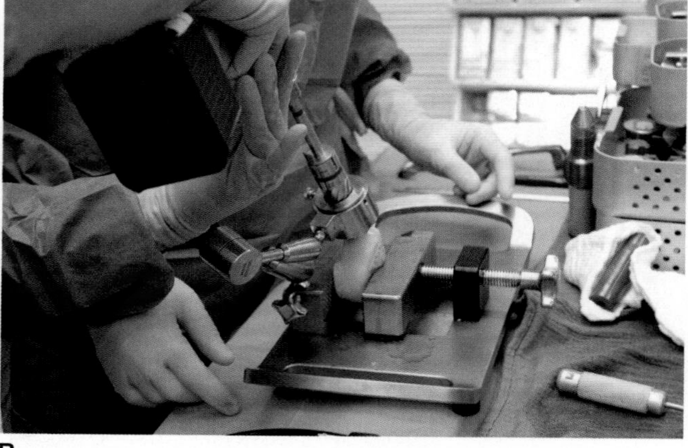

B

Figure 59-6 | A, B. Fresh hemicondyle allograft secured on graft table, with appropriate sizing tube placed in position in preparation for core reaming.

- The appropriately size-matched coring reamer is used to ream at full speed with simultaneous saline irrigation to prevent thermal necrosis (Fig. 59-7).

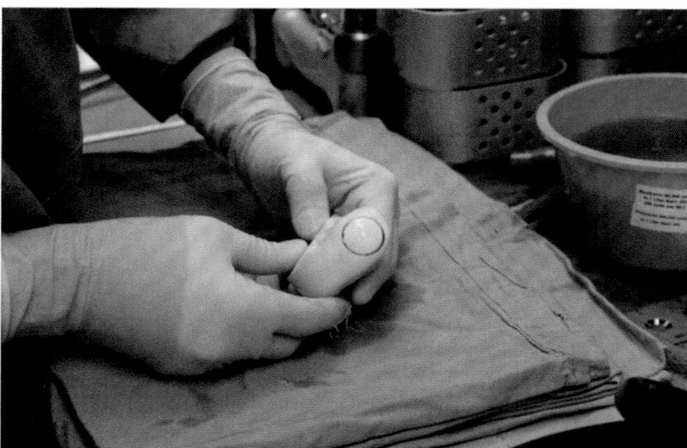

Figure 59-7 | Graft after core reaming has been completed.

- Once drilled to the previously determined depth, a microsagittal saw is used to release the graft core "plug" from the femoral condyle. The saw is placed perpendicular to the long axis of the graft core and at a depth greater than the intended graft depth.
- We use a marker to identify the 12 o'clock position on the articular surface of the plug, and using a ruler, mark out the appropriate depths of the graft at the corresponding 12 o'clock, 4 o'clock, and 8 o'clock positions, as measured earlier.
- A graft-holding clamp is used to grasp the plug at the marked positions circumferentially. A microsagittal saw is used to cut the plug along the plane of the clamp. This step is akin to cutting a patella during total knee arthroplasty (Fig. 59-8).
- Once complete, the corners of the graft are gently beveled to allow easy insertion into the recipient site. In addition, the bony side of the osteochondral plug (opposite the articular cartilage) is gently etched 1 to 2 mm deep in a "pound" sign pattern on the cancellous base to allow for differential stiffness of the graft. If the plug sits proud during insertion, this allows collapse of the cancellous bone to allow the plug to sit flush.
- The plug is soaked in a shallow well of BMAC as the recipient site is re-exposed (Fig. 59-9).

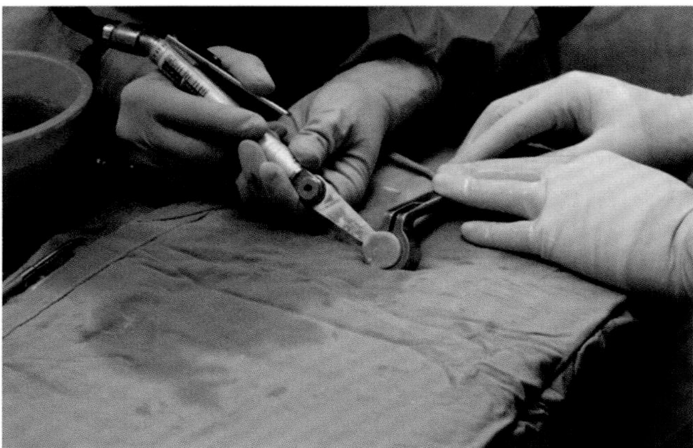

Figure 59-8 | Appropriate depth of the graft measured at each position and cut along the face of the graft holder to size graft to the corresponding recipient size.

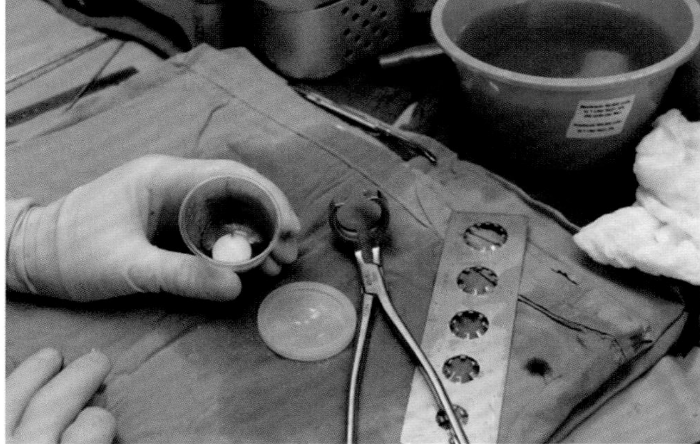

Figure 59-9 | Fresh osteochondral allograft plug soaking in bone marrow aspirate concentrate.

Graft insertion

- The lesion is re-exposed, and the recipient cancellous bone bed is multiply perforated with a small Kirschner wire or drill. Any remaining BMAC is injected into the base of the defect.
- The donor graft is held perpendicular to the defect and provisionally placed in the recipient site. Manual pressure is applied to seat the graft. With the graft nearly fully seated and only a few millimeters proud, an impactor is positioned such that half of the impactor contacts the graft and the other half contacts the recipient condyle. This helps prevent countersinking of the graft.
  - Care is taken to gently impact the graft because excess force can damage the articular cartilage and lead to chondrocyte death.
- The graft is typically stable with press-fit fixation, and no supplemental fixation is required (Fig. 59-10).

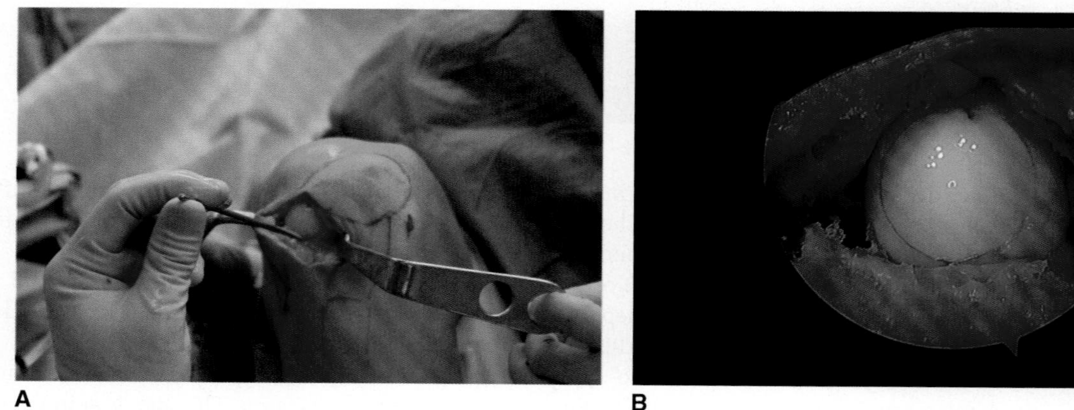

Figure 59-10 | Open **(A)** and arthroscopic **(B)** views of osteochondral allograft once impacted into place.

Closure

- The wound is irrigated thoroughly, the tourniquet is deflated, and hemostasis is achieved (often the fat pad may be a source of bleeding).
- Wound closure is done with standard technique.

Postoperative Protocol

- Patients typically are discharged on the same day as surgery.
- Toe-touch weight bearing with the knee held in extension is continued for a week.
- Range of motion from 0 to 90 degrees is allowed after the 1st week.
- A gradual transition to weight bearing is begun as tolerated after 4th week.

References

1. Langer F, Czitrom A, Pritzker KP, et al. The immunogenicity of fresh and frozen allogeneic bone. *J Bone Joint Surg Am.* 1975;57(2):216-220.
2. Dean CS, Chahla J, Serra Cruz R, et al. Fresh osteochondral allograft transplantation for treatment of articular cartilage defects of the knee. *Arthrosc Tech.* 2016;5(1):e157-e161.
3. Richter DL, Tanksley JA, Miller MD. Osteochondral autograft transplantation: a review of the surgical technique and outcomes. *Sports Med Arthrosc.* 2016;24(2):74-78.
4. Sherman SL, Garrity J, Bauer K, et al. Fresh osteochondral allograft transplantation for the knee: current concepts. *J Am Acad Orthop Surg.* 2014;22(2):121-133.
5. Ball ST, Amiel D, Williams SK, et al. The effects of storage on fresh human osteochondral allografts. *Clin Orthop Relat Res.* 2004;418:246-252.

Chapter 60
Autologous Chondrocyte Implantation

SCOTT D. GILLOGLY
ANGUS F. BURNETT

Overview

- Autologous chondrocyte implantation (ACI) is a two-stage procedure
  - Autologous biopsy (ACI stage 1)
  - Autologous cell implantation/transplantation (ACI stage 2)

ACI Stage 1—Index Arthroscopy and Chondral Biopsy for Cell Culture

- Index arthroscopy is done to assess cartilage defect(s) and any concomitant knee pathology. Considerations include
  - location of defect(s), size of defect(s), defect depth, bone involvement, opposing cartilage surfaces, status of menisci/ligaments, and patellofemoral tracking

Sterile Instruments/Equipment

- Biopsy tools: arthroscopic-ready small gouge and/or small ring curette
- Biopsy medium and containers
- Shipping specimen process or storage arrangements

Patient Positioning

- The setup is identical to that used for routine arthroscopy.
- The patient is placed supine on the operating table.
- Maximal knee flexion should be possible.
- A tourniquet should be available but is not routinely used.

Cartilage Biopsy Surgical Approach

- Biopsy is harvested from lesser or non–weight bearing, nonarticulating surfaces.
  - Superior lateral cartilage margin of lateral femoral condyle
  - Superior medial cartilage margin of medial femoral condyle
  - Intercondylar trochlear notch
- A ring curette or curved notchplasty gouge is used.
- Cartilage biopsy is "peeled off" with the harvest tool and is left attached on one edge.
- A grasper is used to break away the remaining attachment of the cartilage biopsy (prevents specimen from becoming a loose body).

- Two to three slivers of full-thickness normal appearing cartilage tissue (measuring 4 to 5 mm × 7 to 9 mm) are removed down to subchondral bone.
- The approximate weight of specimen is 200 to 300 g.
- The biopsy specimen is placed in sterile medium, and the container is properly marked with all appropriate patient information.
- With ex vivo culture, a 12-fold increase in total autologous chondrocytes takes about 3 to 4 weeks, although culture can be cryopreserved to allow optimal patient timing for reimplantation.

ACI Stage 2—Chondrocyte Implantation with Collagen Membrane or Matrix Membrane

Sterile Instruments/Equipment

- Cultured chondrocytes (delivery arranged and verified)
- Fibrin glue preparation
- Specialty absorbable sutures (6-0 Vicryl)
- Small curettes
- Fine instrument needle holder, scissors, nontoothed pickups
- Absorbable type I/III collagen membrane, sterile packaged, 50 × 40 mm
- Available micro-absorbable anchors that can be reloaded with absorbable 5-0 Vicryl sutures

Patient Positioning

- Standard supine positioning for knee arthrotomy.
- Maximal knee flexion should be possible.
- A tourniquet should be available; it is used only during exposure and defect debridement and then is let down (<60 minutes at lowest pressure possible).

Surgical Approach

- Depends on defect location
- Influenced by any concomitant procedures

Exposure

- Adequate exposure is vital for any successful cartilage repair; however, the degree of exposure varies by defect location, size, and chondrocyte implantation technique.
- Medial or lateral parapatellar incision and arthrotomy can be used.
- An incision is created that could be extended and reused for future procedures such as total knee arthroplasty.
- The patella is everted for more posterior condyle lesions or multiple lesions.
- For patellofemoral lesions, the tubercle can be detached as part of a concomitant realignment procedure and reflected proximally by cutting the fat pad just anterior to the transverse intermeniscal ligament and performing lateral retinacular lengthening and medial capsular incision superiorly up to the vastus medialis obliquus (VMO) without violating its insertion.

Defect Preparation

- Fibrous tissue and damaged chondral tissue are removed with small curettes down to the level of subchondral bone (Fig. 60-1).
- Once exposure is obtained, the defect is demarcated by scoring the periphery of the defect with a no. 15 blade.
  - This creates a delineation between damaged, injured cartilage, and healthier surrounding cartilage tissue.
  - The cut should be to bone level and should create a distinct 90-degree wall at the defect margin (Fig. 60-2).

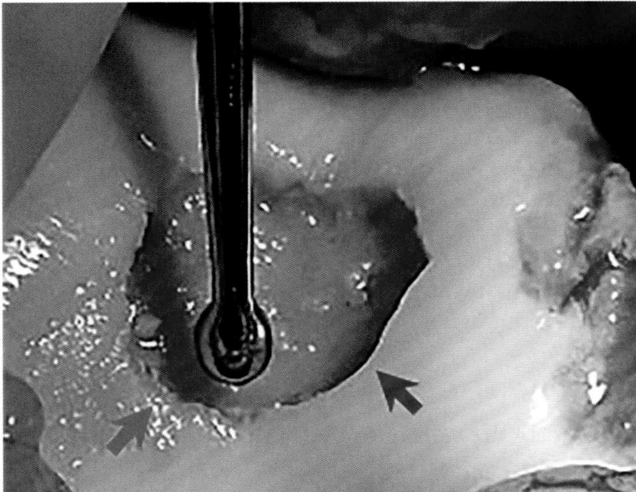

Figure 60-1 | A small curette is used to debride the remaining fibrous tissue and calcified cartilage down to subchondral bone. Note the desired sharp demarcation of the healthy cartilage edge (*blue arrow*) versus the still indistinct edge (*red arrow*).

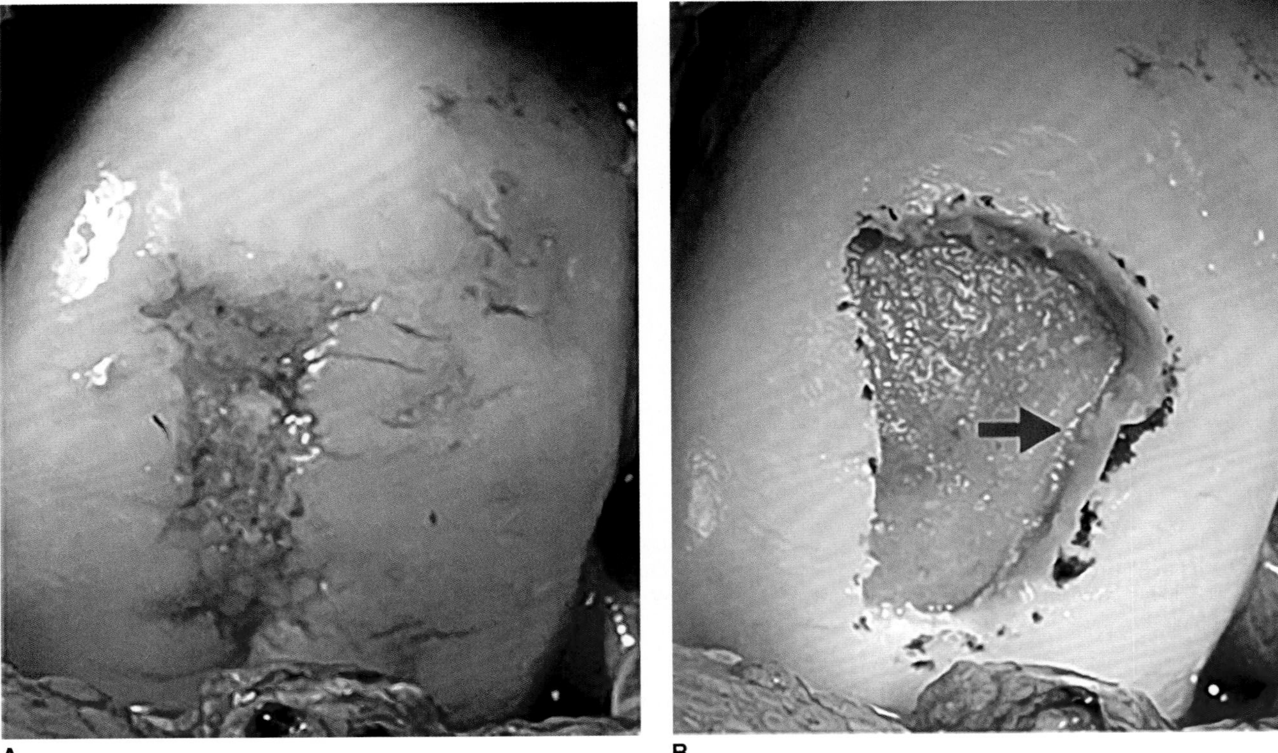

Figure 60-2 | **A.** Defect prior to debridement with fissures and partial delamination of the defect edges. **B.** After debridement and demarcation, the edges are distinct and create a 90-degree angle (*blue arrow*) with the subchondral bone. This will insure containment of the chondrocytes.

- Small curettes are used to debride the defect to remove the calcified cartilage, fibrocartilage, and damaged cartilage.
- Penetration or damage to the subchondral bone should be avoided.
- Because blood may dilute the concentration of chondrocytes, any bleeding from the base of the defect needs to be controlled.
  - Thrombin spray and/or epinephrine soaked neuropatty sponges with pressure
  - Gelfoam hemostatic sponge and fibrin glue
  - Electrocautery with needle point and low voltage

- The goal of this preparation is to have a dry bed of clean subchondral bone and a firm healthy-appearing, sharply demarcated, surrounding cartilage border at the periphery.
- Intralesional osteophytes
  - These typically occur after a previous microfracture of the lesion.
  - The prominent osteophyte acting as a stress riser and the abnormal bony bed (often includes a sclerotic surface from bony overgrowth in response to microfracture) should be avoided.
  - The osteophyte is gently debrided with a high-speed burr, avoiding cancellous bone penetration.
  - One layer at a time is removed so as to not inadvertently plunge into soft cancellous bone.
  - Hemostasis of any bleeding from the abraded osteophyte is controlled as described.
- If not already done, the tourniquet is let down at this point, and the knee and wound are irrigated, and hemostasis is obtained throughout the wound.

Collagen Membrane Preparation

- When the defect is fully debrided, it is measured and the size of the membrane graft is determined (Fig. 60-3A).
- To correctly size the matrix or collagen membrane graft, a paper template from the sterile glove wrapper can be used (Fig. 60-3A).

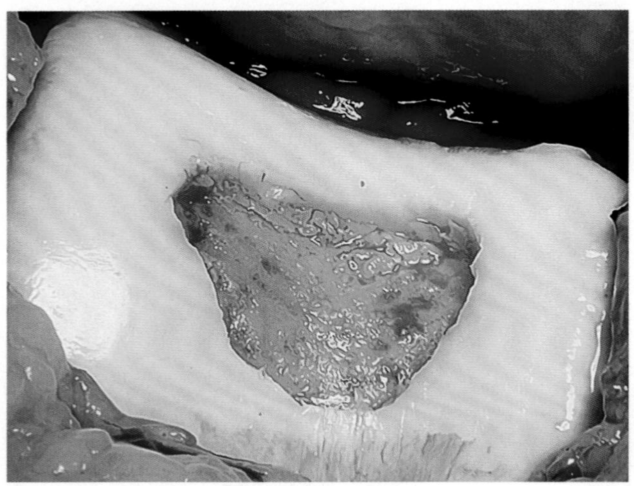
A

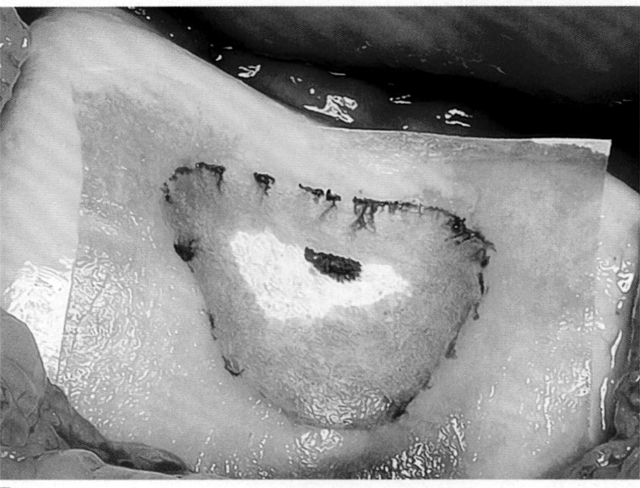
B

Figure 60-3 | A. The trochlear defect has been debrided appropriately. **B.** Sterile glove paper is laid over the defect after saline has remoistened the articular cartilage. Note the easily recognized color change that clearly shows the defect edges. The edges are marked on the paper with a surgical marker, and the paper template can then be cut out. The dot in the superior portion indicates orientation for the membrane graft.

- The edges of the defect are moistened with saline, and a cut piece of glove paper is placed over the defect where an outline of the defect's periphery is easily visible.
- Small dots are placed around the circumference of the defect to create the outline on the paper that will eventually become the template.
- An orientation mark is placed superiorly on the template to keep consistent alignment throughout the steps of implantation.
- The template is cut with scissors, following the dots (Fig. 60-4A).
  - An alternative method is to use a foil suture wrapper pushed gently into the defect, which creates an edge at the defect periphery and allows foil to be cut as a template.
- An absorbable type I/III collagen membrane is used to contain the cells when secured to the defect's periphery.
- The membrane has a smoother outer layer, which will be oriented flush with the articular cartilage, and a rougher undersurface that will be oriented toward subchondral bone (Fig. 60-4B).
- The membrane is freeze dried and is reconstituted with sterile saline.
  - The membrane should be moist and pliable but not saturated.
  - Saline is applied with a small syringe a few drops at a time.

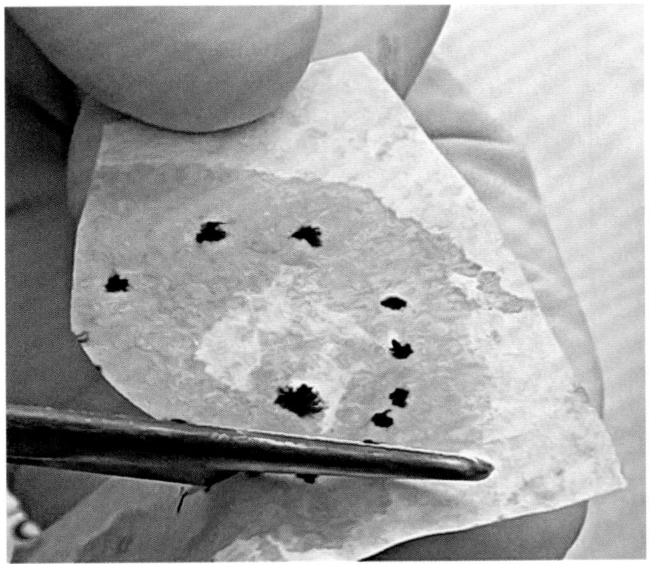
A

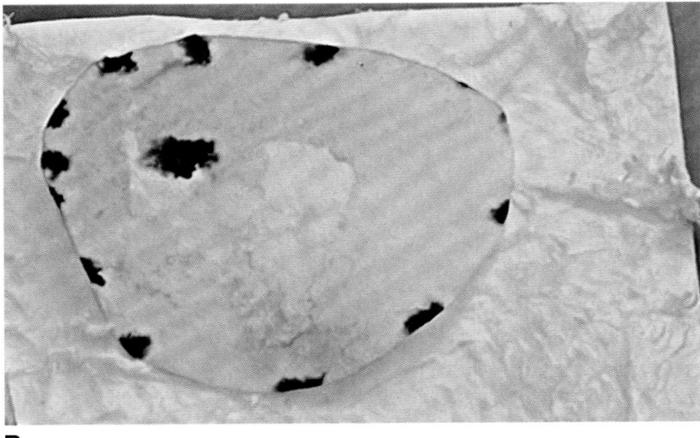
B

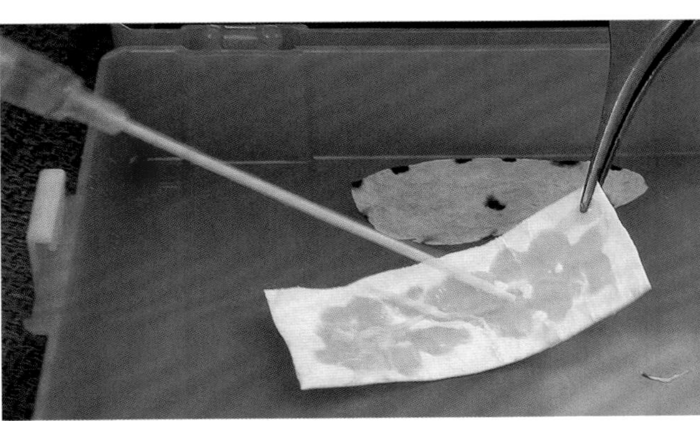
C

Figure 60-4 | **A.** Sterile glove paper template is cut out and then placed on the collagen membrane where **(B)** it is used to cut the membrane to exact size. **C.** Autologous cells placed on the membrane prior to the final cutting using the template.

- With adequate cells available, the deep layer of the membrane is seeded with cells suspended in the serum using the same drop-by-drop method (Fig. 60-4C).
- The template from the defect can be used to ensure that cells are in the area. The membrane is cut around the template.
    - There is no need to oversize the membrane larger than the template because the membrane expands slightly.
    - The orientation of the template should correspond to the correct surface of the membrane *before* it is cut.
    - The template is laid on the smooth surface of the membrane to match the shape of the defect and the rough layer is kept toward the bone.

Collagen Membrane Fixation

- The goal is to create a watertight closure of the defect with the sutured membrane.
- The correctly oriented membrane graft is secured with interrupted sutures, spaced every 2 to 3 mm around the perimeter of the defect with 6-0 Vicryl sutures (Fig. 60-5A and B).
- The needle size is chosen for the depth of surrounding healthy cartilage.
    - Smaller radius of curvature needles are preferable for robust healthy cartilage and require very little grasp of native cartilage.
    - Larger radius of curvature needles do better for thinner remaining cartilage and grasp more of the less robust cartilage to secure the suture.
- Knots are oriented on the graft side rather than over the cartilage.

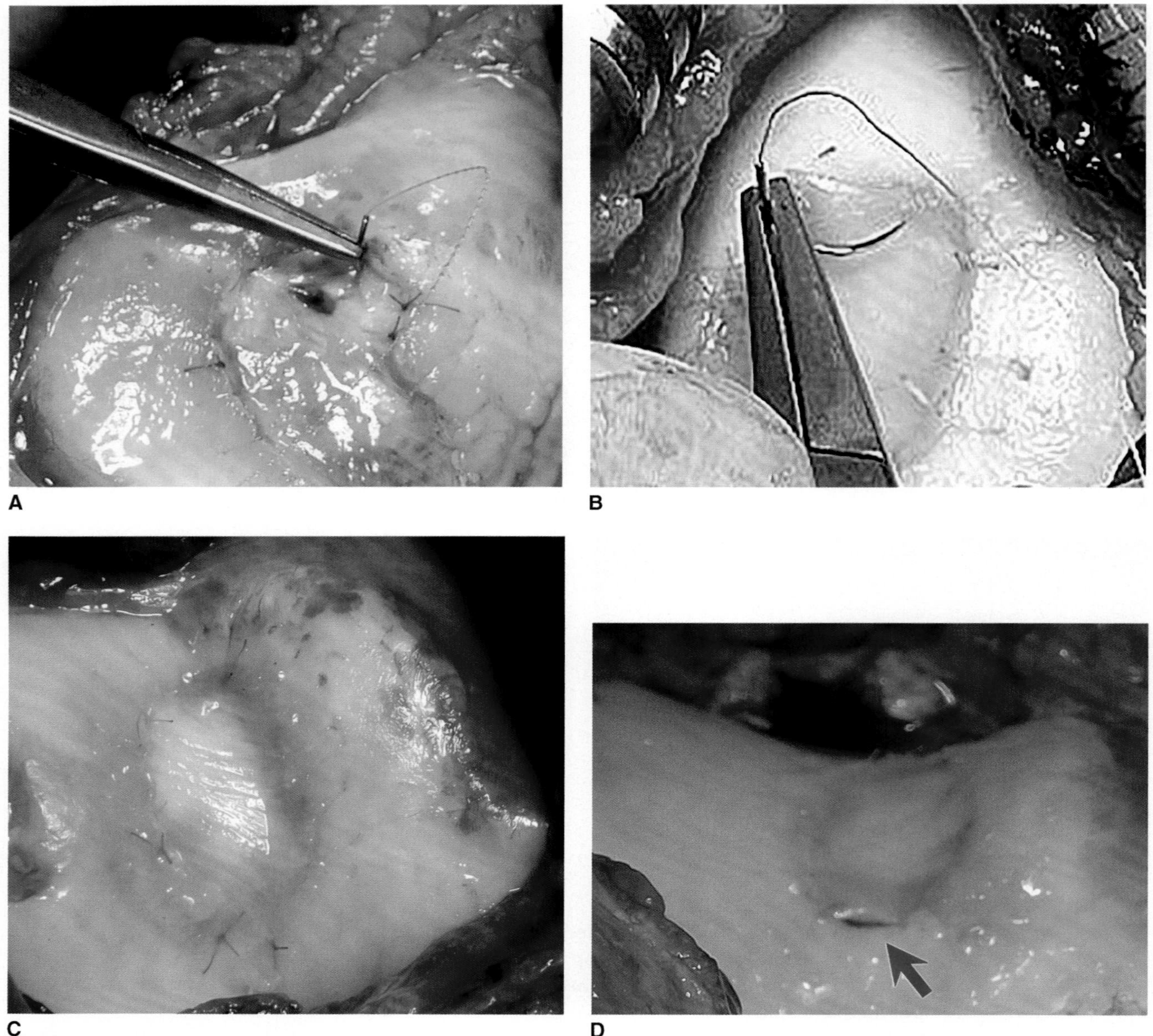

Figure 60-5 | A-C. Collagen membrane is sutured into place with interrupted 6-0 Vicryl sutures re-establishing the normal contour of the articular cartilage. Note that the trochlea defect in **(C)** has the trochlear normal groove contour. **D.** A small opening (*arrow*) is left for the cells to be injected.

- Tension of the graft is adjusted as sequential sutures are put in place to recreate the contour of the articular surface and avoid wrinkles or bunching of the graft by redundant membrane (Fig. 60-5C).
- Excess graft is trimmed with small curved scissors as needed to prevent redundant graft.
  - Care should be taken not to trim too much away.
  - Trimming is done twice to insure sufficient membrane for defect closure.
- Special consideration for any uncontained edges of the defect
  - Uncontained portions can be encountered at
    - The intercondylar notch edge of a large femoral condylar lesion
    - Adult OCD lesions, particularly at the notch side of a medial femoral condylar lesion
    - Chronic lesions with some degree of wear of surrounding cartilage
  - Securing the membrane at areas of uncontainment can be accomplished with
    - Microabsorbable anchors reloaded with absorbable Vicryl sutures, typically 5-0 because it is easier to reload in the anchor

    - Drill holes through the bone edge with suture passed by a Keith needle
    - Attaching membrane to synovium of PCL fibers at the medial notch should be avoided because micromotion occurs and alters the watertight seal
- A small opening is left for injection of the cells under the membrane (Fig. 60-5D).
- The watertight seal is tested by injecting saline with a small syringe and plastic angiocatheter.
  - An additional one to two sutures may be needed in any obvious place of leakage.
  - Caution is needed at this point to not tear the membrane that now has mild tension on it to recreate the articular cartilage surface contour.
- Fibrin glue is applied circumferentially around the suture line once a watertight seal is established with sutures.
- The fibrin glue is allowed to gel, further reinforcing the watertight seal.

Cell Implantation and Closure

- Any concomitant knee procedures are completed before injection of cells to avoid excess manipulation or motion of the knee once the cells are implanted.
- The cells are aspirated from shipping vials with an angiocatheter and 1-cc syringe.
  - Outer shipping vials are nonsterile; only the cells and serum are sterile (as is true for any injectable liquid).
  - Sterile technique is ensured by using a temporarily extra-gloved hand to hold the vial and using the other still sterile hand to aspirate.
  - Once cells are aspirated into the syringe, the vial is passed off and the nonsterile extra glove is removed.
    - The process is repeated for multiple vials of cells.
    - The extra glove of the nonsterile hand is used until complete, and then passed off.
- A new sterile angiocatheter is used to inject the cells through the remaining small opening of the membrane suture line, placing the catheter deep to the membrane.
  - The cell injection is started at the far side under the membrane, and cells are injected as the catheter is slowly retracted.
  - This is repeated for additional cells until the space is fully filled, as evidenced by overflow from the injection opening.
  - The catheter is removed.
- The injection site is sutured with one to two additional 6-0 Vicryl sutures.
- The injection site is sealed with fibrin glue, and the circumference of the defect is touched up with additional glue as needed.
- Once the cells are injected and the site closed/sealed, *no* further knee manipulation is done.
- The knee is gently moved to full extension and left in full extension during closure.
- The wound is closed in layers after the capsule and extensor mechanism are closed.
- Injection of long-acting analgesics into the soft tissues during closure, not intra-articular, should be considered.
- A drain is not routinely used and, if necessary, is kept extra-articular.

Immediate Postoperative Management

- Pain control, ice for patient comfort
- ROM within 24 to 48 hours
- Continuous passive motion up to about 6 hours/day if available
- Leg control exercises
- Touch weight-bearing ambulation
- Advance weight bearing at 4 to 6 weeks
  - Advancement of weight bearing and exercises based on size, characteristics, and location(s) of defect
  - Concomitant procedures rehabilitation is complementary to ACI or matrix ACI (MACI) rehabilitation
- Open chain knee extension exercises are avoided with any patellar or trochlea defect to reduce shear stress

Matrix Autologous Cell Implantation

- Approved by the US FDA in early 2017, MACI cultures the patient's chondrocytes and then seeds them in a 3-D absorbable collagen membrane.
- Because cells are within the membrane and not in liquid suspension, securing the matrix graft into the defect does not require a watertight seal.
- The graft is trimmed to size and secured with fibrin glue and does not require suturing.
- Debridement and demarcation of the defect are essentially identical to ACI; however, the easier fixation with fibrin glue means that less exposure and operative time are required.
- The postoperative course follows the same pathway.

Suggested Readings

Brittberg M, Lindahl A, Nilsson A, et al. Treatment of deep cartilage defects in the knee with autologous chondrocyte transplantation. *New Engl J Med.* 1994;331(14):889-895.

Cortese F, McNicholas M, Janes G, et al. Arthroscopic delivery of matrix-induced autologous chondrocyte implant: international experience and technique recommendations. *Cartilage.* 2012;3(2):156-164.

Gillogly SD, Arnold RM. Autologous chondrocyte implantation and anteromedializaton for isolated patella articular cartilage lesions: 5-11 year follow up. *Am J Sports Med.* 2014;42(4):912-920.

Gillogly SD, Gelven AT. Autologous chondrocyte implantation in the knee. In: Cole B, Sekeiya J, eds. *Surgical Techniques of the Shoulder, Elbow and Knee in Sports Medicine.* 2nd ed. Philadelphia, PA: Saunders-Elsevier; 2013:721-732.

Gillogly SD, Wheeler C. Autologous chondrocyte implantation with collagen membrane. *Sports Med Arthrosc.* 2015;23(3):118-124.

Gomoll AH, Gillogly SD, Cole BJ, et al. Autologous chondrocyte implantation in the patella: a multicenter experience. *Am J Sports Med.* 2014;42(5):1074-1081.

Peterson L, Minas T, Brittberg M, et al. Two- to 9-year outcome after autologous chondrocyte transplantation of the knee. *Clin Orthop Relat Res.* 2000;374:212-234.

Chapter 61
Principles of Ankle Arthroscopy

MICHAEL R. ANDERSON
JUDITH F. BAUMHAUER

Sterile Instruments/Equipment

- Scope
  - The 2.7-mm scope is most frequently used and is our preference.
    - The 2.7-mm scope is ideal for the ankle and allows anterior ankle arthroscopy as well as intra-articular evaluation. Furthermore, the 2.7-mm scope can be safely used for posterior ankle arthroscopy, subtalar arthroscopy, and tendoscopy.
    - Occasionally, the 1.9-mm scope is used in tight ankles and pediatric cases.
    - Some advocate the use of the 4.0-mm scope, which can be useful in anterior ankle arthroscopy but can pose a challenge for intra-articular evaluation.[1]
  - The 30-degree scope is adequate in most situations; however, a 70-degree scope is useful for viewing the posterior joint from anterior portals.
  - Standard arthroscopy tower
    - Monitor, light source, shaver motor, printer.
    - We do not routinely use an arthroscopic pump for fluid inflow, instead we rely on gravity flow from 3-L saline bags.
  - Intra-articular instruments (Fig. 61-1)
    - Commercially available sets designed for ankle arthroscopy incorporate smaller instruments to facilitate safe intra-articular work. These sets generally include the following:
      - Probes
      - Basket forceps in a variety of sizes and angles
        - Useful for creating a "leading edge" in thickened soft tissue or scar tissue that can then be debrided with a motorized shaver. Also useful for the debridement of loose cartilage flaps.
    - Graspers
      - For removal of loose bodies or debris created from the debridement of osteochondral defects.
    - Curettes in a variety of sizes and angles
      - For debridement of osteochondral defects.
    - Microfracture picks in a variety of angles
    - Osteotomes
      - Useful for removal of impinging osteophytes or for removal of cartilage in arthroscopic ankle arthrodesis.
    - Motorized instruments
      - Shavers: Generally a 2.5-mm full-radius shaver is used, although a 3.5-mm shaver can be used as needed.
      - Burrs: 3.0-5.0-mm round burr is useful for debridement of anterior osteophytes or debridement for arthroscopic ankle arthrodesis.

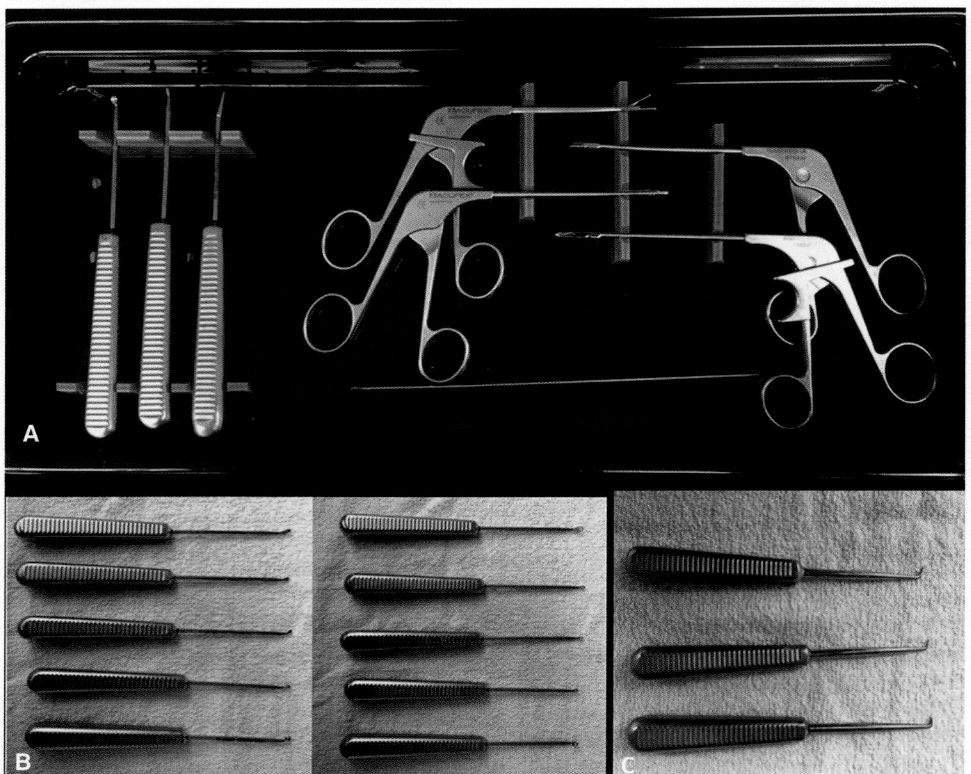

Figure 61-1 | An example of a commercially available ankle/small joint arthroscopy instrument set. **A.** A variety of graspers, basket punches, an osteotome, and curettes. **B.** A variety of open and closed curettes. **C.** Microfracture picks.

Positioning

- Supine
  - Unlike most foot and ankle procedures, the patient's heels are not positioned at the end of the table to accommodate the space required for the noninvasive distraction device. Another option is to use a table rail extender.
- Thigh holder
  - Places the hip in approximately 45 degrees of flexion while the knee is in ~90 degrees of flexion. The proper position allows the heel to gently touch the OR table. We are careful to position the thigh holder proximal to the popliteal fossa to decrease pressure on the vessels in the posterior knee (Fig. 61-2).
- Noninvasive distractor (Fig. 61-3)
  - Noninvasive ankle distraction improves access to the ankle joint.
  - It is important, however, to limit the time distraction is used to decrease both postoperative neurapraxia and compression of the terminal nerve branches at the midfoot.[2,3]
  - Joint distraction can decrease access to the anterior compartment and can be removed during debridement deep to the anterior capsule.[1]
  - As demonstrated in Figure 61-4, the distractor can pull the talus anteriorly and paradoxically decrease access to the ankle joint in unstable ankles. We have found that unstable ankles can often be approached without the use of a distractor.
- Tourniquet
  - A thigh tourniquet can be used at the discretion of the surgeon.

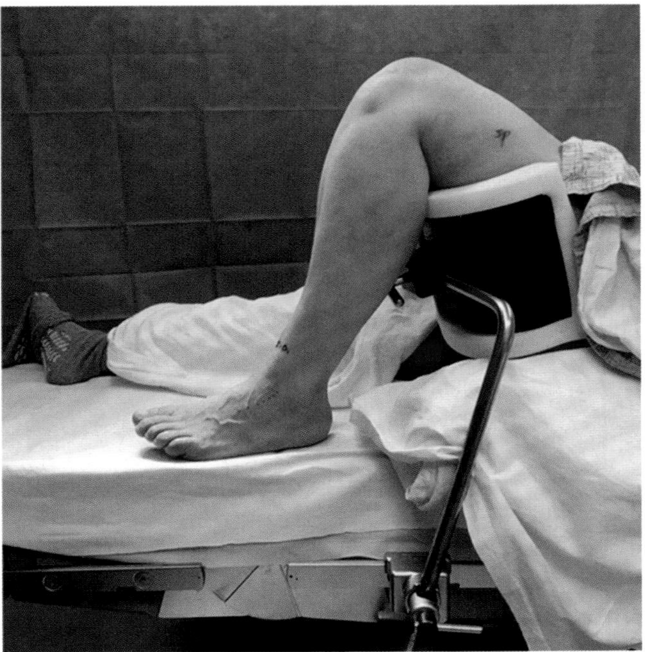

Figure 61-2 | Properly positioned patient. Note the location of the thigh holder slightly proximal to the popliteal fossa and the foot gently resting on the OR table.

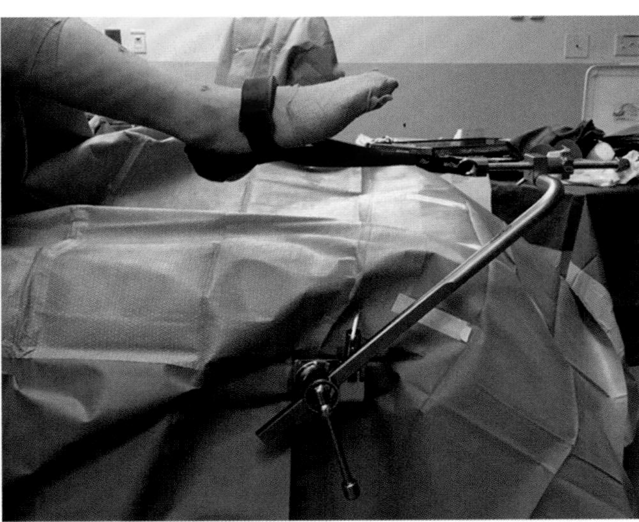

Figure 61-3 | The foot properly placed into a sterile noninvasive distraction device. Note that the clamp is positioned at the level of the toes.

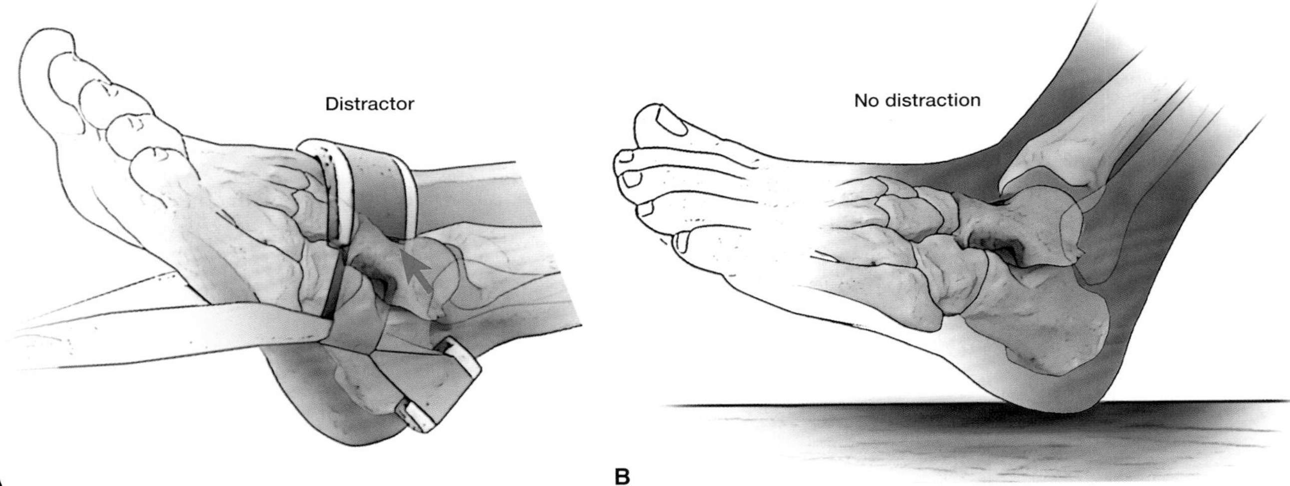

Figure 61-4 | **A.** The talus pulled anteriorly (*red arrow*) by the non invasive distractor in the setting of instability. This can decrease access to the joint. **B.** The talus in an improved position out of distraction facilitating improved access to the ankle joint.

Surgical Anatomy

- Portal placement (Fig. 61-5)
  - Proper placement is crucial given the constrained nature of the ankle joint.
  - The joint is insufflated with 10-15 cc of sterile saline to confirm portals. The needle should easily fall into the joint medially and result in a bulge where the lateral portal will be placed.
  - Portals are created using the "nick and spread" technique to prevent injury to the saphenous nerve and vein medially and the superficial peroneal nerve (SPN) laterally.
  - The anterior portals are used interchangeably for viewing and working.
    - Typically, it is easiest to use the portal nearest the pathology as the working portal.
  - Medial portal
    - Established first and used for the diagnostic portion of the case.

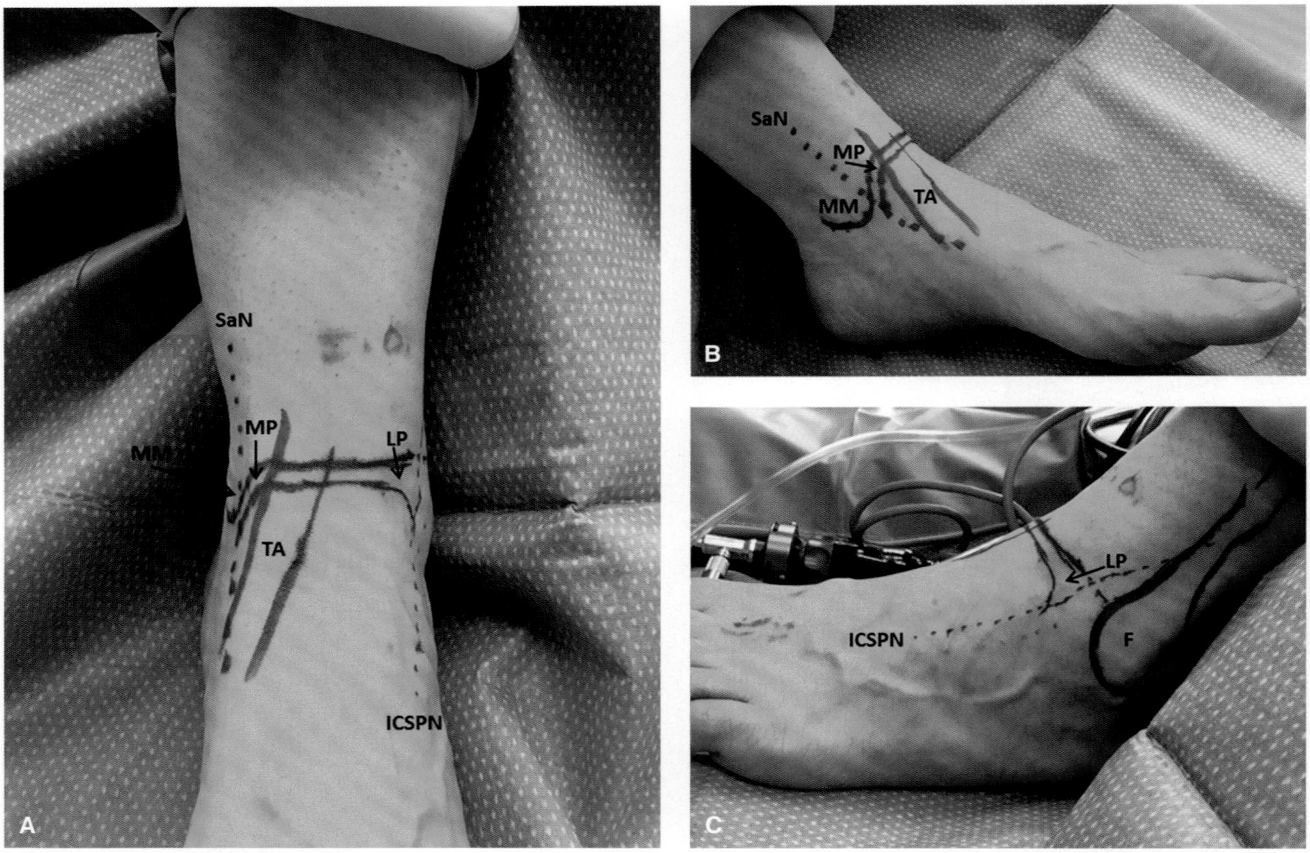

Figure 61-5 | A-C. Surface anatomy aids in the establishment of proper portal placement. MM, medial malleolus; TA, tibialis anterior; SaN, saphenous nerve; MP, medial portal; ICSPN, intermediate cutaneous branch of the superficial peroneal nerve; LP, lateral portal; F, Fibula.

- Placed at the joint line, medial to the anterior tibial tendon.
  - The correct location is typically 1 cm proximal to the tip of the medial malleolus and is characterized by a palpable soft spot.
- Lateral portal
  - Lateral to the extensor digitorum longus tendons or, alternatively, lateral to the peroneus tertius tendon.
  - Localized with a spinal needle under direct visualization (Fig. 61-6).

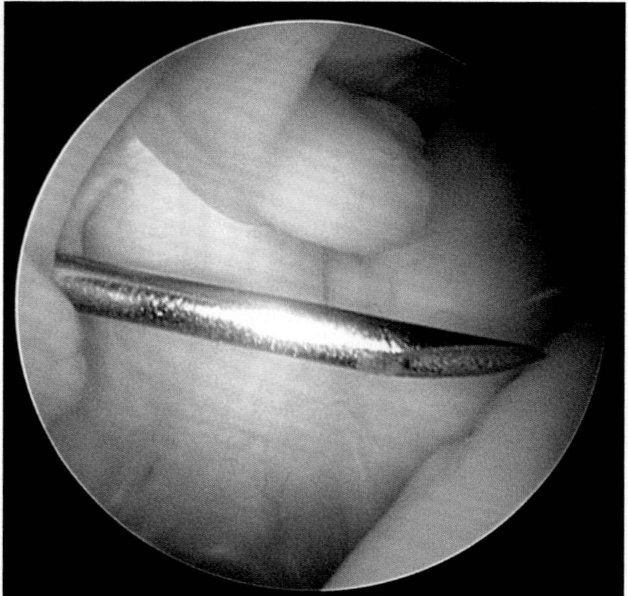

Figure 61-6 | Needle visualization of lateral portal placement ensures a functional portal for intra-articular instruments.

- Careful attention should be paid to the intermediate dorsal cutaneous branch of the SPN, which lies very near a properly placed portal.
    - The nerve can be identified using the fourth toe flexion sign.[4]
- Intra-articular anatomy
    - A routine should be developed to systematically evaluate the ankle joint.
        - Listed below are the structures visualized during ankle arthroscopy.
            - It is often helpful to debride the anterior gutter before a thorough diagnostic arthroscopy.
        - Medial ankle examination (Fig. 61-7)
            - Deltoid ligament—impinging ossicles at the tip of the medial malleolus
            - Medial gutter—loose bodies
            - Medial shoulder of the talus—osteochondral lesions

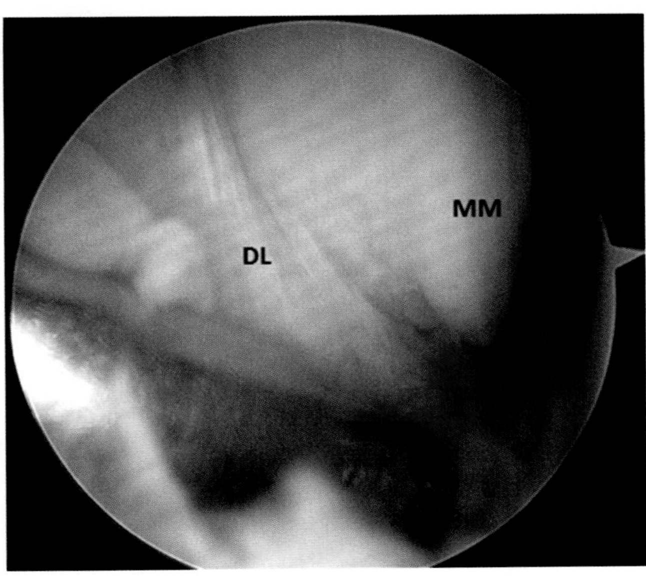

Figure 61-7 | Intra-articular examination of medial ankle. DL, deltoid ligament; MM, medial malleolus.

- Anterior ankle examination
    - Anterior gutter—synovial hypertrophy and loose bodies
        - This area must be carefully debrided to prevent injury to the deep peroneal nerve and anterior tibial artery.[5] It can be helpful to remove traction to allow the neurovascular bundle to relax away from the motorized shaver (Fig. 61-8).
        - Inflamed synovial tissue can bleed and obscure the view if overaggressive debridement is performed.
    - Impinging osteophytes on talar neck and distal tibial plafond (Fig. 61-9)
        - We move the ankle through dorsiflexion and plantar flexion when evaluating for impingement.

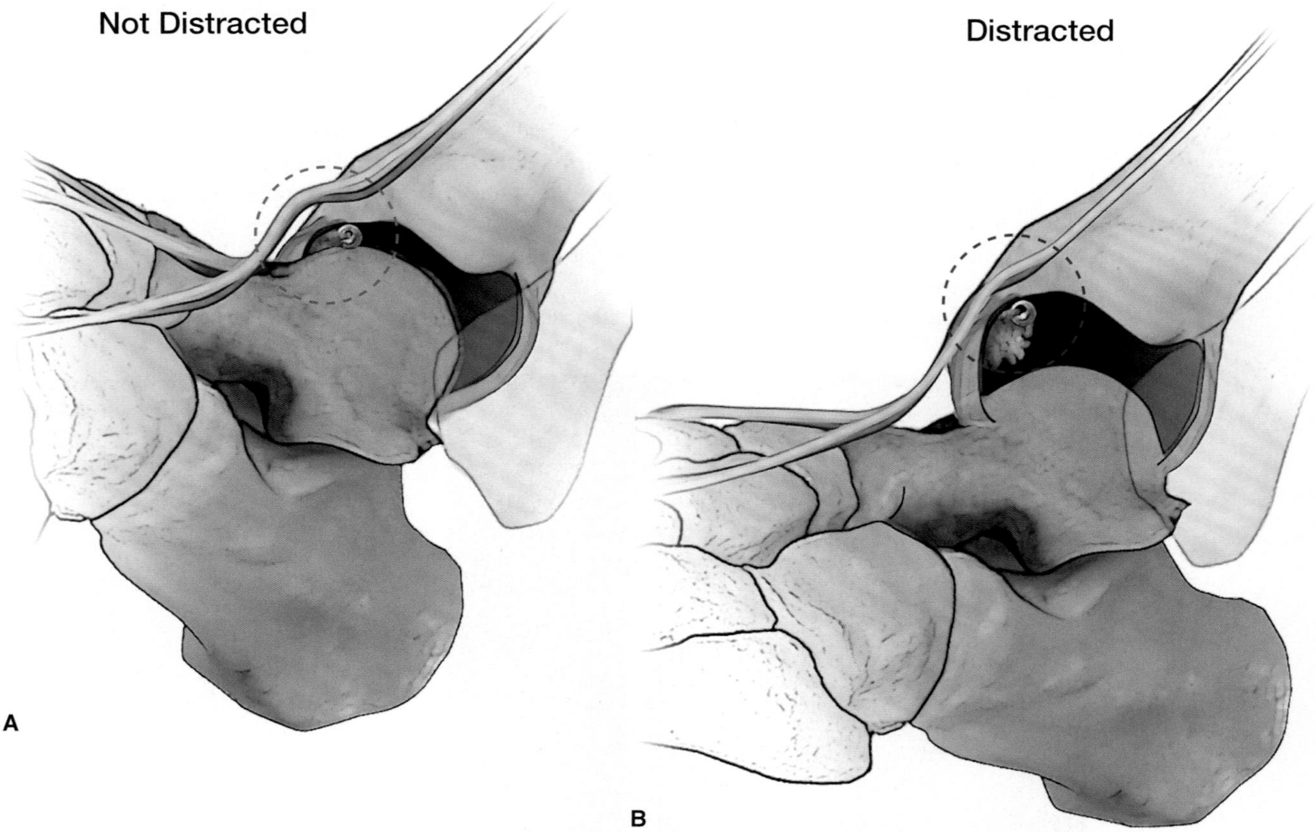

Not Distracted

Distracted

A

B

Figure 61-8 | **A.** Traction can be released to allow the anterior capsule to relax. **B.** The neurovascular bundle is drawn closer to the joint while in traction.

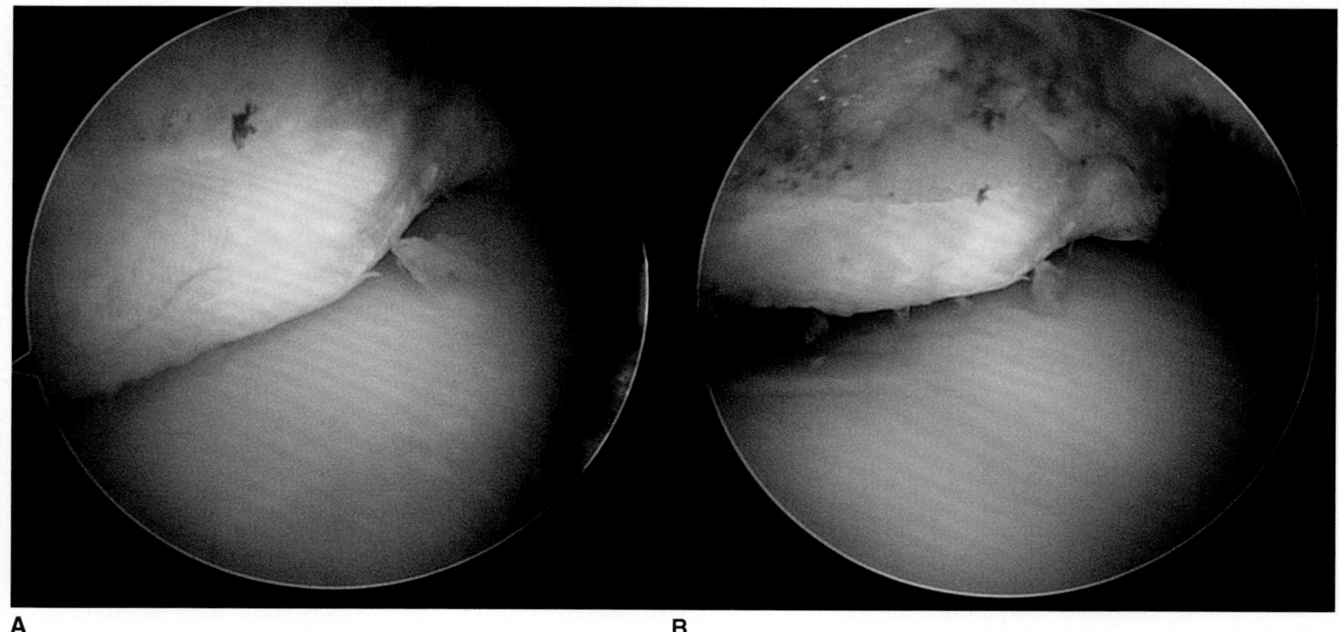

A

B

Figure 61-9 | **A.** Anterior osteophytes on the distal tibia. **B.** Following debridement.

- Lateral ankle examination (Fig. 61-10)
  - Lateral gutter—loose bodies
  - Lateral shoulder of the talus—osteochondral lesions

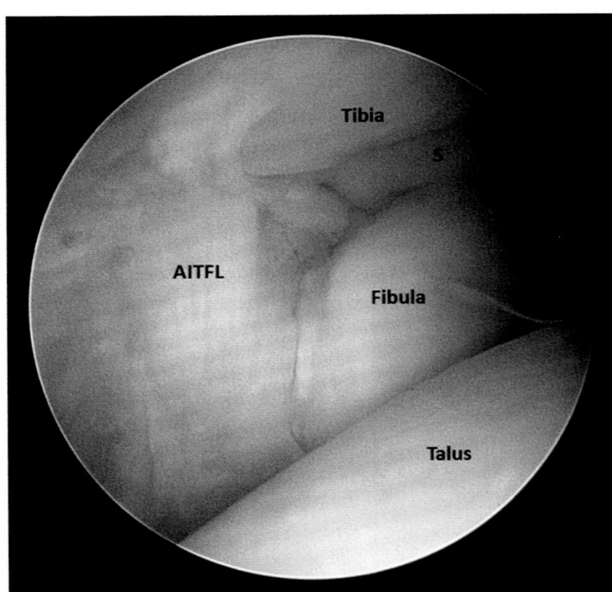

Figure 61-10 | Intra-articular examination of the lateral ankle. S, syndesmosis; AITFL, anterior inferior tibiofibular ligament.

  - "Trifurcation"—the area where the tibial plafond, distal fibula, and talus articulate (Fig. 61-11)
    - Inability to visualize the trifurcation suggests the presence of a Bassett lesion or synovial hypertrophy and should be debrided until this is visible.[6]
    - A probe can be placed in this area to assess competence of the syndesmosis.
  - Anterior inferior tibiofibular ligament

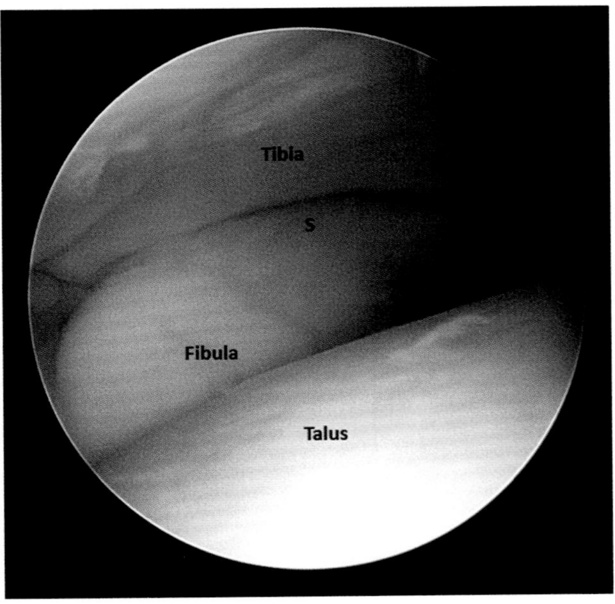

Figure 61-11 | A probe can placed into the trifurcation to stress the syndesmosis (not pictured). S, Intra-articular syndesmosis.

- Posterior ankle examination
  - Posterior inferior tibiofibular ligament and transverse tibiofibular ligament (Fig. 61-12)
  - Extensor hallucis longus tendon
  - Loose bodies can "hide" in the posterior ankle because of the posterior slope of the joint. A gentle squeeze anterior to the Achilles tendon can decrease space in the posterior ankle and bring loose bodies into the visual field of the scope.

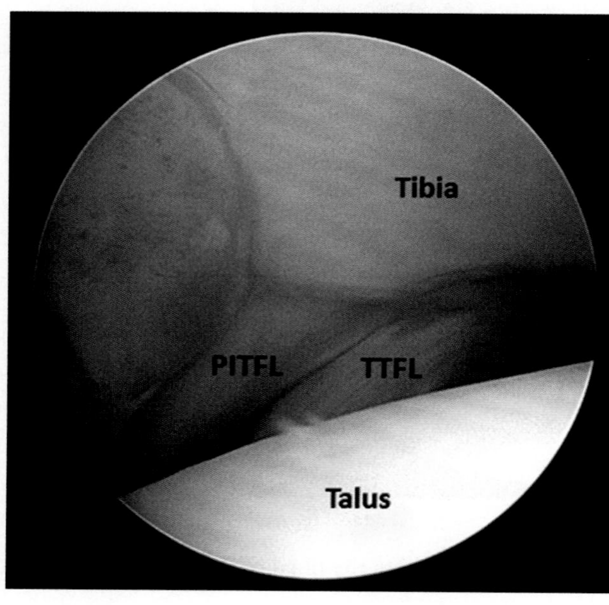

Figure 61-12 | Posterior structures of the ankle as viewed through an anterior portal. PITFL, posterior inferior talofibular ligament; TTFL, transverse tibiofibular ligament.

References

1. van Dijk NC, van Bergen CJ. Advancements in ankle arthroscopy. *J Am Acad Orthop Surg.* 2008;16:635-646.
2. Dowdy PA, Watson BV, Amendola A. Noninvasive ankle distraction: relationship between force, magnitude of distraction, and nerve conduction abnormalities. *Arthroscopy.* 1996;12:64-69.
3. Young BH, Flanigan RM, DiGiovanni BF. Complications of ankle arthroscopy utilizing a contemporary noninvasive distraction technique. *J Bone Joint Surg Am.* 2001;93:963-968.
4. Stephens MM, Kelly PM. Fourth toe flexion sign: a new clinical sign for identification of the superficial peroneal nerve. *Foot Ankle Int.* 2000;21:800-863.
5. Darwish A, Ehsan O, Marynissen H, et al. Pseudoaneurysm of the anterior tibial artery after ankle arthroscopy. *Arthroscopy.* 2004;20:e63-e64.
6. Bassett FH, Gates HS, Billys JB, et al. Talar impingement by the anteroinferior tibiofibular ligament. *J Bone Joint Surg Am.* 1990;72:55-59.

Suggested Readings

Amendola A, Stone JW. *AANA Advanced Arthroscopy: the Foot and Ankle.* Philadelphia, PA: Elsevier; 2010.
Ferkel RD. *Foot and Ankle Arthroscopy.* 2nd ed. Philadelphia, PA: Wolters Kluwer; 2017.

Chapter 62

Arthroscopic Treatment of Osteochondral Lesions of the Talus

G. ANDREW MURPHY
JANE C. YEOH

Introduction

Osteochondral lesions of the talus (OLT) or osteochondritis dissecans of the talus was originally described as transchondral fractures of the talus by Berndt and Harty[1]. After the initial classification by Berndt and Harty[1], several authors further classified OLTs by computed tomography (CT) imaging findings, magnetic resonance imaging (MRI) findings, and arthroscopic findings. OLTs can be symptomatic or asymptomatic. Asymptomatic OLTs should not be treated operatively.

Treatment of OLTs by arthroscopic débridement and bone marrow stimulation techniques has demonstrated good long-term outcomes. Van Bergen et al.[2] demonstrated that 94% (46 of 49) patients returned to work and 88% (37 of 42) patients returned to sport at an average follow-up of 141 ± 34 months. The majority of patients had good or excellent clinical outcomes, measured by the Ogilvie-Harris score (20% excellent, 58% good, 22% fair, 0% poor), AOFAS score (mean 88), and SF-36 (71 ± 16 mean physical component and 94 ± 22 emotional component.[2] When assessed for radiographic progression, 67% (32 of 48) patients showed no radiographic progression of osteoarthritis and 33% (16 of 48) patients showed osteoarthritis progression by one stage.[2]

Classification Systems

Several classification systems exist to grade OLTs by radiographs,[3] MRI,[4] and arthroscopic findings.[5,6] Giannini et al.[7] devised a classification that guides treatment of OLTs (Table 62-1).

Preoperative Planning

- Detailed history and physical examination
  - Clinical findings confirmed with imaging findings.
    - Only 30% (15 of 50) ankles with nonoperatively treated OLTs had ankle tenderness corresponding to the location of the OLT.[7]
  - Pathologies that should be treated alongside the OCL of the talus (e.g., chronic ankle instability)
    - 48% (24 of 50) ankles with nonoperatively treated OLT had subjective instability.[8]

Table 62-1 | Classification of osteochondral lesions based on radiographics, MRI, and arthroscopy

Radiographic Classification	MRI Revised Classification	Arthroscopic Classification	Arthroscopic Grade Based on Articular Cartilage
Berndt and Harty[1]	**Hepple et al.[8]**	**Dipaola et al.[4]**	**Ferkel et al.[6]**
Stage 0[a] Not visible on radiographs *Stage 1* Trabecular compression of subchondral bone	*Stage 1* Articular cartilage damage only	*Stage I* Irregularity and softening of articular cartilage, no definable fragment	*Grade A* Smooth, intact cartilage, but soft and ballottable *Grade B* Rough articular cartilage surface
Stage 2 Partially detached osteochondral fragment	*Stage 2a* Cartilage injury with underlying fracture and surrounding bony edema *Stage 2b* Cartilage injury with underlying fracture without surrounding bony edema	*Stage II* Articular cartilage breached, definable fragment, not displaceable	*Grade C* Articular cartilage has fibrillations and fissures *Grade D* Articular cartilage flap present or bone exposed
Stage 3 Detached and undisplaced osteochondral fragment	*Stage 3* Detached and undisplaced osteochondral fragment	*Stage III* Articular cartilage breached, definable fragment, displace-able, but attached by some overlying articular cartilage	*Grade E* Loose, undisplaced fragment
Stage 4 Detached and displaced osteochondral fragment	*Stage 4* Detached and displaced osteochondral fragment *Stage 5* Osteochondral lesion with subchondral cyst formation	*Stage IV* Detached and displaced osteochondral fragment (loose body)	*Grade F* Loose, displaced fragment

[a]*Stage 0* not part of original classification.

- Obtain weight-bearing AP, lateral, and oblique plain radiographs of the ankle (Fig. 62-1).
- Obtain cross-sectional imaging.
  - MRI cross-sectional imaging (Figs. 62-2 and 62-3)
    - MRI is preferred for visualization of bone marrow edema, soft tissue, and articular cartilage details.

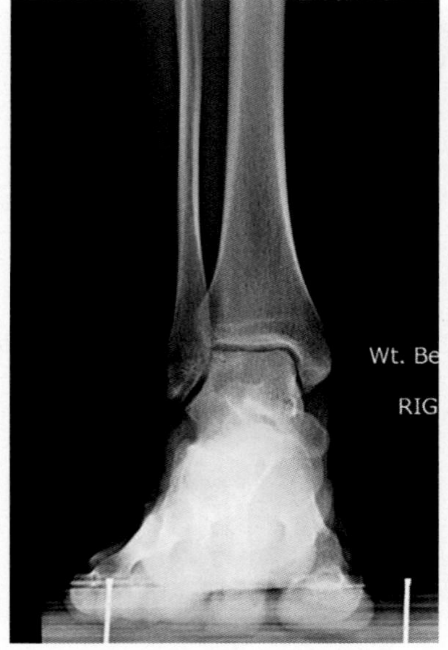

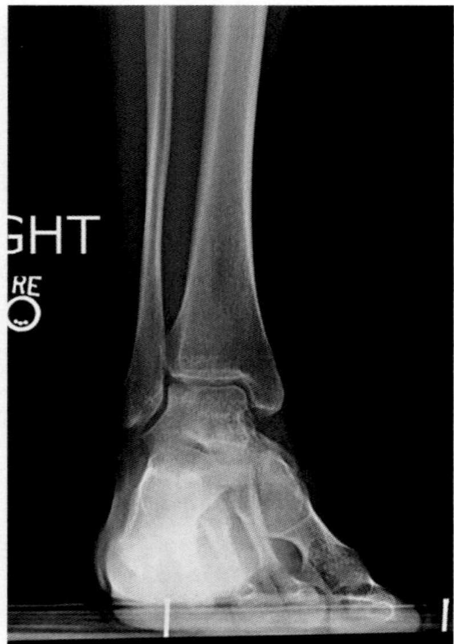

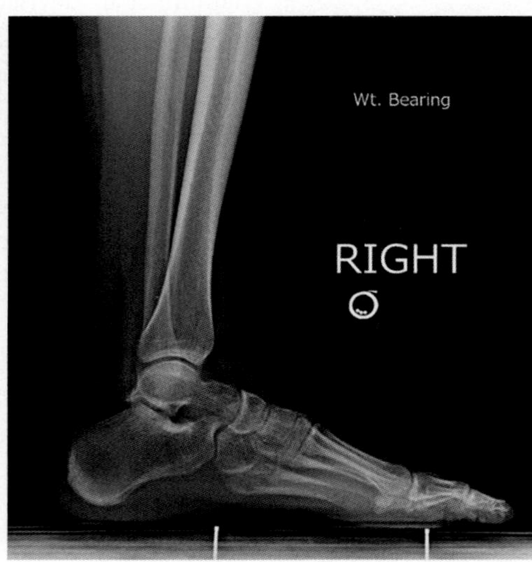

Figure 62-1 | AP, mortise, and lateral weight-bearing radiographs of a lateral OLT in a 17-year-old woman.

- Spiral CT or weight-bearing CT (PEDCAT) (Figs. 62-2 and 62-3)
  - CT is preferred for determining size of the lesion.

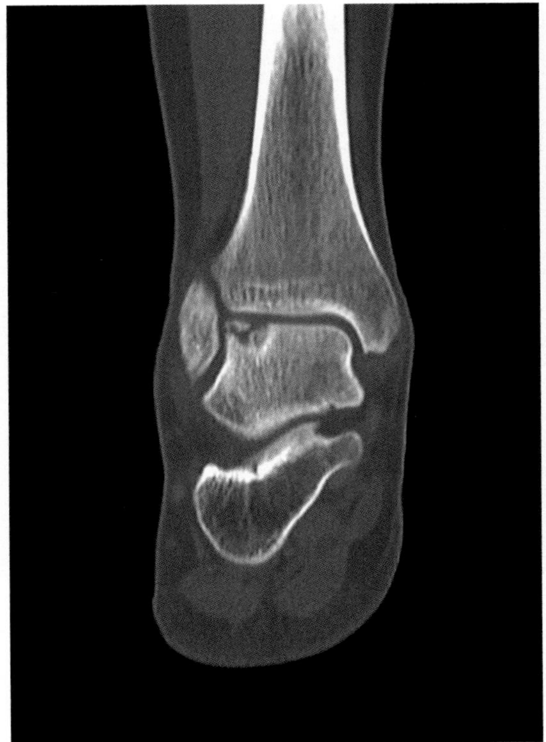

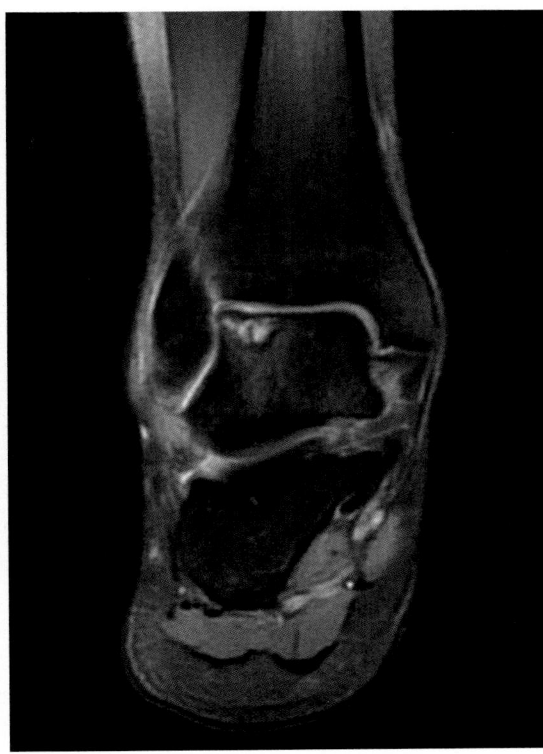

Figure 62-2 | Coronal CT and MR images of a lateral cystic subchondral OLT in a 17-year-old woman (same patient as in Fig. 62-1).

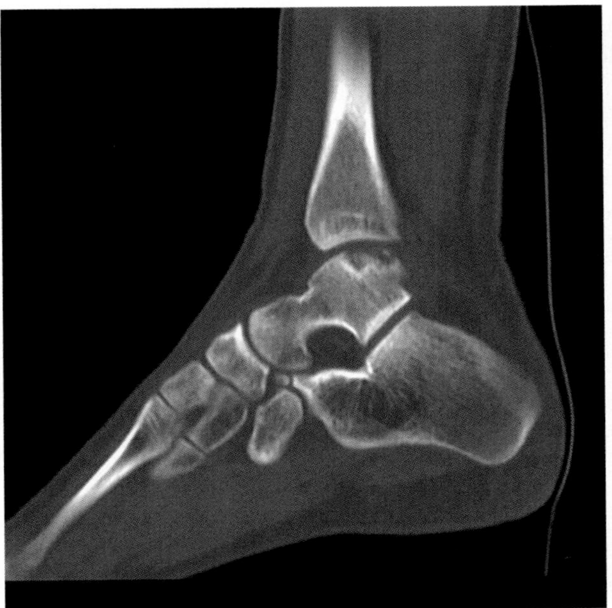

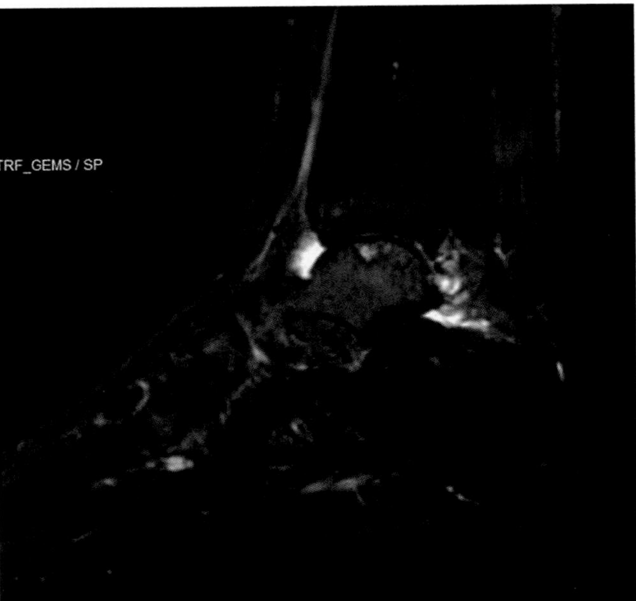

Figure 62-3 | Sagittal CT and MR images of a lateral cystic subchondral OLT (same patient as in Figs. 62-1 and 62-2).

- A comparison of these different imaging modalities can help the physician better understand the osteochondral lesion (Fig. 62-4).

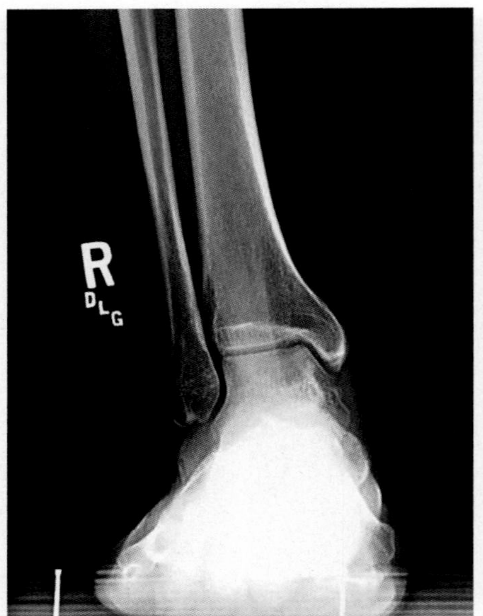

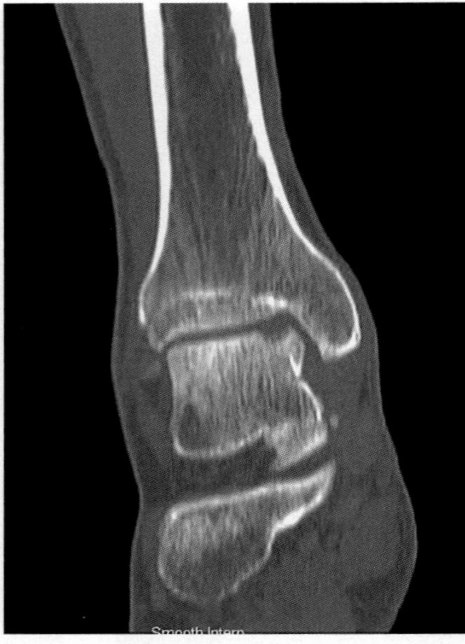
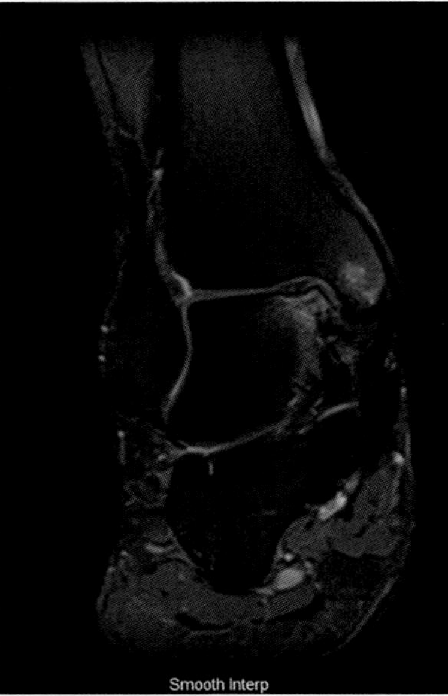

Figure 62-4 | Mortise radiograph, coronal CT image, and coronal MR image of a medial OLT in a 36-year-old man. Note the clear delineation of the bony border of the OLT in the CT image and note the bone marrow edema apparent in the medial talus and medial malleolus on the MRI.

Decision Making

- Primary vs revision surgery
  - The gold standard of primary treatment of small OLTs < 1.5 cm^2 is arthroscopic débridement and bone marrow stimulation or microfracture.
  - Revision surgery or primary surgery of large lesions could include cartilage replacement procedures including osteoarticular transplantation system (OATS), autologous cartilage implantation (ACI), juvenile hyaline cartilage allograft, and bulk osteochondral allograft.
    - Lesions ≥1.5 cm^2 treated with arthroscopic débridement and bone marrow stimulation are associated with increased risk of poor outcome.[9] Therefore, lesions ≥1.5 cm^2 can be treated with arthroscopic débridement and bone marrow stimulation or cartilage replacement procedures.
- Cartilage or surface intact vs damaged[7]
  - Surface completely intact—consider retrograde drilling
  - Cartilage damage—see below
- Size of OCL talus and chronicity determined by Giannini et al.[7]
  - <1 cm^2 acute—débridement
  - ≥1 cm^2 acute—fixation
  - <1.5 cm^2 chronic—microfracture
  - ≥1.5 cm^2 chronic—cartilage replacement (OAT or ACI) ± bone graft (if >5 mm deep)
  - Massive size (≥3.0 cm^2)—bulk osteochondral allograft
- Presence of cyst and size of cyst
  - Noncystic and small subchondral cystic OLTs treated with microfracture have comparable and good clinical outcomes[2]
  - Some experts recommend that larger cystic lesions (>6 mm depth)[6] should be treated with bone grafting; however, bone grafting in this scenario has not been shown to be definitively beneficial in scientific literature.
- This chapter describes the treatment of a full-thickness OLT treated with arthroscopic débridement and microfracture. It also describes particulated arthroscopic juvenile hyaline cartilage allograft implantation. ACI, OATS, or bulk osteochondral graft are not discussed in detail in this chapter.

Sterile Instruments/Equipment (Figs. 62-5 to 62-7)

- Although arthroscopes described range from 30-degree angle, 25-degree angle, and 70-degree angle 2.5- to 4.5-mm arthroscopes, the authors prefer a small joint 2.7-mm 30-degree arthroscope
- Inflow pump set to 30-60 mm Hg
- Shaver 2.5 mm
- Dissector 3 mm

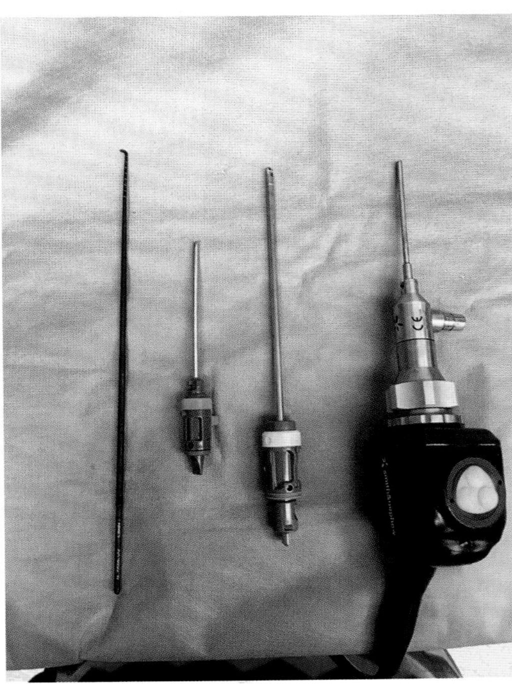

Figure 62-5 | **Left to Right.** Probe, small 2.5-mm shaver, 3-mm burr, and 2.7-mm 30-degree arthroscope.

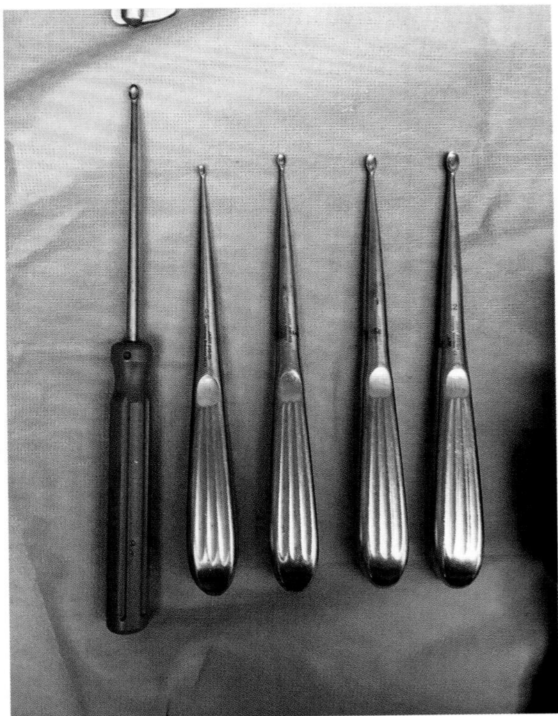

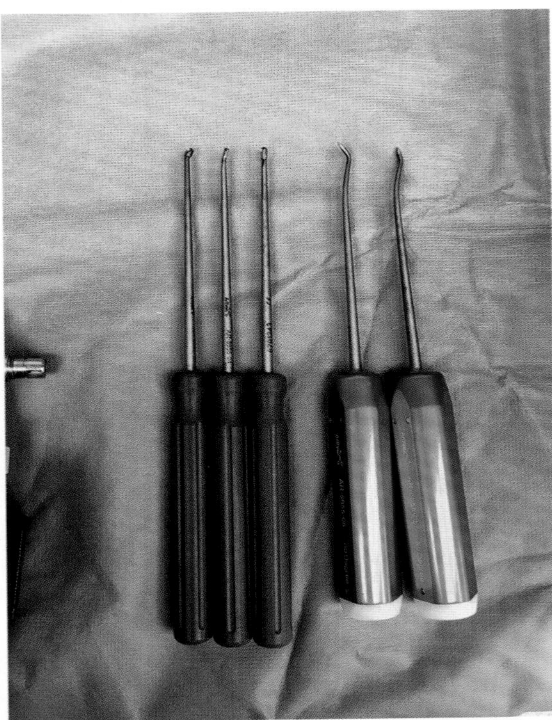

Figure 62-6 | **Left to Right.** Straight curettes of varying sizes, angled ring curettes, and angled microfracture awls.

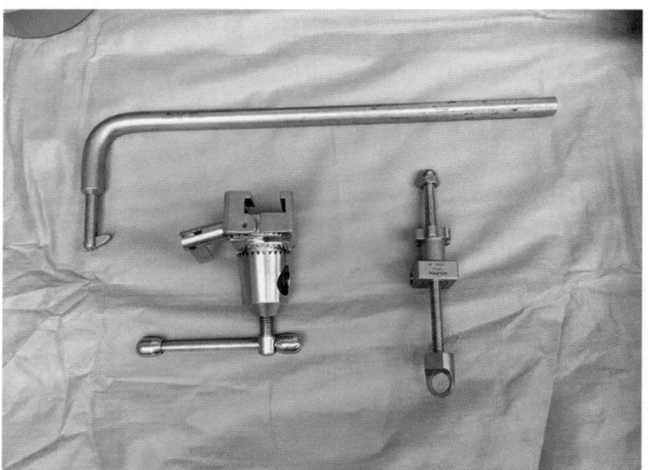

Figure 62-7 | Sterilized foot holder and bed clamp.

- Burr 3 or 4 mm
- Resector 2.7 or 3.5 mm radius
- Microfracture awls
  - Straight and curved
  - Different angulations 30 degrees, 60 degrees, and 90 degrees
- Straight and angled regular curettes
- Several sizes and angles of ring curettes
- Arthroscopy set including
  - Graspers, punches, osteotomes, elevators, chondral picks
- Kirschner wires for drilling if needed 1.1, 1.6, 2.4 mm
- Anterograde or retrograde drilling guide
- Fluoroscopic imaging if needed
- Distraction device if needed
  - Noninvasive distraction device
  - Although methods are available to attach the noninvasive distraction device to the surgeon, the authors prefer a sterile ankle distractor strap attached to a sterilized foot holder and bed clamp

Positioning (Fig. 62-8)

- General anesthesia
- Thigh tourniquet
- Supine with bump under ipsilateral hip so the transmalleolar axis is parallel to the ground
- Hip and knee slightly flexed with leg holder
- Limb exsanguinated before sterile preparation (Fig. 62-8)

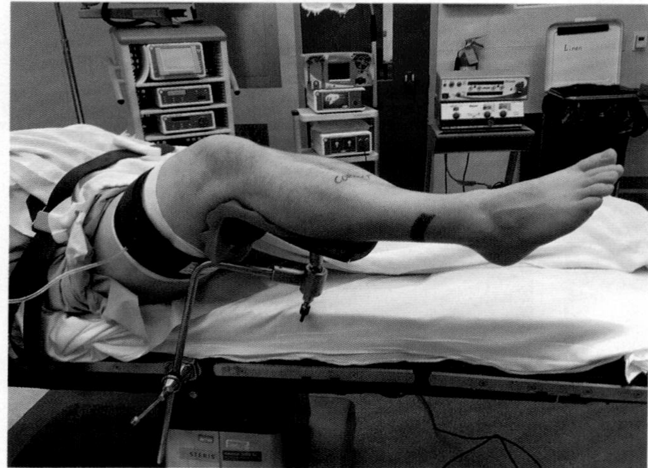

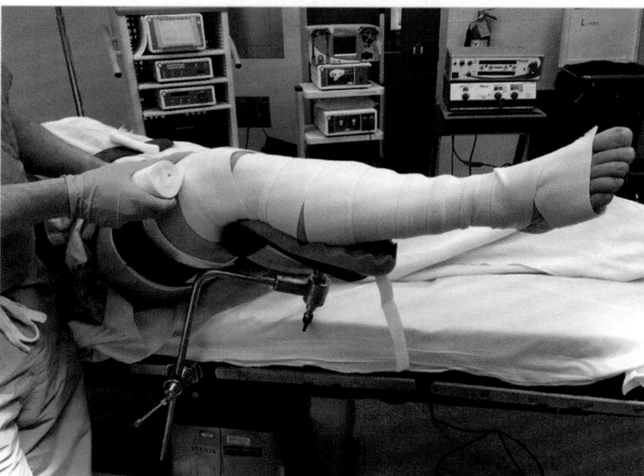

Figure 62-8 | Patient extremity in leg holder with hip and knee slightly flexed, and thigh tourniquet. The author prefers exsanguination of limb prior to sterile preparation.

- The patient is positioned at a height so that the surgeon can rest the foot on his or her chest or abdomen
  - Pearl: The chest or abdomen can be used to extend or dorsiflex ankle to allow anterior capsule relaxation and visualization of the anterior compartment
- Distraction
  - Pearl: Immediate distraction is not needed; distractor is kept sterile and attached to lateral bed rail on top of drape until use.

Portals

- Before sterile prep
  - While plantar flexing and inverting the ankle, the surgeon can identify the medial dorsal cutaneous branch and intermediate dorsal cutaneous branch of the superficial peroneal nerve. Plantar flexion of the fourth toe accomplishes this as well (Fig. 62-9)
  - We use the back of a pen to palpate this nerve and its course as it crosses the ankle joint (Fig. 62-9)
  - Before arthroscopy, the joint is insufflated with 5-10 cc of Marcaine with epinephrine through anteromedial portal (Fig. 62-10)

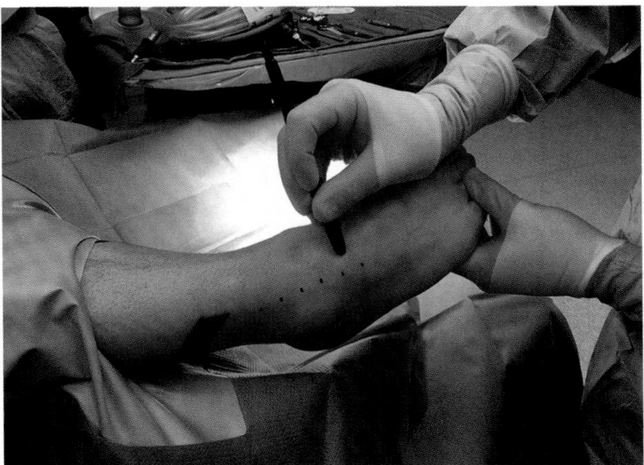
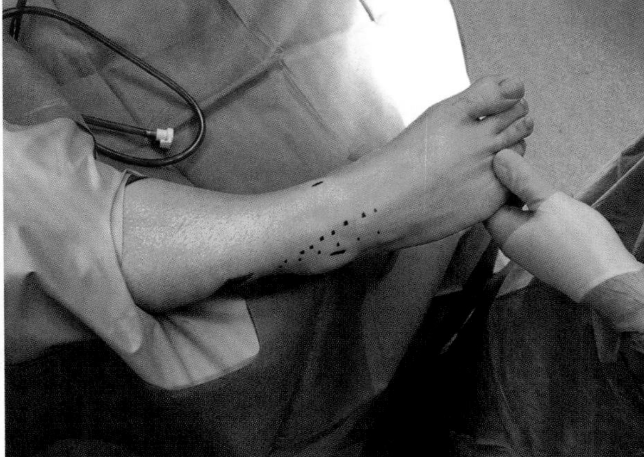

Figure 62-9 | Identification of medial dorsal cutaneous branch and intermediate dorsal cutaneous branch of the superficial peroneal nerve by palpation with the back of a pen while plantar flexing and inverting the ankle. Note that the surgeon plantar flexes the fourth toe to position the ankle for this maneuver.

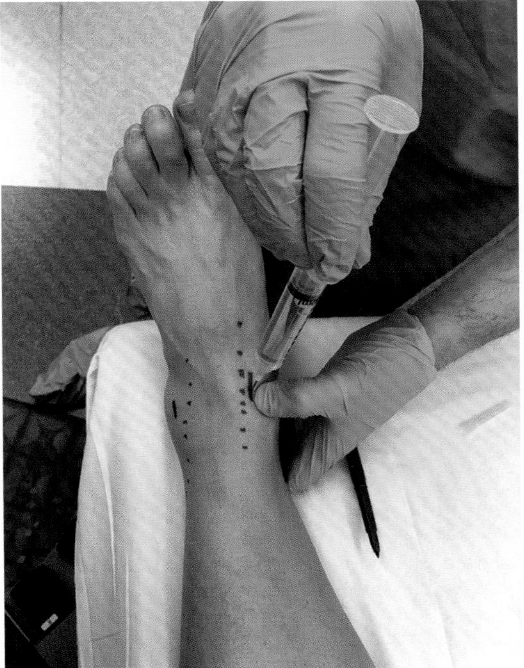
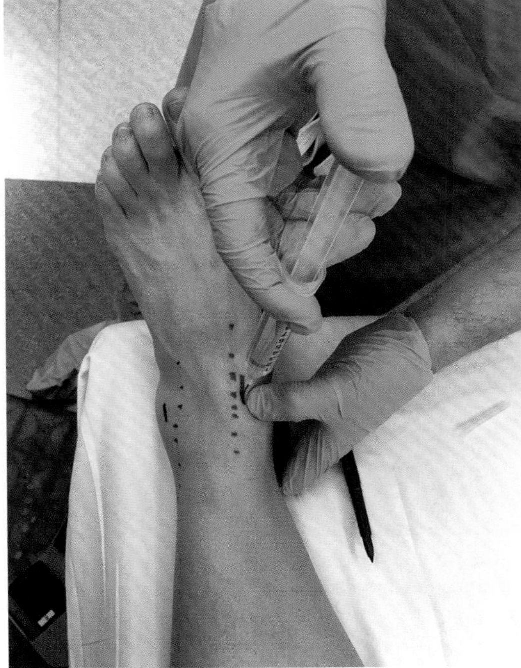

Figure 62-10 | Insufflation of the joint with 5-10 cc of Marcaine with epinephrine with an 18-G needle. Easy flow and backflow ensure intra-articular placement.

- Use of an 18-G needle will provide tactile feedback when entering the joint. The fluid will flow easily and should have backflow; this ensures intra-articular placement.
- This can be done before or after sterile preparation and draping of the extremity.

- Standard portals
  - Anteromedial portal
    - The anteromedial portal is established first because there is less chance of being too proximal or too distal on the anteromedial portal.
    - Between the anterior tibial tendon and medial malleolus, just medial to anterior tibial tendon, at level of joint line (or 0.5-1.0 cm below level of joint line)
    - Small incision 5-8 mm through skin (Fig. 62-11)
    - Subcutaneous layer divided with small hemostat (Fig. 62-12).

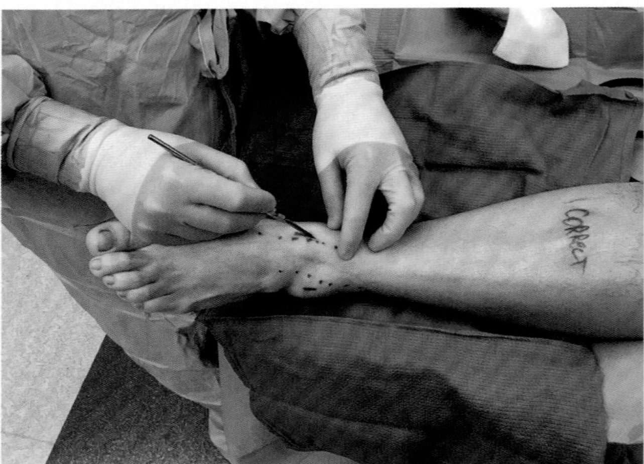

Figure 62-11 | In the anteromedial portal, a small 5- to 8-mm incision is made through skin.

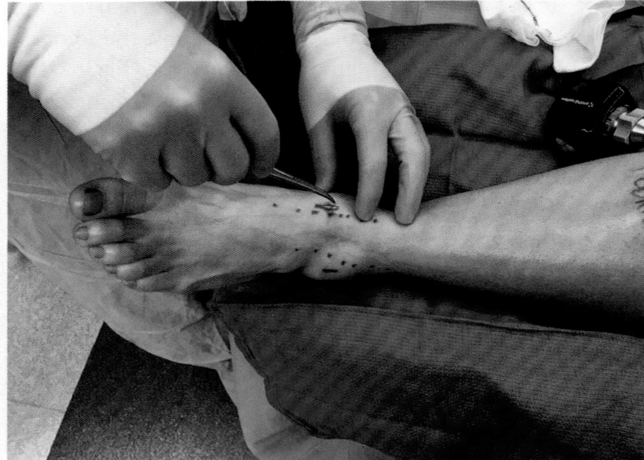

Figure 62-12 | Blunt dissection is performed through the subcutaneous layer with a small hemostat.

- Blunt trocar is placed gently into the joint with the ankle in dorsiflexion (Fig. 62-13).
- The cannula is removed, and an egress of fluid (synovial fluid and saline) indicates that the trocar is correctly placed (Fig. 62-14).
- Arthroscope is placed into trocar.

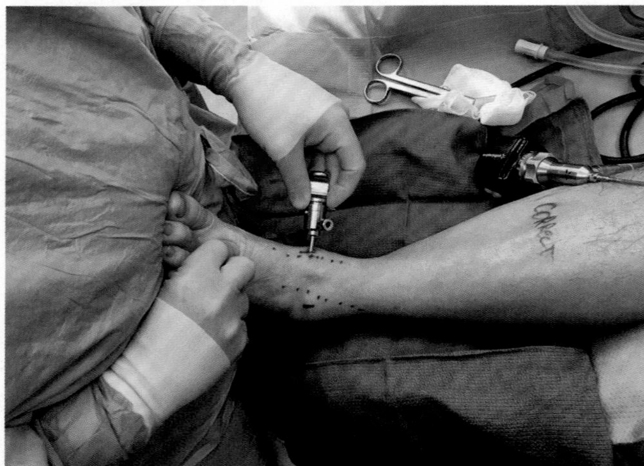

Figure 62-13 | A blunt trocar is placed gently into the anterior space with the ankle in dorsiflexion.

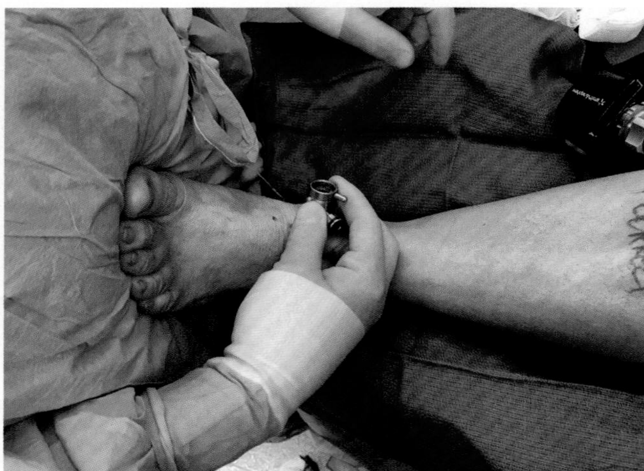

Figure 62-14 | When the cannula is removed, an egress of fluid (synovial fluid and saline) indicates that the trocar is correctly placed.

- Anterolateral portal
  - Before start of procedure, the surgeon can stretch the ankle in plantar flexion and inversion. This sometimes exposes the intermediate branch of the superficial peroneal nerve as it passes the ankle joint and is best done before insufflation of the joint
  - Landmark between extensor tendons (peroneus tertius) and distal fibula just lateral to peroneus tertius at the level of or slightly above the level of the joint
  - This anterolateral portal is entered under direct visualization using the arthroscope in the anteromedial portal. Transillumination with the arthoscope can also help guide the location of this portal.
  - An 18-G needle is placed at the desired location under direct visualization (Fig. 62-15).
  - A small incision (5-8 mm) is made through the skin.

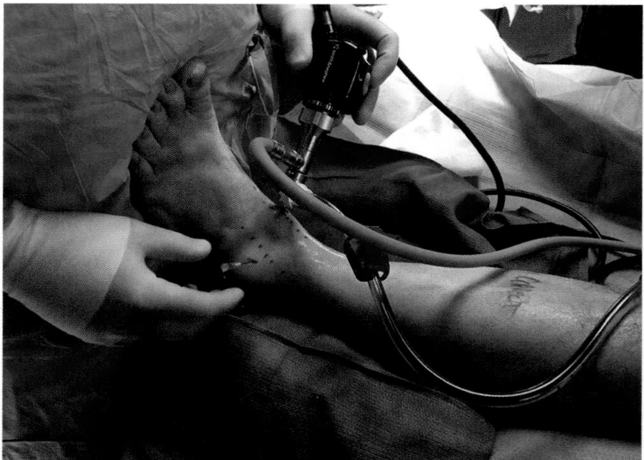

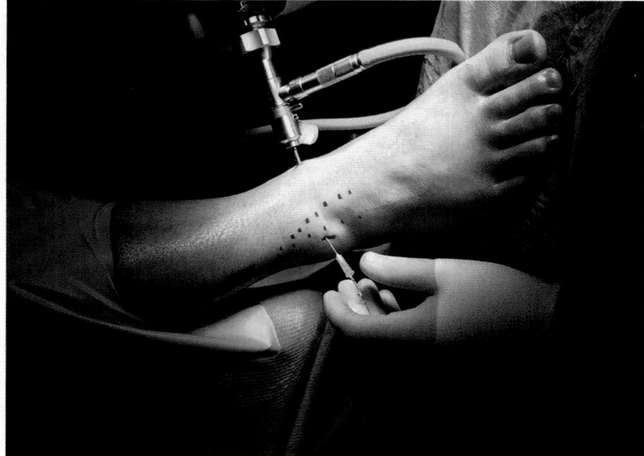

Figure 62-15 | Fluid exiting from 18-G needle, and direct visualization confirms appropriate position of the anterolateral portal.

  - The subcutaneous layer is divided with small hemostat and the joint capsule is entered under direct observation (Fig. 62-16).
  - The ankle joint is entered through the anterolateral portal with probe, shaver, or other tool (Fig. 62-17).

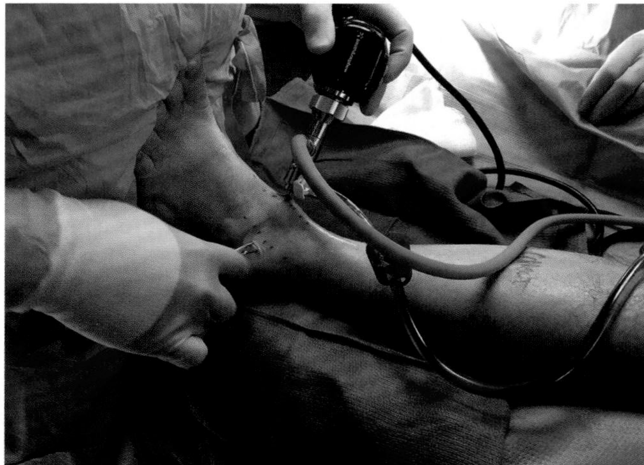

Figure 62-16 | In the anterolateral portal, divide the subcutaneous layer with small hemostat and enter the joint capsule under direct observation.

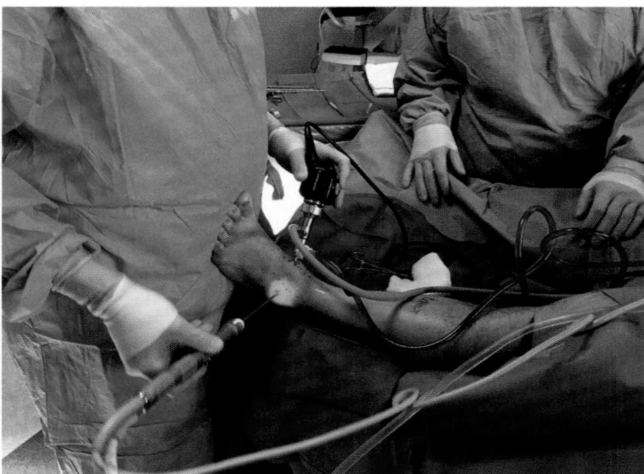

Figure 62-17 | A shaver is placed through the anterolateral portal.

- Arthroscopy from the anterolateral portal allows the tools to be used at the anteromedial portal (Fig. 62-18).

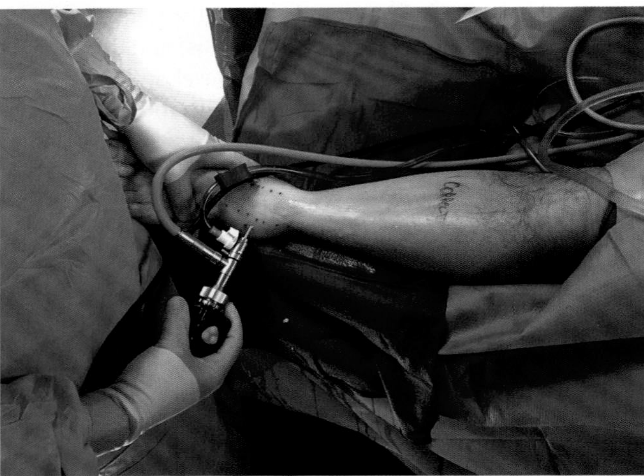

Figure 62-18 | Arthroscopy is performed at the anterolateral portal to allow tools to be used at the anteromedial portal.

- Additional portals
  - Posterolateral portal
    - Location of the portal is between the lateral border of the Achilles tendon and distal fibula, specifically just lateral to Achilles tendon, 1-1.5 cm proximal to the tip of the distal fibula.
    - Under direct visualization using the arthroscope through the anteromedial portal, an 18-G needle is placed toward the medial malleolus.
    - A small incision 5-8 mm is made through skin
    - The subcutaneous layer is divided with small hemostat and the joint capsule is entered with a blunt trocar under direct observation.
  - Other portals, including anterocentral and transmalleolar portals, have been described but are not detailed in this article.

Treatment of OLTs: Arthroscopy, Débridement, and Microfracture

- Diagnostic arthroscopy is done looking at talar neck, medial gutter, lateral gutter syndesmosis, tibial surface, anterior talar dome, and posterior talar dome.
- Arthroscopy of the anterior compartment without distraction is done first. The surgeon can use the chest or abdomen to extend the ankle and relax the anterior capsule.
- Anterior impingement lesions on medial talus are removed first, before defining the OLT because the impinging lesion may block visualization of the OLT.
- Posterior talar dome plantar flexion and distraction can be observed with the help of a noninvasive distractor (Figs. 62-7 and 62-19).
- Both anteromedial and anterolateral portals can be used interchangeably for arthroscopy and preparation.
- The posterior gutter is milked to ensure no loose bodies are present.
- The lesion is defined with a probe.
  - Soft cartilage and delamination indicate an underlying OLT (Fig. 62-20).
  - Grossly unstable or flipped cartilage must be removed to stable perpendicular edges (Figs. 62-21 and 62-22).
  - If the cartilage is completely intact, this patient may be a candidate for retrograde drilling.

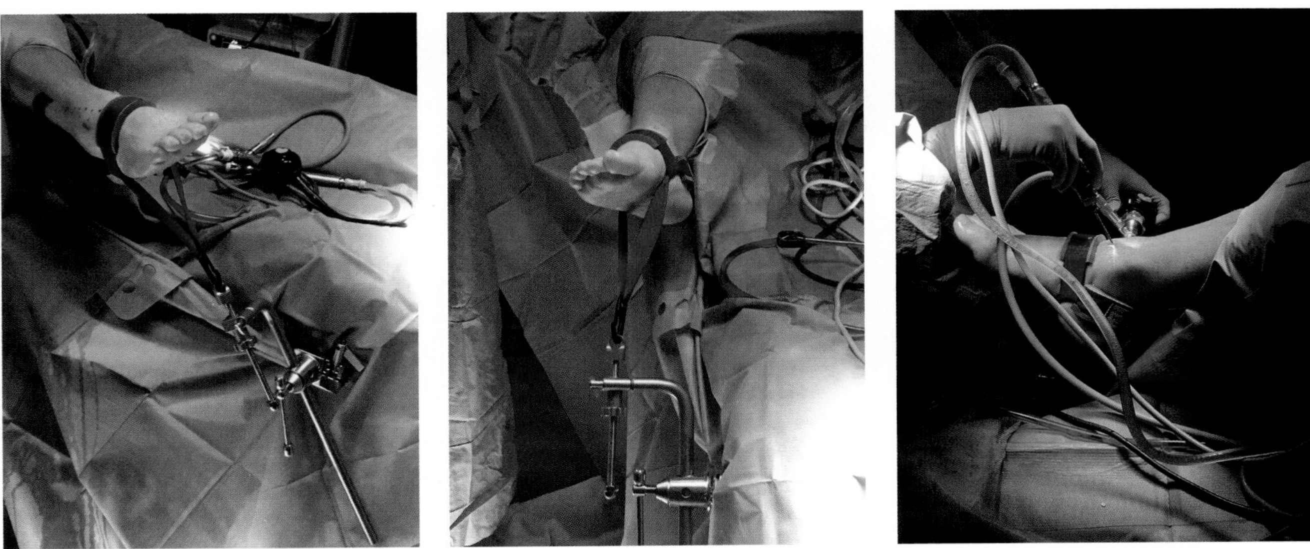

Figure 62-19 | Noninvasive distractor with sterile ankle distractor strap, sterilized foot holder, and bed clamp.

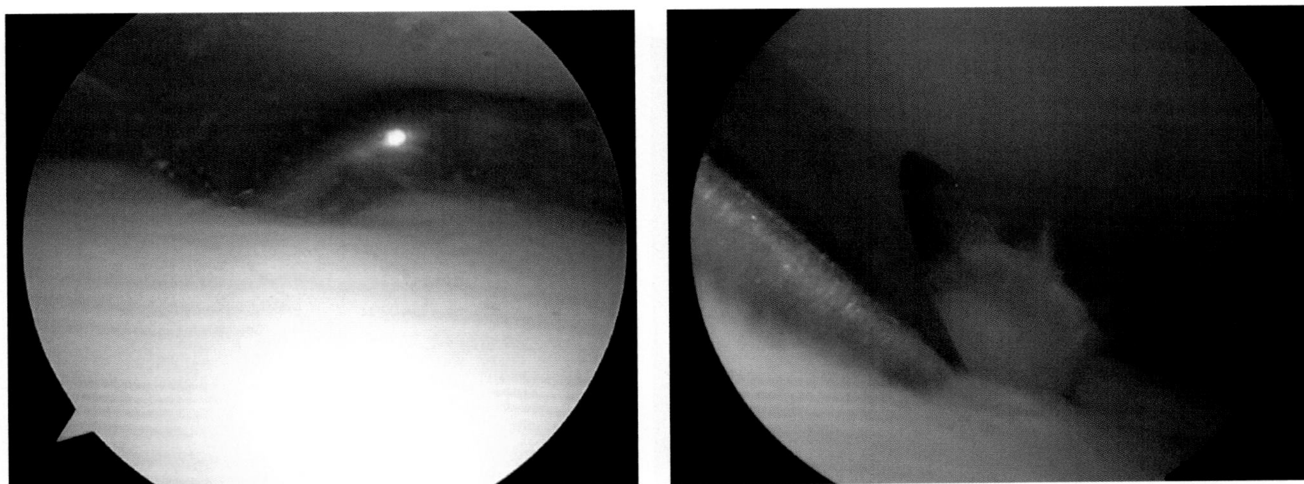

Figure 62-20 | **Left.** Probing soft cartilage indicates an underlying OLT. **Right.** Curette soft and delaminating cartilage overlying OLT.

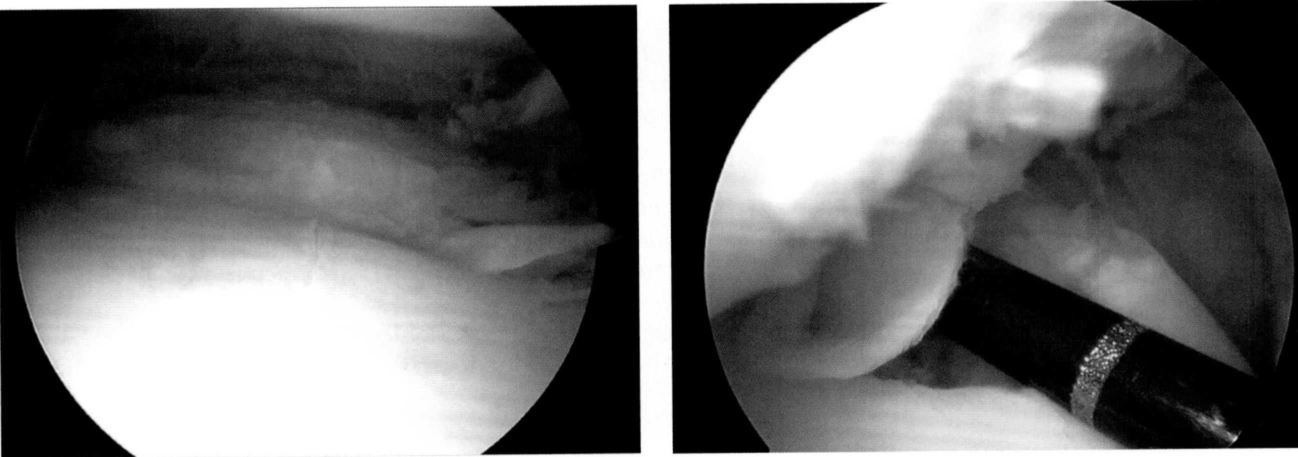

Figure 62-21 | **Left.** Grossly unstable OLT visualized on ankle arthroscopy. **Right.** Probing the unstable cartilage demonstrates that the cartilage flips easily.

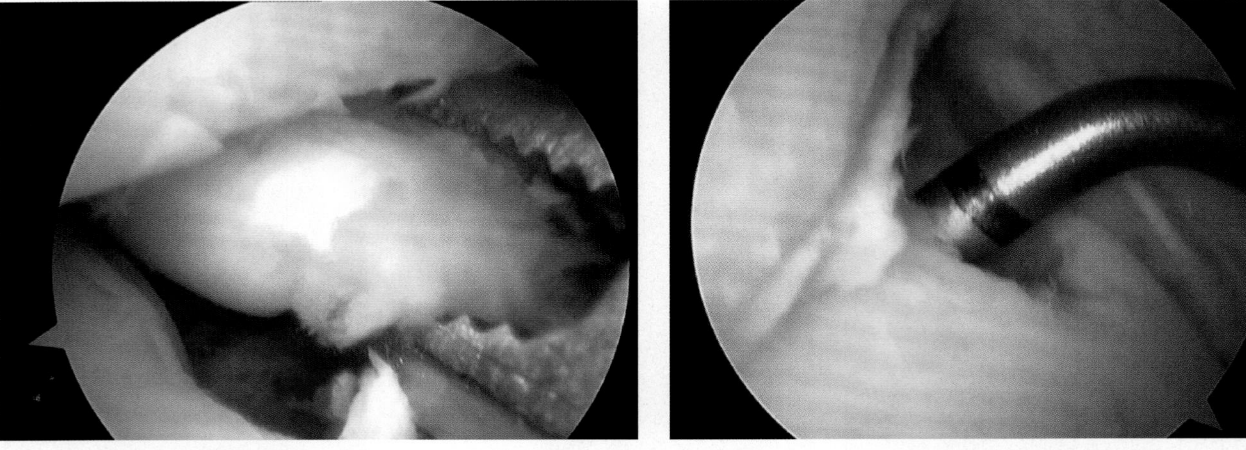

Figure 62-22 | Left. Removal of unstable cartilage with grasper. After the cartilage has been removed and debrided to stable edges, the bony OLT is debrided and **(Right)** bone marrow stimulation is performed with angled pick.

- Cartilage and bony lesions are prepared with a shaver, curettes, and soft tissue punches to remove unstable cartilage flaps to stable, perpendicular edges (Fig. 62-23).
  - Bony preparation may require a small burr.

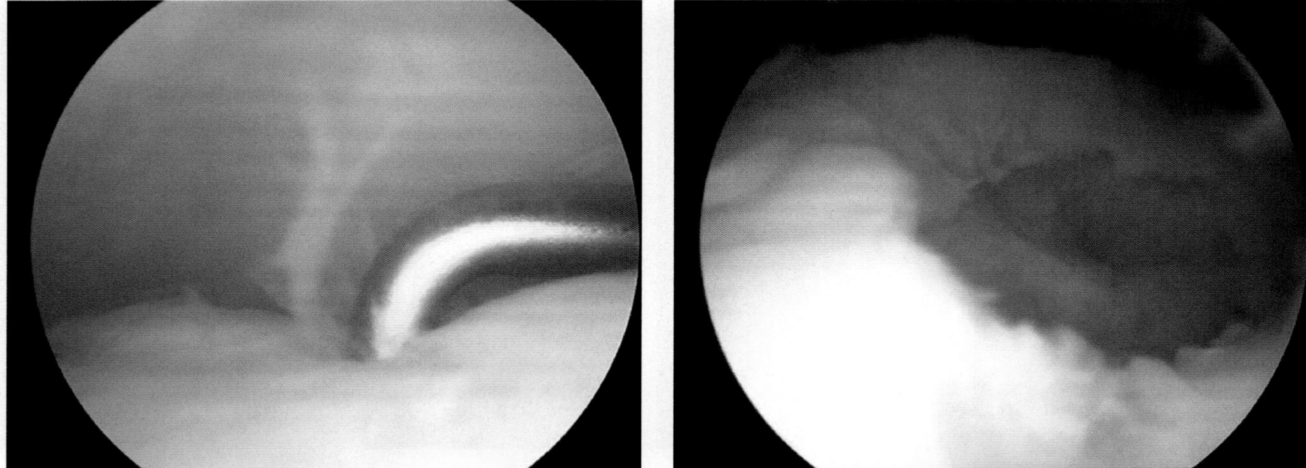

Figure 62-23 | Left. Probing of cartilage overlying OLT demonstrated unstable cartilage and underyling OLT. **Right.** Débridement of cartilage to stable, perpendicular edges. [Two images same case.]

- Straight or angulated picks, awls, or 1.1- or 1.6-mm K-wires are used to microfracture to subchondral bone, ensuring an adequate depth of 2-4 mm.
- Fat droplets can be visualized at the time of microfracture and indicate adequate depth.
- The tourniquet is let down and bleeding is observed with the arthroscope.
- Cysts
  - The arthroscope is used to visualize into cysts.
  - Necrotic or soft tissues existing inside cyst are debrided.
  - Microfracture tools or burs are used to disrupt sclerotic bone overlying cysts.
  - Cysts <6 mm in depth can be treated with débridement, microfracture without bone grafting (Lee et al.[10]).
- If required, posterolateral portals can be used for posterior lesions.
- If treating a central or central-posterior OLT, a noninvasive distractor is placed and the foot is plantar flexed to access OLT.

Arthroscopic Option for Large or Revision OLTs: Particulated Juvenile Hyaline Cartilage Allograft Implantation

- Juvenile hyaline cartilage allograft implantation[11] is an arthroscopic option for large (≥1.5 cm^2) OLTs or revision OLTs that do not require an open procedure or involve harvest site morbidity issues
- Ideally, ≥50% to 60% of the OLT should be contained by native cartilage to allow adequate graft fixation.
- The OLT is prepared by debriding cartilage to stable edges and debriding bone bed (Fig. 62-24).
- Creation of an accessory or "extended" portal may be required to deliver the fibrin and juvenile cartilage fragments.
- The tourniquet is released, and the fluid is removed from the joint.
- During "dry" arthroscopy, the bony bed is suctioned, wicked, and dried.
- The bony base of the OLT is covered with fibrin glue (Fig. 62-25).

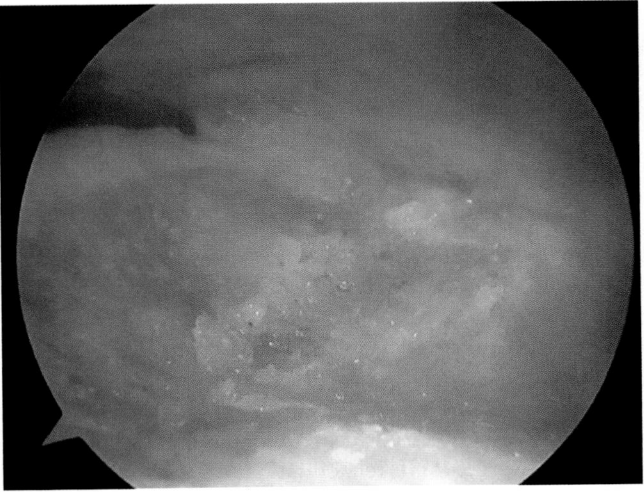

Figure 62-24 | OLT after débridement of cartilage and preparation and débridement of bony bed in preparation for particulated juvenile hyaline cartilage implantation.

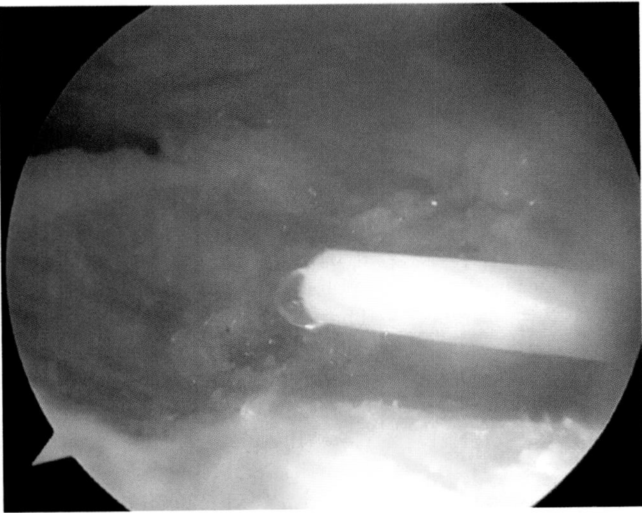

Figure 62-25 | The bony base of the OLT is covered with fibrin glue.

- Particulated juvenile cartilage fragments are delivered to OLT site through a cannula (Fig. 62-26).
- A Freer elevator is used to smooth and spread cartilage fragments (Fig. 62-27).

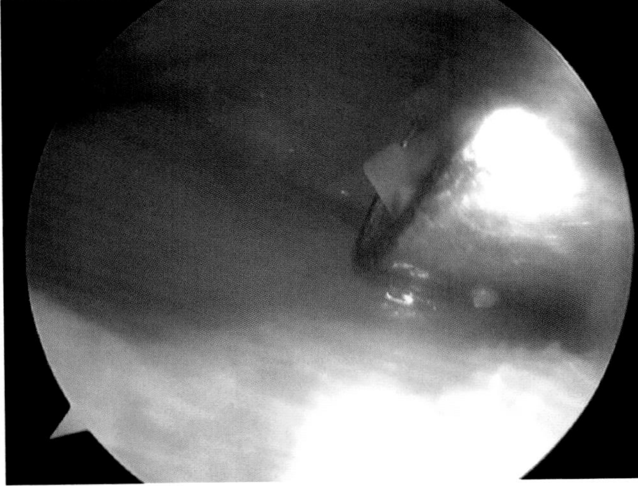

Figure 62-26 | Particulated juvenile cartilage fragments are delivered to OLT site through a cannula.

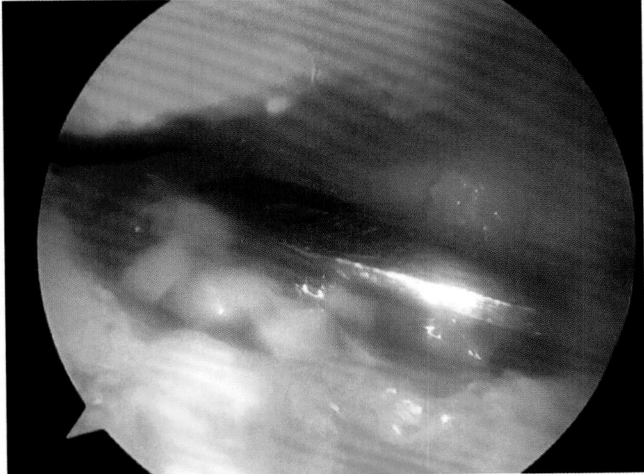

Figure 62-27 | A Freer elevator is used to smooth and spread cartilage fragments.

- After the fibrin base with juvenile cartilage fragments are allowed to set, further fibrin is added to secure juvenile cartilage fragments (Fig. 62-28).

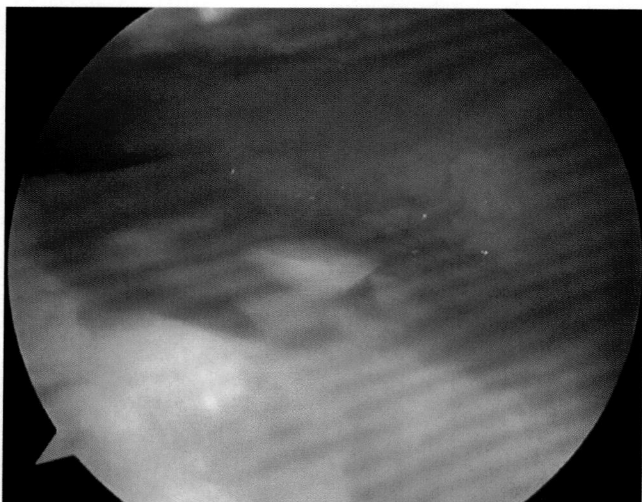

Figure 62-28 | After the fibrin base with juvenile cartilage fragments is allowed to set, further fibrin is added to secure the fragments.

Postoperative Care

- If arthroscopy, débridement, and microfracture alone are performed, a sterile, bulky soft dressing is applied at the time of surgery
- The patient is instructed to be non–weight bearing or toe-touch weight bearing for 4 weeks and allowed immediate gentle postoperative ROM depending on lesion and chronicity.
- Sutures are removed at first follow-up in 2 weeks.
- Gradual weight bearing is allowed at 4 weeks with rehabilitation program.
- Note: If concurrent ligamentous repair or reconstruction is performed, a below-knee splint with medial/lateral struts is applied, and a weight-bearing and rehabilitation protocol is followed according to the ligament repair/reconstruction.

References

1. Berndt AL, Harty M. Transchondral fractures (osteochondritis dissecans) of the talus. *J Bone Joint Surg Am.* 1959;41A: 988-1020.
2. Van Bergen CJ, Kox LS, Maas M, et al. Arthroscopic treatment of osteochondral defects of the talus, outcomes at eight to twenty years of follow-up. *J Bone Joint Surg Am.* 2013; 95-A(6):519-525.
3. Cuttica DJ, Smith WB, Hyer CF, et al. Osteochondral lesions of the talus: predictors of clinical outcome. *Foot Ankle Int.* 2011;32(11):1045-1051.
4. Dipaola JD, Nelson DW, Colville MR. Characterizing osteochondral lesions by magnetic resonance imaging. *Arthroscopy.* 1991;7(1):101-104.
5. El Shazly O, Abou El Soud MM, Nasef Abdelatif NM. Arthroscopic intralesional curettage for large benign talar dome cysts. *SICOT J.* 2015:1-32.
6. Ferkel RD, Zanotti RM, Komenda GA, et al. Arthroscopic treatment of chronic osteochondral lesions of the talus. *Am J Sports Med.* 2008;36(9):1750-1762.
7. Giannini S, Buda R, Faldini C, et al. Surgical treatment of osteochondral lesions of the talus in young active patients. *J Bone Joint Surg Am.* 2005;87(Suppl 2):28-41.
8. Hepple S, Winson IG, Glew D. Osteochondral lesions of the talus: A Revised Classification. *Foot Ankle Int.* 1999;20(12):789-793.
9. Klammer G, Maquieira GJ, Spahn S, et al. Natural history of nonoperatively treated osteochondral lesions of the talus. *Foot Ankle Int.* 2015;36(1):24-31.
10. Lee KB, Park HW, Cho HJ, et al. Comparison of arthroscopic microfracture for osteochondral lesions of the talus with and without subchondral Cyst. *Am J Sports Med.* 2015; 43(8):1951-1956.
11. Zimmer Orthobiologics. DeNovo® NT Natural Tissue Graft, Arthroscopically-Assisted Surgical Technique for Ankle Cartilage Repair. Pages 1-8.

Chapter 63
Achilles Tendon Repair

ANDREW J. ROSENBAUM
ANDREW J. ELLIOTT
MARTIN J. O'MALLEY

Open Repair

Sterile Instruments/Equipment

- Tourniquet
- Number 2 FiberWire suture (Arthrex, Inc., Naples, FL)
- 3-0 Prolene suture (Ethicon, Inc., Somerville, NJ)
- 3-0 Vicryl suture (Ethicon, Inc., Somerville, NJ)
- 4-0 Vicryl suture (Ethicon, Inc., Somerville, NJ)
- 4-0 Ethilon suture (Ethicon, Inc., Somerville, NJ)

Positioning

- The patient is positioned prone.
  - All bony prominences are carefully padded.
- Both legs are prepared and draped (Fig. 63-1).
  - The nonoperative leg will be used to set the tension of the repair.

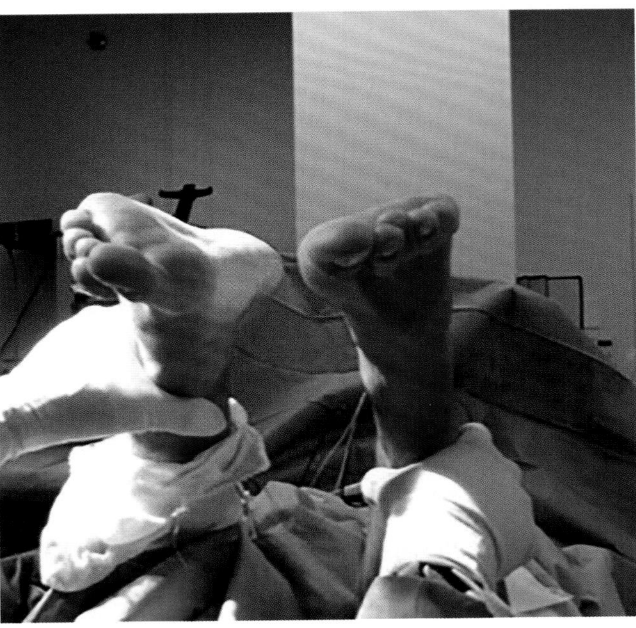

Figure 63-1 | Patient positioning for an Achilles tendon repair. Both legs are prepared so that resting tension of the nonoperative side can be assessed during surgery.

Surgical Approach

- A longitudinal incision is made over the medial border of the tendon (Fig. 63-2).
  - This avoids the sural nerve and allows access to the plantaris tendon if needed.

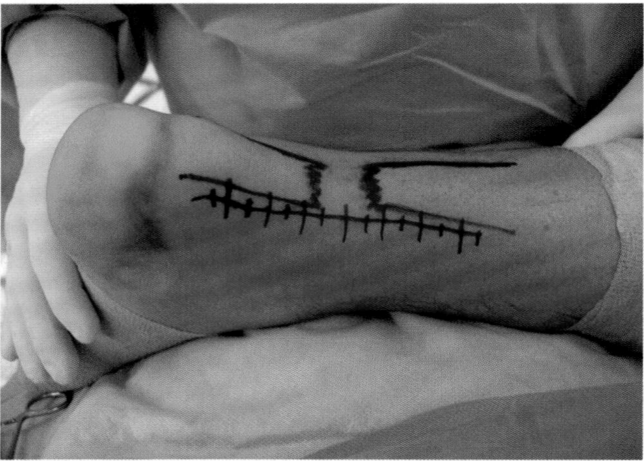

Figure 63-2 | Longitudinal incision over the medial border of the Achilles tendon (*left leg*). (Borrowed from Chapter 110 of *Operative Techniques in Foot and Ankle Surgery* [Technique Figure 1]).

- The skin and subcutaneous layer are mobilized laterally.
  - The paratenon is preserved.
- The sural nerve and lesser saphenous vein are protected as they course lateral to the paratenon.
- A midline incision is made through the paratenon, away from the skin incision.
- The fascia is released just anterior to the Achilles tendon (Fig. 63-3) to allow a less tensioned wound closure.

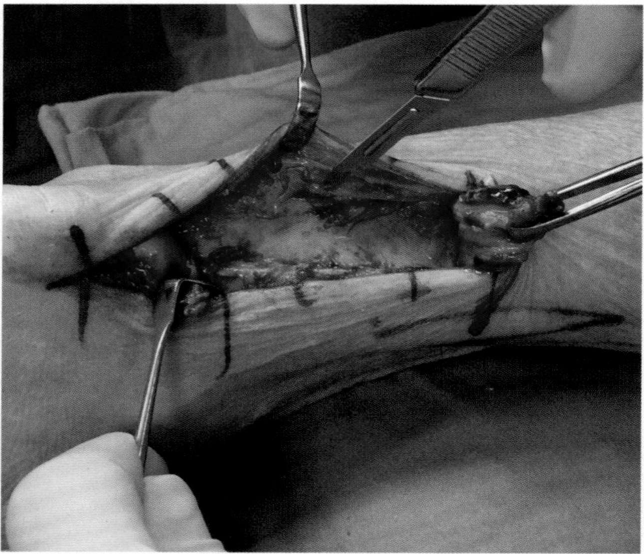

Figure 63-3 | Exposure of the fascia anterior to the Achilles tendon. Releasing this fascia will allow a less tensioned closure of the incision.

Repair Technique

- Limited debridement of the ruptured tendon ends is performed (Fig. 63-4).
- Two no. 2 FiberWire sutures (Arthrex, Inc., Naples, FL) are used.
  - On each tendon end, four loop Krackow locking sutures are passed on the medial side and four on the lateral side[1] (Fig. 63-5).

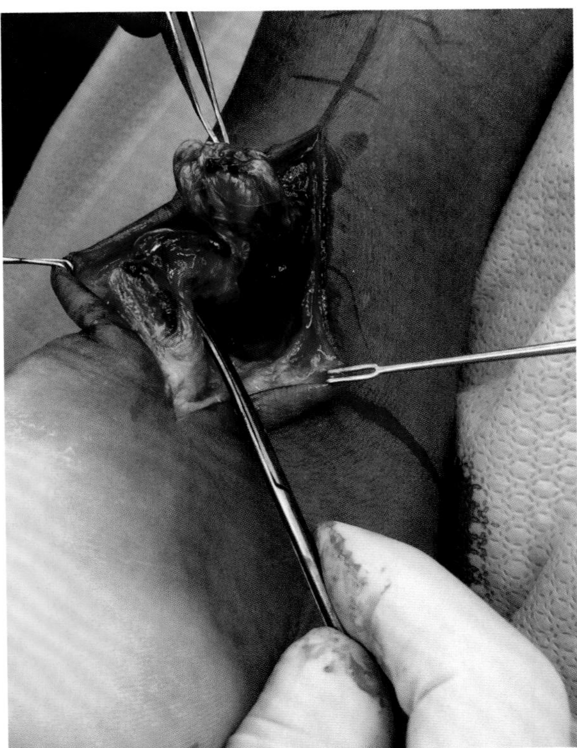

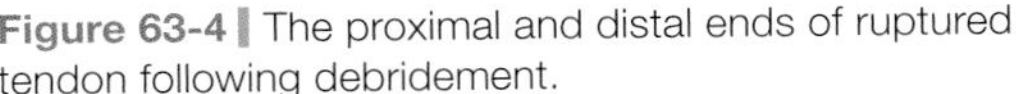

Figure 63-4 | The proximal and distal ends of ruptured tendon following debridement.

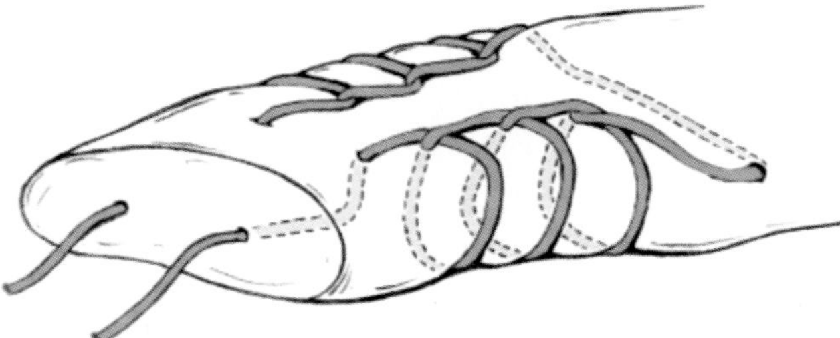

Figure 63-5 | The Krackow locking stitch. (Borrowed from Chapter 110 of *Operative Techniques in Foot and Ankle Surgery* [Technique Figure 2A]).

- The surgical knots are tied while the foot is held at resting tension.
    - This is based on intraoperative evaluation of the contralateral limb.
- An epitendinous repair is performed with 3-0 Prolene suture (Ethicon, Inc., Somerville, NJ) in a figure-of-8 formation (Fig. 63-6).

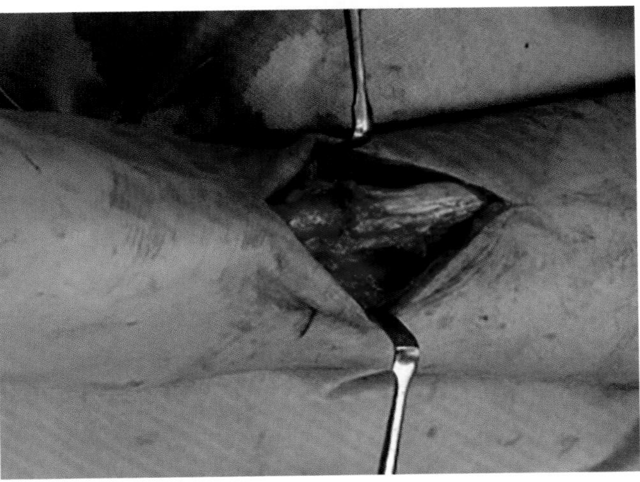

Figure 63-6 | Appearance of Achilles tendon after placement of the epitendinous suture.

- Platelet-rich plasma (PRP) can be injected directly into tendon at the rupture site following epitendinous repair (Fig. 63-7) and may accelerate early healing.[2]
- Meticulous repair of the paratenon is performed next with 3-0 Vicryl suture (Ethicon, Inc., Somerville, NJ).
    - If the paratenon is taut, the ankle can be plantar flexed to relax the tendon and paratenon tissue.
- Subcutaneous closure is done with 4-0 Vicryl suture (Ethicon, Inc., Somerville, NJ).

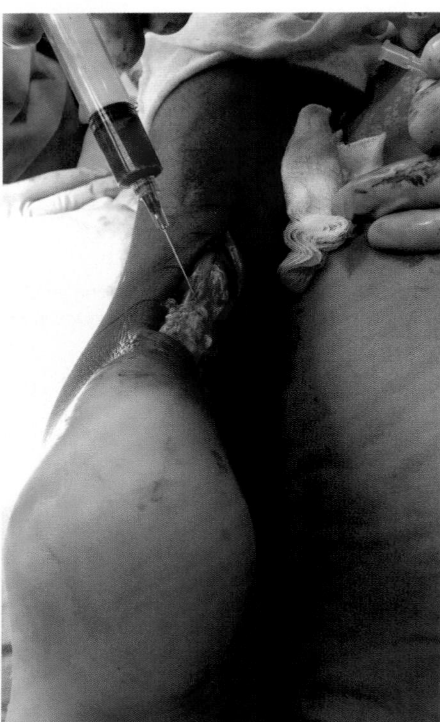

Figure 63-7 | Injection of PRP into rupture site following repair.

- The skin is closed with horizontal mattress 4-0 Ethilon sutures (Fig. 63-8).
- A splint is applied with the foot in resting equinus position.

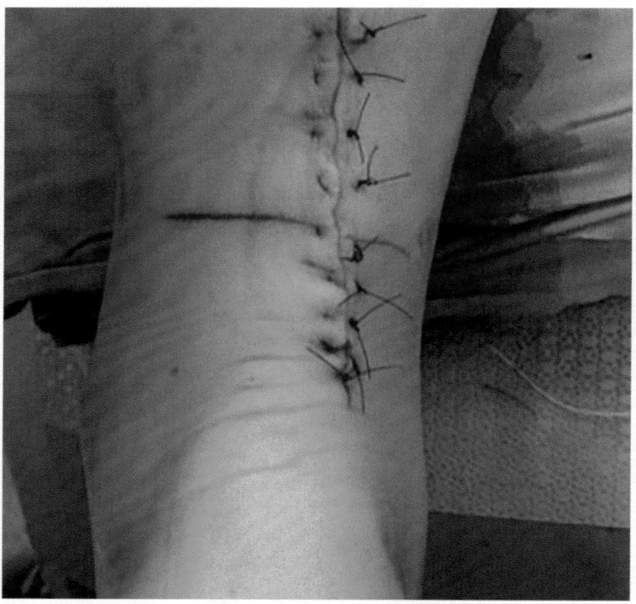

Figure 63-8 | Skin closure with a horizontal mattress suture.

Percutaneous Repair

Sterile Instruments/Equipment

- Tourniquet
- 0 Vicryl suture (Ethicon, Inc., Somerville, NJ)
- 3-0 Vicryl suture (Ethicon, Inc., Somerville, NJ)
- 4-0 Vicryl suture (Ethicon, Inc., Somerville, NJ)
- 4-0 Ethilon suture (Ethicon, Inc., Somerville, NJ)
- PARS Achilles Jig System (Arthrex, Inc., Naples, FL)

Chapter 64
Modified Broström Procedure

DANNY ARORA
ANNUZIATO (NED) AMENDOLA

Introduction

- Ankle sprains are common injuries in both athletes and the general population.[1–4]
- Most ankle sprains occur in sports, with a considerable economic and social impact.[1,4]
- The most common mechanism of injury is an inversion twist of the ankle, which injures the lateral ligament complex.[2–4]
- The surgical options include anatomic repair (Broström technique and modifications), anatomic reconstruction with autograft or allograft, and nonanatomic reconstructions (also known as checkrein procedures) such as the Watson-Jones, Evans, and Chrisman-Snook procedures.[5–12]
- Anatomic repairs have the advantage of restoring the anatomy and kinematics of the ankle while preserving subtalar joint motion.[13–15]

Positioning and Preparation

- The patient is positioned supine on the operating table, and intravenous antibiotics are administered.
- A bump is placed under the ipsilateral hip.
- A proximal thigh tourniquet is preferred.
- The lower leg is prepared and draped in a standard fashion.
- We usually perform a diagnostic ankle arthroscopic examination (21-point as described by Ferkel)[16] before the ligament repair to ensure a thorough evaluation of the ankle and appropriate treatment of incidental lesions. These may include chondral injury and tibiotalar impingement, which may cause pain after returning to sport, if not treated. All pertinent landmarks are drawn out before the start of the procedure: medial and lateral malleoli, anterior tibial tendon, intermediate dorsal cutaneous branch of the superficial peroneal nerve, and standard arthroscopic portals.
- An Esmarch bandage can be used to exsanguinate the limb, and the tourniquet is inflated.

Surgical Approach

- For the skin incision, we prefer a standard curved incision just anterior to the lateral malleolus, extending from the ankle joint to the peroneal tendon sheath.
- An extended lateral incision posterior to the lateral malleolus, along the peroneal tendons, is used when peroneal tendon pathology is highly suspected, or for revision surgery using graft tissue (Fig. 64-1).

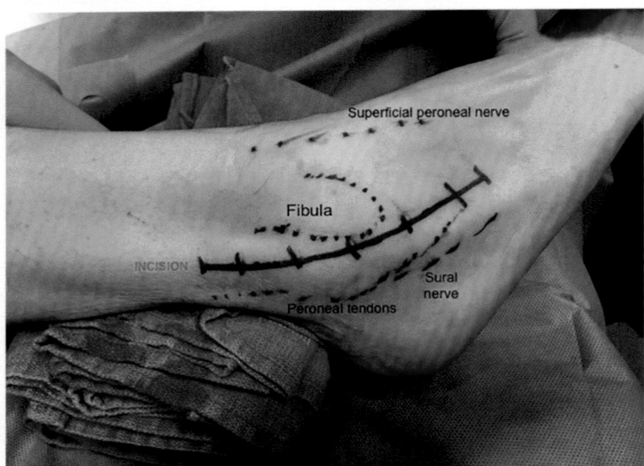

Figure 64-1 | Mapped out relevant anatomy and skin incision.

- Elevation of full-thickness flaps anteriorly allows access to the inferior extensor retinaculum and the anterior tibiofibular ligament (ATFL), as well as the peroneal tendons and calcaneal tuberosity.
- The extensor retinaculum is retracted for later repair and the peroneal sheath is incised, exposing the peroneus longus and brevis tendons distal to the superior peroneal retinaculum (SPR). The peroneal tendons are then retracted distally to expose the calcaneofibular ligament (CFL) underneath.
- The status of the native ATFL and CFL are examined, as well as ankle laxity.
- An arthrotomy is made along the anterior edge of the fibula incising the anterolateral capsule to expose the talofibular joint. The joint is inspected for pathology.
- Flaps are created from the residual ATFL and/or the CFL as well as the periosteum from the underlying fibula for later repair.
- The ATFL and CFL are trimmed and prepared for reattachment and tensioning. Reattachment of the tissue to bone is the preferred method.
- The anterior and distal superficial surface of the fibula is prepared with a rongeur or burr before placement of anchors. Generally, 2 or 3 anchors are placed with a high-strength suture or suture tape, 1 or 2 on the anterior distal fibula for the ATFL attachment site, and 1 at the tip of the fibula for the CFL attachment site (Fig. 64-2).

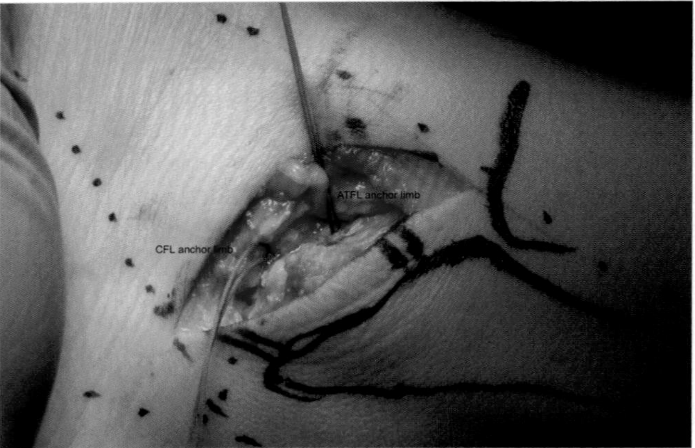

Figure 64-2 | Fibular anchor placement for both ATFL and CFL limbs.

- The sliding sutures from the anchors are used in a baseball stitch fashion to lock one of the strands into the ligamentous tissue; the other strand is used to tension and pull the ligament to bone and tied. The sutures are secured down to bone with the ankle in neutral position. Suture anchors are not always necessary but are preferred.
- The periosteal sleeve developed above on the fibula is then imbricated to the tissue on the edge of the bone; this can be done with a pants-over-vest technique or other type of tight imbrication to overlap the tissue a tight fashion.

At this point, there are two layers of suture, one to bone from the anchors and the overlying periosteal sleeve as the second layer (Fig. 64-3).

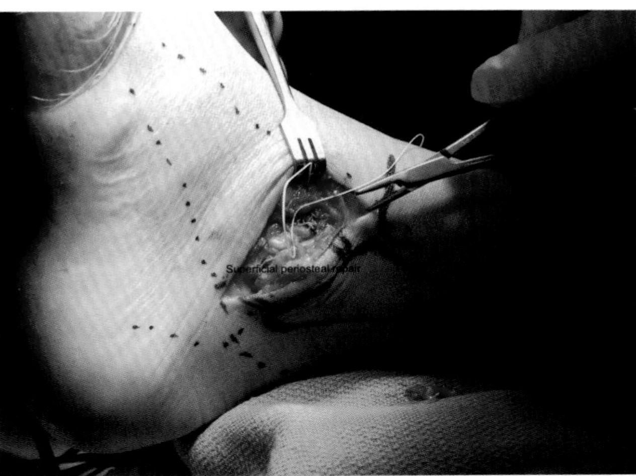

Figure 64-3 | Two-layer repair. First, deep layer closure down to bone with suture anchors. Second, superficial periosteal layer closure.

- The Gould modification (the 3rd layer of tissue) is then performed, in which the mobilized inferior extensor retinaculum (IER) is repaired and advanced to the distal fibula, superficial to the previous two layers of suture, again using a high-strength suture. In essence, this allows a 3-layer closure: (1) bone, (2) periosteal flap, and (3) extensor retinaculum (Figs. 64-4 and 64-5). This layer also covers the knots of the anchor sutures, which sometimes are palpable over the edge of the fibula because there is not much subcutaneous tissue in this area.

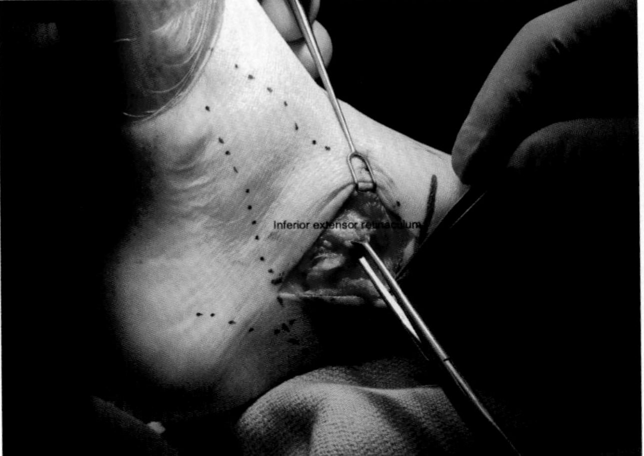

Figure 64-4 | Inferior retinaculum advancement for Gould modification of repair.

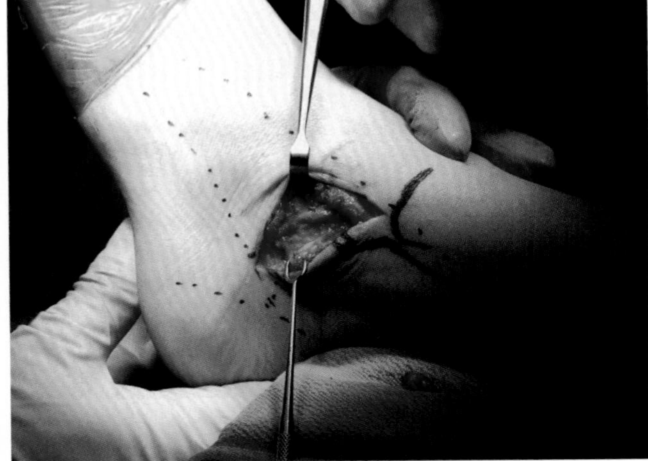

Figure 64-5 | Gould modification of repair.

- A layered tissue closure is performed, with 2-0 Vicryl for the subcutaneous tissues and 3-0 Nylon for the skin. Sterile dressings are applied, and the ankle is well padded and placed into a 3-sided plaster splint. The ankle is immobilized in neutral dorsiflexion and slight eversion.

Postoperative Care

- Patients remain in the splint or cast for 2 weeks, touch weight bearing with crutches.
- At the 2-week follow-up, the splint is removed, a wound check is performed, the dressing is changed, and the leg is placed into a splint or cast for another 2 weeks, touch weight bearing.

- At 4 weeks, the patient is put into an Aircast (DJO, Vista, CA) or other soft brace. Patients can then be progressed to weight bearing as tolerated and start range-of-motion exercises with no inversion until week 6. At that point, patients can progress to strengthening, ROM as tolerated in the soft lace-up brace.
- Physical therapy progresses with mobility and strengthening. At weeks 8-12, sport-specific exercises are begun, with ground-based training.
- Return to sport usually is permitted around 12 weeks with the use of the lace-up brace.

Why Does This Surgery Fail?

- Failure to identify and treat all pathology at the index procedure (eg, ankle joint, peroneal tendons)
- Residual medial ankle instability
- Recurrent ankle laxity
- Bony malalignment (eg, hindfoot varus, forefoot valgus)

Special Considerations

- *Isolated ATFL +/– CFL tear versus combined with peroneal tendon injury*
  - For an isolated ATFL +/– CFL tear, we proceed with the surgical technique described above. The peroneal tendons are inspected for any pathology that requires further surgery. For example, if a peroneal longus or brevis has a split tear, that is repaired directly.
  - If an actual complete tendon tear is identified, a tendon transfer (brevis to longus) is performed.
  - The incision described allows much versatility if any additional procedures are deemed warranted (see Fig. 64-6A and B).

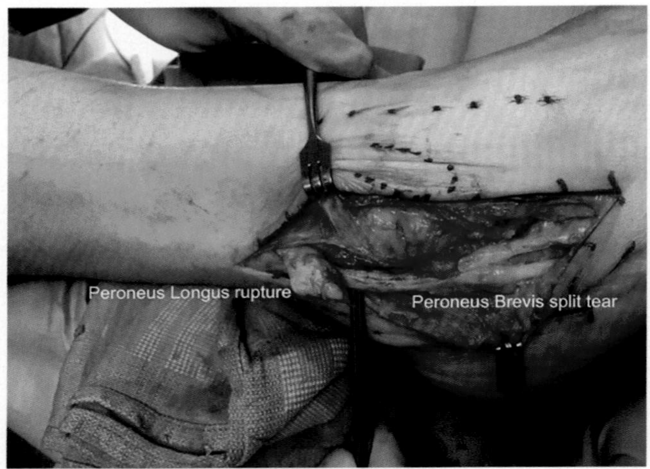

A

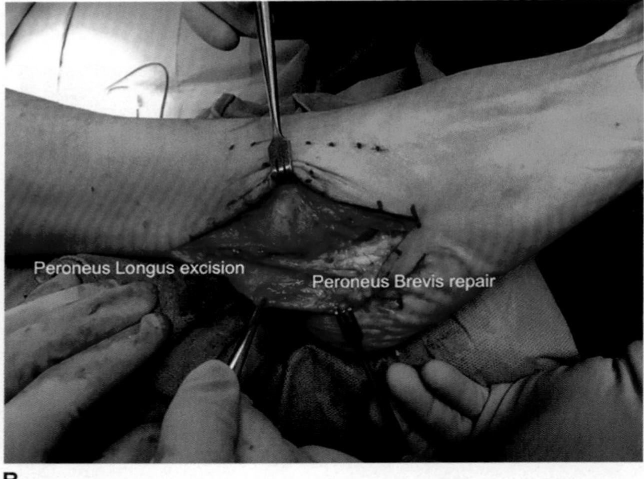

B

Figure 64-6 | A. Peroneus longus tendon rupture and peroneus brevis tendon split tear identified after exploration **B.** Peroneus longus tendon tear excision and peroneus brevis tendon repair.

- *ATFL tear combined with anterolateral impingement*
  - Before the ligament repair, any bony impingement is debrided/excised arthroscopically in the usual fashion.
- *Presence of fibular ossicle/avulsed fragment*
  - If a fibular ossicle or fibular fracture nonunion is present, we prefer to excise that fragment and reattach the tissue (CFL) to the distal fibula with 1 or 2 suture anchors.
- *Revision Broström surgery, severe or chronic ligament instability*
  - During revision Broström surgery or even severe/chronic instability, ligament repair augmentation is used. We usually augment the ATFL repair, but if limited tissue is available for CFL repair or if the ankle is extremely lax, the CFL repair also is augmented.
  - Allograft tendon is preferred for tissue augmentation, but free autografts have also been used (see Fig. 64-7A-C).[17]

- The guidewire is advanced in line with the medullary canal on all fluoroscopic views until it is past the fracture (Fig. 65-3A and B).

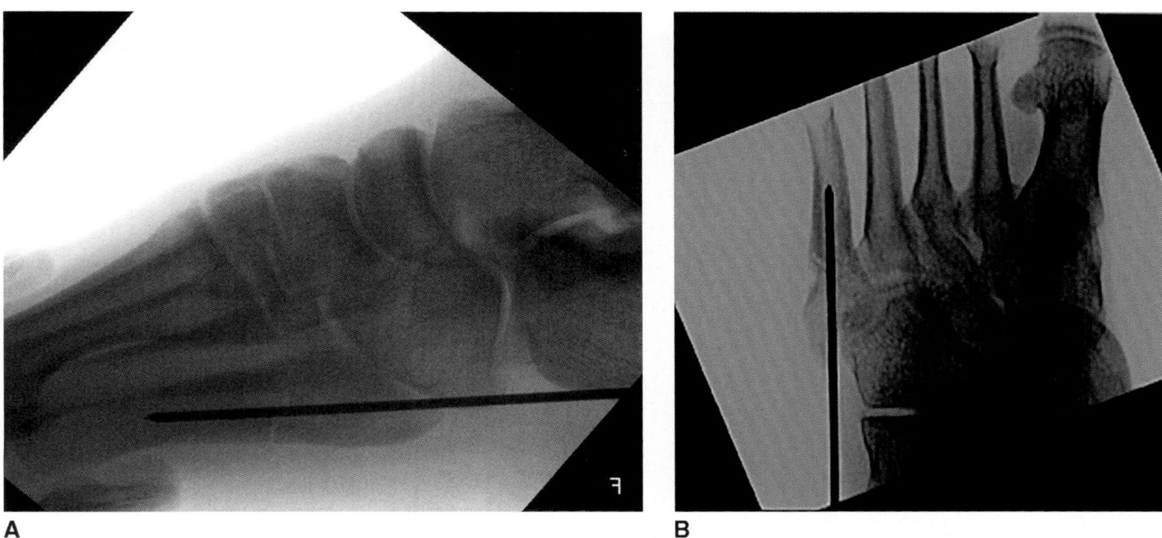

Figures 65-3 | Fluoroscopic images demonstrating placement of the guidewire for medullary screw placement with an acceptable starting point and trajectory in line with the medullary canal on AP **(A)** and lateral **(B)** views.

- A 3.2-mm drill bit is advanced over the guidewire to just past the fracture.
- A cannulated 4.5-mm tap is then advanced over the wire to engage the diaphysis distal to the fracture (Fig. 65-4A and B).

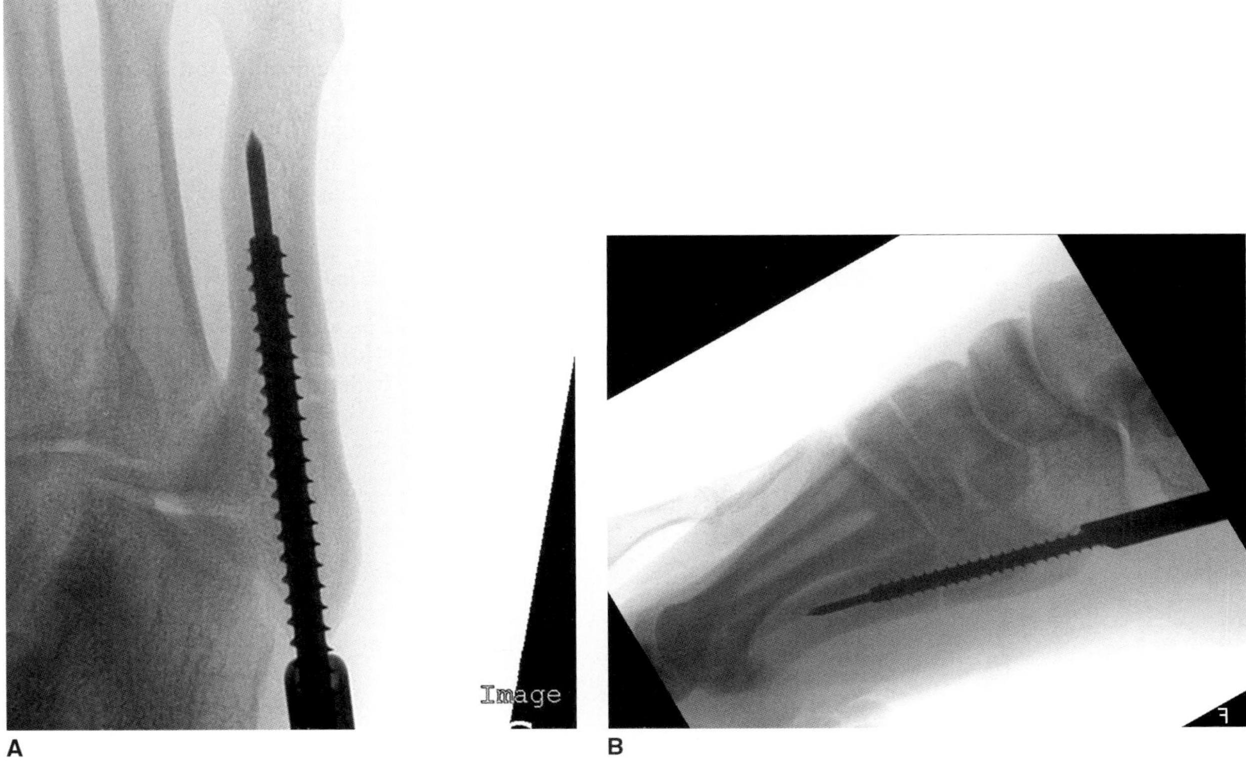

Figure 65-4 | Fluoroscopic images demonstrating the cannulated 4.5-mm tap engaging the diaphysis distal to the fracture site on both oblique **(A)** and lateral **(B)** views.

- The tap is increased by 1-mm increments until adequate endosteal purchase is achieved (Fig. 65-5A and B).
  - This is based on tactile feedback and observation of rotation of the fifth digit with rotation of the tap.

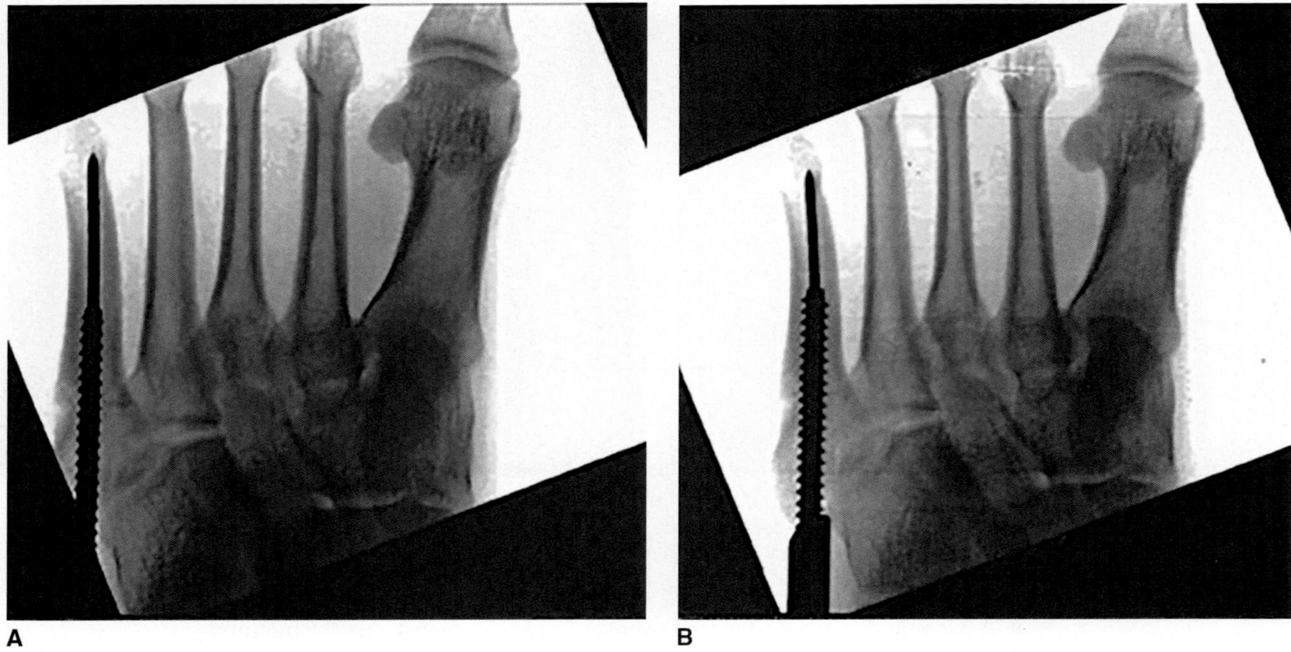

Figure 65-5 | Fluoroscopic images demonstrating increasing the tap diameter from a 4.5-mm **(A)** to a 5.5-mm **(B)** tap to create improved endosteal purchase.

- A screw of appropriate length and diameter is essential to ensure optimal outcome.
  - Preoperative measurements of the intramedullary canal width and anticipated screw length can help with appropriate screw selection.
    - A screw that is too short will have threads crossing the fracture and will not achieve interfragmentary compression.
    - A screw that is more than 60% of the metatarsal length will lead to straightening of the curved metatarsal with gapping of the lateral cortex, increasing the risk of nonunion.[2]
  - Fluoroscopic imaging of the screw adjacent to the metatarsal can help determine appropriate length (Fig. 65-6).

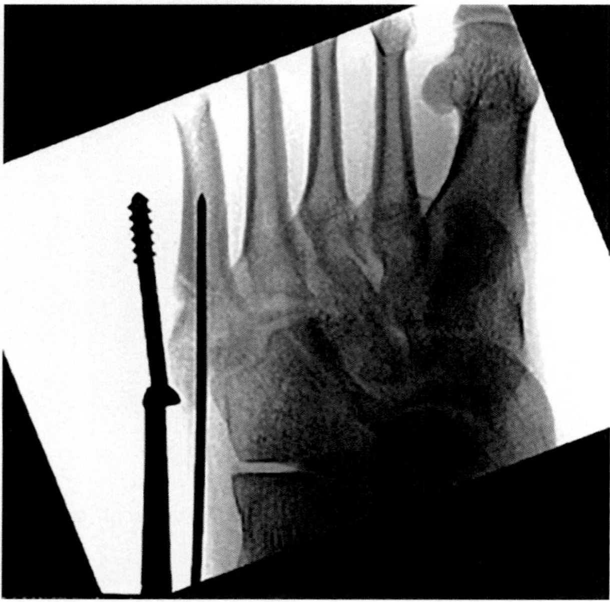

Figure 65-6 | AP image demonstrating overlay of the screw prior to final placement to ensure that the screw threads will cross the fracture site.

- The goal is placement of the most proximal threads of the screw just distal to the fracture site.
- Screw diameter is based on preoperative planning and tactile feedback with use of the tap.
  - We attempt to achieve fixation with a screw of >4.5-mm diameter whenever possible to limit bending and torsional stress at the fracture site.[3]
- The wire is then removed, and the screw is inserted until compression is achieved (Fig. 65-7A and B).

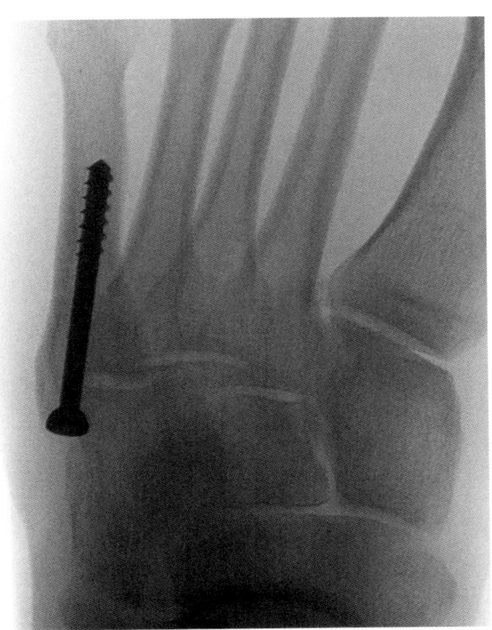

A

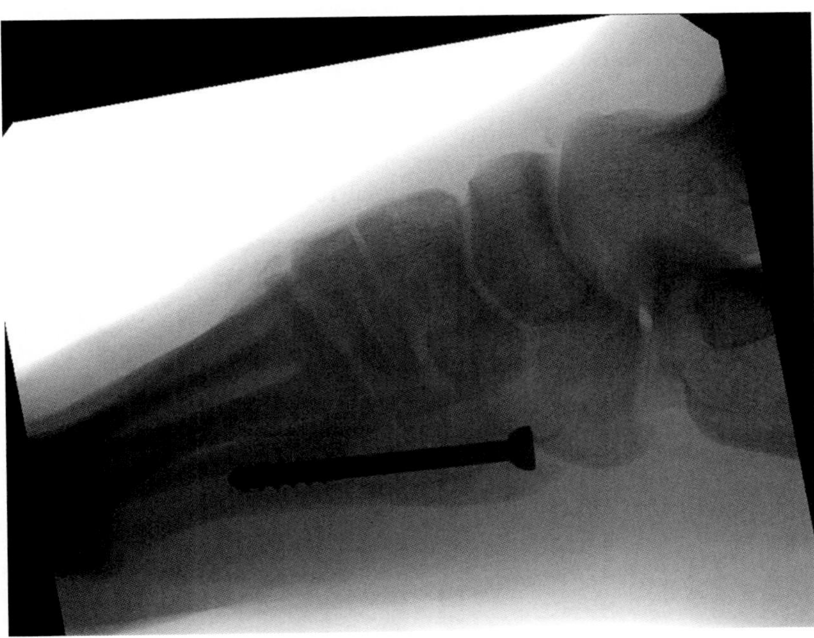

B

Figure 65-7 | AP **(A)** and lateral **(B)** fluoroscopic images demonstrating final medullary screw placement with compression across the fracture site.

- Care should be taken not to overcompress and fragment the metaphyseal segment of the fracture.
- Rotational malunion for a "tighter fit" screw can be eliminated by firmly grasping the fifth metatarsal head and preventing rotation of the metatarsal.

- Open reduction and internal fixation
  - This typically is used in cases of delayed union, nonunion, or failed percutaneous screw fixation with refracture (Fig. 65-8A and B).

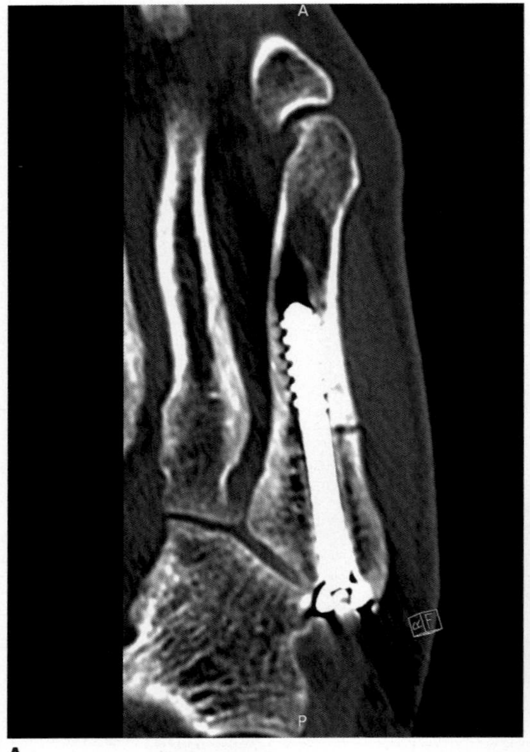

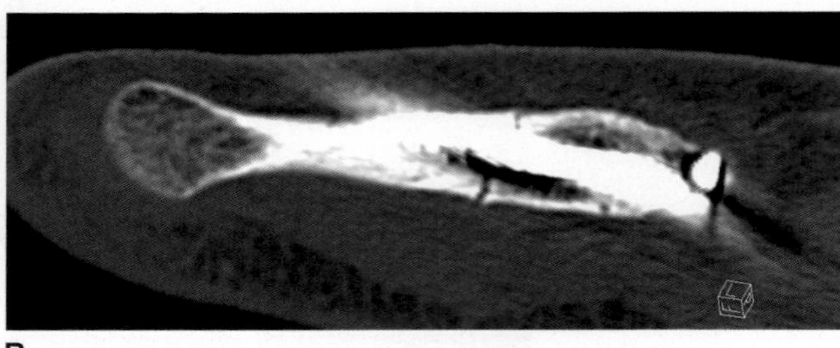

A B

Figures 65-8 | Axial (A) and sagittal **(B)** CT images demonstrating refracture following screw fixation.

  - The nonunion or fracture is exposed and debrided of fibrous tissue, with care taken to avoid heat necrosis at the nonunion site (use of manual instruments).
  - Cancellous autograft bone from the ipsilateral calcaneus is gently impacted (Fig. 65-9A and B).

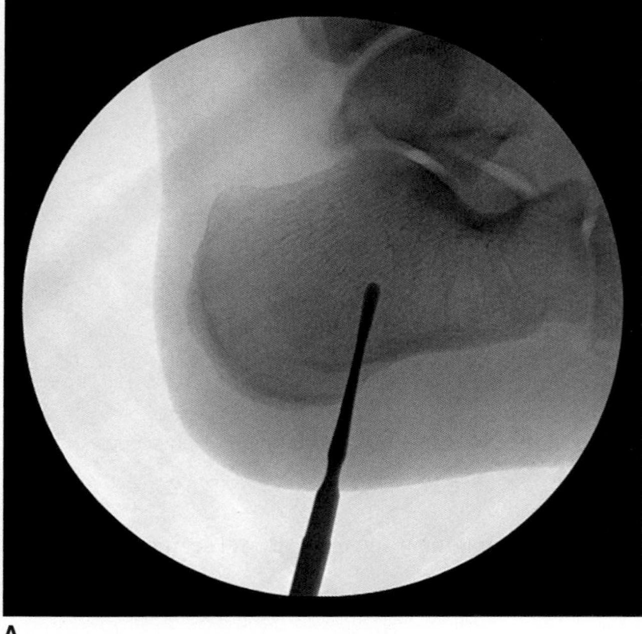

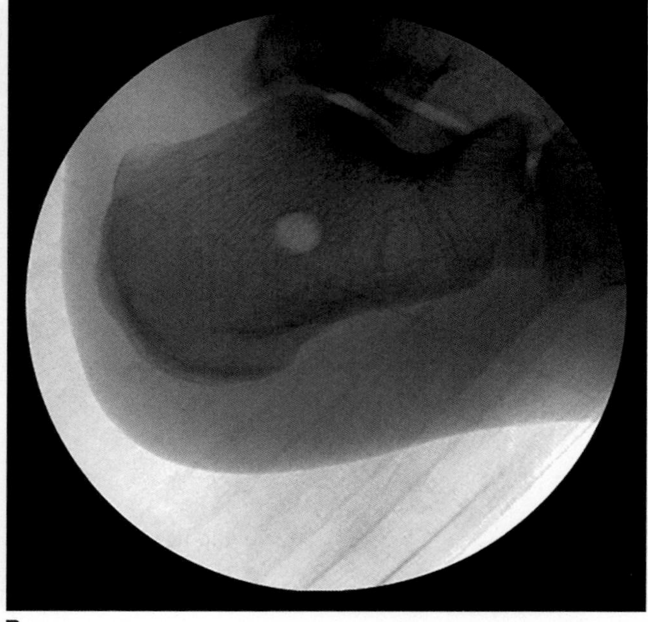

A B

Figure 65-9 | A, B. Successive fluoroscopic images demonstrating the harvest of calcaneal bone graft in a case of refracture of the fifth metatarsal.

Chapter 66
Internal Fixation of Tarsal Navicular Fractures

GABRIELLA ODE
ROBERT ANDERSON

Sterile Instruments/Equipment

- 4.0-mm partially threaded cannulated screws (titanium preferred to allow for future MRI)
- Dental picks
- Small pointed reduction clamps
- Freer elevator
- 2.0-mm drill bit
- Kirschner wires (0.045, 0.054, and 0.062 in)
- Image intensifier/fluoroscopy (mini C-arm)

Patient Positioning

- Supine
- Radiolucent table
- Padded bump underneath the ipsilateral buttock
- Esmarch supramalleolar tourniquet or pneumatic thigh tourniquet

Dorsal Approach[1]

- Indications
  - Advantageous for stress fractures in the mid to lateral third of the navicular bone.
- Exposure
  - Dorsal longitudinal incision centered over the navicular bone, as localized with fluoroscopic imaging.
  - The neurovascular structures (dorsalis pedis artery and superficial peroneal nerve branches) are identified and retracted medially.
  - The extensor tendons (extensor hallics longus medially and extensor hallucis brevis laterally) are retracted.
  - The periosteum of the navicular and the talonavicular joint capsule is incised to aid in identification of the fracture.
  - It often is necessary to remove the dorsal cortical surface and any associated exostoses from the dorsum of the talonavicular joint to clearly identify the fracture site (Fig. 66-1).
  - The fracture site is debrided, with care taken to preserve the articular joint surfaces (Fig. 66-2).
  - A small drill bit or Kirschner wire can be used to perforate the exposed bone surfaces within the fracture itself and is recommended in chronic cases where sclerosis is present (Fig. 66-3).

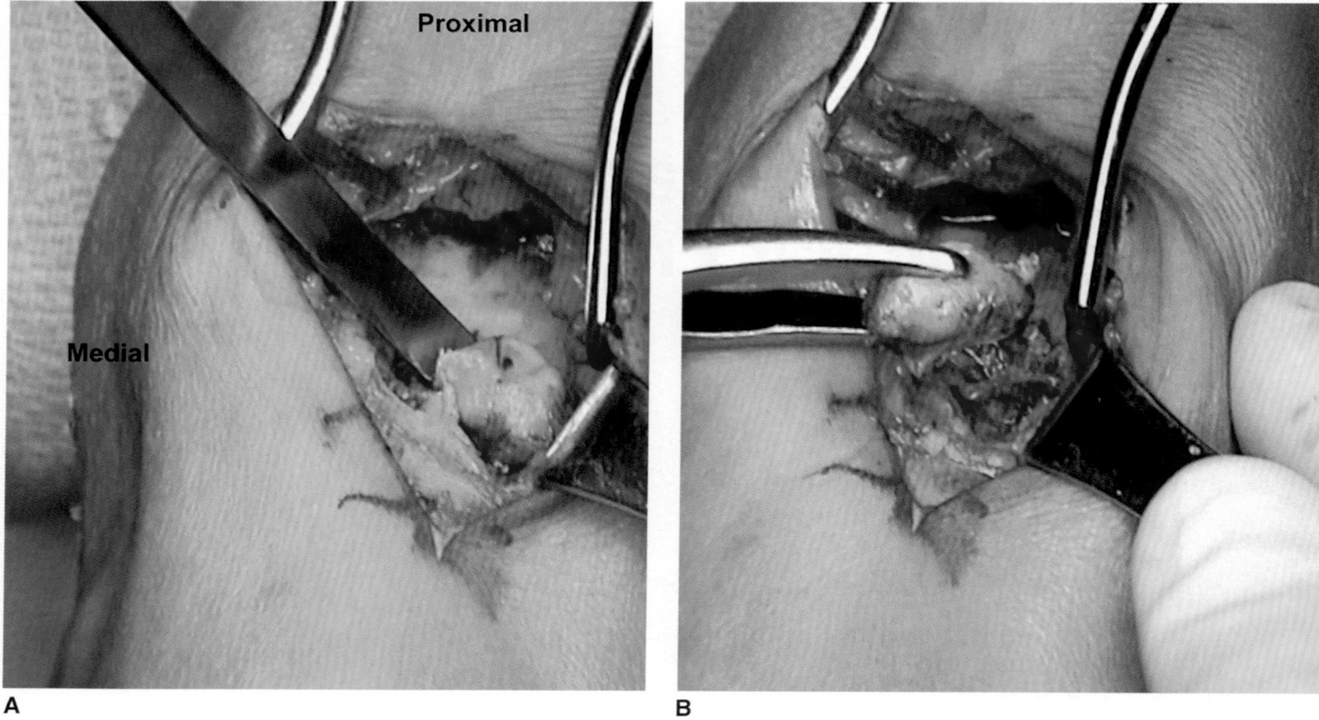

Figure 66-1 | Dorsal approach to navicular fracture with mobilization of dorsal exostosis using an osteotome **(A)** followed by removal using a small rongeur **(B)**.

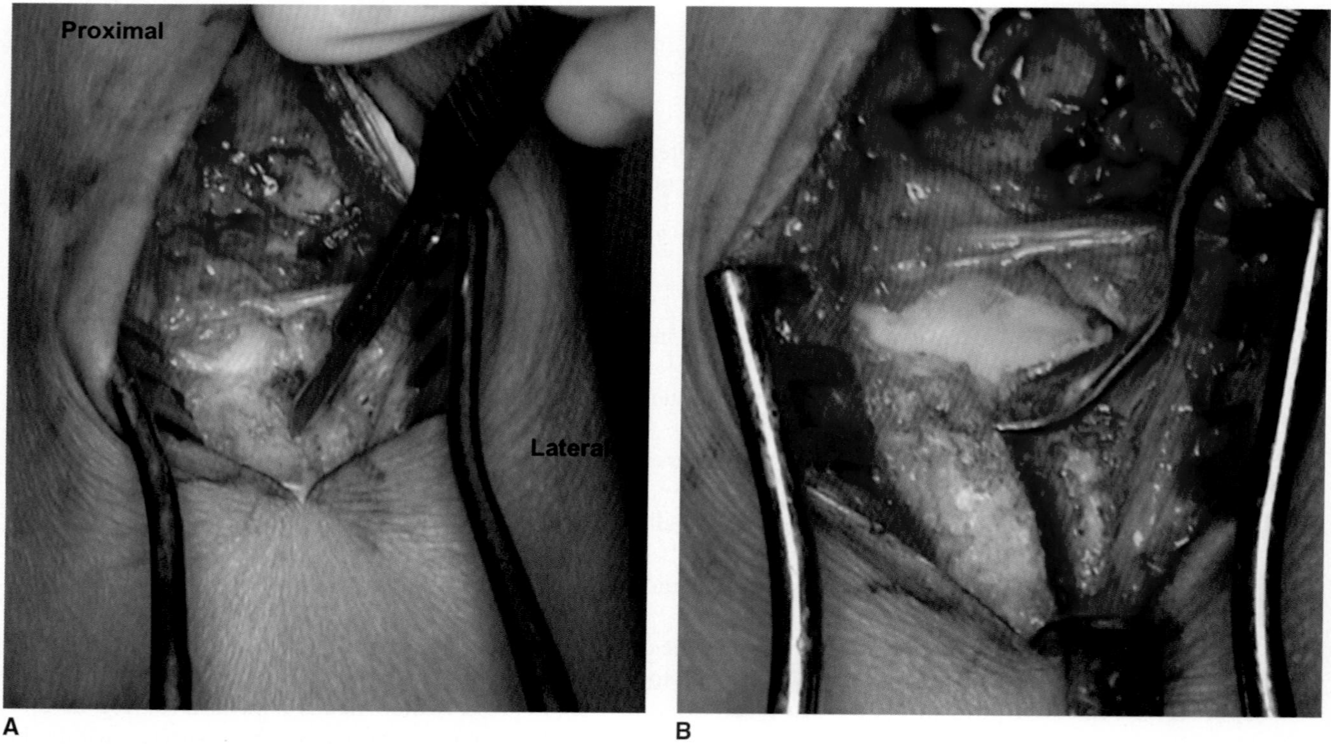

Figure 66-2 | Careful exposure **(A)** and debridement **(B)** of navicular fracture site.

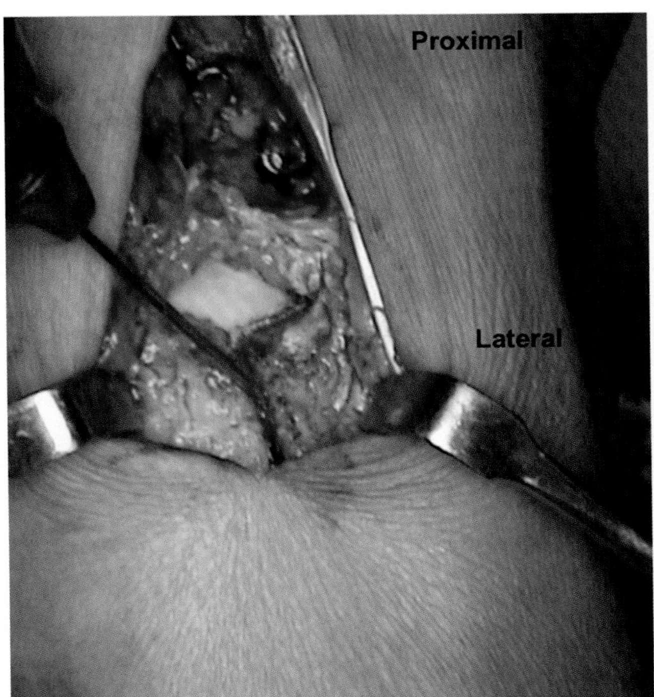

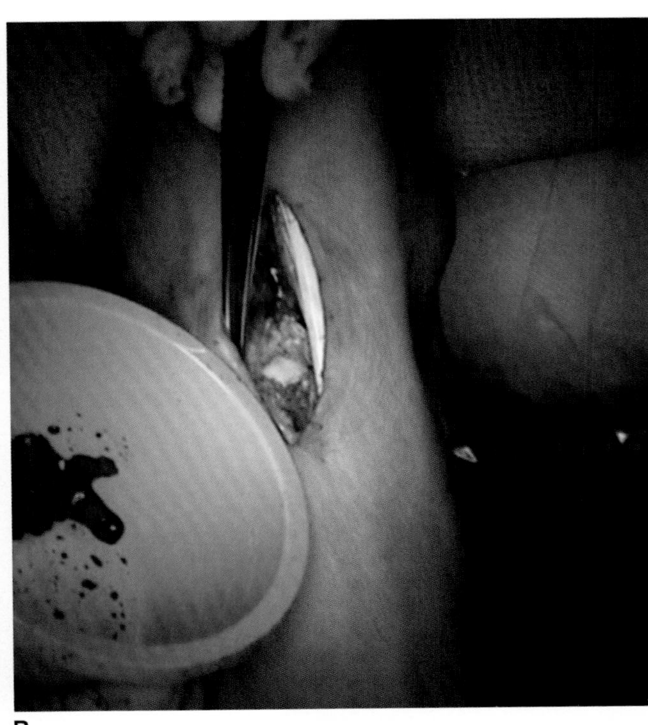

A B

Figure 66-3 | Preparation of the fracture site with K-wire perforation **(A)** followed by application of autologous bone graft **(B)**.

- Reduction and fixation techniques
  - Autologous cancellous bone graft can be harvested from the calcaneal posterior tuberosity or iliac crest and impacted into the fracture site.
    - Under image intensification, displaced fractures are reduced with pointed reduction clamps. The navicular bone is stabilized with two guidewires placed perpendicularly through the fracture site from lateral to medial.
    - The first pin is placed proximally and directed dorsolateral to plantar medial. The second pin is placed parallel in a slightly more distal and plantar location. Care should be taken not to penetrate the far cortex. The pin depth is measured.
    - A cannulated drill bit is advanced across the fracture site over the guidewire.
    - Two partially threaded 4.0-mm screws are placed with fluoroscopy to ensure that the screw does not exit the far cortex. Excessive screw length may injure the anterior or posterior tibial tendon (Fig. 66-4).
  - The wound is closed in layers.
  - The foot is placed in a neutral position in a well-padded splint.
  - Healing is evaluated at 3 months with radiographs and CT imaging (Fig. 66-5).

Medial Approach[2]

- Indications
  - Indicated for higher energy axial load fractures of the navicular (Sangeorzan types 2-4)
- Exposure
  - A medial longitudinal incision is centered over the navicular bone between the anterior and posterior tibial tendons.
  - The saphenous nerve and vein are identified and retracted.
  - The medial retinaculum and the underlying anterior tibial tendon, which is retracted anteriorly, are identified and released.

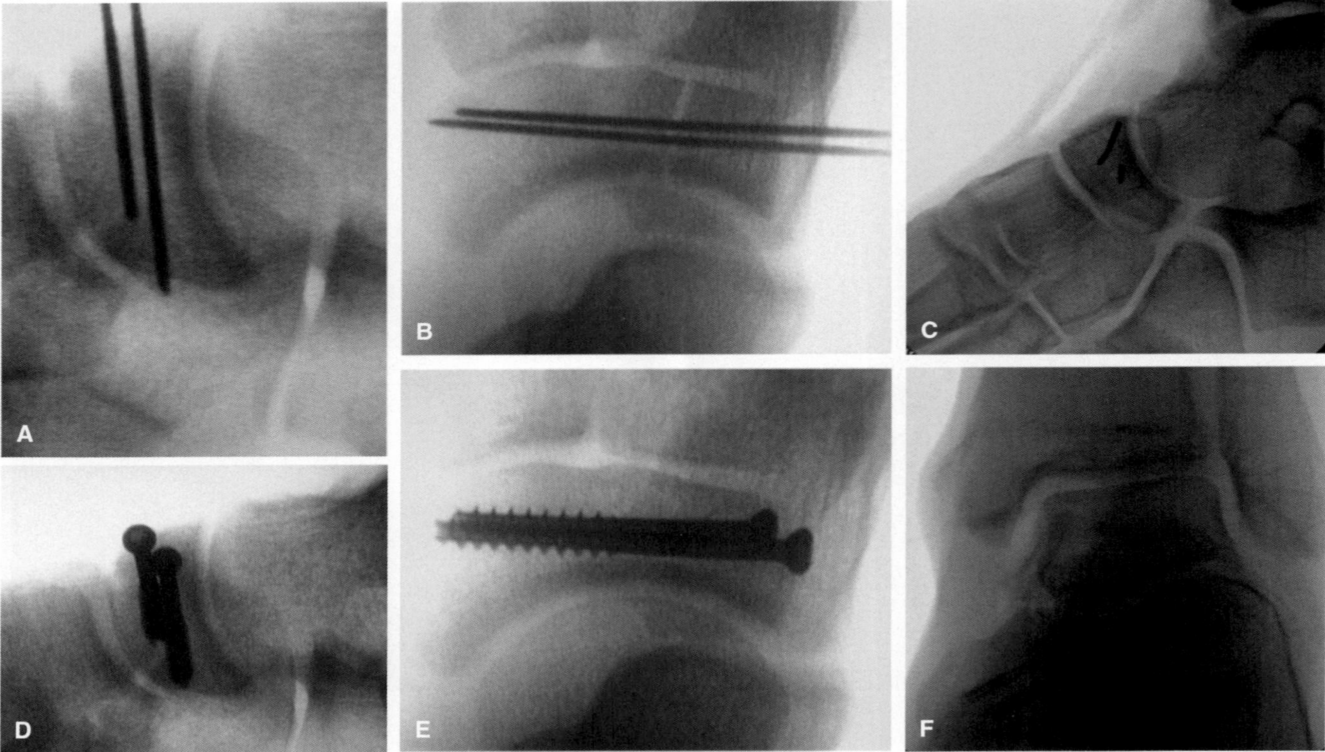

Figure 66-4 | Fluoroscopic imaging of provisional Kirschner wire fixation **(A-C)** followed by placement of two cannulated screws for definitive fixation **(D-F)**.

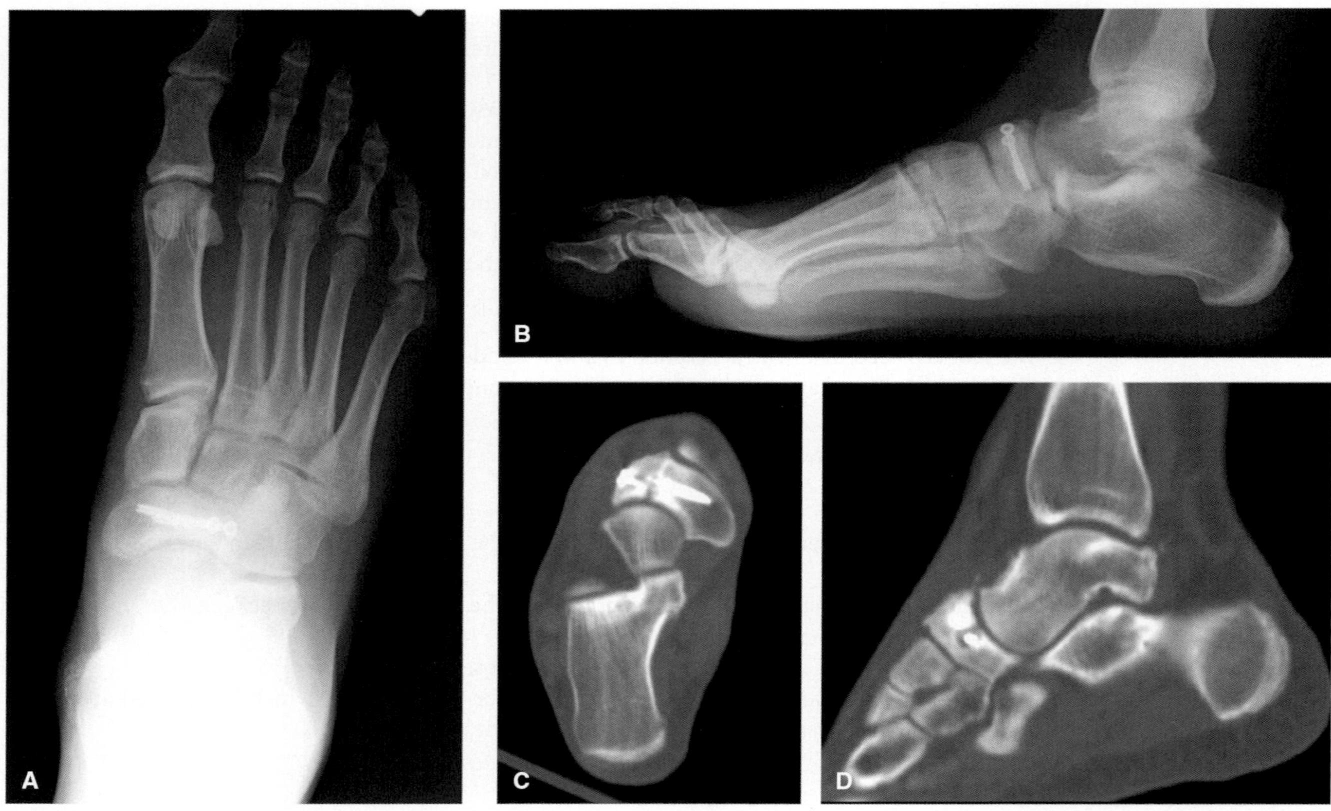

Figure 66-5 | Final radiographs **(A-B)** and CT imaging **(C-D)** at 3 months of dorsal screw fixation construct.

- The medial talonavicular joint capsule is incised to aid identification of the fracture.
- The fracture site is debided, with care taken to preserve the articular joint surfaces.

- Reduction and fixation techniques
  - Under image intensification, displaced fractures are reduced with pointed reduction clamps. Comminuted fractures may require temporary Kirschner wire fixation. The navicular bone is stabilized with two parallel guidewires placed perpendicularly across the fracture site.
  - The pin depth is determined, a cannulated drill bit is advanced across the fracture site over the guidewire, and appropriately sized screws are placed.
  - For fractures with comminution or tenuous fixation, a spanning external fixation device can be placed on the medial aspect of the foot extending from the cuneiform to the talus (Fig. 66-6).

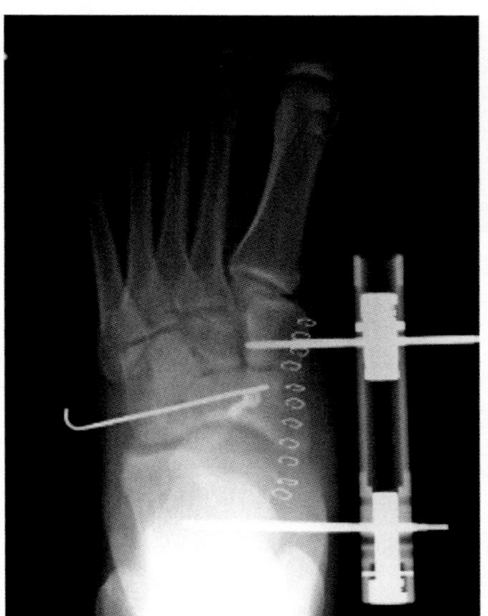

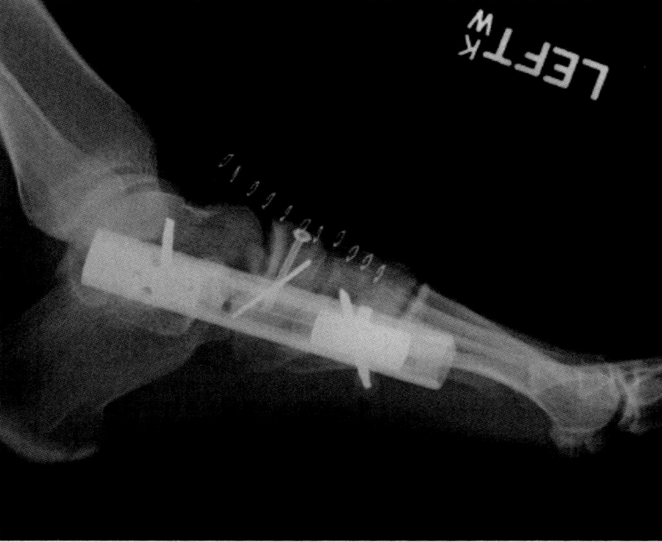

Figure 66-6 | Medial approach with spanning external fixation device.

  - If necessary, autologous cancellous bone graft can be impacted into the fracture site.
    - The wound is closed in layers.
    - The foot is placed in a neutral position in a well-padded splint.

Percutaneous Approach

- Indications
  - Indicated for persistent or progressive incomplete fracture or nondisplaced complete fracture (without sclerosis).
  - May be preferred in competitive collegiate or professional athletes desiring quicker return to sport or reduced risk of recurrent stress fracture.[3]
- Reduction and fixation techniques
  - Two percutaneous Kirschner wires are placed perpendicular to the fracture site (dorsal or medial) and parallel to each other as previously described.
  - The pin depth is determined and then a cannulated drill bit is advanced across the fracture site over the guidewire, and appropriately sized screws are inserted.
  - Care should be taken not to overcompress the screws because of the risk of tendon injury (anterior tibial tendon from dorsal insertion or posterior tibial tendon from medial insertion) or nerve injury (medial plantar nerve from medial approach) (Fig. 66-7).

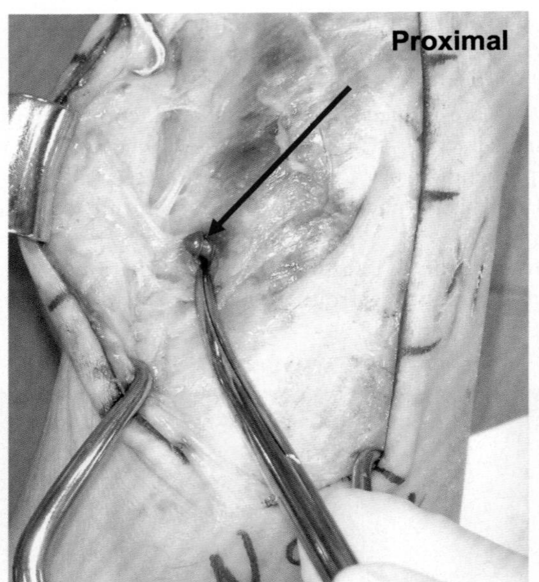

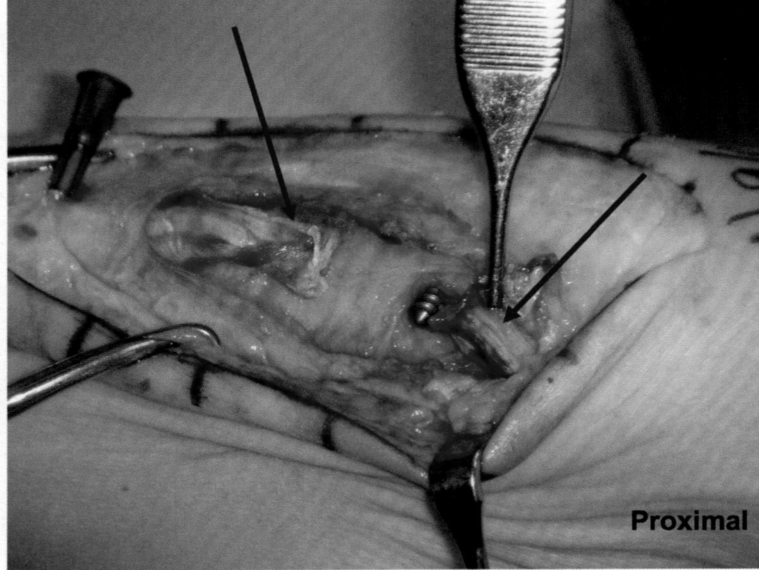

Figure 66-7 | Anterior tibial tendon rupture (*blue arrows*) seen 3 months after percutaneous screw fixation due to penetration of the medial cortex.

References

1. Lee S, Anderson RB. Stress fractures of the tarsal navicular. *Foot Ankle Clin.* 2004;9(1):85-104. doi:10.1016/S1083-7515(03)00151-7.
2. Choi LE, Chou LB. Surgical treatment of tarsal navicular stress fractures. *Oper Tech Sports Med.* 2006;14(4):248-251. doi:10.1053/j.otsm.2006.05.003.
3. Mann JA, Pedowitz DI. Evaluation and treatment of navicular stress fractures, including nonunions, revision surgery, and persistent pain after treatment. *Foot Ankle Clin.* 2009;14(2):187-204. doi:10.1016/j.fcl.2009.01.003.

Index

I

J

K

L

CCS0518

DRAKE MEMORIAL LIBRARY
WITHDRAWN
THE COLLEGE AT BROCKPORT